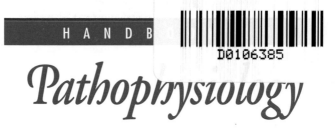

HANDB

Pathophysiology

Second Edition

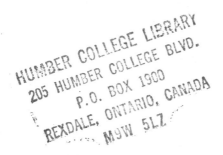

HANDBOOK OF

Pathophysiology

Second Edition

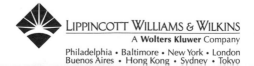

LIPPINCOTT WILLIAMS & WILKINS
A **Wolters Kluwer** Company

Philadelphia • Baltimore • New York • London
Buenos Aires • Hong Kong • Sydney • Tokyo

STAFF

Executive Publisher
Judith A. Schilling McCann, RN, MSN

Editorial Director
William J. Kelly

Clinical Director
Joan M. Robinson, RN, MSN

Senior Art Director
Arlene Putterman

Editorial Project Manager
Ann E. Houska

Clinical Project Manager
Maryann Foley, RN, BSN

Editors
Carol Koetke, Rita M. Doyle

Copy Editors
Kimberly Bilotta (supervisor),
Amy Furman, Dona Hightower Perkins,
Carolyn Petersen, Irene Pontarelli,
Kelly Taylor, Dorothy Terry,
Pamela Wingrod

Designer
Marcia Biderman (design project manager)

Digital Composition Services
Diane Paluba (manager), Joyce Rossi Biletz,
Donna S. Morris

Manufacturing
Patricia K. Dorshaw (director),
Beth J. Welsh

Editorial Assistants
Megan L. Aldinger, Tara L. Carter-Bell,
Linda K. Ruhf

Indexer
Barbara E. Hodgson

The clinical treatments described and recommended in this publication are based on research and consultation with nursing, medical, and legal authorities. To the best of our knowledge, these procedures reflect currently accepted practice. Nevertheless, they can't be considered absolute and universal recommendations. For individual applications, all recommendations must be considered in light of the patient's clinical condition and, before administration of new or infrequently used drugs, in light of the latest package insert information. The authors and publisher disclaim any responsibility for any adverse effects resulting from the suggested procedures, from any undetected errors, or from the reader's misunderstanding of the text.

HBOP2 – D N
06 05 04   10 9 8 7 6 5 4 3 2 1

**Library of Congress
Cataloging-in-Publication Data**
Handbook of pathophysiology.—2nd ed.
    p. ; cm.
  Includes bibliographical references and index.
  1. Physiology, Pathological—Handbooks, manuals, etc. I. Lippincott Williams & Wilkins.
  [DNLM: 1. Disease—Handbooks. 2. Pathology—Handbooks. 3. Physiology—Handbooks. QZ 39 H2359 2005]
  RB113.H24 2005
  616.07--dc22
  ISBN 1-58255-302-5 (hard cover, pbk. : alk. paper)   2004020500

CONTENTS

CONTRIBUTORS AND CONSULTANTS

Margaret Hamilton Birney, RN, PhD
Associate Professor
University of Delaware
Newark

Cheryl L. Brady, RN, MSN
Nursing Instructor
Mercy College of Northwest Ohio
Youngstown

Karen T. Bruchak, RN, MSN, MBA
Principal Consultant, Oncology Global
    Solutions
Siemens Corporation
Malvern, Pa.

Concha Carillo, MS, APN, CGRN, CNP
Gastroenterology Nurse Practitioner
Sterling Rock Falls Clinic
Sterling, Ill.

Sandra H. Clark, RN, MSN
Assistant Professor
Armstrong Atlantic State University
Savannah, Ga.

Yvette P. Conley, PhD
Assistant Professor
University of Pittsburgh

Louise Diehl-Oplinger, RN, MSN,
    APRN, BC, CCRN, CLNC
Advanced Practice Nurse
Warren Hospital
Phillipsburg, N.J.

Shelba Durston, RN, MSN, CCRN
Nursing Instructor
San Joaquin Delta College
Stockton, Calif.

Ellie Z. Franges, RN, MSN, CNRN
Clinical Nurse Specialist, Neuroscience
St. Luke's Hospital and Health Network
Bethlehem, Pa.

Linda Fuhrman, RN, MSN, ANP
Nurse Practitioner
San Francisco Veterans Administration

Julie A. Grant, BA, MSPA-C
Physician Assistant, Division of Allergy
    and Immunology
University of Iowa Hospitals and Clinics
Iowa City

Nancy H. Haynes, RN, PhD(c), CCRN
Assistant Professor
Saint Luke's College
Kansas City, Mo.

Lorenz O. Lutherer, MD, PhD
Professor, Department of Physiology and
    Internal Medicine
Texas Tech University Health Sciences
    Center
Lubbock

Sally R. Russell, RN,BC, MN
Director, Education Services
Anthony J. Jannetti, Inc.
Pitman, N.J.

Mary Clare Shafer, RN, MS, ONC
Infection Control Nurse/Osteoporosis
    Program Coordinator
Tenet-Graduate Hospital
Philadelphia

Mary A. Stahl, RN, MSN, APRN,BC,
   CCRN
Clinical Nurse Specialist
Saint Luke's Hospital
Kansas City, Mo.

Tamara D. Thell, RN, BSN, PHN
Nurse Educator/Nursing Instructor
Anoka-Hennepin Technical College
Anoka, Minn.

David Toub, MD, FACOG
Medical Director
Med Cases, Inc.
Philadelphia

*We extend special thanks to the following
people who contributed to the previous
edition.*

Gary J. Arnold, MD, FACS

Deborah Becker, MSN, CCRN, CRNP, CS

Marcy S. Caplin, RN, MSN

Susan B. Dickey, RNC, PhD

Kay Gentieu, RN, MSN, CRNP

H. Dean Krimmel, RN, MSN

Nancy LaPlante, RN, BSN

Kay Luft, RN, CCRN, TNCC

Elaine Mohn-Brown, RN, EdD

Roger M. Morrell, MD, PhD, FACP, FAIC

Tracey S. Weintraub, RN, MSN, CNS

Patricia A. Wessels, RN, MSN

FOREWORD

Because of the rapid growth in the field of pathophysiology—the study of body function changes caused by disease—staying current can be a constant challenge. Biomedicine made great strides recently with the complete sequencing of the human genome. As more and more becomes known about various pathophysiologic conditions, the base of knowledge will expand exponentially in coming years. "How can I possibly remember all this information so I can give the best patient care?" you may ask.

You probably cannot remember it all. However, now you can carry a portable powerhouse of information, the *Handbook of Pathophysiology,* Second Edition. This volume covers over 450 diseases—their causes, signs and symptoms, and treatment—with clearly written, well-organized entries. The book's consistent format lets you retrieve the facts you need fast.

You will find 32 full-color pages illustrating what happens in metabolic syndrome, coronary artery disease, osteoporosis, ulcers, diabetes, carpal tunnel syndrome, and more. Your understanding is further enhanced by the all-new *Closer look* logo, which draws your eye to quick-reference diagrams, photographs, and illustrations, for a more detailed explanation of a broader subject.

Other time-saving logos include *Age alert, Cultural diversity,* and *Disrupting disease.* The *Age alert* logo provides important facts about a disease that involves a specific age-group, from elderly patients to neonates. Under the *Cultural diversity* logo, you will discover how a disorder is dealt with differently by patients and family members from various cultures. In *Disrupting disease,* you will

see flowcharts that show the points at which a disease process can be interrupted.

The opening chapters start by explaining basic normal cellular and physiological principles and progress through the changes incurred by diseases caused by cancer, infection, genetics, and fluid and electrolyte imbalances. The rest of the book categorizes each disease alphabetically, according to the body system it affects. The appendices contain a table of more than 100 less common, but nonetheless important, disorders such as Creutzfeldt-Jakob disease.

Health care professionals in all stages of their careers and in all work settings always need rapid access to accurate and timely patient care information. This handbook belongs in your hands—at all nursing stations, in hospital conference rooms, and wherever else comprehensive patient care references are needed.

Carrie J. Merkle, RN, PhD, FAAN
Associate Professor
College of Nursing, University of Arizona
Scientific Investigator
Southern Arizona Veterans Administration Health Care System
Tucson

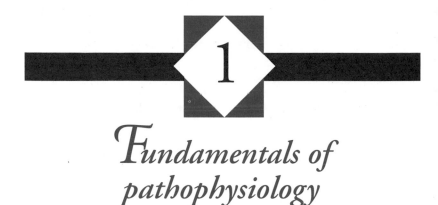

Fundamentals of pathophysiology

An understanding of pathophysiology requires a review of normal physiology—how the body functions day to day, minute to minute—at the levels of cells, tissues, organs, and the whole organism.

HOMEOSTASIS

Every cell in the body is involved in maintaining a dynamic, steady state of internal balance called *homeostasis*. Any cellular change or damage can affect the entire body. When an external stressor, such as injury, lack of nutrients, or invasion by parasites or other organisms, disrupts homeostasis, disease may occur. *Pathophysiology* can be described as what happens when normal defenses against these stressors fail.

Maintaining balance

Three structures in the brain maintain the body's homeostasis:
- *medulla oblongata* is the part of the brain stem linked to vital functions such as respiration and circulation
- *pituitary gland* regulates the function of other glands to determine a person's growth, maturation, and reproduction
- *reticular formation* is a network of nerve cell nuclei and fibers in the brain stem and spinal cord that helps control vital reflexes

such as cardiovascular function and respiration.

Homeostasis is sustained by two kinds of self-regulating feedback mechanisms:
- A *positive* feedback mechanism moves the system away from homeostasis by enhancing a change in the system. For example, the heart pumps at increased rate and force when a person is in shock. If the shock progresses, the heart action may require more oxygen than is available, which results in heart failure.
- A *negative* feedback mechanism restores homeostasis by correcting a deficit in the system. An effective negative feedback mechanism must sense a change in the body—such as a high glucose level—and try to return body functions to normal. In the case of a high glucose level, the effector mechanism triggers increased insulin production by the pancreas, returning glucose levels to normal and restoring homeostasis.

Each of the feedback mechanisms has three components:
- a sensor that detects disruptions in homeostasis (caused by nerve impulses or changes in hormone levels)
- a central nervous system (CNS) control center that receives signals from the sensor and regulates the body's response to those disruptions (by starting the effector mechanism)
- an effector that restores homeostasis.

DISEASE AND ILLNESS

Although *disease* and *illness* are commonly used interchangeably, they aren't synonyms. Disease occurs when homeostasis isn't maintained. Illness occurs when a person is no longer in a state of perceived "normal" health. For example, a person may have a disease (such as coronary artery disease, diabetes, or asthma) but not feel ill because his body has adapted to the disease. In such a situation, a person can perform necessary activities of daily living. Illness usually refers to subjective symptoms that may indicate the presence of disease.

The course and outcome of a disease are influenced by genetic factors (such as a tendency toward obesity), unhealthy behaviors (such as smoking), attitudes (such as having a "type A" personality), and even the person's view of the disease (such as acceptance or denial). Diseases are dynamic and may show themselves in various ways, depending on the patient or his environment.

Causes of disease

The cause of disease may be intrinsic (such as inheritance, age, or sex) or extrinsic (such as an infectious agent or behaviors, including inactivity, smoking, or illegal drug abuse). Diseases that have no known cause are called *idiopathic*.

Development of disease

A disease's development is called its *pathogenesis*. Unless identified and successfully treated, most diseases progress according to a typical pattern of symptoms. Some diseases are self-limiting, resolving quickly with little or no intervention; others are chronic and never resolve. Patients with chronic diseases may undergo periodic remissions and exacerbations.

A disease is usually detected when it causes a change in metabolism or cell division that causes signs and symptoms. Evidence of disease includes hypofunction (such as constipation), hyperfunction (such as increased mucus production), or increased mechanical function (such as a seizure).

The causative agent and the affected cells, tissues, and organs determine how cells respond to disease. The resolution of disease depends on many factors functioning over time, such as extent of disease and the simultaneous presence of other diseases.

Common stress-related disorders

A person's failure to respond adequately to a physiologic or psychological stressor may cause or worsen a disease or condition. Common stress-related disorders and conditions include:

- acute stress disorder
- angina (chest pain)
- anxiety
- depression
- eating disorders
- eczema
- fainting
- headaches (migraine and tension)
- heart palpitations
- hypertension
- inflammatory bowel syndrome
- insomnia or hypersomnia
- irritable bowel syndrome
- menstrual irregularities
- muscle weakness or spasms
- panic attacks
- peptic ulcer disease
- posttraumatic stress disorder
- rash
- sexual dysfunction
- shortness of breath or chest discomfort
- substance use and abuse.

Physical response to stress

According to Hans Selye's General Adaptation Model, the body reacts to stress in the stages shown below.

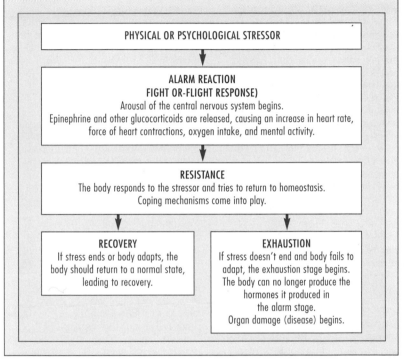

Stages of disease

Typically, diseases progress through these stages:

■ *Exposure or injury*—Target tissue is exposed to a causative agent or is injured.

■ *Latency or incubation period*—The patient has no signs or symptoms.

■ *Prodromal period*—Signs and symptoms are usually mild and nonspecific.

■ *Acute phase*—The disease reaches its full intensity, possibly resulting in complications. This phase is called the *subclinical acute phase* if the patient can still function as though the disease weren't present.

■ *Remission*—A second latent phase occurs in some diseases and is usually followed by another acute phase.

■ *Convalescence*—The patient progresses toward recovery after the disease ends.

■ *Recovery*—The patient regains health or normal functioning. No signs or symptoms of disease remain.

Stress and disease

When a stressor such as a life change occurs, a person may either adapt successfully or fail to adapt. Failure to adapt adequately to stress may result in disease. (See *Common stress-related disorders*.)

Hans Selye, a pioneer in the study of stress and disease, describes the following stages of adaptation to a stressful event: alarm, resistance, and recovery or exhaustion (see *Physical response to stress*). In the alarm stage, the body senses stress and arouses the CNS. The body releases chemicals to mobilize the fight-or-flight response. The sympathoadrenal medullary response causes the release of epinephrine, and the hypothalamic pituitary adrenal axis causes the release of glucocorticoids. These systems work together to let the body respond to stressors. The effect of these chemicals is sometimes described as the "adrenaline rush" of panic or aggression. In the resistance stage, the body responds to the stressor and tries to adapt. Coping mechanisms come into play during this stage. If the stress ceases or the body adapts, recovery begins. If stress continues and the body fails to adapt, the exhaustion state begins. Hormones produced in the alarm stage are no longer produced. As a result, organ damage occurs, leading to disease.

The stress response is controlled by actions in the cells of the nervous and endocrine systems. These actions try to redirect energy to the organ that's most affected by the stress, such as the heart, lungs, or brain.

Stressors may be physiologic or psychological. Physiologic stressors, such as exposure to a toxin, may elicit a harmful response, leading to an identifiable disease or set of signs and symptoms. Psychological stressors, such as the death of a loved one, may also cause a maladaptive response. Stressful events can worsen some chronic diseases, such as diabetes or multiple sclerosis. Effective coping strategies can often prevent or reduce the harmful effects of stress.

CELL PHYSIOLOGY

The cell is the smallest living component of a living organism. Organisms may be made up of a single cell, such as bacteria, or billions of cells, such as human beings. In large organisms, highly specialized *cells* that perform an identical function are organized into *tissue* (such as epithelial tissue, connective tissue, nerve tissue, and muscle tissue). Tissues, in turn, form *organs* (such as skin, skeleton, brain, and

heart), which are integrated into *body systems* (such as the CNS, cardiovascular system, and musculoskeletal system).

Cell components

Like organisms, cells are complex organizations of specialized components, each component having its own function. A normal cell's largest components are the cytoplasm, the nucleus, and the cell membrane, which surrounds the internal components and holds the cell together. (See *A look at cell components*.)

CYTOPLASM

The gel-like cytoplasm consists primarily of *cytosol*, a viscous, semitransparent fluid that's 70% to 90% water and 10% to 30% various proteins, salts, and sugars. Suspended in the cytosol are many tiny structures called *organelles*.

Organelles are the cell's metabolic machinery. Each performs a function to maintain the cell's life. Organelles include mitochondria, ribosomes, endoplasmic reticulum, Golgi apparatus, lysosomes, peroxisomes, cytoskeletal elements, centrosomes, microfilaments, and microtubules.

- *Mitochondria* are spherical or rod-shaped structures that produce most of the body's adenosine triphosphate (ATP). ATP contains high-energy phosphate chemical bonds that fuel many cellular activities. Mitochondria are the sites of cellular respiration — the metabolic use of oxygen to produce energy, carbon dioxide, and water.
- *Ribosomes* are the sites of protein synthesis.
- The *endoplasmic reticulum* is an extensive network of two varieties of membrane-enclosed tubules. The rough endoplasmic reticulum is covered with ribosomes. The smooth endoplasmic reticulum contains enzymes that synthesize lipids.
- The *Golgi apparatus* synthesizes carbohydrate molecules that combine with protein produced by the rough endoplasmic reticulum and lipids produced by the smooth endoplasmic reticulum to form such products as lipoproteins, glycoproteins, and enzymes.

A look at cell components

Tho illustration below shows a cell's components and structures. Each part plays a role in maintaining the cell's life and homeostasis; these functions are shown in parentheses

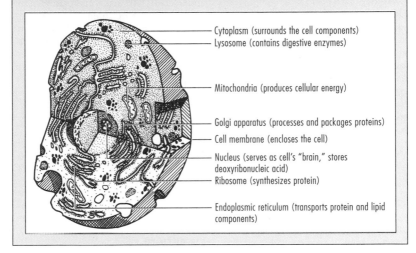

Cytoplasm (surrounds the cell components)
Lysosome (contains digestive enzymes)

Mitochondria (produces cellular energy)

Golgi apparatus (processes and packages proteins)
Cell membrane (encloses the cell)
Nucleus (serves as cell's "brain," stores deoxyribonucleic acid)
Ribosome (synthesizes protein)

Endoplasmic reticulum (transports protein and lipid components)

■ *Lysosomes* are digestive bodies that break down nutrients and foreign or damaged material in cells. A membrane surrounding each lysosome separates its digestive enzymes from the rest of the cytoplasm. The enzymes digest nutrients brought into the cell by *endocytosis*, in which a portion of the cell membrane surrounds and engulfs matter to form a membrane-bound intracellular vesicle. The membrane of the lysosome fuses with the membrane of the vesicle surrounding the endocytosed material. The lysosomal enzymes then digest the engulfed material. Lysosomes digest the foreign matter ingested by white blood cells (WBCs) by a similar process called *phagocytosis*.

■ *Peroxisomes* contain oxidases, which are enzymes that chemically reduce oxygen to hydrogen peroxide and hydrogen peroxide to water.

■ *Cytoskeletal elements* form a network of protein structures that maintain the cell's shape.

■ *Centrosomes* contain centrioles, which are short cylinders adjacent to the nucleus that take part in cell division.

■ *Microfilaments* and *microtubules* enable the movement of intracellular vesicles (allowing axons to transport neurotransmitters) and the formation of the mitotic spindle, the framework for cell division.

NUCLEUS
The cell's control center is the nucleus, which plays a role in cell growth, metabolism, and reproduction. Within the nucleus, one or more *nucleoli* (dark-staining intranuclear structures) synthesize ribonucleic acid (RNA), a complex polynucleotide that controls protein synthesis. The nucleus also stores deoxyribonucleic acid (DNA), the double helix structure that carries genetic material and is responsible for cellular reproduction or division.

CELL MEMBRANE
The semipermeable cell membrane forms the cell's external boundary, separating it

from other cells and from the external environment. The cell membrane consists of a double layer of phospholipids with protein molecules embedded in it. These protein molecules act as receptors, ion channels, or carriers for specific substances.

Cell division

Each cell must replicate itself for life to continue. Cells replicate by division in one of two ways: *mitosis* (division that results in two daughter cells with the same DNA and chromosome content as the original cell) or *meiosis* (division that creates four gametocytes, each containing one-half the number of chromosomes of the original cell). Most cells undergo mitosis; meiosis occurs only in reproductive cells.

MITOSIS

Mitosis, the type of cell division that leads to tissue growth, creates an equal division of material in the nucleus (karyokinesis) followed by division of the cell body (cytokinesis). This process yields two duplicates of the original cell. (See chapter 5, Genetics, for a detailed discussion of mitosis and meiosis.)

Cell functions

A cell's basic functions are movement, conduction, absorption, secretion, excretion, respiration, and reproduction. The human body has some cells that perform a specialized function; for example, muscle cells are responsible for movement. Respiration and reproduction occur in all cells.

MOVEMENT

Some cells, such as muscle cells, work together to produce movement of a specific body part, the contents within an organ, or the entire organism. Muscle cells attached to bone move the extremities. When muscle cells that envelop hollow organs or cavities contract, they produce movement of contents, as in the peristaltic movement of the intestines or the ejection of blood from the heart.

CONDUCTION

Conduction is the transmission of a stimulus — such as a nerve impulse, heat, or sound wave — from one body part to another.

ABSORPTION

The absorption process occurs as substances move through a cell membrane. For example, food is broken down into amino acids, fatty acids, and glucose in the digestive tract. Specialized cells in the intestine then absorb the nutrients and carry them to blood vessels, which take them to other cells of the body. These target cells, in turn, absorb the substances, using them as energy sources or as building blocks to form or repair structural and functional cellular components.

SECRETION

Some cells, such as those in the glands, release substances that are used in another part of the body. The beta cells of the islets of Langerhans of the pancreas, for example, secrete insulin, which is carried by the blood to its target cells, where the insulin helps move glucose across cell membranes.

EXCRETION

Cells excrete the waste generated by normal metabolic processes. This waste includes carbon dioxide, certain acids, and nitrogen-containing molecules.

RESPIRATION

Cellular respiration occurs in the mitochondria, where ATP is produced. The cell absorbs oxygen; it then uses the oxygen and releases carbon dioxide during cellular metabolism. The energy stored in ATP is used in other reactions that require energy.

REPRODUCTION

New cells need to replace older cells for tissue and body growth. Most cells divide and reproduce through mitosis, but some cells, such as nerve and muscle cells, typically lose their ability to reproduce after birth.

Cell types

Each of the four types of tissue (epithelial, connective, nerve, and muscle) consists of several specialized cell types, which perform specific functions.

EPITHELIAL CELLS

Epithelial cells line most of the body's internal and external surfaces, such as the skin's epidermis, the internal organs, blood vessels, body cavities, glands, and sensory organs. The functions of epithelial cells include support, protection, absorption, excretion, and secretion.

CONNECTIVE TISSUE CELLS

Connective tissue cells are found in the skin, bones and joints, artery walls, nerves, body fat, and fascia around organs. The types of connective tissue cells include fibroblasts (which form collagen, elastin, and reticular fibers), adipose (fat) cells, mast cells (which release histamines and other substances during inflammation), and bone cells. The major functions of connective tissues are protection, metabolism, support, temperature maintenance, and elasticity.

NERVE CELLS

Two types of cells — neurons and neuroglial cells — make up the nervous system. *Neurons* have a cell body, dendrites, and an axon. The dendrites carry nerve impulses to the cell body from the axons of other neurons. Axons carry impulses away from the cell body to other neurons or organs. A myelin sheath around the axon facilitates rapid conduction of impulses by keeping them within the nerve cell. Neurons perform the following functions:
- generate electrical impulses
- conduct electrical impulses
- influence other neurons, muscle cells, and cells of glands by transmitting those impulses.

Neuroglial cells support, nourish, and protect the neurons. There are four types:
- Oligodendroglia produce myelin in the CNS.
- Astrocytes provide essential nutrients to neurons and help neurons maintain the proper bioelectrical potentials for impulse conduction and synaptic transmission.
- Ependymal cells help produce cerebrospinal fluid.
- Microglia ingest and digest tissue debris when nerve tissue is damaged.

MUSCLE CELLS

Muscle cells contract to produce movement or tension. The intracellular proteins actin and myosin interact to form cross-bridges that result in muscle contraction. An increase in intracellular calcium is necessary for muscle to contract. The increase occurs when the muscle cell is stimulated. This causes depolarization of the muscle cell and creates an action potential that leads to the release of intracellular calcium from its storage sites in the sarcoplasmic reticulum.

There are three basic types of muscle cells:
- Skeletal (striated) muscle cells are long, cylindrical cells that extend along the entire length of the skeletal muscles. These muscles, which attach directly to the bone or are connected to the bone by tendons, are responsible for voluntary movement. By contracting and relaxing, striated muscle cells alter the muscle's length. Contraction shortens the muscle; relaxation permits the muscle to return to its resting length.
- Smooth (nonstriated) muscle cells are spindle-shaped cells found in the walls of hollow internal organs, such as in the GI and genitourinary tracts, and of blood vessels and bronchioles. Unlike striated muscle cells, smooth muscle cells contract involuntarily. By contracting and relaxing, they change the hollow structure's luminal diameter and thereby move substances through the organ.
- Cardiac muscle cells branch out across the smooth muscle of the heart's chambers. Although they are striated, they contract involuntarily. They produce and transmit cardiac action potentials, which cause cardiac muscle cells to contract. Impulses travel from cell to cell as though no cell membrane existed.

 CLINICAL ALERT
In older adults, skeletal muscle cells become smaller and many are replaced by fibrous connective tissue. The result is loss of muscle strength and mass.

ℙATHOPHYSIOLOGIC CHANGES

The cell faces several challenges through its life. Stressors, changes in the body's health, disease, and other extrinsic and intrinsic factors can change the cell's normal functioning (homeostasis).

Cell adaptation

Cells can usually continue functioning despite changing conditions or stressors, but severe or prolonged stress or changes may injure or even destroy cells. When cell integrity is threatened—for example, by hypoxia, anoxia, chemical injury, infection, or temperature extremes—the cell reacts in one of two ways:
- by drawing on its reserves to keep functioning
- by adaptive changes or cellular dysfunction.

If enough cellular reserve is available and the body doesn't detect abnormalities, the cell adapts by atrophy, hypertrophy, hyperplasia, metaplasia, or dysplasia. (See *Adaptive cell changes*.) If cellular reserve is insufficient, the cell dies (necrosis). Necrosis is usually localized and easily identifiable.

ATROPHY

Atrophy is a reduction in the size of a cell or organ that may occur when cells face disuse or reduced workload, insufficient blood flow, malnutrition, or reduced hormonal or nerve stimulation. Examples of atrophy include loss of muscle mass and tone after prolonged bed rest.

HYPERTROPHY

In contrast, hypertrophy is an increase in the size of a cell or organ due to an increase in workload. The three basic types of hypertrophy are *physiologic*, *compensatory*, and *pathologic*.
- Physiologic hypertrophy reflects an increase in workload that isn't caused by disease—for example, the increase in muscle size caused by hard physical labor or weight training.

- Compensatory hypertrophy takes place when cell size increases to take over for other, nonfunctioning cells. For instance, one kidney will enlarge when the other isn't functioning or is removed.
- Pathologic hypertrophy is a response to disease. An example is thickening of the heart muscle as the muscle pumps against increasing resistance in a patient with hypertension.

HYPERPLASIA

Hyperplasia is an increase in the number of cells caused by increased workload, hormonal stimulation, or decreased tissue density. Like hypertrophy, hyperplasia may be *physiologic*, *compensatory*, or *pathologic*.
- Physiologic hyperplasia is an adaptive response to normal changes. An example, in women, is the monthly increase in number of uterine cells that occurs in response to estrogen stimulation of the endometrium after ovulation.
- Compensatory hyperplasia occurs in some organs to replace tissue that has been removed or destroyed. For example, liver cells regenerate when part of the liver is removed.
- Pathologic hyperplasia is a response to either excessive hormonal stimulation or abnormal production of hormonal growth factors. Examples include endometrial hyperplasia, in which excessive secretion of estrogen causes heavy menstrual bleeding and possibly malignant changes, and acromegaly, in which excessive growth hormone production causes bones to enlarge.

METAPLASIA

Metaplasia is the replacement of one cell type with another cell type (one that can better endure the change or stressor). A common cause of metaplasia is constant irritation or injury that starts an inflammatory response. The new cell type can better endure the stress of chronic inflammation. Metaplasia may be either *physiologic* or *pathologic*.
- Physiologic metaplasia is a normal response to changing conditions and is usually transient. For example, in the body's normal response to inflammation, mono-

cytes that migrate to inflamed tissues change into macrophages.

■ Pathologic metaplasia is a response to an extrinsic toxin or stressor and is usually irreversible. For example, after years of exposure to cigarette smoke, stratified squamous epithelial cells replace the normal ciliated columnar epithelial cells of the bronchi. Although the new cells can better withstand smoke, they don't secrete mucus or have cilia to protect the airway. If exposure to cigarette smoke continues, the squamous cells can become cancerous.

DYSPLASIA

In dysplasia, abnormal differentiation of dividing cells results in cells that are abnormal in size, shape, and appearance. Although dysplastic cell changes aren't cancerous, they can precede cancerous changes. Common examples include dysplasia of epithelial cells of the cervix or the respiratory tract.

Cell injury

Injury to any cellular component can lead to disease as the cells lose their ability to adapt. One early indication of cell injury is a biochemical lesion that forms on the cell at the point of injury. For example, in a patient with chronic alcoholism, biochemical lesions on the cells of the immune system may increase the patient's susceptibility to infection, and cells of the pancreas and liver are affected in a way that prevents their reproduction. These cells can't return to normal functioning.

CAUSES OF CELL INJURY

Cell injury may result from any of several intrinsic or extrinsic causes:

■ *Toxins* — Substances that originate in the body (endogenous factors) or outside the body (exogenous factors) can cause toxic injuries. Common endogenous toxins include products of genetically determined metabolic errors, gross malformations, and hypersensitivity reactions. Exogenous toxins include alcohol, lead, carbon monoxide, and drugs that alter cellular function. Examples of such drugs are chemotherapeutic agents used for cancer and immunosuppressants used to prevent rejection in organ transplant recipients.

CLOSER LOOK
Adaptive cell changes

Cells adapt to changing conditions and stressors within the body in the ways shown below.

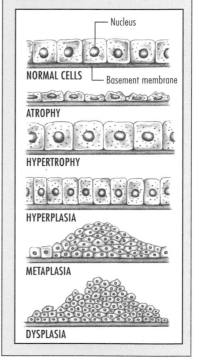

NORMAL CELLS
— Nucleus
— Basement membrane

ATROPHY

HYPERTROPHY

HYPERPLASIA

METAPLASIA

DYSPLASIA

■ *Infection* — Viruses, fungi, protozoa, and bacteria can cause cell injury or death. These organisms affect cell integrity, usually by interfering with cell division, producing nonviable, mutant cells. For example, human immunodeficiency virus alters the cell when the virus is replicated in the cell's RNA.

■ *Physical injury* — A disruption in the cell or in the relationships of the intracellular organelles causes physical injury. Two major types of physical injury are thermal and mechanical. Causes of thermal injury include burns, radiation therapy for cancer, X-rays, and ultraviolet radiation. Causes of mechanical injury include surgery, trauma from motor vehicle accidents, and frostbite.

■ *Deficit injury*—When a deficit of water, oxygen, or nutrients occurs, or if constant temperature and adequate waste disposal aren't maintained, normal cellular metabolism can't take place. A lack of just one of these basic requirements can cause cell disruption or death. Causes of deficit include hypoxia (inadequate oxygen), ischemia (inadequate blood supply), and malnutrition.

Irreversible cell injury occurs when the cell membrane or the organelles can no longer function.

Cell degeneration

Degeneration is a type of cell damage that usually occurs in the cytoplasm and does not affect the nucleus. Degeneration, which usually affects organs with metabolically active cells, such as the liver, heart, and kidneys, may be caused by:
■ increased water in the cell or cellular swelling
■ fatty infiltrates
■ atrophy
■ autophagocytosis (that is, the cell absorbs some of its own parts)
■ pigment changes
■ calcification
■ hyaline infiltration
■ hypertrophy
■ hyperplasia
■ dysplasia (related to chronic irritation).

When cell changes are identified, prompt health care can slow degeneration and prevent cell death. An electron microscope can help identify cellular changes, and thus diagnose a disease, before the patient complains of any symptoms. Unfortunately, many cell changes remain unidentifiable even under a microscope, making early detection of disease impossible. An example of reversible degenerative change is cervical dysplasia; examples of irreversible degenerative diseases include Huntington's disease and amyotrophic lateral sclerosis.

Cell aging

During the normal process of aging, cells lose structure and function. Atrophy, a decrease in size or a wasting away, may indicate loss of cell structure. Hypertrophy or hyperplasia is characteristic of lost cell function.

Cell aging can be affected by intrinsic or extrinsic factors. Intrinsic factors can be congenital, degenerative, immunologic, inherited, metabolic, neoplastic, nutritional, or psychogenic. Examples include:
■ degenerative—loss of lubricating fluids, as in joints
■ immunologic—altered levels of immunoglobulins
■ metabolic—decreased hormonal secretion
■ nutritional—decreased oxygen, inadequate amino acids

Extrinsic factors can be physical or infectious. Physical extrinsic agents include:
■ chemicals
■ electricity
■ force
■ humidity
■ radiation
■ temperature.

Infectious extrinsic agents include:
■ bacteria
■ fungi
■ insects
■ protozoa
■ viruses
■ worms.

All body systems show signs of aging. Diminished blood vessel elasticity, reduced bowel motility, and reduced muscle mass and subcutaneous fat are examples. Cell aging can slow down or speed up, depending on the number and extent of injuries and the amount of wear and tear on the cell.

The cell aging process limits the human life span (of course, most people die of disease before they reach the maximum life span of about 110 years). Several theories have been proposed to explain why cells age. (See *Biological theories of aging*.)

Cell death

Like disease, cell death may be caused by internal (intrinsic) factors that limit the cell's life span or external (extrinsic) factors

Biological theories of aging

Various theories have been proposed to explain the process of normal aging. Biological theories attempt to explain physical aging as an involuntary process that eventually leads to cumulative changes in cells, tissues, and fluids.

THEORY	SOURCES	RETARDANTS
CROSS-LINK THEORY Strong chemical bonding between organic molecules in the body causes increased stiffness, chemical instability, and insolubility of connective tissue and DNA.	Lipids, proteins, carbohydrates, and nucleic acids	Restricting calories and sources of lathyrogens (antilink agents) such as chickpeas
FREE RADICAL THEORY An increased number of unstable free radicals produce effects harmful to biological systems, such as chromosomal changes, pigment accumulation, and collagen alteration.	Environmental pollutants; oxidation of dietary fats, proteins, carbohydrates, and elements	Improving environmental monitoring; decreasing intake of free-radical-stimulating foods; Increasing intake of vitamins A and C (mercaptans) and vitamin E
IMMUNOLOGIC THEORY Because the aging immune system is less able to distinguish body cells from foreign cells, it attacks and destroys body cells as if they were foreign. This may explain the adult onset of such conditions as diabetes mellitus, rheumatic heart disease, and arthritis. Theorists have speculated about the existence of several erratic cellular mechanisms that can trigger attacks on various tissues through autoaggression or immunodeficiencies.	Alteration of B and T cells of the humoral and cellular systems	Immunoengineering — selective alteration and replenishment or rejuvenation of the immune system
WEAR-AND-TEAR THEORY Body cells, structures, and functions wear out or are overused through exposure to internal and external stressors. Effects of the residual damage accumulate, the body can no longer resist stress, and death occurs.	Repeated injury or overuse; internal and external stressors (physical, psychological, social, and environmental), including trauma, chemicals, and buildup of naturally occurring wastes	Reevaluating and possibly adjusting lifestyle

that contribute to cell damage and aging. When a stressor is severe or prolonged, the cell can no longer adapt and it dies.

Cell death, or necrosis, may occur in different ways, depending on the tissues or organs involved.

■ Apoptosis is genetically programmed cell death. This accounts for the constant cell turnover in the skin's outer keratin layer and the eye's lens.

■ Liquefaction necrosis occurs when a lytic (lysosomal), or dissolving, enzyme liquefies necrotic cells. This type of necrosis is common in the brain, which has a rich supply of lytic enzymes.

■ In caseous necrosis, the necrotic cells disintegrate but the cellular pieces remain undigested for months or years. This type of necrotic tissue gets its name from its crumbly, cheeselike (caseous) appearance. It commonly occurs in pulmonary tuberculosis.

■ In fat necrosis, enzymes called lipases break down intracellular triglycerides into free fatty acids. These free fatty acids combine with sodium, magnesium, or calcium ions to form soaps. The tissue becomes opaque and chalky white.

■ Coagulative necrosis commonly occurs when the blood supply to any organ (except the brain) is interrupted. It typically affects the kidneys, heart, and adrenal glands. Lytic (lysosomal) enzyme activity in the cells is inhibited, so that the necrotic cells maintain their shape, at least temporarily.

■ Gangrenous necrosis, a form of coagulative necrosis, typically results from a lack of blood flow and is complicated by an overgrowth and invasion of bacteria. It commonly occurs in the lower legs as a result of arteriosclerosis or in the GI tract. Gangrene can occur in one of three forms: dry, moist (or wet), or gas.

– *Dry gangrene* occurs when bacterial invasion is minimal. It's marked by dry, wrinkled, dark brown or blackened tissue on an extremity.

– *Moist (or wet) gangrene* develops with liquefaction necrosis that includes extensive lytic activity from bacteria and WBCs to produce a liquid center in an affected area. It can occur in the internal organs as well as the extremities.

– *Gas gangrene* develops when anaerobic *Clostridium* bacteria infect tissue. It's more likely to occur with severe trauma and may be fatal. The bacteria release toxins that kill nearby cells and the gas gangrene rapidly spreads. Release of gas bubbles from affected muscle cells indicates that gas gangrene is present.

NECROTIC CHANGES

When a cell dies, enzymes inside the cell are released, and these enzymes start to dissolve cellular components. This process triggers an acute inflammatory reaction in which WBCs migrate to the necrotic area and begin to digest the dead cells. At this point, the dead cells — primarily the nuclei — begin to change morphologically in one of three ways:

■ pyknosis, in which the nucleus shrinks, becoming a dense mass of genetic material with an irregular outline

■ karyorrhexis, in which the nucleus breaks up, strewing pieces of genetic material throughout the cell

■ karyolysis, in which hydrolytic enzymes released from intracellular structures called lysosomes dissolve the nucleus.

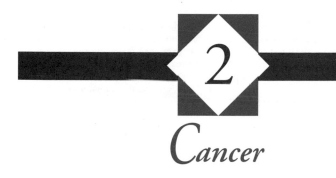

Cancer

Cancer, or *malignant neoplasia,* is a group of more than 100 diseases characterized by deoxyribonucleic acid (DNA) damage that causes abnormal cell growth and development. Malignant cells have two defining characteristics: They can no longer divide and differentiate normally, and they have acquired the ability to invade surrounding tissues and travel to distant sites.

In the United States, cancer causes more than a half million deaths each year, second only to cardiovascular disease. However, a 1999 review of the Healthy People 2010 cancer objectives by the U.S. Department of Health and Human Services had encouraging results: reversal of a 20-year trend of increasing cancer incidence and deaths. The rates for all cancers combined and for most of the top 10 cancer sites declined between 1990 and 1996.

Worldwide, the most common cancers are skin cancer, leukemias, lymphomas, and cancers of the breast, bone, GI tract and associated structures, thyroid, lung, urinary tract, and reproductive tract. (See *Reviewing common cancers,* pages 39 to 50.) In the United States, the most common forms of cancer are lung, breast, prostate, and colorectal. Some cancers, such as ovarian germ-cell tumors and retinoblastoma, occur predominantly in younger patients, but more than two-thirds of the patients who develop cancer are over age 65.

HOW DOES CANCER DEVELOP?

Most of the numerous theories about carcinogenesis suggest that it involves three steps: initiation, promotion, and progression.

Initiation

Initiation refers to the damage to or mutation of DNA that occurs when the cell is exposed to an initiating substance or event (such as chemicals, virus, or radiation) during DNA replication (transcription). Usually, enzymes detect errors in transcription and remove or repair them. Sometimes, however, an error is missed. If regulatory proteins recognize the error and block further division, then the error may be repaired or the cell may self-destruct. If these proteins miss the error, it becomes a permanent mutation that's passed on to future generations of cells.

Promotion

Promotion involves the mutated cell's exposure to factors (*promoters*) that enhance its growth. This exposure may occur shortly after initiation or years later.

Promoters may be hormones such as estrogen, food additives such as nitrates, or drugs such as nicotine. Promoters can affect the mutated cell by altering one or more of the following:

- function of genes that control cell growth and duplication
- cell response to growth stimulators or inhibitors
- intercellular communication.

Progression

Some investigators believe that progression is a late promotion phase in which the tumor invades, metastasizes, and becomes resistant to drugs. This step is irreversible.

CAUSES

The healthy body is well equipped to defend itself against cancer. Only when the immune system and other defenses fail does cancer prevail.

Current evidence suggests that cancer develops from a complex interaction of exposure to carcinogens and accumulated mutations in several genes. Researchers have identified approximately 100 cancer genes. Some cancer genes, called *oncogenes*, activate cell division and influence embryonic development. Other cancer genes, the *tumor-suppressor genes*, halt cell division. Normal human cells typically contain proto-oncogenes (oncogene precursors) and tumor-suppressor genes, which remain dormant unless they're transformed by genetic or acquired mutation. Common causes of acquired genetic damage are viruses, radiation, environmental and dietary carcinogens, and hormones. Other factors that interact to increase a person's likelihood of developing cancer are age, nutritional status, hormonal balance, response to stress, and genetic predisposition; these are discussed below as risk factors.

Genetic predisposition

Some cancers and precancerous lesions may result directly or indirectly from genetic predisposition. Direct cause occurs when a single gene is responsible for the cancer, as in Wilms' tumor and retinoblastoma, for example. Indirect carcinogenesis is associated with inherited conditions, such as Down syndrome or immunodeficiency diseases. Common characteristics of genetically predisposed cancer include:

- early onset of malignant disease
- increased incidence of bilateral cancer in paired organs (breasts, adrenal glands, kidneys, and eighth cranial nerves [acoustic neuroma])
- increased incidence of multiple primary cancers in nonpaired organs
- abnormal chromosome complement in tumor cells.

Viruses

Viral proto-oncogenes typically contain DNA that's identical to that of human oncogenes. In animal studies of viral ability to transform cells, some viruses that infect people have shown the potential to cause cancer. For example, the Epstein-Barr virus, which causes infectious mononucleosis, has been linked to Burkitt's lymphoma and nasopharyngeal carcinoma.

Failure of immunosurveillance

Research suggests that cancer cells develop continually but that the immune system recognizes these cells as foreign and destroys them. This defense mechanism, termed immunosurveillance, has two major components: cell-mediated immune response and humoral immune response. These two components interact to promote antibody production, cellular immunity, and immunologic memory. Researchers believe that an intact immune system is responsible for spontaneous regression of tumors. Thus, cancer development is a concern for patients who must take immunosuppressants.

Cell-mediated immune response

Cancer cells carry cell-surface antigens (specialized protein molecules that trigger an immune response) called *tumor-associated antigens (TAAs)* and *tumor-specific antigens (TSAs)*. The cell-mediated immune response begins when T lymphocytes encounter a TAA or a TSA and become sensitized to it. After repeated contacts, the sensitized T cells release chemical factors called *lymphokines*, some of which begin to destroy the antigen. This reaction triggers the transformation of a different population of T lymphocytes into "killer T lymphocytes" targeted to cells carrying the specific antigen—in this case, cancer cells.

Humoral immune response

The humoral immune response reacts to a TAA by triggering the release of antibodies from plasma cells and activating the serum-complement system to destroy the antigen-bearing cells. However, an opposing immune factor, a "blocking antibody," may enhance tumor growth by protecting malignant cells from immune destruction.

Disruption of the immune response

Immunosurveillance isn't a fail-safe system. If the immune system fails to recognize tumor cells as foreign, the immune response won't activate. The tumor will continue to grow until it's beyond the immune system's ability to destroy it. In addition to this failure of surveillance, other mechanisms may come into play.

The tumor cells may suppress the immune defenses. The tumor antigens may combine with humoral antibodies to form complexes that essentially hide the antigens from the normal immune defenses. These complexes could also depress further antibody production. Tumors also may change their antigenic "appearance" or produce substances that impair usual immune defenses. The tumor growth factors not only promote the growth of the tumor but also increase the person's risk of infection. Finally, prolonged exposure to a tumor antigen may deplete the patient's lymphocytes and further impair the ability to mount an appropriate response.

The patient's supply of suppressor T lymphocytes may be inadequate to defend against malignant tumors. Suppressor T lymphocytes usually help to regulate antibody production; they also signal the immune system when an immune response is no longer needed. Certain carcinogens, such as viruses or chemicals, may weaken the immune system by destroying or damaging suppressor T cells or their precursors, and subsequently allow for tumor growth.

Theoretically, cancer develops when any of several factors disrupts the immune response:

■ *Aging cells.* As cells age, errors in copying genetic material during cell division may cause mutations. If the aging immune system doesn't recognize these mutations as foreign, the mutated cells may proliferate and form a tumor.

■ *Cytotoxic drugs or steroids.* These agents can decrease antibody production and can destroy circulating lymphocytes.

■ *Extreme stress or certain viral infections.* These conditions may depress the immune response, thus allowing cancer cells to proliferate.

■ *Suppression of the immune system.* Radiation, cytotoxic drug therapy, and lymphoproliferative and myeloproliferative diseases (such as lymphatic and myelocytic leukemia) depress bone marrow production and impair leukocyte function.

■ *Acquired immunodeficiency syndrome.* This condition weakens the cell-mediated immune response.

■ *Cancer.* The disease itself is immunosuppressive. Advanced disease exhausts the immune system, leading to anergy (the absence of immune reactivity).

*R*ISK FACTORS

Many cancers are related to specific environmental and lifestyle factors that predispose a person to develop cancer. Accumulating data suggest that some of these risk factors start carcinogenesis, others promote the disease process, and some do both.

Air pollution

Air pollution has been linked to the development of cancer, particularly lung cancer. People who live near industries that release toxic chemicals have an increased cancer risk. Many outdoor air pollutants—such as arsenic, benzene, hydrocarbons, polyvinyl chlorides, and other industrial emissions, as well as vehicle exhaust—have been studied for their carcinogenic properties.

Indoor air pollution, such as from cigarette smoke and radon, also increases cancer risk. In fact, indoor air pollution may be more carcinogenic than outdoor air pollution.

Tobacco

Cigarette smoking increases the risk of lung cancer more than 10-fold over that of nonsmokers by late middle age. Tobacco smoke contains nitrosamines and polycyclic hydrocarbons, two carcinogens that are known to cause mutations. The risk of lung cancer from cigarette smoking correlates directly with the duration of smoking and the number of cigarettes smoked per day. Tobacco smoke is also linked to laryngeal cancer and contributes to cancer of the bladder, pancreas, kidney, and cervix. Research also shows that a person who stops smoking decreases his risk of lung cancer.

Although the cancer risk from pipe and cigar smoking is similar to that of cigarette smoking, some evidence suggests that the effects are less severe. Smoke from cigars and pipes is more alkaline. This alkalinity decreases nicotine absorption in the lungs and is more irritating to the lungs, so that the smoker doesn't inhale as readily.

Inhalation of "second-hand" smoke, or passive smoking, by nonsmokers also increases the risk of lung and other cancers. Use of smokeless tobacco, in which the oral tissue directly absorbs nicotine and other carcinogens, may cause oral cancers that seldom occur in people who don't use the product.

Alcohol

Alcohol consumption, especially in conjunction with cigarette smoking, is commonly associated with cirrhosis of the liver, a precursor to hepatocellular cancer. The risk of breast and colorectal cancers also increases with alcohol consumption. Possible mechanisms for breast cancer development include impaired removal of carcinogens by the liver, impaired immune response, and interference with cell membrane permeability of the breast tissue. Alcohol stimulates rectal cell proliferation in rats, a finding that may help explain its role in the increased incidence of colorectal cancer.

Heavy use of alcohol and cigarette smoking together increase the incidence of cancers of the mouth, larynx, pharynx, and esophagus more than either one would alone. Alcohol probably acts as a solvent for the carcinogenic substances found in smoke, enhancing their absorption.

Sexual and reproductive behavior

Sexual practices have been linked to specific types of cancer. Early age of first sexual intercourse and the number of sexual partners are positively correlated with a woman's risk of cervical cancer. Furthermore, a woman who has had only one sexual partner is at higher risk if that partner has had multiple partners. The suspected underlying mechanism here involves virus transmission, most likely human papillomavirus (HPV), specifically types 16, 18, 31, and 33. Other types of HPV have been linked to cervical dysplasia or carcinoma in situ of the cervix.

Occupation

Because of exposure to specific substances, workers in certain occupations face an increased risk of cancer. People exposed to asbestos, such as insulation installers and miners, are at risk for a type of lung cancer called *mesothelioma*. Asbestos may also promote other carcinogens. Workers involved in the production of dyes, rubber, paint, and beta-naphthylamine are at increased risk for bladder cancer.

Ultraviolet radiation

Exposure to ultraviolet radiation, or sunlight, causes genetic mutation in the P53 control gene. Sunlight also releases tumor necrosis factor alpha in exposed skin, possibly diminishing the immune response. Ultraviolet sunlight is a direct cause of basal and squamous cell cancers of the skin. The amount of exposure to ultraviolet radiation also relates to the type of cancer that develops. For example, cumulative exposure to ultraviolet sunlight is linked to basal and squamous cell skin cancer, and severe episodes of burning and blistering at a young age are linked to melanoma.

Ionizing radiation

Ionizing radiation (such as X-rays) is linked to acute leukemia; thyroid, breast,

ACS guidelines: Diet, nutrition, and cancer prevention

Because of the numerous aspects of diet and nutrition that may contribute to the development of cancer, the American Cancer Society (ACS) has developed a list of guidelines to reduce cancer risk in people age 2 and older.
◆ Choose most of the foods you eat from plant sources.
◆ Eat five or more servings of fruits and vegetables each day.
◆ Eat other foods from plant sources, such as breads, cereals, grain products, rice, pasta, or beans, several times each day.

◆ Limit your intake of high-fat foods, particularly from animal sources.
◆ Choose low-fat foods.
◆ Limit consumption of meats, especially high-fat and red meats.
◆ Be physically active and achieve and maintain a healthy weight.
◆ Be at least moderately active for 60 minutes or more on most days of the week.
◆ Stay within your healthy weight range.
◆ Limit your consumption of alcoholic beverages, if you drink at all.

lung, stomach, colon, and urinary tract cancers; and multiple myeloma. Low doses can cause DNA mutations and chromosomal abnormalities, and large doses can inhibit cell division. This damage can directly affect carbohydrate, protein, lipid, and nucleic acids (macromolecules), or it can act on intracellular water to produce free radicals that damage the macromolecules.

Ionizing radiation can also enhance the effects of genetic abnormalities. For example, it further increases the risk of cancer in people with a genetic abnormality that affects DNA repair mechanisms. Other factors include the part and percentage of the body that is exposed, the person's age, hormonal balance, prescribed drugs, and preexisting or concurrent conditions.

Hormones

Hormones — specifically the sex steroid hormones estrogen, progesterone, and testosterone — have been implicated as promoters of breast, endometrial, ovarian, and prostate cancer.

Estrogen, which stimulates the proliferation of breast and endometrial cells, is considered a promoter for breast and endometrial cancers. Prolonged exposure to estrogen, as in women with early menarche and late menopause, increases the risk of breast cancer. Likewise, long-term use of estrogen replacement without progesterone supplementation for menopausal symptoms increases a woman's risk of endometrial cancer. Progesterone may play a

protective role, counteracting estrogen's stimulatory effects.

The male sex hormones stimulate the growth of prostatic tissue. However, research fails to show an increased risk of prostatic cancer in men who take exogenous androgens.

Diet

Numerous aspects of diet are linked to an increase in cancer, including:
■ obesity (in women only, possibly related to production of estrogen by fatty tissue), which is linked to a suspected increased risk of endometrial cancer
■ high consumption of dietary fat, which is linked to endometrial, breast, prostatic, ovarian, and rectal cancers
■ high consumption of smoked foods and salted fish or meats and foods containing nitrites, which may be linked to gastric cancer
■ naturally occurring carcinogens (such as hydrazines and aflatoxin) in foods, which are linked to liver cancer
■ carcinogens produced by microorganisms stored in foods, which are linked to stomach cancer
■ diet low in fiber (resulting in slow transport through the gut), which is linked to colorectal cancer.

The American Cancer Society (ACS) has developed specific nutritional guidelines for cancer prevention. (See *ACS guidelines: Diet, nutrition, and cancer prevention.*)

$\mathcal{P}$ATHOPHYSIOLOGIC CHANGES

Cancer's characteristic features are rapid, uncontrollable proliferation of cells and independent spread from a primary site (site of origin) to other tissues where it establishes secondary foci (metastases). This spread occurs through circulation in the blood or lymphatic fluid, by unintentional transplantation from one site to another during surgery, and by local extension. Because of their growth and development, cell size, shape, number, differentiation, and function of cancer cells differ from those of normal cells. In addition, cancer cells can travel to distant tissues and organ systems. (See *Cancer cell characteristics*.)

Cell growth

Typically, each of the billions of cells in the human body has an internal clock that tells the cell when it's time to reproduce. Mitotic reproduction occurs in a sequence called the *cell cycle*. Normal cell division occurs in direct proportion to cells lost, thus providing a mechanism for controlling growth and differentiation. These controls are absent in cancer cells, and cell production exceeds cell loss. Consequently, cancer cells enter the cell cycle more fre-

quently and at different rates. They're usually found in the synthesis and mitosis phases of the cell cycle, and they spend very little time in the resting phase.

Normal cells reproduce at a rate controlled by the activity of specific control or regulator genes (called *proto-oncogenes* when they function normally). These genes produce proteins that act as "on" and "off" switches. There is no generalized control gene; different cells respond to specific control genes. The P53 and c-myc genes are two examples of control genes: P53 can stop deoxyribonucleic acid (DNA) replication if the cell's DNA has been damaged; c-myc helps start DNA replication, and if it senses an error in DNA replication, it can cause the cell to self-destruct.

Hormones, growth factors, and chemicals released by neighboring cells or by immune or inflammatory cells can affect control gene activity. These substances bind to specific receptors on the cell membranes and send out signals causing the control genes to stimulate or suppress cell reproduction. Examples of hormones and growth factors that affect control genes include:
- interleukin 10, which suppresses cytokine production by helper T cells
- tumor necrosis factor, which mediates inflammation and catabolism
- interferon (alpha and beta), which suppresses viral activity
- erythropoietin, which stimulates red blood cell (RBC) proliferation
- epidermal growth factor, which stimulates epidermal cell proliferation
- insulin-like growth factor, which stimulates fat and connective tissue proliferation.

Substances released by injured or infected nearby cells or by cells of the immune system also affect cellular reproduction. For example, interleukin, released by immune cells, stimulates cell proliferation and differentiation. Interferon, released from virus-infected and immune cells, may affect the cell's rate of reproduction.

Also, cells that are close to one another appear to communicate with each other through gap junctions (channels through which ions and small molecules pass).

Cancer cell characteristics

Cancer cells, which grow and develop uncontrollably, typically exhibit these characteristics:
- ◆ Vary in size and shape
- ◆ Undergo abnormal mitosis
- ◆ Function abnormally
- ◆ Don't resemble the cell of origin
- ◆ Produce substances not usually associated with the original cell or tissue
- ◆ Aren't encapsulated
- ◆ Can spread to other sites

commonly lodges in the first capillary bed it encounters. For example, blood from most organs next enters the capillaries of the lungs, which are the most common site of metastasis.

Once lodged, the tumor cells develop a protective coat of fibrin, platelets, and clotting factors to evade detection by the immune system. Then they become attached to the epithelium, ultimately invading the vessel wall, interstitium, and the parenchyma of the target organ. (See *How cancer metastasizes*.) To survive, the new tumor develops its own vascular network and may ultimately spread again.

Lymphatic spread. The lymphatic system is the most common route for distant metastasis. Tumor cells enter the lymphatic vessels through damaged basement membranes and are transported to regional lymph nodes. The tumor becomes trapped in the first lymph node it encounters. The consequent enlargement, possibly the first evidence of metastasis, may be due to the increased tumor growth within the node or a localized immune reaction to the tumor. The lymph node may filter out or contain some of the tumor cells, limiting further spread. The cells that escape can enter the blood from the lymphatic circulation through plentiful connections between the venous and lymphatic systems.

Metastatic sites. Typically, the first capillary bed, whether lymphatic or vascular, that the circulating tumor mass encounters determines the location of the metastasis. For example, because the lungs receive all of the systemic venous return, they're frequent sites for metastasis. In breast cancer, the axillary lymph nodes, which are close to the breast, are a common site of metastasis. Other types of cancer seem most likely to spread to specific organs. This organ tropism (movement of the cancer toward a specific organ) may result from growth factor or hormones secreted by the target organ or chemotactic factors that attract the tumor. (See *Common sites of metastasis*, page 24.)

CLOSER LOOK

How cancer metastasizes

Cancer usually spreads through the bloodstream to other organs and tissues, as shown here.

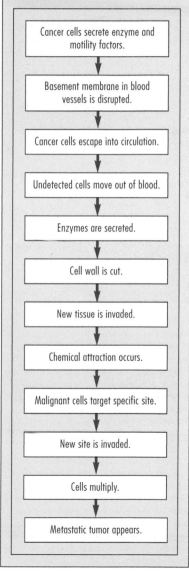

Cancer cells secrete enzyme and motility factors.

↓

Basement membrane in blood vessels is disrupted.

↓

Cancer cells escape into circulation.

↓

Undetected cells move out of blood.

↓

Enzymes are secreted.

↓

Cell wall is cut.

↓

New tissue is invaded.

↓

Chemical attraction occurs.

↓

Malignant cells target specific site.

↓

New site is invaded.

↓

Cells multiply.

↓

Metastatic tumor appears.

Common sites of metastasis

The table below lists some of the more common sites of metastasis for selected cancers.

ORIGINAL SITE	METASTASIS SITE
Breast	Axillary lymph nodes, lung, liver, bone, brain
Colorectal	Liver, lung, peritoneum
Lung	Liver, brain, bone
Ovarian	Peritoneum, diaphragm, liver, lungs
Prostate	Bone
Testicular	Lungs, liver

SIGNS AND SYMPTOMS

In most patients, the earlier the cancer is found, the more effective the treatment is likely to be and the better the prognosis. Some cancers may be diagnosed on a routine physical examination, even before the person develops signs or symptoms. Others may display early warning signals. The American Cancer Society developed a mnemonic device to identify cancer warning signs. (See *Cancer's seven warning signs.*)

Unfortunately, a person may not notice or heed the warning signs. These patients may present with some of the commoner signs and symptoms of advancing disease, such as fatigue, cachexia, pain, anemia, leukopenia and thrombocytopenia, and infection. These signs and symptoms are nonspecific and can be attributed to many other disorders.

Fatigue

Patients commonly describe fatigue as feelings of weakness, being tired, and lacking energy or the ability to concentrate. The underlying mechanism for fatigue isn't known, but it's believed to be the combined result of several pathophysiologic mechanisms.

The very existence of the tumor may contribute to fatigue. A malignant tumor needs oxygen and nutrients to grow. Thus, it depletes the surrounding tissues of blood and oxygen. For example, a vascular tumor can cause lethargy from inadequate oxygen supply to the brain. Lung cancer can interfere with gas exchange and oxygen supply to the heart and peripheral tissues. Accumulating waste products and muscle loss from the release of toxic products of metabolism or other substances from the tumor further add to the fatigue.

Other factors also play a role in fatigue. Pain can be physically and emotionally draining. Stress, anxiety, and other emotional factors further compound the problem. If the person lacks the energy required for self-care, then malnutrition, consequent lack of energy reserves, and anemia can contribute to fatigue.

Cachexia

Cachexia, a generalized wasting of fat and protein, is common in an individual with cancer. A person with cachexia typically appears emaciated and wasted, and experiences an overall deterioration in physical status. Cachexia is characterized by anorexia (loss of appetite), alterations in taste perception, early satiety, weight loss, anemia, marked weakness, and altered metabolism of proteins, carbohydrates, and lipids. Anorexia may accompany pain or adverse reactions to chemotherapy or radiation therapy. Diminished perception of sweet, sour, or salty sensations also contribute to anorexia. Food that once seemed seasoned and palatable now tastes bland.

Protein-calorie malnutrition may cause hypoalbuminemia, edema (the lack of serum proteins, which usually keep fluid in the blood vessels, allows fluid to escape into the tissues), muscle wasting, and immunodeficiency.

The high metabolic activity of malignant tumor cells carries with it the need for nutrients above those required for normal metabolism. As cancer cells appropriate nutrients to fuel their growth, normal tissue becomes starved and depleted, and wasting begins. Under normal circumstances, when starvation occurs, the body spares protein, relying on carbohydrates and fats for energy production. However, cancer cells metabolize both protein and fatty acids to produce energy.

The patient with cancer usually feels sated after eating only a few bites of food. This feeling is believed to be the result of metabolites released from the tumor. Also, tumor necrosis factor produced by the body in response to cancer contributes to cachexia.

Pain

In cancer's early stages, pain is typically absent or mild; as cancer progresses, however, the pain's severity usually increases. When it occurs, pain usually results from one or more of the following:
- pressure or compression
- obstruction
- invasion of sensitive tissue
- visceral surface stretching
- tissue destruction
- inflammation.

Pressure on or obstruction of nerves, blood vessels, or other tissues and organs leads to tissue hypoxia, accumulation of lactic acid, and possibly cell death. In areas where space for the tumor to grow is limited, such as in the brain or bone, compression is a common cause of pain. Also, pain occurs when the viscera, which is usually hollow, is stretched by a tumor, as in GI cancer.

Cancer cells also release proteolytic enzymes that directly injure or destroy neighboring cells. This injury sets up a painful inflammatory response.

Anemia

Cancer of the blood-forming cells, white blood cells or red blood cells may directly cause anemia. Anemia in patients with metastatic cancer is commonly the result of chronic bleeding, severe malnutrition, or chemotherapy or radiation.

Cancer's seven warning signs

The American Cancer Society has developed an easy way to remember the seven warning signs of cancer. Each letter in the word CAUTION represents a possible warning sign that should spur a person to see a physician.

Change in bowel or bladder habits
A sore that doesn't heal
Unusual bleeding or discharge
Thickening or lump in the breast or elsewhere
Indigestion or difficulty swallowing
Obvious change in a wart or mole
Nagging cough or hoarseness

Leukopenia and thrombocytopenia

Typically, leukopenia and thrombocytopenia occur when cancer invades the bone marrow. Chemotherapy and radiation therapy to the bones also can cause leukopenia.

Leukopenia greatly increases the patient's risk of infection; thrombocytopenia increases his risk of hemorrhage. Even when the platelet count is normal, platelet function may be impaired in certain hematologic cancers.

Infection

Infection is common in the patient with advanced cancer, particularly those with myelosuppression from treatment, direct invasion of the bone marrow, development of fistulas, or immunosuppression from hormone release in response to chronic stress. Malnutrition and anemia further increase the patient's risk of infection. Also, obstructions, effusions, and ulcerations may develop, creating a favorable environment for microbial growth.

DIAGNOSIS

A thorough history and physical examination should precede sophisticated diagnostic tests. The choice of diagnostic tests is determined by the patient's signs and symptoms and the suspected body system involved. Diagnostic tests serve several purposes, including:
- establishing tumor presence and extent of disease
- determining possible sites of metastasis
- evaluating affected and unaffected body systems
- identifying the stage and grade of tumor.

Useful tests for early detection and staging of tumors include screening tests, X-rays, radioactive isotope scanning (nuclear medicine imaging), computed tomography (CT) scanning, ultrasonography, magnetic resonance imaging (MRI), positron emission tomography (PET) scanning and endoscopy. The single most important diagnostic tool is the biopsy for direct histologic study of the tumor tissue.

Screening tests

Screening tests are perhaps the most important diagnostic tools in the prevention and early detection of cancer. They may provide valuable information about the possibility of cancer even before the patient develops signs and symptoms. The American Cancer Society has recommended specific screening tests to aid in the early detection of cancer. (See *ACS guidelines: Early cancer detection.*)

Diagnosis by imaging

Imaging studies, such as radiography, nuclear medicine scans, CT and ultrasonography, are commonly used to diagnose cancer. Tests, such as MRI and PET, provide highly distinct images of the body area being scanned.

X-RAY EXAMINATION
Typically, X-rays are ordered to identify and evaluate changes in tissue densities.

The type and location of the X-ray is determined by the patient's signs and symptoms and the suspected location of the tumor or metastasis. For example, a chest X-ray may be used to identify lung cancer if the patient is an older smoker or to rule out lung metastasis in a patient with colorectal cancer.

Some X-rays, such as those of the GI tract (with barium enema) and the urinary tract (excretory urography), involve the use of contrast agents. Radiopaque substances can also be injected into the lymphatic system, and their flow can be monitored by lymphangiography. This specialized X-ray technique is helpful in evaluating tumors of the lymph nodes and metastasis. Because lymphangiography is invasive and may be difficult to interpret, CT scans and MRI have largely replaced that method.

RADIOACTIVE ISOTOPE SCANNING
With radioactive isotope scanning, a specialized camera detects radioactive isotopes that are injected into the bloodstream or ingested. The radiologist evaluates their distribution (uptake) throughout tissues, organs, and organ systems. This type of scanning provides a view of organs and regions within the organ that can't be seen with a simple X-ray. The area of uptake is termed a hot spot or a cold spot (an area of decreased uptake). Typically, tumors are revealed as cold spots; the exception is the bone scan, in which hot spots indicate the presence of disease. Examples of organs commonly evaluated with radioactive isotope scanning include thyroid, liver, spleen, brain, and bone.

COMPUTED TOMOGRAPHY SCANNING
CT scanning evaluates successive layers of tissue by using narrow-beam X-ray to provide a cross-sectional view of the structure. It can also reveal different characteristics of tissues within a solid organ. CT images are commonly obtained of the brain and head, body, and abdomen to assess for neurologic, pelvic, abdominal, and thoracic cancers.

ACS guidelines: Early cancer detection

Everyone should have a general cancer-related check-up (including health counseling and specific examinations for malignant and non-malignant disorders) every 3 years for ages 20 to 40 and every year for age 40 and older. The following recommendations from the American Cancer Society (ACS) focus on five common cancers whose survival rates can be improved if the cancer is detected early.

SCREENING AREA AND TEST	FREQUENCY AND POPULATION
BREAST	
◆ Mammogram	◆ Every year for age 40 and older
◆ Clinical breast examination	◆ Part of every woman's health examination; every year for age 40 and older; every 3 years for ages 20 to 39
◆ Breast self-examination	◆ Optional; suggested monthly for age 20 and older*
COLON AND RECTUM	
◆ Fecal occult blood test (FOBT)	◆ Every year for age 50 and older**
◆ Flexible sigmoidoscopy	◆ Every 5 years for age 50 and older**
◆ Colonoscopy	◆ Every 10 years for age 50 and older
◆ Double-contrast barium enema	◆ Every 5 years for age 50 and older
PROSTATE	
◆ Prostate-specific antigen	◆ Annually for men younger than age 50 at high risk and men age 50 and older with life expectancy of at least 10 years
◆ Digital rectal examination	◆ Annually for men younger than age 50 at high risk and men age 50 and older with life expectancy of at least 10 years
CERVIX	
◆ Papanicolaou (Pap) test	◆ Annually for sexually active women and women age 18 and older; women ages 30 to 70, with three or more consecutive satisfactory examinations with normal findings, every 2 to 3 years; women age 70 and older with three or more consecutive satisfactory examinations and no abnormal Pap tests in the last 10 years, screening may stop
ENDOMETRIUM	
◆ Tissue sampling	◆ Annually, beginning at age 35, for women at risk for hereditary nonpolyposis colon cancer

* Women in their 20s should be instructed about the benefits and limitations of breast self-examination; women have the option of not performing breast self-examination or performing it only occasionally.
** Most clinicians prefer the combination of FOBT and flexible sigmoidoscopy over either of the two tests alone.

ULTRASONOGRAPHY
Ultrasonography uses high-frequency sound waves to detect tissue density changes that are difficult or impossible to determine by radiology or endoscopy. Ultrasound helps differentiate cysts from solid tumors and is commonly used to provide information about abdominal and pelvic cancer.

MAGNETIC RESONANCE IMAGING

MRI uses magnetic fields and radio frequencies to view a cross-section of the body organs and structures. Like CT scanning, it's commonly used to evaluate neurologic, pelvic, abdominal, and thoracic cancers.

POSITRON EMISSION TOMOGRAPHY SCANNING

PET scanning uses radioisotope technology to create a picture of the body in action. PET scanning uses computers to construct images from the emission of positive electrons (positrons) by radioactive substances administered to the patient. Unlike other diagnostic methods that simply create images of how the body looks, PET scanning provides real-time three-dimensional imaging of the body while it functions. Using PET scanning to study the spread of cancer involves injecting the cancer patient with a small amount of radioactive glucose. Cancerous cells metabolize sugar more quickly than healthy cells, so the PET images show cancer cells as having a greater concentration of sugar.

Endoscopy

Endoscopy provides a direct view of a body cavity or passageway to detect abnormalities. Common endoscopic sites include the upper and lower GI tract, and bronchial tree. During endoscopy, the physician can excise small tumors, aspirate fluid, or obtain tissue specimens for histologic examination.

Biopsy

A biopsy, the removal of a portion of suspicious tissue, is the only definitive method to diagnose cancer. Biopsy tissue specimens can be taken by curettage, fluid aspiration (pleural effusion), fine-needle aspiration (breast), dermal punch (skin or mouth), endoscopy (rectal polyps and esophageal lesions), and surgical excision (visceral tissue and nodes). The tissue specimen then undergoes laboratory analysis for cell type and characteristics to provide information about the grade and stage of the cancer.

Tumor cell markers

Some cancer cells release substances that usually aren't present in the body or are present only in small quantities. These substances, called *tumor markers* or *biological markers,* are produced by the cancer cell's genetic material during growth and development or by other cells in response to the presence of cancer. (See *Common tumor cell markers.*)

Markers may be found on the tumor's cell membrane or in the blood, cerebrospinal fluid, or urine. Tumor cell markers include hormones, enzymes, genes, antigens, and antibodies. Tumor cell markers have many clinical uses, such as:

■ screening people who are at high risk for cancer
■ diagnosing a specific type of cancer in conjunction with clinical manifestations
■ monitoring therapy's effectiveness
■ detecting cancer recurrence.

Tumor cell markers provide a method for detecting and monitoring the progression of certain types of cancer. Unfortunately, several disadvantages of tumor cell markers may preclude their use alone. For example:

■ By the time the tumor cell marker level is elevated, the disease may be too far advanced to treat.
■ Most tumor cell markers aren't specific enough to identify one specific type of cancer.
■ Some nonmalignant diseases, such as pancreatitis or ulcerative colitis, are also linked to tumor cell markers.

Perhaps the worst drawback is that the absence of a tumor cell marker doesn't mean that a person is free from cancer. For example, mucinous ovarian cancer tumors typically don't express the ovarian cancer marker CA 125, so that a normal test result doesn't eliminate the possibility of ovarian cancer.

Common tumor cell markers

Tumor cell markers may be used to detect, diagnose, or treat cancer. Alone, however, they aren't enough for a diagnosis. Tumor cell markers may also be caused by benign (nonmalignant) conditions. The chart below highlights some of the more commonly used tumor cell markers and their associated malignant and nonmalignant conditions.

MARKER	MALIGNANT CONDITIONS	NONMALIGNANT CONDITIONS
Alpha fetoprotein	◆ Endodermal sinus tumor ◆ Liver cancer ◆ Ovarian germ cell cancer ◆ Testicular germ cell cancer (specifically embryonal cell carcinoma)	◆ Ataxia-telangiectasia ◆ Cirrhosis ◆ Hepatitis ◆ Pregnancy ◆ Wiskott-Aldrich syndrome
Carcinoembryonic antigen	◆ Bladder cancer ◆ Breast cancer ◆ Cervical cancer ◆ Colorectal cancer ◆ Kidney cancer ◆ Liver cancer ◆ Lung cancer ◆ Lymphoma ◆ Melanoma ◆ Ovarian cancer ◆ Pancreatic cancer ◆ Stomach cancer ◆ Thyroid cancer	◆ Inflammatory bowel disease ◆ Liver disease ◆ Pancreatitis ◆ Tobacco use
CA 15-3	◆ Breast cancer (usually advanced) ◆ Lung cancer ◆ Ovarian cancer ◆ Prostate cancer	◆ Benign breast disease ◆ Benign ovarian disease ◆ Endometriosis ◆ Hepatitis ◆ Lactation ◆ Pelvic inflammatory disease ◆ Pregnancy
CA 19-9	◆ Bile duct cancer ◆ Colorectal cancer ◆ Pancreatic cancer ◆ Stomach cancer	◆ Cholecystitis ◆ Cirrhosis ◆ Gallstones ◆ Pancreatitis
CA 27-29	◆ Breast cancer ◆ Colon cancer ◆ Kidney cancer ◆ Liver cancer ◆ Lung cancer ◆ Ovarian cancer ◆ Pancreatic cancer ◆ Stomach cancer ◆ Uterine cancer	◆ Benign breast disease ◆ Endometriosis ◆ Kidney disease ◆ Liver disease ◆ Ovarian cysts ◆ Pregnancy (first trimester)

(continued)

Common tumor cell markers *(continued)*

MARKER	MALIGNANT CONDITIONS	NONMALIGNANT CONDITIONS
CA 125	◆ Colorectal cancer ◆ Gastric cancer ◆ Ovarian cancer ◆ Pancreatic cancer	◆ Endometriosis ◆ Liver disease ◆ Menstruation ◆ Pancreatitis ◆ Pelvic inflammatory disease ◆ Peritonitis ◆ Pregnancy
Human chorionic gonadotropin	◆ Choriocarcinoma ◆ Embryonal cell carcinoma ◆ Gestational trophoblastic disease ◆ Liver cancer ◆ Lung cancer ◆ Pancreatic cancer ◆ Specific dysgerminomas of the ovary ◆ Stomach cancer ◆ Testicular cancer	◆ Marijuana use ◆ Pregnancy
Lactate dehydrogenase	◆ Almost all cancers ◆ Ewing's sarcoma ◆ Leukemia ◆ Non-Hodgkin's lymphoma ◆ Testicular cancer	◆ Anemia ◆ Heart failure ◆ Hypothyroidism ◆ Liver disease ◆ Lung disease
Neuron-specific enolase	◆ Kidney cancer ◆ Melanoma ◆ Neuroblastoma ◆ Pancreatic cancer ◆ Small-cell lung cancer ◆ Testicular cancer ◆ Thyroid cancer ◆ Wilms' tumor	◆ Unknown
Prostatic acid phosphatase	◆ Prostate cancer	◆ Benign prostatic conditions
Prostate-specific antigen	◆ Prostate cancer	◆ Benign prostatic hyperplasia ◆ Prostatitis

Tumor Classification

Tumors are first classified as benign or malignant, depending on the specific features exhibited by the tumor. Benign tumors are usually well differentiated; that is, their cells closely resemble those of the tissue of origin. Commonly encapsulated, with well-defined borders, benign tumors grow slowly, usually displacing but not infiltrating surrounding tissues and causing only slight damage. Benign tumors don't metastasize.

Conversely, most malignant tumors are undifferentiated to varying degrees, having cells that may differ considerably from those of the tissue of origin. They're seldom encapsulated and are usually poorly delineated. They rapidly expand in all directions, causing extensive damage as they infiltrate surrounding tissues. Most malignant tumors metastasize through the blood or lymph to secondary sites.

Malignant tumors are further classified by tissue type, degree of differentiation (grading), and extent of the disease (staging). High-grade tumors are poorly differentiated and are more aggressive than low-grade tumors. Early-stage cancers carry a more favorable prognosis than later-stage cancers that have metastasized.

Tissue type

Histologically, the type of tissue in which the growth originates classifies malignant tumors. Three cell layers form during the early stages of human embryonic development:

■ Ectoderm primarily forms the external embryonic covering and the structures that will come into contact with the environment.

■ Mesoderm forms the circulatory system, muscles, supporting tissue, and most of the urinary and reproductive system.

■ Endoderm gives rise to the internal linings of the embryo, such as the epithelial lining of the pharynx and the respiratory and GI tracts.

Carcinomas are tumors of epithelial tissue. They may originate in the endodermal tissues, which develop into internal structures, such as the stomach and intestine, or in ectodermal tissues, which develop into external structures such as the skin. Tumors arising from glandular epithelial tissue are commonly called *adenocarcinomas*.

Sarcomas originate in the mesodermal tissues, which develop into supporting structures, such as the bone, muscle, fat, or blood. Sarcomas may be further classified based on the specific cells involved. For example, malignant tumors arising from pigmented cells are called *melanomas*; from plasma cells, *myelomas*; and from lymphatic tissue, *lymphomas*.

Grading

Histologically, malignant tumors are classified by their degree of differentiation. The greater their differentiation, the greater the tumor cells' similarity to the tissue of origin. Typically, a malignant tumor is graded on a scale of 1 to 4, in order of increasing clinical severity.

■ *Grade 1:* Well differentiated; cells closely resemble the tissue of origin and maintain some specialized function.

■ *Grade 2:* Moderately well differentiated; cells vary somewhat in size and shape with increased mitosis.

■ *Grade 3:* Poorly differentiated; cells vary widely in size and shape with little resemblance to the tissue of origin; mitosis is greatly increased.

■ *Grade 4:* Undifferentiated; cells exhibit no similarity to tissue of origin.

Staging

Malignant tumors are staged (classified anatomically) by the extent of the disease. The most commonly used method for staging is the TNM staging system, which evaluates *t*umor size, *n*odal involvement, and *m*etastatic progress. This classification system provides an accurate tumor description that's adjustable as the disease progresses. TNM staging enables reliable comparison of treatments and survival rates among large population groups; it also identifies nodal involvement and metastasis to other areas. (See *Understanding TNM staging,* page 32.)

Understanding TNM staging

The TNM (tumor, node, and metastasis) system developed by the American Joint Committee on Cancer provides a consistent method for classifying malignant tumors based on the extent of the disease. It also offers a convenient structure to standardize diagnostic and treatment protocols. Differences in classification may occur, depending on the primary cancer site.

T FOR PRIMARY TUMOR
The anatomic extent of the primary tumor depends on its size, depth of invasion, and surface spread. Tumor stages progress from TX to T4 as follows:
TX — Primary tumor can't be assessed
T0 — No evidence of primary tumor
Tis — Carcinoma in situ
T1, T2, T3, T4 — Increasing size or local extent (or both) of primary tumor

N FOR NODAL INVOLVEMENT
Nodal involvement reflects the tumor's spread to the lymph nodes as follows:
NX — Regional lymph nodes can't be assessed
N0 — No evidence of regional lymph node metastasis
N1, N2, N3 — Increasing involvement of regional lymph nodes

M FOR DISTANT METASTASIS
Metastasis denotes the extent (or spread) of disease. Levels range from MX to M4 as follows:
MX — Distant metastasis can't be assessed
M0 — No evidence of distant metastasis
M1 — Single, solitary distant metastasis
M2, M3, M4 — Multiple foci or multiple organ metastasis

TREATMENT

Cancer treatments include surgery, radiation therapy, chemotherapy, immunotherapy (also called *biotherapy*), and hormonal therapy. Each may be used alone or in combination (called *multimodal therapy*), depending on the tumor's type, stage, localization, and responsiveness and on limitations imposed by the patient's clinical status. Cancer treatment has four goals:
■ cure, to eradicate the cancer and promote long-term patient survival
■ control, to arrest tumor growth
■ palliation, to alleviate symptoms when the disease is beyond control
■ prophylaxis, to provide treatment when no tumor is detectable but the patient is known to be at high risk for tumor development or recurrence.

Cancer treatment is further categorized by type according to when it's used, as follows:
■ primary, to eradicate the disease

■ adjuvant, in addition to primary, to eliminate microscopic disease and promote cure or improve the patient's response
■ salvage or palliative, to manage recurrent disease.

As with any treatment regimen, complications may arise. Indeed, many complications of cancer are related to the adverse effects of treatment, such as fluid and electrolyte imbalances resulting from anorexia, vomiting, or diarrhea; bone marrow suppression, including anemia, leukopenia, thrombocytopenia, and neutropenia; and infection. Hypercalcemia is the most common metabolic abnormality experienced by cancer patients. Pain, which accompanies all progressing cancers, can reach intolerable levels.

Certain complications are life-threatening and require prompt intervention. These oncologic emergencies may result from the tumor's effects or its by-products, secondary involvement of other organs caused by disease spread, or adverse effects of treatment. (See *Common cancer emergencies,* pages 34 and 35.)

Surgery

Surgery, once the mainstay of cancer treatment, is now typically combined with other therapies. It may be performed to diagnose the disease, initiate primary treatment, or achieve palliation, and it's sometimes done for prevention. The surgical biopsy procedure is diagnostic surgery, and additional surgery then removes the bulk of the tumor. When used as primary treatment, surgery is an attempt to remove the entire tumor (or as much as possible, by a procedure called *debulking*), along with surrounding tissues, including lymph nodes.

A common method of surgical removal of a small tumor mass is called "wide and local excision." The tumor mass is removed along with a small or moderate amount of easily accessible surrounding tissue that's normal. A radical or modified radical excision removes the primary tumor along with lymph nodes, nearby involved structures, and surrounding structures that may be at high risk for disease spread. Typically, a radical excision results in some degree of disfigurement and altered functioning. Today's less radical surgical procedures such as a lumpectomy instead of mastectomy are more acceptable to the patient. The health care professional and the patient should discuss the type of surgery. Ultimately, the choice belongs to the patient.

Palliative surgery is used to relieve complications, such as pain, ulceration, obstruction, hemorrhage, or pressure. Examples include a cordotomy to relieve intractable pain and bowel resection or ostomy to remove a bowel obstruction. Also, surgery may be performed to remove hormone-producing glands, thereby limiting the growth of a hormone-sensitive tumor.

Prophylactic surgery involves removal of nonvital tissues or organs with a high potential for developing cancer in patients with personal or familial risk factors for a particular type of cancer. One example is prophylactic mastectomy. This type of surgery is controversial because of it possible long-term physiologic and psychological effects, although potential benefits may significantly outweigh the disadvantages.

Radiation therapy

Radiation therapy uses high-energy radiation to treat cancer. Used alone or with other therapies, it aims to destroy dividing cancer cells while damaging normal cells as little as possible. Two types of radiation are used to treat cancer: ionizing radiation and particle beam radiation. Both target the cellular deoxyribonucleic acid (DNA). Ionizing radiation deposits energy that damages the genetic material inside the cancer cells. Normal cells are also affected but can recover. Particle beam radiation uses a special machine and fast-moving particles to treat the cancer. The particles can cause more cell damage than ionizing radiation does.

The guiding principle for radiation therapy is that the dose be large enough to eradicate the tumor but small enough to minimize the adverse effects to the surrounding normal tissue. How well the treatment meets this goal is the *therapeutic ratio*.

Radiation interacts with oxygen in the nucleus to break strands of DNA and interacts with water in body fluids (including fluid in the cells) to form free radicals, which also damage the DNA. If this damage isn't repaired, the cells die, immediately or when they try to divide. Radiation may also make tumor cells unable to enter the cell cycle. Thus, cells most vulnerable to radiation therapy are those that divide frequently, for example, cells of the bone marrow, lymph, GI epithelium, and gonads.

Therapeutic radiation can be delivered by external beam radiation or by intracavitary or interstitial implants. Use of implants requires an inpatient stay, and anyone who comes in contact with the patient while the internal radiation implants are in place must wear radiation protection. High-dose-rate remote brachytherapy, a temporary form of radiation implantation (it's in place for only a few minutes), delivers powerful radiation directly to the tumor through several hollow catheters, while minimizing damage to the surrounding tissues. This therapy is typically done on an outpatient basis. It has been used to treat breast, cervical, esophageal, lung, pancreatic, and prostatic cancers.

Common cancer emergencies

The following chart lists certain oncologic emergencies that may arise and the associated malignancy.

EMERGENCIES AND CAUSE	ASSOCIATED MALIGNANCY
CARDIAC TAMPONADE ◆ Fluid accumulation around pericardial space or pericardial thickening caused by radiation therapy	◆ Breast cancer ◆ Leukemia ◆ Lymphoma ◆ Melanoma
HYPERCALCEMIA ◆ Increased bone resorption from bone destruction or tumor-related elevation of parathyroid hormone, osteoclast-activating factor, or prostaglandin levels	◆ Breast cancer ◆ Lung cancer ◆ Multiple myeloma ◆ Renal cancer
DISSEMINATED INTRAVASCULAR COAGULATION ◆ Widespread clotting in arterioles and capillaries and simultaneous hemorrhage	◆ Hematologic cancer ◆ Mucin-producing adenocarcinomas
MALIGNANT PERITONEAL INFUSION ◆ Seeding of tumor into the peritoneum, excess intraperitoneal fluid production or release of humoral factors by the tumor	◆ Ovarian cancer
MALIGNANT PLEURAL EFFUSION ◆ Implantation of cancer cells on pleural surface, tumor obstruction of lymphatic channels or pulmonary veins, shedding of necrotic tumor cells into the pleural space, or thoracic duct perforation	◆ Breast cancer ◆ GI tract cancer ◆ Leukemia ◆ Lung cancer (most common) ◆ Lymphoma ◆ Testicular cancer
SPINAL CORD COMPRESSION ◆ Encroachment on spinal cord or cauda equina caused by metastasis or vertebral collapse and displacement of bony elements	◆ Cancer of lung, breast, kidney, GI tract, prostate, or cervix ◆ Melanoma
SUPERIOR VENA CAVA SYNDROME ◆ Impaired venous return caused by occlusion of vena cava	◆ Breast cancer ◆ Lung cancer ◆ Lymphoma

Common cancer emergencies *(continued)*

EMERGENCIES AND CAUSE	ASSOCIATED MALIGNANCY
SYNDROME OF INAPPROPRIATE ANTIDIURETIC HORMONE ◆ Ectopic production by tumor; abnormal stimulation of hypothalamus-pituitary axis; mimicking or enhanced effects on kidney; may result from chemotherapy	◆ Bladder cancer ◆ GI tract cancer ◆ Hodgkin's disease ◆ Prostate cancer ◆ Sarcomas ◆ Small-cell lung cancer
TUMOR LYSIS SYNDROME ◆ Rapid cell destruction and turnover caused by chemotherapy or rapid tumor growth	◆ Leukemias ◆ Lymphomas

Normal and malignant cells respond to radiation differently, depending on blood supply, oxygen saturation, previous irradiation, and immune status. Generally, normal cells recover from radiation faster than malignant cells. Success of treatment and damage to normal tissue also vary with the radiation's intensity. Although a large, single dose of radiation has greater cellular effects than fractions of the same amount delivered sequentially, the longer schedule allows time for normal tissue to recover between doses.

ADVERSE EFFECTS
Radiation may be used palliatively to relieve pain, obstruction, malignant effusions, cough, dyspnea, ulcerations, and hemorrhage. It can also promote healing of pathologic fractures after surgical stabilization and delay metastasis.

Combining radiation and surgery can minimize the need for radical surgery, prolong survival, and preserve anatomic function. For example, preoperative doses of radiation shrink a large tumor to operable size while preventing further spread of the disease during surgery. After the wound heals, postoperative doses prevent residual cancer cells from multiplying or metastasizing.

Radiation therapy has local and systemic adverse effects because it affects normal cells along with malignant cells. Systemic adverse effects — such as weakness, fatigue, anorexia, nausea, vomiting, and anemia — may respond to antiemetics, steroids, frequent small meals, fluid maintenance, and rest. The effects are seldom severe enough to require stopping radiation, but they may make a dosage adjustment necessary. (For localized adverse effects, see *Radiation's adverse effects,* page 36.)

Patients receiving radiation therapy must have frequent blood tests to check blood counts, particularly white blood cells and platelets if the target site involves areas of bone marrow production. Radiation also requires special skin care measures, such as covering the irradiated area with loose cotton clothing to protect it from light and avoiding deodorants, colognes, and other topical agents during treatment.

Chemotherapy

Chemotherapy includes a wide range of antineoplastic drugs, which may induce regression of a tumor and suppress its metastasis. It's particularly useful in controlling residual disease and as an adjunct to surgery or radiation therapy. It can induce long remissions and sometimes bring about cure, especially in a patient with childhood leukemia, Hodgkin's disease,

Radiation's adverse effects

Radiation therapy can cause local adverse effects depending on the area irradiated. The chart below highlights some of the more commonly seen local effects and the measures to manage them.

AREA IRRADIATED	ADVERSE EFFECT	MANAGEMENT
Head and neck	◆ Alopecia	◆ Gentle combing and grooming of scalp ◆ Soft head cover
	◆ Mucositis	◆ Cool carbonated drinks ◆ Ice, ice pops ◆ Soft, nonirritating diet ◆ Non-alcohol-based mouthwash with viscous lidocaine ◆ Soft toothbrushes or swabs
	◆ Xerostomia (dry mouth)	◆ Good oral hygiene ◆ Oral saliva replacement
	◆ Dental caries	◆ Gingival care ◆ Prophylactic fluoride to teeth
Chest	◆ Lung tissue irritation	◆ Avoidance of people with upper respiratory infections ◆ Humidifier if necessary ◆ Steroid therapy
	◆ Pericarditis ◆ Myocarditis	◆ Antiarrhythmics
	◆ Esophagitis	◆ Analgesia ◆ Fluid maintenance ◆ Total parenteral nutrition
Kidneys	◆ Anemia ◆ Azotemia ◆ Edema ◆ Headache ◆ Hypertensive neuropathy ◆ Lassitude ◆ Nephritis	◆ Fluid and electrolyte maintenance ◆ Monitoring for signs of renal failure
Abdomen and pelvis	◆ Cramps ◆ Diarrhea	◆ Fluid and electrolyte maintenance ◆ Loperamide and diphenoxylate with atropine ◆ Low-residue diet

choriocarcinoma, or testicular cancer. As a palliative treatment, chemotherapy aims to improve the patient's quality of life by temporarily relieving pain and other symptoms.

Every dose of a chemotherapeutic agent destroys only a percentage of tumor cells.

Therefore, regression of the tumor requires repeated doses of drugs. The goal is to eradicate enough of the tumor so that the immune system can destroy the remaining malignant cells.

Tumor cells that are in the active phase of cell division (called the *growth fraction*) are the most sensitive to chemotherapeutic agents. Nondividing cells are the least sensitive and thus are the most potentially dangerous. They must be destroyed to eradicate a malignancy. Therefore, repeated cycles of chemotherapy are used to destroy nondividing cells as they enter the cell cycle to begin active proliferation.

Depending on the type of cancer, one or more different categories of chemotherapeutic agents may be used. The most commonly used types of chemotherapeutic agents are:

■ *Alkylating agents and nitrosoureas* inhibit cell growth and division by reacting with DNA at any phase of the cell cycle. They prevent cell replication by breaking and cross-linking DNA.

■ *Antimetabolites* prevent cell growth by competing with metabolites in the production of nucleic acid, substituting themselves for purines and pyrimidines, which are essential for DNA and ribonucleic acid (RNA) synthesis. They exert their effect during the S phase of the cell cycle.

■ *Antitumor antibiotics* block cell growth by binding with DNA and interfering with DNA-dependent RNA synthesis. Acting in any phase of the cell cycle, they bind to DNA and generate toxic oxygen free radicals that break one or both strands of DNA.

■ *Plant (Vinca) alkaloids* prevent cellular reproduction by disrupting mitosis. Acting primarily in the M phase of the cell cycle, they interfere with the formation of the mitotic spindle by binding to microtubular proteins.

■ *Hormones and hormone antagonists* impair cell growth by one or both of two mechanisms. They may alter the cell environment, thereby affecting the cell membrane's permeability, or they may inhibit the growth of hormone-susceptible tumors by changing their chemical environment. These agents include adrenocorticosteroids, androgens, gonadotropin inhibitors, and aromatase inhibitors.

Other chemotherapeutic agents include podophyllotoxins and taxanes (which, like plant alkaloids, interfere with formation of the mitotic spindle) and miscellaneous agents, such as hydroxyurea and L-asparaginase (which seem to be cell-cycle-specific agents but whose mode of action is unclear). (See *Chemotherapy's action in the cell cycle,* page 38.)

A combination of drugs from different categories may be used to kill the most tumor cells. Combination therapy typically includes drugs with different toxicities and synergistic actions. Use of combination therapy also helps prevent the development of drug-resistant mechanisms by the tumor cells.

ADVERSE EFFECTS

Chemotherapy causes numerous adverse effects that reflect the drugs' mechanism of action. Although antineoplastic agents are toxic to cancer cells, they can also cause transient changes in normal tissues, especially those with proliferating cells. For example, antineoplastic agents typically cause anemia, leukopenia, and thrombocytopenia (because they suppress bone marrow function); vomiting (because they irritate the GI epithelial cells); and alopecia and dermatitis (because they destroy hair follicles and skin cells). Many antineoplastic agents are given I.V., and they can cause venous sclerosis and pain when administered. If when administered they escape or discharge from the vein directly into the tissue (are extravasated), they may cause deep cutaneous necrosis, requiring debridement and skin grafting. To minimize the risk of extravasation, most drugs with the potential for direct tissue injury are now given through a central venous catheter.

The pharmacologic action of a given drug determines whether it's administered orally, subcutaneously, I.M., I.V., intracavitarily, intrathecally, or by arterial infusion. Dosages are calculated according to the patient's body surface area, with adjustments for the patient's general condition and the degree of myelosuppression.

DISRUPTING DISEASE
Chemotherapy's action in the cell cycle

Some chemotherapeutic drugs are cell-cycle specific, impairing cellular growth by causing changes in the cell during specific phases of the cell cycle. Other drugs are cell-cycle nonspecific, affecting the cell at any phase during the cell cycle. The illustration below shows where the cell-cycle specific drugs work to disrupt cancer cell growth.

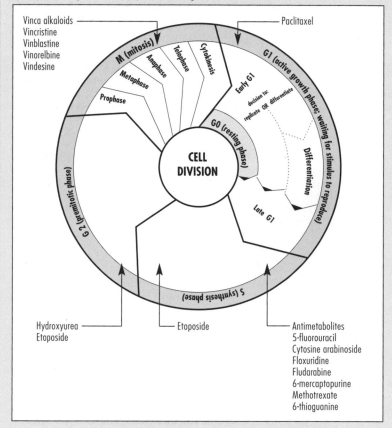

Vinca alkaloids
Vincristine
Vinblastine
Vinorelbine
Vindesine

Paclitaxel

M (mitosis)
Cytokinesis
Telophase
Anaphase
Metaphase
Prophase

G1 (active growth phase; waiting for stimulus to reproduce)

Early G1

decision to:
replicate OR differentiate

G0 (resting phase)

Differentiation

Late G1

CELL DIVISION

G 2 (premitotic phase)

S (synthesis phase)

Hydroxyurea
Etoposide

Etoposide

Antimetabolites
5-fluorouracil
Cytosine arabinoside
Floxuridine
Fludarabine
6-mercaptopurine
Methotrexate
6-thioguanine

Many patients approach chemotherapy apprehensively. They need to be allowed to express their concerns and be provided with simple and truthful information. Explanations about what to expect, including possible adverse effects, can help minimize fear and anxiety.

Hormonal therapy

Hormonal therapy is based on studies showing that certain hormones can inhibit the growth of certain cancers. For example, the luteinizing hormone–releasing hormone analogue, leuprolide, is used to treat prostate cancer. With long-term use, this hormone inhibits testosterone release and tumor growth. Tamoxifen, an anti-estrogen hormonal agent, blocks estrogen receptors in breast tumor cells that require estrogen to thrive. Also, women at high risk for breast cancer can take tamoxifen prophylactically. Adrenocortical steroids are effective in treating leukemias and lymphomas because they suppress lymphocytes.

Adverse effects of these hormonal agents include hot flashes, sweating, impotence, decreased libido, nausea and vomiting, and, with tamoxifen, blood disorders (dyscrasias).

Biotherapy

Biotherapy (also known as *immunotherapy*) relies on treatment agents known as biological response modifiers. Biological agents are usually combined with chemotherapeutic drugs or radiation therapy. Much of the work done in biotherapy is still experimental, but the Food and Drug Administration has approved several new drugs that are providing promising results. For example, rituximab—a monoclonal antibody—is effective in treating relapsed or refractory B-cell non-Hodgkin's lymphoma.

The main biotherapy agent classifications are interferons, interleukins, hematopoietic growth factors, and monoclonal antibodies. Interferons have antiviral, antiproliferative, and immunomodulary effects. Interleukins exert their effects on the T lymphocytes. Monoclonal antibodies such as rituximab provide the most tumor-specific therapy for cancer by selectively binding to tumor cell surfaces. Although not used to treat cancer directly, hematopoietic growth factors are used to increase the patient's blood counts when chemotherapy or radiation reduces them.

Adverse effects of biotherapeutic agents mimic the body's normal immune response, with flulike symptoms being the most common.

Reviewing common cancers

The table below highlights the important signs and symptoms and diagnostic test results for some of the most common cancers.

TYPE AND FINDINGS	DIAGNOSTIC TEST RESULTS
ACUTE LEUKEMIA	
◆ Sudden onset of high fever resulting from bone marrow invasion and cellular proliferation within bone marrow ◆ Thrombocytopenia and abnormal bleeding caused by bone marrow suppression ◆ Weakness, lassitude linked to anemia from bone marrow invasion ◆ Pallor and weakness linked to anemia ◆ Chills and recurrent infections caused by proliferation of immature nonfunctioning white blood cells (WBCs) ◆ Bone pain from leukemic infiltration of bone ◆ Neurologic manifestations including headache, papilledema, facial palsy, blurred vision, and meningeal irritation caused by leukemic infiltration or cerebral bleeding ◆ Liver, spleen, and lymph node enlargement from leukemic cell infiltration	◆ Bone marrow aspiration reveals proliferation of immature WBCs. ◆ Complete blood count (CBC) shows thrombocytopenia and neutropenia. ◆ Differential WBC count reveals cell type. ◆ Lumbar puncture reveals leukemic infiltration to cerebrospinal fluid (CSF).

(continued)

Reviewing common cancers *(continued)*

TYPE AND FINDINGS	DIAGNOSTIC TEST RESULTS

BASAL CELL CARCINOMA

- Noduloulcerative lesions usually on face (forehead, eyelid regions, and nasolabial folds) appearing as small, smooth, pinkish, and translucent papules with telangiectatic vessels crossing surface; occasionally pigmented; depressed centers with firm elevated borders with enlargement resulting from basal cell proliferation in the deepest layer of epidermis with local invasion
- Superficial basal cell epitheliomas, commonly on chest and back, appearing as oval or irregularly shaped, lightly pigmented scaly plaques with sharply defined, threadlike elevated borders resembling psoriasis or eczema resulting from basal cell proliferation
- Sclerosing basal cell epitheliomas occurring on the head and neck and appearing as waxy, sclerotic yellow to white plaques without distinct borders resulting from basal cell proliferation

- All types diagnosed by clinical appearance, incisional or excisional biopsy, and histologic study.

BLADDER CANCER

Early stages
- Commonly produces no symptoms

Later stages
- Gross painless intermittent hematuria caused by tumor invasion
- Suprapubic pain after voiding from pressure exerted by the tumor or obstruction
- Bladder irritability and frequency related to tumor compression and invasion

- Cystoscopy and biopsy confirm cell type.
- Urinalysis reveals hematuria and malignant cytology.
- Excretory urography identifies large early stage tumor or infiltrating tumor.
- Retrograde cystography reveals changes in bladder structure and bladder wall integrity.
- Pelvic arteriography confirms tumor invasion into bladder wall.
- Computed tomography (CT) scan reveals thickened bladder wall and enlarged retroperitoneal lymph nodes.
- Ultrasonography detects metastasis beyond bladder; differentiates presence of tumor from cyst.

BONE CANCER

- Possibly producing no symptoms
- Bone pain especially at night from tumor disruption of normal structural integrity and pressure on surrounding tissues
- Tender, swollen, possibly palpable mass resulting from tumor growth

- Incisional or aspiration biopsy confirms cell type.
- Bone X-rays, radioisotope bone scan, and CT scan reveal tumor size.
- Elevated alkaline phosphatase level.

Reviewing common cancers *(continued)*

TYPE AND FINDINGS	DIAGNOSTIC TEST RESULTS

BONE CANCER *(continued)*

- Pathologic fractures caused by tumor invasion and destruction of bone causing weakening
- Hypercalcemia from ectopic parathyroid hormone production by the tumor or increased bone resorption
- Limited mobility (late in the disease) from continued tumor growth and disruption of bone strength

BREAST CANCER

- Hard stony mass in the breast related to cellular growth
- Change in symmetry of breast caused by growth of tumor on one side
- Skin thickening or dimpling, scaly skin around nipple or changes in nipple, edema, or ulceration related to tumor cell infiltration to surrounding tissues
- Warm, hot, pink area from inflammation and infiltration of surrounding tissues
- Unusual discharge or drainage indicating tumor invasion and infiltration into the ductal system
- Pain related to advancement of tumor and subsequent pressure
- Hypercalcemia or pathologic fractures caused by metastasis to bone

- Breast examination reveals lump or mass in breast.
- Mammography reveals presence of mass and location.
- Needle or surgical biopsy confirms the cell type.
- Ultrasonography reveals solid tumor differentiating it from a fluid-filled cyst.
- Bone scan and CT scan reveal metastasis.
- Elevated alkaline phosphatase levels, liver biopsy, and liver function studies reveal liver metastasis.
- Hormonal receptor assay identifies tumor as hormonal dependent.

CERVICAL CANCER

- No symptoms or other clinically apparent changes in preinvasive cervical cancer
- Abnormal vaginal bleeding with persistent vaginal discharge and postcoital pain and bleeding related to cellular invasion and erosion of the cervical epithelium
- Pelvic pain caused by pressure on surrounding tissues and nerves from cellular proliferation
- Vaginal leakage of urine and feces from fistulas caused by erosion and necrosis of cervix
- Anorexia, weight loss, and anemia related to the hypermetabolic activity of cellular proliferation and increased tumor growth needs

- Papanicolaou (Pap) test reveals malignant cellular changes.
- Colposcopy identifies the presence and extent of early lesions.
- Biopsy confirms cell type.
- CT scan, nuclear imaging scan, and lymphangiography identify metastasis.

(continued)

Reviewing common cancers *(continued)*

TYPE AND FINDINGS	DIAGNOSTIC TEST RESULTS

CHRONIC LYMPHOCYTIC LEUKEMIA

- Slow onset of fatigue related to anemia
- Splenomegaly caused by increased numbers of lysed red blood cells being filtered
- Hepatomegaly and lymph node enlargement from infiltration by leukemic cells
- Bleeding tendencies caused by thrombocytopenia
- Infections related to deficient humoral immunity

- CBC reveals:
  - numerous abnormal lymphocytes with mild but persistently elevated WBC count
  - granulocytopenia common but WBC count increasing as disease progresses
  - hemoglobin levels below 11 g/dl
  - neutropenia (under 1,500/µl)
  - lymphocytosis (over 10,000/µl)
  - thrombocytopenia (under 150,000/µl).
- Serum globulin levels are decreased.
- Bone marrow aspiration and biopsy show lymphocytic invasion.

COLORECTAL CANCER

Tumor on right colon
- Black tarry stools caused by tumor erosion and necrosis of the intestinal lining
- Anemia caused by increased tumor growth needs and bleeding resulting from necrosis and ulceration of mucosa
- Abdominal aching, pressure, or cramps caused by pressure from tumor
- Weakness, fatigue, anorexia, weight loss caused by increased tumor growth needs
- Vomiting as disease progresses related to possible obstruction.

Tumor on left colon
- Intestinal obstruction including abdominal distention, pain, vomiting, cramps, and rectal pressure related to increasing tumor size and ulceration of mucosa
- Constipation, diarrhea, or ribbon- or pencil-shaped stools as disease progresses.
- Dark red or bright red blood in stools caused by erosion and ulceration of mucosa

- Digital rectal examination (DRE) reveals mass.
- Hemoccult test (guaiac) detects blood in stools.
- Proctoscopy or sigmoidoscopy reveals tumor mass.
- Colonoscopy visualizes tumor location up to the ileocecal valve.
- CT scan reveals areas of possible metastasis.
- Barium X-ray shows location and size of lesions not manually or visually detectable.
- Carcinoembryonic antigen (tumor marker) may be elevated.

Reviewing common cancers (continued)

TYPE AND FINDINGS	DIAGNOSTIC TEST RESULTS

ESOPHAGEAL CANCER

- ◆ No early symptoms
- ◆ Dysphagia secondary to tumor interfering with passageway
- ◆ Weight loss resulting from dysphagia, tumor growth and increasing obstruction, and anorexia related to tumor growth needs
- ◆ Ulceration and subsequent hemorrhage from erosive effects (fungating and infiltrative) of the tumor
- ◆ Fistula formation and possible aspiration secondary to continued erosive tumor effects

- ◆ Esophageal X-ray with barium swallow and motility studies reveals structural and filling defects and reduced peristalsis.
- ◆ Endoscopic examination with punch and brush biopsies confirms cancer cell type.

HODGKIN'S DISEASE

- ◆ Painless swelling in one of the lymph nodes (usually the cervical region) with a history of upper respiratory tract infection
- ◆ Persistent fever, night sweats, fatigue, weight loss, and malaise related to hypermetabolic state of cellular proliferation and defective immune function
- ◆ Pruritus that becomes acute as the disease progresses
- ◆ Finger and toe pain, nerve irritation, or absence of pulse caused by rapid enlargement of lymph nodes
- ◆ Pericardial friction rub, pericardial effusion, and jugular vein engorgement caused by direct invasion from mediastinal lymph nodes
- ◆ Enlargement of retroperitoneal nodes, spleen, and liver related to progression of disease and cellular infiltration

- ◆ Lymph node biopsy confirms presence of Reed-Sternberg cells, nodular fibrosis, and necrosis.
- ◆ Bone marrow, liver, mediastinal, lymph node, and spleen biopsies reveal histologic presence of cells.
- ◆ Chest X-ray, abdominal CT scan, lung scan, bone scan, and lymphangiography detect lymph and organ involvement.
- ◆ Hematologic tests show:
  – mild to severe normocytic anemia
  – normochromic anemia
  – elevated, normal, or reduced WBC count
  – differential with any combination of neutrophilia, lymphocytopenia, monocytosis, and eosinophilia.
- ◆ Elevated alkaline phosphatase level indicates bone or liver involvement.

LARYNGEAL CANCER

- ◆ Hoarseness persisting longer than 3 weeks related to encroachment on the true vocal cord
- ◆ Lump in the throat or pain or burning when drinking citrus juice or hot liquids related to tumor growth
- ◆ Dysphagia caused by increasing pressure and obstruction with tumor growth
- ◆ Dyspnea and cough related to progressive tumor growth and metastasis
- ◆ Enlargement of cervical lymph nodes and pain radiating to ear related to invasion of lymphatic tissue and subsequent pressure

- ◆ Laryngoscopy shows presence of tumor.
- ◆ Xeroradiography, biopsy, laryngeal tomography, CT scan, or laryngography identifies borders of the lesion.
- ◆ Chest X-ray reveals metastasis.

(continued)

Reviewing common cancers *(continued)*

TYPE AND FINDINGS	DIAGNOSTIC TEST RESULTS

LIVER CANCER

◆ Mass in right upper quadrant with a tender nodular liver on palpation caused by tumor cell growth
◆ Severe pain in epigastrium or right upper quadrant related to tumor size and increased pressure on surrounding tissue
◆ Bruit, hum, or rubbing sound if tumor involves a large part of the liver
◆ Weight loss, weakness, anorexia related to increased tumor growth needs
◆ Dependent edema caused by tumor invasion and obstruction of portal veins

◆ Needle or open biopsy of the liver confirms cell type.
◆ Serum glutamic-oxaloacetic transaminase, serum glutamic-pyruvic transaminase, alkaline phosphatase, lactic dehydrogenase, and bilirubin are elevated, indicating abnormal liver function.
◆ Alpha fetoprotein levels are elevated.
◆ Chest X-ray reveals possible metastasis.
◆ Liver scan may show filling defects.
◆ Serum electrolyte studies reveal hypernatremia and hypercalcemia; serum laboratory studies reveal hypoglycemia, leukocytosis, or hypocholesterolemia.

LUNG CANCER

◆ Cough, hoarseness, wheezing, dyspnea, hemoptysis, and chest pain linked to local infiltration of pulmonary membranes and vasculature
◆ Fever, weight loss, weakness, anorexia linked to increased tumor growth needs from hypermetabolic state of cellular proliferation
◆ Bone and joint pain from cartilage erosion caused by abnormal production of growth hormone
◆ Cushing's syndrome linked to abnormal production of adrenocorticotropic hormone
◆ Hypercalcemia from abnormal production of parathyroid hormone or bone metastasis
◆ Hemoptysis, atelectasis, pneumonitis, and dyspnea from bronchial obstruction linked to increasing growth
◆ Shoulder pain and unilateral paralysis of diaphragm from phrenic nerve involvement
◆ Dysphagia from esophageal compression
◆ Venous distention, facial, neck, and chest edema caused by obstruction of vena cava
◆ Piercing chest pain, increasing dyspnea, severe arm pain caused by invasion of the chest wall

◆ Chest X-ray shows an advanced lesion, including size and location.
◆ Sputum cytology reveals possible cell type.
◆ CT scan of the chest delineates tumor size and relationship to surrounding structures.
◆ Bronchoscopy locates tumor; washings reveal malignant cell type.
◆ Needle lung biopsy confirms cell type.
◆ Mediastinal and supraclavicular node biopsies reveal possible metastasis.
◆ Thoracentesis shows malignant cells in pleural fluid.
◆ Bone scan, bone marrow biopsy, and CT scan of brain and abdomen reveal metastasis.

Reviewing common cancers *(continued)*

TYPE AND FINDINGS	DIAGNOSTIC TEST RESULTS

MALIGNANT BRAIN TUMORS

- Headache, dizziness, vertigo, nausea and vomiting, and papilledema from increased intracranial pressure from tumor invasion and compression of surrounding tissues
- Cranial nerve dysfunction from tumor invasion or compression of cranial nerves
- Focal deficits including motor deficits (weakness, paralysis, or gait disorders) and sensory disturbances (anesthesia, paresthesia, or disturbances of vision or hearing) caused by tumor invasion or compression of motor or sensory control areas of the brain
- Disturbances of higher function including defects in cognition, learning, and memory

Local
- Dementia, personality or behavioral changes, gait disturbances, seizures, language disorders
- Sensory loss, hemianopia, cranial nerve dysfunction, ataxia, pupillary abnormalities, nystagmus, hemiparesis, and autonomic dysfunction depending on location of tumor

- Stereotactic tissue biopsy confirms cell type.
- Neurologic assessment reveals manifestations of lesion affecting specific lobe.
- Skull X-ray, CT scan, MRI, and cerebral angiography identify location of mass.
- Brain scan reveals area of increased uptake in location of tumor.
- Lumbar puncture shows increased pressure and protein levels, decreased glucose levels, and, occasionally, tumor cells in CSF.

MELANOMA

- Enlargement of skin lesion or nevus with color changes, inflammation or soreness, itching, ulceration, bleeding, or textural changes caused by malignant transformation of melanocytes in the basal layer of the epidermis or within the aggregated melanocytes of an existing nevus

Superficial spreading melanoma
- Red, white, and blue color over a brown or black background with an irregular, notched margin typically on areas of chronic irritation

Nodular melanoma
- Polypoidal nodule with uniformly dark discoloration appearing as a blackberry but possibly flesh colored with flecks of pigment around base

Lentigo maligna melanoma
- Large flat freckle of tan, brown, black, whitish, or slate color with irregularly scattered black nodules on surface

- Skin biopsy with histologic examination confirms cell type and tumor thickness.
- Chest X-ray, CT scan of chest and abdomen, or CT of brain reveals metastasis.
- Bone scan reveals bone metastasis.

(continued)

Reviewing common cancers *(continued)*

TYPE AND FINDINGS	DIAGNOSTIC TEST RESULTS

MULTIPLE MYELOMA

- ◆ Severe, constant back and rib pain that increases with exercise because of invasion of bone
- ◆ Arthritic symptoms including achiness, joint swelling, and tenderness possibly from vertebral compression
- ◆ Pathologic fractures resulting from invasion of bone causing loss of structural integrity and strength
- ◆ Azotemia from tumor proliferation to the kidney and pyelonephritis because of subsequent tubular damage from large amounts of Bence Jones protein, hypercalcemia, and hyperuricemia
- ◆ Anemia, bleeding, and infections because of tumor effects on bone marrow cell production
- ◆ Thoracic deformities and increasing vertebral complaints because of extension of tumor and continued vertebral compression
- ◆ Loss of 5" (12.7 cm) or more of body height caused by vertebral collapse

- ◆ CBC shows moderate to severe anemia; differential may show 40% to 50% lymphocytes but seldom more than 3% plasma cells.
- ◆ Differential smear reveals rouleaux formation from elevated erythrocyte sedimentation rate.
- ◆ Urine studies reveal Bence Jones protein and hypercalciuria.
- ◆ Bone marrow aspiration detects myelomatoid cells (abnormal number of immature plasma cells).
- ◆ Serum electrophoresis shows elevated globulin spike that is electrophoretically and immunologically abnormal.
- ◆ Bone X-rays early reveal diffuse osteoporosis; in later stages, they show multiple sharply circumscribed osteolytic lesions, particularly in the skull, pelvis, and spine.

NON-HODGKIN'S LYMPHOMA

- ◆ Swelling of the lymph glands, enlarged tonsils and adenoids, and painless, rubbery nodes in the cervical supraclavicular areas from cellular proliferation
- ◆ Dyspnea and coughing linked to lymphocytic infiltration of oropharynx
- ◆ Abdominal pain and constipation because of mechanical obstruction of surrounding tissues

- ◆ Lymph node biopsy reveals cell type.
- ◆ Biopsy of tonsils, bone marrow, liver, bowel, or skin reveals malignant cells.
- ◆ CBC may show anemia.
- ◆ Uric acid level may be elevated or normal.
- ◆ Serum calcium levels are elevated if bone lesions are present.
- ◆ Serum protein levels are normal.
- ◆ Bone and chest X-rays, lymphangiography, liver and spleen scans, abdominal CT scan, and excretory urography show evidence of metastasis.

Reviewing common cancers (continued)

TYPE AND FINDINGS	DIAGNOSTIC TEST RESULTS

OVARIAN CANCER

- ◆ Vague abdominal discomfort, dyspepsia and other mild GI complaints from increasing size of tumor exerting pressure on nearby tissues
- ◆ Urinary frequency, constipation from obstruction resulting from increased tumor size
- ◆ Pain from tumor rupture, torsion, or infection
- ◆ Feminizing or masculinizing effects because of cellular type
- ◆ Ascites linked to invasion and infiltration of the peritoneum
- ◆ Pleural effusions linked to pulmonary metastasis

- ◆ Pap test may be normal.
- ◆ Abdominal ultrasound, CT, or X-ray delineates tumor presence and size.
- ◆ CBC may show anemia.
- ◆ Excretory urography reveals abnormal renal function and urinary tract abnormalities or obstruction.
- ◆ Chest X-ray reveals pleural effusion with distant metastasis.
- ◆ Barium enema shows obstruction and size of tumor.
- ◆ Lymphangiography reveals lymph node involvement.
- ◆ Mammography is normal to rule out breast cancer as the primary site.
- ◆ Liver functions studies are abnormal with ascites.
- ◆ Paracentesis fluid aspiration reveals malignant cells.
- ◆ Tumor markers, such as carcinoembryonic antigen and human chorionic gonadotropin, are positive.

PANCREATIC CANCER

- ◆ Jaundice with clay-colored stools and dark urine because of obstruction of bile flow from tumor in head of pancreas
- ◆ Recurrent thrombophlebitis from tumor cytokines acting as platelet aggregating factors
- ◆ Nausea and vomiting because of duodenal obstruction
- ◆ Weight loss, anorexia, and malaise, caused by effects of increased tumor growth needs
- ◆ Abdominal or back pain caused by tumor pressure
- ◆ Blood in the stools from ulceration of GI tract or ampulla of Vater

- ◆ Laparotomy with biopsy confirms cell type.
- ◆ Ultrasound identifies location of mass.
- ◆ Angiography reveals vascular supply of the tumor.
- ◆ Endoscopic retrograde cholangiopancreatography visualizes tumor area.
- ◆ CT scan and MRI identify tumor location and size.
- ◆ Serum laboratory tests reveal increased serum bilirubin, serum amylase, and serum lipase.
- ◆ Prothrombin time (PT) is prolonged.
- ◆ Elevations of aspartate aminotransferase and alanine aminotransferase indicate necrosis of liver cells.
- ◆ Marked elevation of alkaline phosphatase indicates biliary obstruction.
- ◆ Plasma insulin immunoassay shows measurable serum insulin in the presence of islet cell tumors.
- ◆ Hemoglobin and hematocrit may show mild anemia.
- ◆ Fasting blood glucose may reveal hypoglycemia or hyperglycemia.

(continued)

Reviewing common cancers *(continued)*

TYPE AND FINDINGS	DIAGNOSTIC TEST RESULTS

PROSTATE CANCER

- Symptoms appearing only in late stages
- Difficulty starting a urinary stream, dribbling, urine retention caused by obstruction of urinary tract from tumor growth
- Hematuria (rare) from infiltration of bladder

- Biopsy confirms cell type.
- Digital rectal examination reveals a small hard nodule.
- Prostate-specific antigen is elevated.
- Serum acid phosphatase levels are elevated.
- MRI, CT scan, and excretory urography identify tumor mass.
- Elevated alkaline phosphatase levels and positive bone scan indicate bone metastasis.

RENAL CANCER

- Pain resulting from tumor pressure and invasion
- Hematuria caused by tumor spreading to renal pelvis
- Smooth, firm, nontender mass palpable over affected kidney caused by tumor growth
- Possible fever from hemorrhage or necrosis
- Hypertension from compression of renal artery with renal parenchymal ischemia and renin excess
- Polycythemia caused by erythropoietin excess
- Hypercalcemia from ectopic parathyroid hormone production by the tumor or bone metastasis
- Urinary retention caused by obstruction of urinary flow
- Pulmonary embolism caused by renal venous obstruction

- CT scan, I.V. and retrograde pyelography, ultrasound, cystoscopy (to rule out associated bladder cancer) and nephrotomography, and renal angiography identify presence of tumor and help differentiate it from a cyst.
- Liver function tests show increased levels of alkaline phosphatase, bilirubin, alanine aminotransferase, and aspartate aminotransferase, and PT is prolonged.
- Urinalysis reveals gross or microscopic hematuria.
- CBC shows anemia, polycythemia, and increased erythrocyte sedimentation rate.
- Serum calcium levels are elevated.

SQUAMOUS CELL CARCINOMA

- Lesions on skin of the face, ears, dorsa of hands and forearms from cell proliferation in sun-damaged areas
- Induration and inflammation as cell changes from nonmalignant to malignant cell
- Ulceration and invasion of underlying tissues from continued cell proliferation

- Excisional biopsy confirms cell type.

Reviewing common cancers *(continued)*

TYPE AND FINDINGS	DIAGNOSTIC TEST RESULTS

STOMACH CANCER

- ◆ Chronic dyspepsia and epigastric discomfort linked to tumor growth in gastric cells and destruction of mucosal barrier
- ◆ Weight loss, anorexia, feelings of fullness after eating, anemia, and fatigue caused by increased tumor growth needs
- ◆ Blood in stools from erosion of gastric mucosa by tumor

- ◆ Barium X-ray with fluoroscopy shows tumor or filling defects in outline of stomach, loss of flexibility and distensibility, and abnormal mucosa with or without ulceration.
- ◆ Gastroscopy with fiber-optic endoscopy visualizes gastric mucosa including presence of gastric lesions for biopsy.
- ◆ CT scans, X-rays, liver and bone scans, and liver biopsy reveal metastasis.

TESTICULAR CANCER

- ◆ Firm, painless, smooth testicular mass and occasional complaints of heaviness caused by tumor growth
- ◆ Gynecomastia and nipple tenderness linked to tumor production of chorionic gonadotropin or estrogen
- ◆ Urinary complaints linked to ureteral obstruction
- ◆ Cough, hemoptysis, and shortness of breath from invasion of the pulmonary system

- ◆ Testicular palpation reveals detectable mass.
- ◆ Transillumination of testicles reveal tumor that does not transilluminate.
- ◆ Surgical excision and biopsy reveal cell type; inguinal exploration determines the extent of nodal involvement.
- ◆ Excretory urography detects ureteral deviation from para-aortic node involvement.
- ◆ Serum alpha fetoprotein and beta human chorionic gonadotropin levels as tumor markers are elevated.
- ◆ Lymphangiography, ultrasound, and abdominal CT scan reveal mass and possible metastasis.

THYROID CANCER

- ◆ Painless nodule or hard nodule in an enlarged thyroid gland or palpable lymph nodes with thyroid enlargement reflecting tumor growth
- ◆ Hoarseness, dysphagia, and dyspnea from increased tumor growth and pressure on surrounding structures
- ◆ Hyperthyroidism from excess thyroid hormone production from tumor
- ◆ Hypothyroidism caused by tumor destruction of the gland

- ◆ Thyroid scan reveals hypofunctional nodes or cold spots.
- ◆ Needle biopsy confirms cell type.
- ◆ CT scan, ultrasound, and chest X-ray reveal medullary cancer.

(continued)

Reviewing common cancers *(continued)*

TYPE AND FINDINGS	DIAGNOSTIC TEST RESULTS

UTERINE (ENDOMETRIAL) CANCER

◆ Uterine enlargement caused by tumor growth
◆ Postmenopausal bleeding or persistent and unusual premenopausal bleeding from erosive effects of tumor growth
◆ Pain and weight loss linked to progressive infiltration and invasion of tumor cells and continued cellular proliferation

◆ Endometrial, cervical, and endocervical biopsies are positive for malignant cells, revealing cell type.
◆ Dilatation and curettage identifies malignancy in patients whose biopsies were negative.
◆ Multiple cervical biopsies and endocervical curettage pinpoint cervical involvement.
◆ Schiller's test reveals cervix resistant to staining (indicating cancerous tissues).
◆ Chest X-ray and CT scan reveal metastasis.
◆ Barium enema identifies possible bladder or rectal involvement.

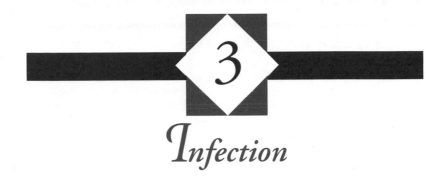

3

Infection

The 20th century saw astonishing advances in treating and preventing infection—potent antibiotics, complex immunizations, and modern sanitation—yet infection remains the most common cause of human disease. Even in countries with advanced medical care, infectious disease remains a major cause of serious illness. In developing countries, infection is one of the most critical health problems.

WHAT IS INFECTION?

Infection is the invasion and multiplication of microorganisms in or on body tissue that produce signs and symptoms and an immune response. Infection injures the host by causing cell damage from microorganism-produced toxins or from intracellular multiplication, or by competing with host metabolism. Infectious diseases range from relatively mild illnesses to debilitating and lethal conditions, from the common cold through chronic hepatitis to acquired immunodeficiency syndrome. The severity of infection varies with the pathogenicity and number of the invading microorganisms and the strength of host defenses. Very young and very old people are especially susceptible.

For infection to be transmitted, there must be a causative agent, susceptible host, infectious reservoir, portal of entry into the host, mode of transmission, and a por-

tal of exit. (See *Chain of infection,* pages 52 and 53.)

RISK FACTORS

A healthy person can usually ward off infections with the body's own built-in defense mechanisms. However, if an imbalance develops, the potential for infection increases. Risk factors for the development of infection include weakened defense mechanisms, environmental and developmental factors, and pathogen characteristics. The body's built-in defenses include:
- intact skin
- normal flora that inhabit the skin and various organs (see *How microbes interact with the body,* page 54)
- lysozymes (enzymes that can kill microorganisms or microbes) secreted by eyes, nasal passages, glands, stomach, and genitourinary organs
- defensive structures such as the cilia that sweep foreign matter from the airways
- a healthy immune system.

Weakened defense mechanisms
The body has many defense mechanisms for resisting entry and multiplication of microbes. However, a weakened immune system makes it easier for these pathogens to invade the body and launch an infec-

Chain of infection

An infection can occur only if the six components depicted here are present. Removing one link in the chain prevents infection.

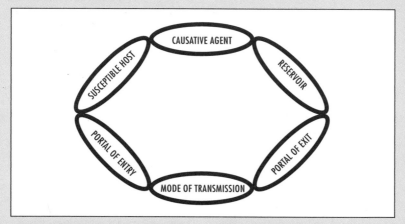

CAUSATIVE AGENT
A *causative agent* for infection is any microbe that can produce disease.

RESERVOIR
The *reservoir* is the environment or object in or on which a microbe can survive and, in some cases, multiply. Inanimate objects, human beings, and other animals can all serve as reservoirs, providing the essential requirements for a microbe to survive at specific stages in its life cycle.

PORTAL OF EXIT
The *portal of exit* is the path by which an infectious agent leaves its reservoir. Usually, this portal is the site where the organism grows. Common portals of exit associated with human reservoirs include the respiratory, genitourinary, and GI tracts; the skin and mucous membranes; and the placenta (in transplacental disease transmission from mother to fetus). Blood, sputum, emesis, stool, urine, wound drainage, and genital secretions also serve as portals of exit. The portal of exit varies from one infectious agent to the next.

tious disease. This weakened state is called *immunodeficiency* or *immunocompromise*.

Impaired function of white blood cells and low levels of T and B cells characterize immunodeficiencies. An immunodeficiency may be congenital (caused by a genetic defect and present at birth) or acquired (developed after birth). Acquired immunodeficiency may result from infection, malnutrition, chronic stress, or pregnancy. Diabetes, renal failure, and cirrhosis can suppress the immune response, as can drugs such as corticosteroids and chemotherapeutic agents.

Regardless of the cause, the result of immunodeficiency is the same: The body's ability to recognize and fight pathogens is impaired. People who are immunodeficient are more susceptible to all infections, are more acutely ill when they become infected, and require a much longer time to recover.

MODE OF TRANSMISSION

The *mode of transmission* is the means by which the infectious agent passes from the portal of exit in the reservoir to the susceptible host. Infections can be transmitted through one of four modes: contact, airborne, enteric, and vector-borne. Some organisms use more than one transmission mode to get from the reservoir to a new host. As with portals of exit, the transmission mode varies with the specific microbe.

Contact transmission is subdivided into direct contact, indirect contact, and droplet spread (contact with droplets that enter the environment).

Direct contact refers to person-to-person spread of organisms through physical contact.

Indirect contact occurs when a susceptible person comes in contact with a contaminated object.

Droplet spread results from contact with contaminated respiratory secretions. It differs from airborne transmission in that the droplets don't remain suspended in the air but settle to surfaces.

Airborne transmission occurs when fine particles containing pathogens remain suspended in the air for a prolonged period, and then are spread widely by air currents and inhaled.

Enteric (oral-fecal) transmission occurs when infecting organisms found in feces are ingested by susceptible victims, in many cases through fecally contaminated food or water.

Vector-borne transmission occurs when an intermediate carrier, or vector, such as a flea or a mosquito, transfers a microbe to another living organism. Vector-borne transmission is of most concern in tropical areas, where insects commonly transmit disease.

PORTAL OF ENTRY

Portal of entry refers to the path by which an infectious agent invades a susceptible host. Usually, this path is the same as the portal of exit.

SUSCEPTIBLE HOST

A *susceptible host* is also required for the transmission of infection to occur. The human body has many defense mechanisms for resisting the entry and multiplication of pathogens. When these mechanisms function normally, infection doesn't occur. However, in a weakened host, an infectious agent is more likely to invade the body and launch an infectious disease.

Environmental factors

Other conditions that may weaken a person's immune defenses include poor hygiene, malnutrition, inadequate physical barriers to prevent microbial invasion, emotional and physical stressors, chronic diseases, medical and surgical treatments, and inadequate immunization.

Good hygiene promotes normal host defenses; poor hygiene increases the risk of infection. Unclean skin harbors microbes and offers an environment for them to colonize, and untended skin is more likely to allow invasion. Frequent washing removes surface microbes and maintains an intact barrier to infection, but it may damage the skin. To maintain skin integrity, lubricants and emollients may be used to prevent cracks and breaks.

The body needs a balanced diet to provide the nutrients, vitamins, and minerals that an effective immune system needs. Protein malnutrition inhibits the production of antibodies, and without antibodies

How microbes interact with the body

Microbes interact with their host in various ways.

DOUBLE BENEFIT
Some of the microorganisms of the normal human flora interact with the body in ways that mutually benefit both parties. *Escherichia coli* organisms, part of the normal intestinal flora, obtain nutrients from the human host; in return, they secrete vitamin K, which the human body needs for blood clotting.

SINGLE BENEFIT
Other microbes of the normal flora have a commensal interaction with the human body — an interaction that benefits one party (in this case, the microbes) without affecting the other.

PARASITIC INTERACTION
Some pathogenic microbes such as helminths (worms) are parasites. This means that they harm the host while they benefit from their interaction with the host.

the body can't mount an effective attack against microbe invasion. Malnutrition is directly related to incidence of nosocomial infections (infections that a patient acquires in the hospital). Along with a balanced diet, the body needs adequate vitamins and minerals for processing nutrients.

Dust can facilitate transportation of pathogens. For example, dust-borne spores of the fungus *aspergillus* transmit the infection. If inhaled spores become established in the lungs, they're difficult to expel. Fortunately, people with intact immune systems can usually resist infection with *aspergillus,* which is usually dangerous only in the presence of severe immunosuppression.

Developmental factors

Very young and very old people are at higher risk for infection. The human immune system doesn't fully develop until about age 6 months. An infant exposed to an infectious agent usually develops an infection. The most common type of infection in toddlers affects the respiratory tract. When young children put toys and other objects into their mouths, their exposure to various pathogens increases.

Exposure to communicable diseases continues throughout childhood, as children progress from day-care facilities to schools. Such skin diseases as impetigo and lice infestation commonly pass from one child to another at this age. Accidents are common in childhood as well, and broken or abraded skin opens the way for bacterial invasion. Lack of immunization also contributes to incidence of childhood diseases.

Advancing age, on the other hand, is linked to a declining immune system, partly as a result of decreasing thymus function. Chronic diseases, such as diabetes and atherosclerosis, can weaken defenses by impairing blood flow and nutrient delivery to body systems.

Pathogen characteristics

Enough microbes must be present to cause a disease in a healthy human. The number needed to cause a disease varies from one microbe to the next and from host to host, and may be affected by the mode of transmission. The severity of an infection depends on several factors, including the microbe's pathogenicity — that is, the likelihood that it will cause pathologic changes or disease. Factors that affect pathogenicity include the microbe's specificity, invasiveness, quantity, virulence, toxigenicity, adhesiveness, antigenicity, and viability.
■ Specificity is the range of hosts to which a microbe is attracted. Some microbes may be attracted to a wide range of humans and animals, whereas others select only human or only animal hosts.
■ Invasiveness (sometimes called *infectivity*) is a microbe's ability to invade and multiply in the host tissues. Some microbes can enter through intact skin;

others can enter only if the skin or mucous membrane is broken. Some microbes produce enzymes that enhance their invasiveness.

■ Quantity refers to the number of microbes that succeed in invading and reproducing in the body.

■ Virulence is the severity of the disease a pathogen can produce. Virulence can vary depending on the host defenses; any infection can be life-threatening in an immunodeficient patient. Infection with a pathogen known to be particularly virulent needs early diagnosis and treatment.

■ Toxigenicity is related to virulence. It describes a pathogen's potential to damage host tissues by producing and releasing toxins.

■ Adhesiveness is the ability of the pathogen to attach to host tissue. Some pathogens secrete a sticky substance that helps them adhere to tissue while protecting them from the host's defense mechanisms.

■ Antigenicity is the degree to which a pathogen can induce a specific immune response. Microbes that invade and localize in tissue initially stimulate a cellular response; those that disseminate quickly throughout the host's body generate an antibody response.

■ Viability is the ability of a pathogen to survive outside its host. Most microbes can't live and multiply outside a reservoir.

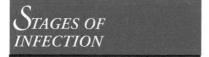

STAGES OF INFECTION

Development of an infection usually proceeds through four stages. The first stage, *incubation*, may be rapid or it may last for years. During incubation, the pathogen is replicating, the disease is contagious, and the patient can transmit the disease. During stage two, the *prodromal stage*, the still-contagious host begins to feel vaguely unwell. In stage three, *acute disease*, microbes are actively destroying host cells and affecting specific host systems. The patient recognizes which area of the body is affect-

ed and may voice complaints that are more specific. Finally, the *convalescent stage,* stage four, begins when the body's defense mechanisms have confined the microbes and are healing damaged tissue.

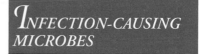

INFECTION-CAUSING MICROBES

Microbes responsible for infectious diseases include bacteria, viruses, fungi, parasites, mycoplasmas, rickettsiae, and chlamydiae.

Bacteria

Bacteria are simple one-celled microorganisms with a cell wall that protects them from many of the human body's defense mechanisms. Although they lack a nucleus, bacteria possess all the other mechanisms they need to survive and rapidly reproduce.

Bacteria can be classified according to shape—spherical cocci, rod-shaped bacilli, and spiral-shaped spirilla. Bacteria can also be classified according to their need for oxygen (aerobic or anaerobic), their mobility (motile or nonmotile), and their tendency to form protective capsules (encapsulated or nonencapsulated) or spores (sporulating or nonsporulating).

Bacteria damage body tissues by interfering with essential cell function or by releasing exotoxins or endotoxins, which cause cell damage. (See *How bacteria damage tissue,* page 56.) During bacterial growth, the cells release exotoxins, enzymes that damage the host cell, altering its function or killing it. Enterotoxins, a specific type of exotoxin secreted by bacteria, infect the GI tract; they affect the part of the brain that controls vomiting and cause gastroenteritis. Exotoxins also can cause diffuse reactions in the host, such as inflammation, bleeding, clotting, and fever. Endotoxins, found in the cell walls of gram-negative bacteria, are released during lysis of the bacteria.

Examples of bacterial infection include staphylococcal wound infection, cholera,

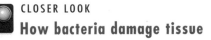

CLOSER LOOK
How bacteria damage tissue

Bacteria and other infectious organisms constantly infect the human body. Some, such as the intestinal bacteria that produce vitamins, are beneficial. Others are harmful, causing illnesses ranging from the common cold to life-threatening septic shock.

To infect a host, bacteria must first enter it. They do this by adhering to the mucosal surface and directly invading the host cell or by attaching to epithelial cells and producing toxins, which invade host cells. To survive and multiply within a host, bacteria or their toxins adversely affect biochemical reactions in cells. The result is a disruption of normal cell function or cell death (see illustration below). For example, the diphtheria toxin damages heart muscle by inhibiting protein synthesis. In addition, as some organisms multiply, they extend into deeper tissue and eventually gain access to the bloodstream.

Some toxins cause blood to clot in small blood vessels. The tissues supplied by these vessels may be deprived of blood and damaged (see illustration below).

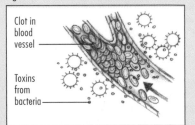

Clot in
blood
vessel

Toxins
from
bacteria

Other toxins can damage the cell walls of small blood vessels, causing leakage. This fluid loss results in decreased blood pressure, which in turn impairs the heart's ability to pump enough blood to vital organs (see illustration below).

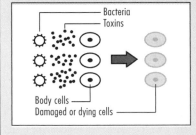

Bacteria
Toxins

Body cells
Damaged or dying cells

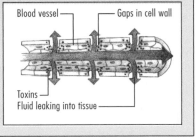

Blood vessel — Gaps in cell wall

Toxins
Fluid leaking into tissue

and streptococcal pneumonia. (See *Gram-positive and gram-negative bacteria*.)

Viruses

Viruses are subcellular organisms made up only of a ribonucleic acid (RNA) nucleus or a deoxyribonucleic acid (DNA) nucleus covered with proteins. They're the smallest known organisms, so tiny that only an electron microscope can make them visible. Independent of the host cells, viruses can't replicate. Rather, they invade a host cell and stimulate it to participate in forming additional virus particles. Some viruses destroy surrounding tissue and release tox-

ins. (See *Viral infection of a host cell,* page 58.) Viruses lack the genes necessary for energy production. They depend on the ribosomes and nutrients of infected host cells for protein production. The estimated 400 viruses that infect humans are classified according to their size, shape, and means of transmission (respiratory, fecal, oral, sexual).

Most viruses enter the body through the respiratory, GI, and genital tracts. A few, such as human immunodeficiency virus (HIV), are transmitted through blood, broken skin, and mucous membranes. Viruses can produce a wide variety

Gram-positive and gram-negative bacteria

This flowchart highlights the different types of gram-positive and gram-negative bacteria.

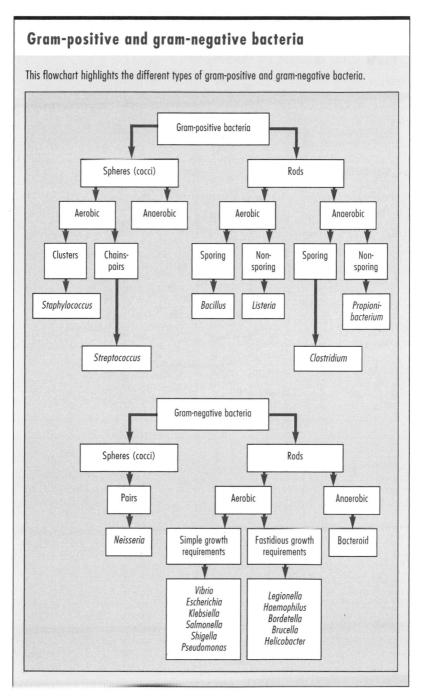

CLOSER LOOK
Viral infection of a host cell

The virion (A) attaches to receptors on the host-cell membrane and releases enzymes (B) that weaken the membrane and enable the virion to penetrate the cell (called *absorption*). The virion removes the protein coat that protects its genetic material (C), replicates (D), matures, and then escapes from the cell by budding from the plasma membrane (E). The infection then can spread to other host cells.

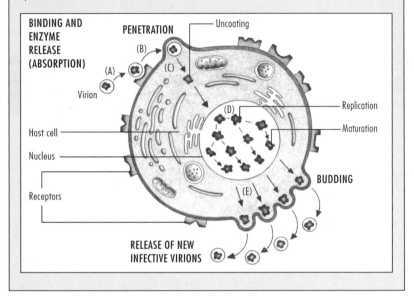

of illnesses, including the common cold, herpes simplex, herpes zoster, chickenpox, infectious mononucleosis, hepatitis B and hepatitis C, and rubella. Signs and symptoms depend on the host cell's status, the specific virus, and whether the intracellular environment provides good living conditions for the virus.

Retroviruses are a unique type of virus that carry their genetic code in RNA rather than the more common carrier, DNA. These RNA viruses contain the enzyme reverse transcriptase, which changes viral RNA into DNA. The host cell then incorporates the alien DNA into its own genetic material. The most notorious retrovirus is HIV.

Fungi

Fungi have rigid walls and nuclei that are enveloped by nuclear membranes. They occur as yeast (single-cell, oval-shaped organisms) or molds (organisms with hyphae, or branching filaments). Depending on the environment, some fungi may occur in both forms. Found almost everywhere on earth, fungi live on organic matter, in water and soil, on animals and plants, and on a wide variety of unlikely materials. They can live inside and outside their host. Superficial fungal infections cause athlete's foot and vaginal infections. *Candida albicans* is part of the body's normal flora, but under certain circumstances it can cause yeast infections of virtually any part of the body. The most common infection sites are the mouth, skin, vagina, and GI tract. For example, antibiotic treatment or a change in the pH of the susceptible tissues (because of a disease such as diabetes or use of certain drugs such as hormonal contraceptives) can wipe out the normal bacteria that keep the yeast population in check.

Parasites

Parasites are unicellular or multicellular organisms that live on or in another organism and obtain nourishment from the host. They take only the nutrients they need and usually don't kill their hosts. Examples of parasites that can produce an infection if they cause cellular damage to the host include helminths, such as pinworms and tapeworms, and arthropods, such as mites, fleas, and ticks. Helminths can infect the human gut; arthropods commonly cause skin and systemic disease.

Mycoplasmas

Mycoplasmas are bacteria-like organisms, the smallest of the cellular microbes that can live outside a host cell, although some may be parasitic. Lacking cell walls, they can assume many different shapes ranging from coccoid to filamentous. The lack of a cell wall makes them resistant to penicillin and other antibiotics that work by inhibiting cell wall synthesis. Mycoplasmas can cause primary atypical pneumonia and many secondary infections.

Rickettsiae

Rickettsiae are gram-negative, bacteria-like organisms that can cause life-threatening illness. They may be coccoid, rod-shaped, or irregularly shaped. Because they're live viruses, rickettsiae require a host cell for replication. They have no cell wall, and their cell membranes are leaky; thus, they must live inside another, better-protected cell. Rickettsiae are transmitted by the bites of arthropod carriers, such as lice, fleas, and ticks, and through exposure to their waste products. Rickettsial infections that occur in the United States include Rocky Mountain spotted fever, typhus, and Q fever.

Chlamydiae

Chlamydiae are smaller than rickettsia and bacteria but larger than viruses. They depend on host cells for replication and are susceptible to antibiotics. Chlamydiae are transmitted by direct contact such as occurs during sexual activity. They're a common cause of infections of the urethra, bladder, fallopian tubes, and prostate gland.

PATHOPHYSIOLOGIC CHANGES

Clinical expressions of infectious disease vary, depending on the pathogen involved and the organ system affected. Most of the signs and symptoms result from host responses, which may be similar or very different from host to host. During the prodromal stage, a person complains of common, nonspecific signs and symptoms, such as fever, muscle aches, headache, and lethargy. In the acute stage, signs and symptoms that are more specific provide evidence of the microbe's target. However, some illnesses remain asymptomatic and are discovered only by laboratory tests.

Inflammation

The inflammatory response is a major reactive defense mechanism in the battle against infective agents. Inflammation may be the result of tissue injury, infection, or allergic reaction. Acute inflammation has two stages: vascular and cellular. In the *vascular stage*, arterioles at or near the injury's site briefly constrict and then dilate, causing fluid pressure to increase in the capillaries. The consequent movement of plasma into the interstitial space causes edema. At the same time, inflammatory cells release histamine and bradykinin, two substances that increase capillary permeability. Red blood cells and fluid flow into the interstitial space, contributing to ede-

DISRUPTING DISEASE
Blocking inflammation

Several substances control inflammation. The flowchart below shows the progression of inflammation and the points ✻ at which drugs can reduce inflammation and pain.

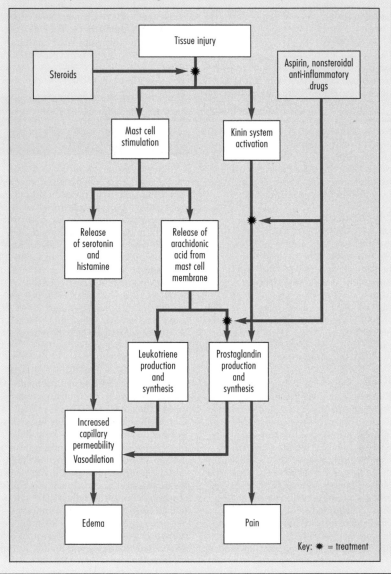

Key: ✻ = treatment

ma. The extra fluid arriving in the inflamed area dilutes microbial toxins.

During the *cellular stage* of inflammation, white blood cells and platelets move toward the damaged cells. Phagocytosis of the dead cells and microorganisms begins. Platelets control any excess bleeding in the area, and mast cells arriving at the site release heparin to maintain blood flow to the area. (See *Blocking inflammation*.)

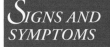

SIGNS AND SYMPTOMS

Acute inflammation is the body's immediate response to cell injury or cell death. The cardinal signs of inflammation include redness, heat, pain, edema, and decreased function of a body part.

■ Redness results when arterioles dilate and circulation to the inflammation site increases. Filling of previously empty or partially distended capillaries causes a localized blush.

■ Heat in the area results from local vasodilation, fluid leakage into the interstitial spaces, and increased blood flow to the area.

■ Pain occurs when pain receptors are stimulated by swollen tissue, local pH changes, and chemicals excreted during the inflammatory process.

■ Edema is caused by local vasodilation, leakage of fluid into interstitial spaces, and the blockage of lymphatic drainage to help wall off the inflammation.

■ Decreased function occurs primarily as a result of edema and pain at the site.

CLINICAL ALERT
Localized infections produce a rapid inflammatory response with obvious signs and symptoms. Disseminated infections have a slow inflammatory response and take longer to identify and treat, thereby increasing morbidity and mortality.

Fever
Fever occurs with the introduction of an infectious agent. An elevated temperature helps fight an infection because many microorganisms can't survive in a hot environment. When the body temperature rises too high, however, body cells can be damaged, particularly those of the nervous system.

Diaphoresis (sweating) is the body's method of cooling itself and returning the temperature to "normal" for that individual. Artificial methods to reduce a slight fever can impair the body's defenses against infection.

Leukocytosis
The body responds to the introduction of pathogens by increasing the number and types of circulating white blood cells (WBCs). This process is called *leukocytosis*. In the acute or early stage, the neutrophil count increases. Bone marrow begins to release immature leukocytes, because existing neutrophils can't meet the body's demand for defensive cells. The immature neutrophils (called "bands" in the differential WBC count) can't serve any defensive purpose.

As the acute phase comes under control and the damage is isolated, the next stage of the inflammatory process takes place. Neutrophils, monocytes, and macrophages begin the process of phagocytosis of dead tissue and bacteria. Neutrophils and monocytes, attracted to the site of infection by chemotaxis, identify the foreign antigen and attach to it. Then they engulf, kill, and degrade the microorganism that carries the antigen on its surface. Macrophages, a mature type of monocyte, arrive at the site later and remain in the area of inflammation longer than the other cells. Besides phagocytosis, macrophages play several other key roles at the site, such as preparing the area for healing and processing antigens for a cellular immune response. An elevated monocyte count is common during resolution of an injury and in chronic infections.

Chronic inflammation

An inflammation reaction lasting longer than 2 weeks is referred to as chronic inflammation. It may follow an acute process. A poorly healed wound or an unresolved infection can lead to chronic inflammation. The body may encapsulate a pathogen that it can't destroy in order to isolate it. An example of such a pathogen is *Mycobacterium tuberculosis*, the cause of tuberculosis; encapsulated mycobacteria appear in X-rays as identifiable spots in the lungs. With chronic inflammation, permanent scarring and loss of tissue function can occur.

DIAGNOSIS

Accurate assessment helps identify infectious diseases, appropriate treatment, and avoidable complications. It begins with obtaining the patient's complete medical history, performing a thorough physical examination, and conducting or ordering appropriate diagnostic tests. Tests that can help identify and gauge the extent of infection include laboratory studies, radiographic tests, and scans.

Typically, the first test is a white blood cell (WBC) count and a differential count. Elevation in the overall number of WBCs is an abnormal result. The differential count is the relative number of each of five types of WBCs — neutrophils, eosinophils, basophils, lymphocytes, and monocytes. It's obtained by classifying 100 or more WBCs in a stained film of peripheral blood. Multiplying the percentage value of each type by the total WBC count gives the absolute number of each type of WBC. This test recognizes only that something has stimulated an immune response. Bacterial infection usually causes an elevation in these numbers; viruses may cause no change or a decrease in normal WBC level.

An erythrocyte sedimentation rate test may be done to reveal that an inflammatory process is occurring within the body.

The next step is to obtain a stained smear from a specific body site to determine the causative agent. Stains that may be used to visualize the microorganism include:

- Gram stain, which identifies gram-negative or gram-positive bacteria
- acid-fast stain, which identifies mycobacteria and *Nocardia*
- silver stain, which identifies fungi, *Legionella,* and *Pneumocystis.*

Although stains provide rapid and valuable diagnostic information, they only tentatively identify a pathogen. Confirmation requires culturing. Any body substance can be cultured. Types of cultures that may be ordered are blood, urine, sputum, throat, nasal, wound, skin, stool, and cerebrospinal fluid.

A specimen obtained for culture must not be contaminated with any other substance. For example, a urine specimen must not contain debris from the perineum or vaginal area. If obtaining a clean urine specimen isn't possible, the patient must be catheterized to make sure that only the urine is being examined. Contaminated specimens may mislead and prolong treatment.

Additional tests that may be requested include magnetic resonance imaging to locate infection sites, chest X-rays to search the lungs for respiratory changes, and gallium scans to detect abscesses.

TREATMENTS

Treatments of infections can vary widely. Vaccines may be given to induce a primary immune response under conditions that won't cause disease. If infection occurs, treatment is tailored to the specific causative organism. Drug therapy should be used only when it's appropriate. Supportive therapy can play an important role in fighting infections.

- Antibiotics work in various ways, depending on the antibiotic class. Their action is bactericidal (killing the bacteria) or bacteriostatic (preventing the bacteria

Antimicrobial drugs and chemicals

The following agents prevent growth of microorganisms or destroy them by a specific action.

MECHANISMS OF ACTION	AGENT
Inhibition of cell-wall synthesis	Bacitracin Carbapenems Cephalosporins Cycloserine Fosfomycin Monobactams Penicillins Vancomycin
Damage to cytoplasmic membrane	Imidazoles Polyene antifungals Polymyxins
Metabolism of nucleic acid	Nitrofurans Nitroimidazoles Quinolones Rifampin
Protein synthesis	Aminoglycosides Chloramphenicol Clindamycin Macrolides Mupirocin Spectinomycin Tetracycline
Modification of energy metabolism	Dapsone Isoniazid Sulfonamides Trimethoprim

from multiplying). Antibiotics may inhibit cell wall synthesis, protein synthesis, bacterial metabolism, or nucleic acid synthesis or activity, or they may increase cell membrane permeability. (See *Antimicrobial drugs and chemicals*.)

■ Antifungal drugs destroy the invading microbe by increasing cell membrane permeability. The antifungal binds sterols in the cell membrane, resulting in leakage of intracellular contents, such as potassium, sodium, and nutrients.

■ Antiviral drugs stop viral replication by interfering with deoxyribonucleic acid synthesis.

The overuse of antimicrobials has created widespread resistance to some drugs. Some pathogens that were once well controlled by medicines are again surfacing with increased virulence. One such pathogen known to cause tuberculosis is *M. tuberculosis*.

Some diseases, including most viral infections, don't respond to available drugs. Supportive care is the only recourse while the host defenses repel the invader. To help the body fight an infection, the patient should:

■ use standard precautions to avoid spreading the infection
■ drink plenty of fluids
■ get plenty of rest
■ avoid people who may have other illnesses
■ take over-the-counter medications appropriate for the symptoms only with full knowledge about dosage, actions, and possible adverse effects or reactions
■ follow the physician's orders for taking prescription drugs and be sure to finish the entire prescription
■ not share the prescription with others.

*I*NFECTIONS

Infection can strike any part of the body. The accompanying chart describes various infections along with their signs and symptoms and appropriate diagnostic tests. (See *Reviewing common infections*, pages 64 to 81.)

Reviewing common infections

INFECTION AND FINDINGS	DIAGNOSIS

BACTERIAL INFECTIONS

Anthrax
Cutaneous anthrax
◆ Small, elevated, itchy lesion that resembles an insect bite, develops into a vesicle, and finally becomes a small, painless ulcer with a necrotic (black) center
◆ Enlarged lymph glands

Inhalational anthrax
◆ Initial flulike symptoms, such as malaise, fever, headache, myalgia, and chills
◆ Progression to severe respiratory difficulties, such as dyspnea, stridor, chest pain, and cyanosis
◆ Onset of shock

Intestinal anthrax:
◆ Nausea and vomiting
◆ Decreased appetite
◆ Fever
◆ Progression to abdominal pain, vomiting blood, and severe diarrhea

◆ Isolation of *Bacilllus anthracis* from cultures of the blood, skin lesions, or sputum confirms the diagnosis.
◆ Specific antibodies may be detected in the blood.

Botulism
◆ Initial signs and symptoms include dry mouth, sore throat, weakness, dizziness, vomiting, and diarrhea
◆ Cardinal sign: acute symmetrical cranial nerve impairment (ptosis, diplopia, and dysarthria)
◆ Descending weakness or paralysis of muscles in the extremities or trunk
◆ Dyspnea from respiratory muscle paralysis

Infant botulism
◆ Generalized muscle weakness, hypotonia, and feeble cry
◆ Constipation
◆ Depressed gag reflex and inability to suck
◆ Flaccid facial expression, ptosis, and ophthalmoplegia due to cranial nerve deficits
◆ Areflexia and loss of head control

◆ Identification of the offending toxin in the patient's serum, stool, gastric content, or the suspected food confirms the diagnosis.
◆ Electromyogram showing diminished muscle action potential after a single supramaximal nerve stimulus is also diagnostic.

Reviewing common infections *(continued)*

INFECTION AND FINDINGS	DIAGNOSIS

BACTERIAL INFECTIONS *(continued)*

Chlamydial infections
Cervicitis
◆ Cervical erosion
◆ Dyspareunia
◆ Mucopurulent discharge
◆ Pelvic pain
Endometritis or salpingitis
◆ Pain and tenderness of the lower abdomen, cervix, uterus, and lymph nodes
◆ Chills, fever
◆ Breakthrough bleeding, bleeding after intercourse, and vaginal discharge
◆ Dysuria
Urethral syndrome
◆ Dysuria, pyuria, and urinary frequency
Urethritis
◆ Dysuria, erythema, tenderness of the urethral meatus
◆ Urinary frequency
◆ Pruritus and urethral discharge (copious and purulent or scant and clear or mucoid
Epididymitis
◆ Painful scrotal swelling
◆ Urethral discharge
Prostatitis
◆ Low back pain
◆ Urinary frequency, nocturia, and dysuria
◆ Painful ejaculation
Proctitis
◆ Diarrhea
◆ Tenesmus
◆ Pruritus
◆ Bloody or mucopurulent discharge
◆ Diffuse or discrete ulceration in the rectosigmoid colon

◆ Swab from site of infection establishes a diagnosis of urethritis, cervicitis, salpingitis, endometritis, or proctitis.
◆ Culture of aspirated material establishes a diagnosis of epididymitis.
◆ Antigen-detection methods are the diagnostic tests of choice for identifying chlamydial infection.
◆ Polymerase chain reaction (PCR) test is highly sensitive and specific.

Conjunctivitis
◆ Hyperemia of the conjunctiva
◆ Discharge
◆ Tearing
◆ Pain
◆ Photophobia (with corneal involvement)
◆ Itching and burning
Note: May also result from viral infection

◆ Culture from the conjunctiva identifies the causative organism.
◆ In stained smears, predominance of lymphocytes indicates viral infection; of neutrophils, bacterial infection; of eosinophils, an allergy-related infection.

(continued)

Reviewing common infections *(continued)*

INFECTION AND FINDINGS	DIAGNOSIS

BACTERIAL INFECTIONS *(continued)*

Gonorrhea
Men
- May be asymptomatic
- Urethritis, including dysuria and purulent urethral discharge, with redness and swelling at the site of infection

Women
- May be asymptomatic
- Inflammation and a greenish yellow discharge from the cervix

Men or women
- Pharyngitis or tonsillitis
- Rectal burning, itching, and bloody mucopuru-lent discharge

Clinical features vary according to the site involved
- Urethra: dysuria, urinary frequency and inconti-nence, purulent discharge, itching, red and ede-matous meatus
- Vulva: occasional itching, burning, and pain due to exudate from an adjacent infected area
- Vagina: engorgement, redness, swelling, and profuse purulent discharge
- Liver: right-upper quadrant pain
- Pelvis: severe pelvic and lower abdominal pain, muscle rigidity, tenderness, and abdominal dis-tention; nausea, vomiting, fever, and tachycar-dia (may develop in patients with salpingitis or pelvic inflammatory disease (PID)

- Culture from the site of infection, grown on a Thayer-Martin or Transgrow medium, establishes the diagnosis by isolating *Neisseria gonorrhoeae.*
- Gram stain shows gram-negative diplococci.
- Complement fixation and immunofluorescent as-says of serum reveal antibody titers four times the normal rate.

Listeriosis
- Commonly causes asymptomatic carrier state
- Malaise
- Chills
- Fever
- Back pain

Fetuses
- Abortion
- Premature delivery or stillbirth
- Organ abscesses

Neonates
- Meningitis, resulting in tense fontanels
- Irritability
- Lethargy
- Seizures
- Coma

- *Listeria monocytogenes* is identified by its diag-nostic tumbling motility on a wet mount of the culture.
- Positive culture of blood, spinal fluid, drainage from cervical or vaginal lesions, or lochia from a mother with an infected infant.

Reviewing common infections *(continued)*

INFECTION AND FINDINGS	DIAGNOSIS

BACTERIAL INFECTIONS *(continued)*

Lyme disease

Stage 1
- Erythema chronicum migrans (ECM): red macule or papule, commonly on the site of a tick bite, which grows to over 20" (50.8 cm), feels hot and itchy, and resembles a bull's eye or target; after a few days, more lesions erupt and a migratory, ringlike rash appears
- Conjunctivitis
- Diffuse urticaria occurs
- Lesions are replaced by small red blotches in 3 to 4 weeks
- Malaise and fatigue
- Intermittent headache
- Neck stiffness
- Fever, chills, and achiness
- Regional lymphadenopathy

Stage 2
- Neurologic abnormalities: fluctuating meningoencephalitis with peripheral and cranial neuropathy; begins weeks to months later
- Facial palsy
- Cardiac abnormalities: brief, fluctuating atrioventricular heart block, left ventricular dysfunction, cardiomegaly

Stage 3
- Arthritis with marked swelling begins weeks or years later
- Neuropsychiatric symptoms such as psychotic behavior, memory loss, dementia, and depression
- Encephalopathic symptoms, such as headache, confusion, and difficulty concentrating
- Ophthalmic manifestations such as iritis, keratitis, renal vasculitis, optic neuritis

- Because *Borrelia burgdorferi* is unusual in humans and indirect immunofluorescent antibody tests are marginally sensitive, diagnosis is usually based on the characteristic ECM lesion and related clinical findings.
- Serology reveals mild anemia and elevated erythrocyte sedimentation rate (ESR), white blood cell (WBC) count, serum immunoglobulin (Ig) M level, and aspartate aminotransferase.
- Cerebrospinal fluid (CSF) analysis reveals presence of antibodies to *B. burgdorferi* if the disease has affected the central nervous system (CNS).

(continued)

Reviewing common infections *(continued)*

INFECTION AND FINDINGS	DIAGNOSIS

BACTERIAL INFECTIONS *(continued)*

Meningitis
- ◆ Fever
- ◆ Chills
- ◆ Headache
- ◆ Nuchal rigidity
- ◆ Vomiting
- ◆ Photophobia
- ◆ Lethargy
- ◆ Coma
- ◆ Positive Brudzinski's and Kernig's signs
- ◆ Exaggerated and symmetrical deep tendon reflexes and opisthotonos
- ◆ Wide pulse pressure
- ◆ Bradycardia
- ◆ Occasional rash
  Note: May also result from viral, protozoal, or fungal infection.

- ◆ Lumbar puncture isolates the infecting organism (usually *Neisseria meningitidis, Haemophilus influenzae* [in children and young adults], or *Streptococcus pneumoniae* [in adults]) from CSF and shows increased CSF cell count and protein level and decreased CSF glucose level.
- ◆ Blood culture isolates the infecting organism.

Otitis media
- ◆ Ear pain
- ◆ Ear drainage
- ◆ Hearing loss
- ◆ Fever
- ◆ Lethargy
- ◆ Irritability
- ◆ Vertigo
- ◆ Signs of upper respiratory tract infection (such as sneezing and coughing)
- ◆ Tinnitus

- ◆ Otoscopy reveals obscured or distorted bony landmarks of the tympanic membrane.
- ◆ Pneumatoscopy can show decreased tympanic membrane mobility.
- ◆ Culture of the ear drainage identifies the causative organism.

Peritonitis
- ◆ Sudden, severe, and diffuse abdominal pain that tends to intensify and localize in the area of the underlying disorder with associated rebound tenderness
- ◆ Weakness and pallor
- ◆ Excessive sweating
- ◆ Cold skin
- ◆ Decreased intestinal motility and paralytic ileus
- ◆ Intestinal obstruction causes nausea, vomiting, and abdominal rigidity
- ◆ Hypotension
- ◆ Tachycardia
- ◆ Fever
- ◆ Abdominal distention

- ◆ Abdominal X-ray shows edematous and gaseous distention of the small and large bowel or in the case of visceral organ perforation, air lying under the diaphragm.
- ◆ Chest X-ray may show elevation of the diaphragm.
- ◆ Blood studies show leukocytosis.
- ◆ Paracentesis reveals bacteria, exudate, blood, pus, or urine.
- ◆ Laparotomy may be necessary to identify the underlying cause.

Reviewing common infections *(continued)*

INFECTION AND FINDINGS	DIAGNOSIS

BACTERIAL INFECTIONS *(continued)*

Plague
Bubonic plague
- Malaise and fever
- Pain or tenderness in regional lymph nodes, possibly associated with swelling
- Painful, inflamed, and possibly suppurative buboes; classic sign is an excruciatingly painful bubo
- Hemorrhagic areas that become necrotic; such areas appear dark, hence the name "black death"
- Restlessness, disorientation, delirium, toxemia, and staggering gait

Primary pneumonic plague
- Acute onset of high fever, chills, severe headache, tachycardia, tachypnea, and dyspnea
- Productive cough (first mucoid sputum, later frothy pink or red)
- Severe prostration, respiratory distress, and usually death

Secondary pneumonic plague
- Pulmonary extension of the bubonic form
- Cough producing bloody sputum
- Severe prostration, respiratory distress, and usually death

Septicemic plague
- Toxicity, hyperpyrexia, seizures, prostration, shock, and disseminated intravascular coagulation
- Widespread nonspecific tissue damage

- Characteristic buboes and a history of exposure to rodents are strongly suggestive of diagnosis.
- Stained smears and cultures of *Yersinia pestis* obtained from a needle aspirate of a small amount of fluid from skin lesions confirm the diagnosis.
- Other laboratory findings include elevated WBC count with increased polymorphonuclear leukocytes and hemoagglutination reaction (antibody titer) studies.
- In pneumonic plague, chest X-ray shows fulminating pneumonia and stained smear and culture of sputum identify *Y. pestis*.
- In septicemic plague, stained smear and blood culture containing *Y. pestis* are diagnostic.
- For a presumptive diagnosis of plague, a fluorescent antibody test may be ordered.

Pneumonia
- High temperature
- Cough with purulent, yellow or bloody sputum
- Dyspnea
- Crackles, and decreased breath sounds
- Pleuritic pain
- Chills
- Malaise
- Tachypnea
  Note: May also result from fungal or protozoal infection.

- Chest X-rays confirm the diagnosis by disclosing infiltrates.
- Sputum specimen, Gram stain and culture, and sensitivity tests help differentiate the type of infection and the drugs that are effective.
- WBC count indicates leukocytosis in bacterial pneumonia, and a normal or low count in viral or mycoplasmal pneumonia.
- Blood cultures reflect bacteremia and are used to determine the causative organism.
- Arterial blood gas (ABG) levels vary, depending on severity of pneumonia and underlying lung state.
- Bronchoscopy or transtracheal aspiration allows the collection of material for culture.
- Pulse oximetry may show a reduced oxygen saturation level
(continued)

Reviewing common infections *(continued)*

INFECTION AND FINDINGS	DIAGNOSIS

BACTERIAL INFECTIONS *(continued)*

Salmonellosis
- ◆ Fever
- ◆ Abdominal pain, severe diarrhea with enterocolitis

Typhoidal infection
- ◆ Headache
- ◆ Increasing fever
- ◆ Constipation

- ◆ Blood cultures isolate the organism in typhoid fever, paratyphoid fever, and bacteremia.
- ◆ Stool cultures isolate the organism in typhoid fever, paratyphoid fever, and enterocolitis.
- ◆ Cultures of urine, bone marrow, pus, and vomitus may show the presence of Salmonella.

Shigellosis
Children
- ◆ High fever
- ◆ Diarrhea with tenesmus
- ◆ Nausea, vomiting, and abdominal pain and distention
- ◆ Irritability
- ◆ Drowsiness
- ◆ Stool may contain pus, mucus, or blood
- ◆ Dehydration and weight loss

Adults
- ◆ Sporadic, intense abdominal pain
- ◆ Rectal irritability
- ◆ Tenesmus
- ◆ Headache and prostration
- ◆ Stool may contain pus, mucus, and blood

- ◆ Microscopic examination of a fresh stool may reveal mucus, red blood cells, and polymorphonuclear leukocytes; direct immunofluorescence with specific antisera may reveal Shigella.
- ◆ Severe infection increases hemagglutinating antibodies.
- ◆ Sigmoidoscopy or proctoscopy may reveal typical superficial ulcerations.

Syphilis
Primary syphilis
- ◆ Chancres (small, fluid-filled lesions) on the anus, fingers, lips, tongue, nipples, tonsils, or eyelids
- ◆ Regional lymphadenopathy

Secondary syphilis
- ◆ Symmetrical mucocutaneous lesions
- ◆ General lymphadenopathy
- ◆ Rash may be macular, papular, pustular, or nodular
- ◆ Headache
- ◆ Malaise
- ◆ Anorexia, weight loss, nausea, and vomiting
- ◆ Sore throat and slight fever
- ◆ Alopecia
- ◆ Brittle and pitted nails

- ◆ Dark field examination of a lesion identifies *Treponema pallidum.*
- ◆ Fluorescent treponemal antibody absorption tests identify antigens of *T. pallidum* in tissue, ocular fluid, CSF, tracheobronchial secretions, and exudates from lesions.
- ◆ Venereal Disease Research Laboratory slide test and rapid plasma reagin test detect nonspecific antibodies.

Reviewing common infections *(continued)*

INFECTION AND FINDINGS	DIAGNOSIS

BACTERIAL INFECTIONS *(continued)*

Syphilis (continued)
Late syphilis
- ◆ Benign — gumma lesion found on any bone or organ
- ◆ Gastric pain, tenderness, enlarged spleen
- ◆ Anemia
- ◆ Involvement of the upper respiratory tract; perforation of the nasal septum or palate; destruction of bones and organs
- ◆ Fibrosis of elastic tissue of the aorta
- ◆ Aortic insufficiency
- ◆ Aortic aneurysm
- ◆ Meningitis
- ◆ Paresis
- ◆ Personality changes
- ◆ Arm and leg weakness

Tetanus
Localized
- ◆ Spasm and increased muscle tone near the wound

Systemic
- ◆ Marked muscle hypertonicity
- ◆ Hyperactive deep tendon reflexes
- ◆ Tachycardia
- ◆ Profuse sweating
- ◆ Low-grade fever
- ◆ Painful, involuntary muscle contractions

Diagnosis column:
- ◆ Diagnosis may rest on clinical features, a history of trauma, and no previous tetanus immunization.
- ◆ Blood cultures and tetanus antibody tests are often negative; only one-third of patients have a positive wound culture.
- ◆ CSF pressure may rise above normal.

Toxic shock syndrome
- ◆ Intense myalgias
- ◆ Fever over 104° F (40° C)
- ◆ Vomiting and diarrhea
- ◆ Headache
- ◆ Decreased level of consciousness (LOC)
- ◆ Rigor
- ◆ Conjunctival hyperemia
- ◆ Vaginal hyperemia and discharge
- ◆ Deep red rash (especially on the palms and soles) that later desquamates
- ◆ Severe hypotension

Diagnosis column:
- ◆ Diagnosis is based on clinical findings and body system involvement.
- ◆ Isolation of *Staphylococcus aureus* from vaginal discharge or lesions.
- ◆ Negative results on blood tests for Rocky Mountain spotted fever, leptospirosis, and measles help rule out these disorders.

(continued)

Reviewing common infections *(continued)*

INFECTION AND FINDINGS	DIAGNOSIS
BACTERIAL INFECTIONS *(continued)*	

Tuberculosis
- Fever and night sweats
- Productive cough lasting longer than 3 weeks
- Hemoptysis
- Malaise
- Adenopathy
- Weight loss
- Pleuritic chest pain
- Symptoms of airway obstruction from lymph node involvement

- Chest X-ray shows nodular lesions, patchy infiltrates (mainly in upper lobes), cavity formation, scar tissue, and calcium deposits.
- Tuberculin skin test reveals infection at some point, but doesn't indicate active disease.
- Stains and cultures of sputum, CSF, urine, drainage from abscesses, or pleural fluid show heat-sensitive, nonmotile, aerobic, acid-fast bacilli.
- CT or MRI scans allow the evaluation of lung damage and may confirm a difficult diagnosis.
- Bronchoscopy shows inflammation and altered lung tissue. It also may be performed to obtain sputum if the patient can't produce an adequate sputum specimen.

Tularemia
- Signs and symptoms appear from 3 to 14 days after exposure
- Reddened skin area progressing to an ulcer
- Inguinal or axillary lymphadenopathy
- Headache
- Muscle pains
- Shortness of breath
- Dry cough
- Hemoptysis
- Fever
- Chills
- Sweating
- Weight loss
- Joint stiffness
- Progressive weakness
- Pneumonia

- Serology is positive for tularemia.
- Blood culture is positive for tularemia.
- Chest X-ray reveals infiltrate pneumonia.

Reviewing common infections *(continued)*

INFECTION AND FINDINGS	DIAGNOSIS

BACTERIAL INFECTIONS *(continued)*

Urinary tract infections
Cystitis
- Dysuria, frequency, urgency, and suprapubic pain
- Cloudy, malodorous, and possibly bloody urine
- Fever
- Nausea and vomiting
- Costovertebral angle tenderness

Acute pyelonephritis
- Fever and shaking chills
- Nausea, vomiting, and diarrhea
- Symptoms of cystitis may be present
- Tachycardia
- Generalized muscle tenderness

Urethritis
- Dysuria, frequency, and pyuria

- ◆ Urine culture reveals microorganism.
- ◆ Urinary microscopy is positive for pyuria, hematuria, or bacteriuria.

Whooping cough (pertussis)
- Irritating, hacking cough characteristically ending in a loud, crowing, inspiratory whoop that may expel tenacious mucus
- Anorexia
- Sneezing
- Listlessness
- Infected conjunctiva
- Low-grade fever

- ◆ Classic clinical findings suggest the disease.
- ◆ Nasopharyngeal swabs and sputum cultures show *Bordetella pertussis*.
- ◆ Fluorescent antibody screening of nasopharyngeal smears is less reliable than cultures.
- ◆ Serology shows an elevated WBC count.

VIRAL INFECTIONS

Chickenpox (varicella)
- Pruritic rash of small, erythematous macules that progresses to papules and then to clear vesicles on an erythematous base
- Slight fever
- Malaise and anorexia
- Congenital varicella: hypoplastic deformity and scarring of a limb, retarded growth, and CNS and eye manifestations
- An immunocompromised patient with progressive varicella: lesions and a high fever for more than 7 days

- ◆ Characteristic clinical signs suggest the virus.
- ◆ Isolation of virus from vesicular fluid helps confirm the virus; Giemsa stain distinguishes varicella-zoster from vaccinia and variola viruses.

(continued)

Reviewing common infections *(continued)*

INFECTION AND FINDINGS	DIAGNOSIS

VIRAL INFECTIONS *(continued)*

Cytomegalovirus infection
◆ Mild, nonspecific complaints
◆ Immunodeficient population: pneumonia, chorioretinitis, colitis, encephalitis, abdominal pain, diarrhea, or weight loss
◆ Infants ages 3 to 6 months appear asymptomatic but may develop hepatic dysfunction, hepatosplenomegaly, spider angiomas, pneumonitis, and lymphadenopathy
◆ Congenital infection: jaundice, petechial rash, hepatosplenomegaly, thrombocytopenia, hemolytic anemia

◆ Virus isolated in urine, saliva, throat, cervix, WBC and biopsy specimens. Complement fixation studies, hemagglutination inhibition antibody tests, and indirect immunofluorescent test for CMV IgM antibody (congenital infections) aid diagnosis.

Herpes simplex
Type 1
◆ Fever
◆ Sore, red, swollen throat
◆ Submaxillary lymphadenopathy
◆ Increased salivation, halitosis, and anorexia
◆ Severe mouth pain
◆ Edema of the mouth
◆ Vesicles (on the tongue, gingiva, and cheeks, or anywhere in or around the mouth) on a red base that eventually rupture, leaving a painful ulcer and then yellow crusting
Type 2
◆ Tingling in the area involved
◆ Malaise
◆ Dysuria
◆ Dyspareunia (painful intercourse)
◆ Leukorrhea (white vaginal discharge containing mucus and pus cells)
◆ Localized, fluid-filled vesicles that are found on the cervix, labia, perianal skin, vulva, vagina, glans penis, foreskin, and penile shaft, mouth or anus; inguinal swelling may be present

◆ Tzanck smear shows multinucleated giant cells.
◆ Herpes simplex virus culture is positive.
◆ Virus is isolated from local lesions.
◆ Tissue biopsy aids diagnosis.
◆ Elevated antibodies and increased WBC count indicate primary infection.

Reviewing common infections *(continued)*

INFECTION AND FINDINGS	DIAGNOSIS

VIRAL INFECTIONS *(continued)*

Herpes zoster
- Pain within the dermatome affected
- Fever
- Malaise
- Pruritus
- Paresthesia or hyperesthesia in the trunk, arms, or legs may also occur
- Small, red, nodular skin lesions on painful areas (nerve specific) that change to pus or fluid-filled vesicles

- Staining antibodies from vesicular fluid and identification under fluorescent light differentiates herpes zoster from localized herpes simplex.
- Examination of vesicular fluid and infected tissue shows eosinophilic intranuclear inclusions and varicella virus.
- Lumbar puncture shows increased pressure; CSF shows increased protein levels and possibly pleocytosis.

Human immunodeficiency virus infection
- Rapid weight loss
- Dry cough
- Recurring fever or profuse night sweats
- Profound and unexplained fatigue
- Swollen lymph glands in the armpits, groin, or neck
- Diarrhea that lasts for more than a week
- White spots or unusual blemishes on the tongue, in the mouth, or in the throat
- Pneumonia
- Red, brown, pink, or purplish blotches on or under the skin or inside the mouth, nose, or eyelids
- Memory loss, depression, and other neurologic disorders

- Two enzyme-linked immunosorbent assays (ELISAs) are positive.
- Western blot test is positive.

Infectious mononucleosis
- Headache
- Malaise and fatigue
- Sore throat
- Cervical lymphadenopathy
- Temperature fluctuations with an evening peak
- Splenomegaly
- Hepatomegaly
- Stomatitis
- Exudative tonsillitis or pharyngitis
- Maculopapular rash

- Monospot test is positive.
- WBC count is abnormally high (10,000 to 20,000/µl) during the second and third weeks of illness. From 50% to 70% of the total count consists of lymphocytes and monocytes, and 10% of the lymphocytes are atypical.
- Heterophil antibodies in serum drawn during the acute phase and at 3- to 4-week intervals increase to four times normal.
- Indirect immunofluorescence shows antibodies to Epstein-Barr virus and cellular antigens.

(continued)

Reviewing common infections *(continued)*

INFECTION AND FINDINGS	DIAGNOSIS

VIRAL INFECTIONS *(continued)*

Mumps
- ◆ Myalgia
- ◆ Malaise and fever
- ◆ Headache
- ◆ Earache aggravated by chewing
- ◆ Parotid gland tenderness and swelling, and pain when chewing or when drinking sour or acidic liquids
- ◆ Swelling of the other salivary glands

- ◆ Virus is isolated from throat washings, urine, blood, or spinal fluid.
- ◆ Serologic antibody testing shows a rise in paired antibodies.
- ◆ Clinical signs and symptoms, especially parotid gland enlargement are characteristic.

Rabies
Prodromal symptoms
- ◆ Local or radiating pain or burning and a sensation of cold, pruritus, and tingling at the bite site
- ◆ Malaise and fever
- ◆ Headache
- ◆ Nausea
- ◆ Sore throat and persistent loose cough
- ◆ Nervousness, anxiety, irritability, hyperesthesia, sensitivity to light and loud noises
- ◆ Excessive salivation, tearing and perspiration
Excitation phase
- ◆ Intermittent hyperactivity, anxiety, apprehension
- ◆ Shallow respirations
- ◆ Altered LOC
- ◆ Ocular palsies
- ◆ Strabismus
- ◆ Asymmetrical pupillary dilation or constriction
- ◆ Absence of corneal reflexes
- ◆ Facial muscle weakness
- ◆ Forceful, painful pharyngeal muscle spasms that expel fluids from the mouth, resulting in dehydration
- ◆ Swallowing problems cause frothy drooling and soon the sight, sound, or thought of water triggers uncontrollable pharyngeal muscle spasms and excessive salivation
- ◆ Nuchal rigidity
- ◆ Seizures
- ◆ Cardiac arrhythmias
Terminal phase
- ◆ Gradual, generalized, flaccid paralysis
- ◆ Peripheral vascular collapse
- ◆ Coma and death

- ◆ Virus is isolated from saliva or throat.
- ◆ Fluorescent rabies antibody (FRA) test is positive.
- ◆ WBC count is elevated.
- ◆ Histologic examination of brain tissue from human rabies victims shows perivascular inflammation of the gray matter, degeneration of neuron, and characteristic minute bodies, called Negri bodies, in the nerve cells.

Reviewing common infections *(continued)*

INFECTION AND FINDINGS	DIAGNOSIS

VIRAL INFECTIONS *(continued)*

Respiratory syncytial virus infection
Mild disease
- Nasal congestion
- Coughing and wheezing
- Malaise
- Sore throat
- Earache
- Dyspnea
- Fever

Bronchitis, bronchiolitis, pneumonia
- Nasal flaring, retraction, cyanosis, and tachypnea
- Wheezes, rhonchi, and crackles
- Signs of CNS infection, such as weakness, irritability, and nuchal rigidity may be observed

- Cultures of nasal and pharyngeal secretions may reveal the virus; however, this infection is so labile that cultures aren't always reliable.
- Serum antibody titers may be elevated.
- Recently developed serologic techniques are the indirect immunofluorescent and ELISA methods.
- Chest X-rays help detect pneumonia.

Rubella
- Maculopapular, mildly itchy rash that usually begins on the face and then spreads rapidly, often covering the trunk and extremities
- Small, red macules on the soft palate (Forchheimer spots)
- Low-grade fever
- Headache
- Malaise
- Anorexia
- Sore throat
- Cough
- Postauricular, suboccipital, and posterior cervical lymph node enlargement

- Clinical signs and symptoms are usually sufficient to make a diagnosis.
- Cell cultures of the throat, blood, urine, and CSF, along with convalescent serum that shows a fourfold rise in antibody titers, confirms the diagnosis.

Rubeola
- Fever
- Photophobia
- Malaise
- Anorexia
- Conjunctivitis, puffy red eyes, and rhinorrhea
- Coryza
- Hoarseness, hacking cough
- Koplik's spots (tiny, bluish white specks surrounded by a red halo), pruritic macular rash that becomes papular and erythematous

- Diagnosis rests on distinctive clinical features.
- Measles virus may be isolated from the blood, nasopharyngeal secretions, and urine during the febrile stage.
- Serum antibodies appear within 3 days.

(continued)

Reviewing common infections *(continued)*

INFECTION AND FINDINGS	DIAGNOSIS

VIRAL INFECTIONS *(continued)*

Severe acute respiratory syndrome (SARS)
Initially
◆ Fever greater than 100.4° F (38° C)
◆ Headache
◆ General discomfort and body aches
After 2 to 7 days
◆ Dry cough
◆ Shortness of breath

◆ Nasopharyngeal or oropharyngeal secretions, blood or stool are positive for virus.
◆ Reverse transcription polymerase chain reaction is positive for RNA of SARS coronavirus (Co-V).
◆ SARS-CoV antibodies are found in the serum obtained more than 28 days after the onset of symptoms.
◆ Cell culture test is positive.

Smallpox
◆ Abrupt onset of chills (and possible seizures in children)
◆ High fever (above 104° F [40° C])
◆ Headache, backache, severe malaise, vomiting (especially in children), and marked prostration
◆ Occasionally, violent delirium, stupor, or coma
◆ Sore throat and cough as well as lesions on the mucous membranes of the mouth, throat, and respiratory tract
◆ Skin lesions progressing from macular to papular, vesicular, and pustular, with eventual desquamation causing intense pruritus and permanently disfiguring scars
◆ In fatal cases, death typically resulting from encephalitic manifestations, extensive bleeding from orifices, or secondary bacterial infections

◆ Most conclusive laboratory test is culture of variola virus isolated from an aspirate of vesicles and pustules.
◆ Microscopic examination of smears from lesion scrapings and complement fixation to detect virus or antibodies to the virus in the patient's blood.

Reviewing common infections *(continued)*

INFECTION AND FINDINGS	DIAGNOSIS

FUNGAL INFECTIONS

Histoplasmosis
Primary acute histoplasmosis
- ◆ May produce no symptoms or may cause symptoms of a mild respiratory illness similar to a severe cold or influenza
- ◆ Fever
- ◆ Malaise
- ◆ Headache
- ◆ Myalgia
- ◆ Anorexia
- ◆ Cough
- ◆ Chest pain
- ◆ Anemia, leukopenia, or thrombocytopenia
- ◆ Oropharyngeal ulcers

Progressive disseminated histoplasmosis
- ◆ Hepatosplenomegaly
- ◆ General lymphadenopathy
- ◆ Anorexia and weight loss
- ◆ Fever and, possibly, ulceration of the tongue, palate, epiglottis, and larynx, with resulting pain, hoarseness, and dysphagia

Chronic pulmonary histoplasmosis
- ◆ Productive cough, dyspnea, and occasional hemoptysis
- ◆ Weight loss
- ◆ Extreme weakness
- ◆ Breathlessness and cyanosis

African histoplasmosis
- ◆ Cutaneous nodules, papules, and ulcers
- ◆ Lesions of the skull and long bones
- ◆ Lymphadenopathy and visceral involvement without pulmonary lesions

- ◆ Culture or histology reveals the organism.
- ◆ Stained biopsies using Gomori's stains or periodic acid-Schiff reaction give a fast diagnosis of the disease.
- ◆ Positive histoplasmin skin test or urine antigen test indicates exposure to histoplasmosis.
- ◆ Rising complement fixation and agglutination titers (more than 1:32) strongly suggest histoplasmosis.

(continued)

Reviewing common infections *(continued)*

INFECTION AND FINDINGS	DIAGNOSIS

PROTOZOAL INFECTIONS

Malaria
Benign form
◆ Chills
◆ Fever
◆ Headache and myalgia
Acute attacks
(occur when erythrocytes rupture)
◆ Chills and shaking
◆ Fever up to 107° F (41.7° C)
◆ Profuse sweating
◆ Hepatosplenomegaly
◆ Hemolytic anemia
Life-threatening form
◆ Persistent high fever
◆ Orthostatic hypotension
◆ Red blood cell (RBC) sludging that leads to capillary obstruction at various sites
◆ Hemiplegia
◆ Seizures
◆ Delirium and coma
◆ Hemoptysis
◆ Vomiting
◆ Abdominal pain, diarrhea, and melena
◆ Oliguria, anuria, uremia

◆ Peripheral blood smears of RBCs identify the parasite.
◆ Indirect fluorescent serum antibody tests are unreliable in the acute phase.
◆ Hemoglobin levels are decreased.
◆ Leukocyte count is normal to decreased.
◆ Protein and leukocytes are present in urine sediment.

Schistosomiasis
◆ Transient pruritic rash at the site of cercariae penetration
◆ Fever
◆ Myalgia
◆ Cough
Later signs and symptoms
◆ Hepatomegaly, splenomegaly, and lymphadenopathy
Schistosoma mansoni *and* S. japonicum
◆ Irregular fever
◆ Malaise, weakness
◆ Weight loss
◆ Diarrhea
◆ Ascites, hepatosplenomegaly
◆ Portal hypertension
◆ Fistulas, intestinal stricture
S. haematobium
◆ Terminal hematuria, dysuria
◆ Ureteral colic

◆ Typical symptoms and a history of travel to endemic areas suggest the diagnosis.
◆ Ova in the urine or stool or a mucosal lesion biopsy confirm diagnosis.
◆ WBC count shows eosinophilia.

Reviewing common infections *(continued)*

INFECTION AND FINDINGS	DIAGNOSIS

PROTOZOAL INFECTIONS *(continued)*

Toxoplasmosis
Ocular toxoplasmosis
- Chorioretinitis
- Yellow-white elevated cotton patches
- Blurred vision
- Scotoma
- Pain
- Photophobia

Acquired toxoplasmosis
- Malaise, myalgia, headache
- Fatigue
- Sore throat
- Fever
- Cervical lymphadenopathy
- Maculopapular rash

Congenital
- Hydrocephalus or microcephalus
- Seizures
- Jaundice
- Purpura and rash

- Identification of *Toxoplasma gondii* in an appropriate tissue specimen confirms diagnosis.
- CT scans and MRI disclose lesions in patients with toxoplasmosis encephalitis.

Trichinosis
Stage 1 (enteric phase)
- Anorexia
- Nausea, vomiting, diarrhea
- Abdominal pain and cramps

Stage 2 (systemic phase) and stage 3 (muscular encystment phase)
- Edema (especially of the eyelids or face)
- Muscle pain
- Itching and burning skin
- Sweating
- Skin lesions
- Fever
- Delirium and lethargy in severe respiratory, cardiovascular, or CNS infection

- Stools may contain mature worms and larvae during the invasion stage.
- Skeletal muscle biopsies can show encysted larvae 10 days after ingestion.
- Skin testing may show a positive histamine-like reactivity.
- Elevated acute and convalescent antibody titers confirm the diagnosis.
- Serology results indicate elevated aspartate aminotransferase, alanine aminotransferase, creatine kinase, and lactate dehydrogenase levels during the acute stages and an elevated eosinophil count.
- Lumbar puncture demonstrates CNS involvement with normal or elevated CSF lymphocytes and increased protein levels.

4

$\mathcal{F}$luids and electrolytes

The body is mostly liquid — various electrolytes dissolved in water. Electrolytes are ions (electrically charged versions) of essential elements — predominantly sodium (Na^+), chloride (Cl^-), oxygen (O_2), hydrogen (H^+), bicarbonate (HCO_3^-), calcium (Ca^{2+}), potassium (K^+), sulfate (SO_4^{2-}), magnesium (Mg^{2+}), and phosphate (PO_4^{3-}). Only ionic forms of elements can dissolve or combine with other elements. The balance of electrolytes in the body must stay within a narrow range for the body to function. The kidneys maintain chemical balance throughout the body by producing and eliminating urine. They regulate the volume, electrolyte level, and acid-base balance of body fluids; detoxify and eliminate wastes; and regulate blood pressure by regulating fluid volume. The skin and lungs also play a role in fluid and electrolyte balance. Sweating results in loss of sodium and water; every breath contains water vapor.

$\mathcal{F}$LUID BALANCE

The kidneys maintain fluid balance in the body by regulating the amount and the components of fluid inside and around the cells.

Intracellular fluid
The fluid *inside* each cell is called intracellular fluid (ICF). Each cell has its own

mixture of components in the ICF, but the amounts of these substances are similar in every cell. ICF contains relatively large amounts of potassium, magnesium, and phosphate ions.

Extracellular fluid
The fluid in the spaces *outside* the cells, called extracellular fluid (ECF), is constantly moving. Normally, ECF includes blood plasma and interstitial fluid (the fluid between cells in tissues); in some pathologic states it accumulates, in a so-called third space, the space around organs in the chest or abdomen.

ECF is rapidly transported through the body by circulating blood and between blood and tissue fluids by fluid and electrolyte exchange across the capillary walls. ECF contains large amounts of sodium, chloride, and bicarbonate ions, plus cell nutrients such as oxygen, glucose, fatty acids, and amino acids. It also contains carbon dioxide that's being transported from the cells to the lungs for excretion and other cellular products that are being transported from the cells to the kidneys for excretion.

The kidneys maintain the volume and composition of ECF and, to a lesser extent, ICF by continually exchanging water and ionic solutes (substances dissolved in the water) — such as hydrogen, sodium, potassium, chloride, bicarbonate, sulfate, and phosphate ions — across the cell membranes of the renal tubules.

Fluid exchange

Two sets of forces determine the exchange of fluid between blood plasma and interstitial fluid. All four forces equalize levels of fluids, electrolytes, and proteins on both sides of the capillary wall.

Forces that tend to move fluid from the vessels to the interstitial fluid include:
- hydrostatic pressure of blood (the outward pressure of plasma against the walls of capillaries)
- osmotic pressure of tissue fluid (pressure exerted by a solute in solution on a semipermeable membrane).

Forces that tend to move fluid into vessels include:
- oncotic pressure of plasma proteins (also called colloid osmotic pressure; the osmotic or pulling force of albumin in the intravascular space that draws fluid into the capillaries; similar to osmosis, but because proteins can't cross the vessel wall, they attract fluid into the area of greater concentration)
- hydrostatic pressure of interstitial fluid (inward pressure against the capillary walls).

Hydrostatic pressure at the arteriolar end of the capillary bed is greater than at the venular end. Oncotic pressure of plasma increases slightly at the venular end as fluid escapes. When the endothelial barrier (capillary wall) is normal and intact, fluid escapes at the arteriolar end of the capillary bed and is replaced at the venular end. The small amount of fluid lost from the capillaries into the interstitial tissue spaces is drained off through the lymphatic system and returned to the bloodstream.

𝒜CID-BASE BALANCE

Regulation of the extracellular fluid environment involves the ratio of acid to base, measured as pH. In physiology, all positively charged ions are acids and all negatively charged ions are bases. To regulate acid-base balance, the kidneys secrete hydrogen ions (acid), reabsorb sodium (acid) and bicarbonate ions (base), acidify phosphate salts, and produce ammonium ions (acid). These processes keep the blood at its normal pH of 7.35 to 7.45. The following are important pH boundaries:
- less than 6.8 = incompatible with life
- less than 7.2 = cell function seriously impaired
- less than 7.35 = acidosis
- 7.35 to 7.45 = normal
- greater than 7.45 = alkalosis
- greater than 7.55 = cell function seriously impaired
- greater than 7.8 = incompatible with life.

𝒫ATHOPHYSIOLOGIC CHANGES IN FLUID AND ELECTROLYTE IMBALANCE

The regulation of intracellular and extracellular electrolyte levels depends on:
- balance between the intake of substances containing electrolytes and the output of electrolytes in urine, feces, and sweat
- transport of fluid and electrolytes between extracellular fluid (ECF) and intracellular fluid (ICF).

Fluid imbalance occurs when regulatory mechanisms can't compensate for abnormal intake or output at any level, from the cell to the organism. Fluid and electrolyte imbalances include edema and isotonic, hypertonic, and hypotonic fluid alterations and electrolyte alterations. Disorders of fluid volume or osmolarity (level of electrolytes in the fluid) result. Many conditions also affect capillary exchange, resulting in fluid shifts.

Edema

Despite almost constant interchange of fluids through the endothelial barrier, the body maintains a steady state of extracellular fluid balance between the plasma and interstitial fluid. An excessive amount of fluid in the interstitial spaces is called *edema*. It's classified as localized or systemic. Obstruction of the veins or lymphatic system or increased vascular permeability usually causes localized edema in the af-

Causes of edema

Excess fluid that accumulates in the interstitial spaces causes edema. This table shows the causes and the associated underlying conditions.

CAUSE	UNDERLYING CONDITIONS
Increased hydrostatic pressure	◆ Heart failure ◆ Constrictive pericarditis ◆ Venous thrombosis ◆ Cirrhosis
Hypoproteinemia	◆ Cirrhosis ◆ Malnutrition ◆ Nephrotic syndrome ◆ Gastroenteropathy
Lymphatic obstruction	◆ Cancer ◆ Inflammatory scarring ◆ Radiation
Sodium retention	◆ Excessive salt intake ◆ Increased tubular reabsorption of sodium ◆ Reduced renal perfusion
Increased endothelial permeability	◆ Inflammation ◆ Burns ◆ Trauma ◆ Allergic or immunologic reactions

fected area, such as the swelling around an injury. Systemic or generalized edema may be caused by heart failure or renal disease. Massive systemic edema is called *anasarca*.

Edema results from abnormal expansion of the interstitial fluid or from the accumulation of excessive fluid in a third space, such as the peritoneum (ascites), pleural cavity (hydrothorax), or pericardial sac (pericardial effusion). (See *Causes of edema*.)

Tonicity

Many fluid and electrolyte disorders are classified according to how they affect osmotic pressure, or tonicity. Tonicity describes the relative levels of electrolytes (osmotic pressure) on both sides of a semipermeable membrane (the cell wall or the capillary wall). (The word *normal* in this context refers to the usual electrolyte concentration of physiologic fluids. Normal saline has a sodium chloride concentration of 0.9%.)

■ Isotonic solutions have the same electrolyte concentration and, therefore, the same osmotic pressure as ECF.

■ Hypertonic solutions have a greater than normal level of some essential electrolytes, usually sodium.

■ Hypotonic solutions have a lower than normal level of some essential electrolytes, usually sodium.

ISOTONIC ALTERATIONS

Isotonic alterations or disorders don't make the cells swell or shrink, because osmosis doesn't take place. These alterations occur when osmotic pressure is equal between intracellular and extracellular fluids but a dramatic change in total-body fluid volume takes place. Examples include blood loss from penetrating trauma or expansion of fluid volume when a patient receives too much normal saline solution.

HYPERTONIC ALTERATIONS

Hypertonic alterations occur when the ECF has a higher concentration of solutes than the ICF. Water flows out of the cell through the semipermeable cell membrane, causing cell shrinkage. This alteration can occur when a patient is given hypertonic (greater than 0.9%) saline, when severe dehydration causes hypernatremia (high sodium concentration in blood), or when renal disease causes sodium retention.

HYPOTONIC ALTERATIONS

When the ECF becomes hypotonic, osmotic pressure forces some ECF into the cells, causing them to swell. Overhydration is the most common cause; as water dilutes the ECF, the ECF becomes hypotonic with respect to the ICF. Water moves into the cells until balance is restored. In extreme hypotonicity, cells may swell until they burst and die.

Alterations in electrolyte balance

The major electrolytes are the *cations* (positively charged ions) sodium, potassium, calcium, and magnesium and the *anions* (negatively charged ions) chloride, phosphate, and bicarbonate. The body continuously tries to maintain intracellular and extracellular balance of electrolytes. Too much or too little of an electrolyte will affect most body systems.

SODIUM AND POTASSIUM

Sodium is the major cation in ECF, and potassium is the major cation in ICF. Especially in nerves and muscles, communication within and between cells involves changes (repolarization and depolarization) in the surface charge on the cell membrane. During repolarization, an active transport mechanism in the cell mem-

brane, called the sodium-potassium pump, continually shifts sodium into and potassium out of cells; during depolarization, the process is reversed.

Physiologic roles of sodium cations include:
- maintaining tonicity of ECF
- regulating acid-base balance by renal reabsorption of sodium ions and excretion of hydrogen ions (acid)
- facilitating nerve conduction and neuromuscular function
- facilitating glandular secretion
- maintaining water balance.

Physiologic roles of potassium include:
- maintaining cell electrical neutrality
- facilitating cardiac muscle contraction and electrical conductivity
- facilitating neuromuscular transmission of nerve impulses
- maintaining acid-base balance.

CHLORIDE

Chloride is mainly an extracellular anion; it accounts for two-thirds of all anions. Secreted by the stomach mucosa as hydrochloric acid, it provides an acid environment for digestion and enzyme activation. Chloride also:
- helps maintain acid-base and water balances
- influences the tonicity of ECF
- facilitates exchange of oxygen and carbon dioxide in red blood cells
- helps activate salivary amylase, which triggers the digestive process.

CALCIUM

Calcium is indispensable in cell permeability, bone and tooth formation, blood coagulation, nerve impulse transmission, and normal muscle contraction. Hypocalcemia can cause tetany and seizures; hypercalcemia can cause cardiac arrhythmias and coma.

MAGNESIUM

Magnesium is present in smaller quantity, but physiologically it's as significant as the other major electrolytes. The major function of magnesium is to enhance neuromuscular communication. Other functions include:

Fluid and electrolyte implications of blood pressure findings

Blood pressure reflects changes in fluid and electrolyte status.

BLOOD PRESSURE	FLUID AND ELECTROLYTE STATUS
Normal	◆ Hemodynamic stability ◆ Initial hemodynamic instability
Hypotension	◆ Fluid volume deficit ◆ Potassium imbalance ◆ Calcium imbalance ◆ Magnesium imbalance ◆ Acidosis
Hypertension	◆ Fluid volume excess ◆ Hypernatremia

- stimulating parathyroid hormone secretion, which regulates intracellular calcium
- activating many enzymes in carbohydrate and protein metabolism
- assisting cell metabolism
- helping transport sodium, potassium, and calcium across cell membranes
- aiding protein transport.

PHOSPHATE
The phosphate anion is involved in cellular metabolism as well as neuromuscular regulation and hematologic function. Phosphate reabsorption in the renal tubules is inversely related to calcium levels, which means that an increase in urinary phosphorous triggers calcium reabsorption and vice versa.

EFFECTS OF ELECTROLYTE IMBALANCE
Electrolyte imbalances can affect all body systems. Too much or too little potassium or too little calcium or magnesium can increase the excitability of the cardiac muscle, causing arrhythmias. Multiple neurologic symptoms can result from electrolyte imbalance, ranging from disorientation or confusion to a completely depressed central nervous system. Too much or too little sodium or too much potassium can cause

oliguria (scanty urine production). Blood pressure may be increased or decreased. (See *Fluid and electrolyte implications of blood pressure findings.*) The GI tract is particularly susceptible to electrolyte imbalance:

- too much potassium — abdominal cramps, nausea, and diarrhea
- too little potassium — paralytic ileus
- too much magnesium — nausea, vomiting, and diarrhea
- too much calcium — nausea, vomiting, and constipation.

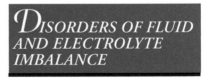

DISORDERS OF FLUID AND ELECTROLYTE IMBALANCE

Fluid and electrolyte balance is essential for health. Many factors — such as illness, injury, medications, surgery, and treatments — can disrupt a person's fluid and electrolyte balance. Even a person with a minor illness is at risk for fluid and electrolyte imbalance. (See *Electrolyte imbalances.*)

(Text continues on page 90.)

Electrolyte imbalances

Signs and symptoms of electrolyte imbalance are often subtle. Blood chemistry tests help diagnose and evaluate electrolyte imbalances.

ELECTROLYTE IMBALANCE	SIGNS AND SYMPTOMS	DIAGNOSTIC TEST RESULTS
Hyponatremia	◆ Muscle twitching and weakness from osmotic swelling of cells ◆ Lethargy, confusion, seizures, and coma from altered neurotransmission ◆ Hypotension and tachycardia from decreased extracellular circulating volume ◆ Nausea, vomiting, and abdominal cramps from edema affecting receptors in the brain or vomiting center of the brain stem ◆ Oliguria or anuria from renal dysfunction	◆ Serum sodium < 135 mEq/L (135 mmol/L) ◆ Decreased urine specific gravity ◆ Decreased serum osmolality ◆ Urine sodium > 100 mEq/24 hours (100 mmol/24 hours) ◆ Increased red blood cell count
Hypernatremia	◆ Agitation, restlessness, fever, and decreased level of consciousness from altered cellular metabolism ◆ Hypertension, tachycardia, pitting edema, and excessive weight gain from water shift from intracellular to extracellular fluid ◆ Thirst, increased viscosity of saliva, and rough tongue from fluid shift ◆ Dyspnea, respiratory arrest, and death from dramatic increase in osmotic pressure	◆ Serum sodium > 145 mEq/L (145 mmol/L) ◆ Urine sodium < 40 mEq/24 hours (40 mmol/24 hours) ◆ High serum osmolality
Hypokalemia	◆ Dizziness, hypotension, arrhythmias, electrocardiogram (ECG) changes, and cardiac arrest from changes in membrane excitability ◆ Nausea, vomiting, anorexia, diarrhea, decreased peristalsis, and abdominal distention from decreased bowel motility ◆ Muscle weakness, fatigue, and leg cramps from decreased neuromuscular excitability	◆ Serum potassium < 3.5 mEq/L (3.5 mmol/L) ◆ Coexisting low serum calcium and magnesium levels not responsive to treatment for hypokalemia usually suggest hypomagnesemia ◆ Metabolic alkalosis ◆ ECG changes include flattened T waves, elevated U waves, depressed ST segment

(continued)

Electrolyte imbalances *(continued)*

ELECTROLYTE IMBALANCE	SIGNS AND SYMPTOMS	DIAGNOSTIC TEST RESULTS
Hyperkalemia	◆ Tachycardia changing to bradycardia, ECG changes, and cardiac arrest from hypopolarization and alterations in repolarization ◆ Nausea, diarrhea, and abdominal cramps from decreased gastric motility ◆ Muscle weakness and flaccid paralysis from inactivation of membrane sodium channels	◆ Serum potassium > 5 mEq/L (5 mmol/L) ◆ Metabolic acidosis ◆ ECG changes include tented and elevated T waves, widened QRS complex, prolonged PR interval, flattened or absent P waves, depressed ST segment
Hypochloremia	◆ Muscle hypertonicity and tetany ◆ Shallow, depressed breathing ◆ Usually hyponatremia with muscle weakness and twitching	◆ Serum chloride < 98 mEq/L (98 mmol/L) ◆ Serum pH > 7.45 (supportive value) ◆ Serum CO_2 > 32 mEq/L (32 mmol/L) (supportive value)
Hyperchloremia	◆ Deep, rapid breathing ◆ Weakness ◆ Diminished cognitive ability, possibly leading to coma	◆ Serum chloride > 108 mEq/L (108 mmol/L) ◆ Serum pH < 7.35, serum CO_2 < 22 mEq/L (22 mmol/L) (supportive values)
Hypocalcemia	◆ Anxiety, irritability, twitching around the mouth, laryngospasm, seizures, positive Chvostek's and Trousseau's signs from enhanced neuromuscular irritability ◆ Hypotension and arrhythmias from decreased calcium influx	◆ Serum calcium < 8.5 mg/dl (2.125 mmol/L) ◆ Low platelet count ◆ ECG shows lengthened QT interval, prolonged ST segment, arrhythmias ◆ Possible changes in serum protein because half of serum calcium is bound to albumin

Electrolyte imbalances *(continued)*

ELECTROLYTE IMBALANCE	SIGNS AND SYMPTOMS	DIAGNOSTIC TEST RESULTS
Hypercalcemia	◆ Drowsiness, lethargy, headaches, irritability, confusion, depression, or apathy from decreased neuromuscular irritability (increased threshold) ◆ Weakness and muscle flaccidity from depressed neuromuscular irritability and decreased release of acetylcholine at the myoneural junction ◆ Bone pain and pathological fractures from calcium loss from bones ◆ Heart block from decreased neuromuscular irritability ◆ Anorexia, nausea, vomiting, constipation, and dehydration from hyperosmolarity ◆ Flank pain from kidney stone formation ◆ Usually hypokalemia and hypocalcemia	◆ Serum calcium > 10.5 mg/dl (2.625 mmol/L) ◆ ECG shows signs of heart block and shortened QT interval ◆ Azotemia ◆ Decreased parathyroid hormone level ◆ Sulkowitch urine test shows increased calcium precipitation
Hypomagnesemia	◆ Hyperirritability, tetany, leg and foot cramps, positive Chvostek's and Trousseau's signs, confusion, delusions, and seizures from alteration in neuromuscular transmission ◆ Arrhythmias, vasodilation, and hypotension from enhanced sodium influx or concurrent effects of calcium and potassium imbalance	◆ Serum magnesium < 1.5 mEq/L (0.62 mmol/L) ◆ Coexisting low serum potassium and calcium levels

(continued)

Electrolyte imbalances (continued)

ELECTROLYTE IMBALANCE	SIGNS AND SYMPTOMS	DIAGNOSTIC TEST RESULTS
Hypermagnesemia	◆ Hypermagnesemia is uncommon, caused by decreased renal excretion (renal failure) or increased intake of magnesium ◆ Diminished reflexes, muscle weakness to flaccid paralysis from suppression of acetylcholine release at the myoneural junction, blocking neuromuscular transmission and reducing cell excitability ◆ Respiratory distress secondary to respiratory muscle paralysis ◆ Heart block, bradycardia from decreased sodium influx ◆ Hypotension from relaxation of vascular smooth muscle and reduction of vascular resistance by displacing calcium from the vascular wall surface	◆ Serum magnesium > 2.4 mEq/L (1.2 mmol/L) ◆ Coexisting elevated potassium and calcium levels
Hypophosphatemia	◆ Muscle weakness, tremor, and paresthesia from deficiency of adenosine triphosphate ◆ Peripheral hypoxia from 2,3-diphosphoglycerate deficiency	◆ Serum phosphate < 2.5 mg/dl (0.8 mmol/L) ◆ Urine phosphate > 1.3 g/24 hours (42 mmol/24 hours)
Hyperphosphatemia	◆ No symptoms, usually, unless condition leads to hypocalcemia, with tetany and seizures	◆ Serum phosphate > 4.5 mg/dl (1.45 mmol/L) ◆ Serum calcium < 9 mg/dl (2.25 mmol/L) ◆ Urine phosphorus < 0.9 g/24 hours (29 mmol/24 hours)

Hypovolemia

Water content of the human body progressively decreases from birth to old age, as follows:

■ in a neonate, as much as 75% of body weight
■ in adults, about 60% of body weight
■ in elderly persons, about 55%.

Most of the decrease occurs in the first 10 years of life. Hypovolemia, or extracellular fluid (ECF) volume deficit, is the isotonic loss of body fluids, that is, relatively equal losses of sodium and water.

AGE ALERT
Infants are at risk for hypovolemia because their bodies need to have a higher proportion of water to total body weight.

CAUSES

Excessive fluid loss, reduced fluid intake, third-space fluid shift, or a combination of these factors can cause ECF volume loss.

Causes of fluid loss include:
■ hemorrhage
■ excessive perspiration

- renal failure with polyuria (excessive excretion of urine)
- abdominal surgery
- vomiting or diarrhea
- nasogastric drainage
- diabetes mellitus with polyuria or diabetes insipidus
- fistulas
- excessive use of laxatives
- excessive diuretic therapy
- fever.
  Possible causes of reduced fluid intake include:
- dysphagia (difficulty in swallowing)
- coma
- environmental conditions preventing fluid intake
- psychiatric illness.
  Fluid shift may be related to:
- burns (during the initial phase)
- acute intestinal obstruction
- acute peritonitis
- pancreatitis
- crushing injury
- pleural effusion
- hip fracture (1.5 to 2 L of blood may accumulate in tissues around the fracture).

PATHOPHYSIOLOGY

Hypovolemia is an isotonic disorder. Fluid volume deficit decreases capillary hydrostatic pressure and fluid transport. Cells are deprived of normal nutrients that provide for energy production, metabolism, and other cellular functions. Decreased renal blood flow triggers the renin-angiotensin system to increase sodium and water reabsorption. The cardiovascular system compensates by increasing heart rate, cardiac contractility, venous constriction, and systemic vascular resistance, thus increasing cardiac output and mean arterial pressure. Hypovolemia also triggers the thirst response, releasing more antidiuretic hormones and producing more aldosterone.

When compensation fails, hypovolemic shock occurs in the following sequence:
- decreased intravascular fluid volume
- diminished venous return
- reduced cardiac output
- decreased mean arterial pressure
- impaired tissue perfusion

- decreased oxygen and nutrient delivery to cells
- multisystem organ failure.

SIGNS AND SYMPTOMS

Signs and symptoms depend on the amount of fluid loss. (See *Estimating fluid loss,* page 92.) These may include:
- orthostatic hypotension caused by increased systemic vascular resistance and decreased cardiac output
- tachycardia (rapid beating of the heart) induced by the sympathetic nervous system to increase cardiac output and mean arterial pressure
- thirst, to prompt ingestion of fluid (increased ECF osmolality stimulates the thirst center in the hypothalamus)
- flattened jugular veins caused by decreased circulating blood volume
- sunken eyeballs caused by decreased volume of total-body fluid and consequent dehydration of connective tissue and aqueous humor
- dry mucous membranes caused by decreased body fluid volume (glands that produce fluids to moisten and protect the vascular mucous membranes fail, and the membranes dry rapidly)
- diminished skin turgor caused by decreased fluid in the dermal layer (making skin less pliant)
- rapid weight loss caused by acute loss of body fluid

AGE ALERT
In hypovolemic infants younger than age 4 months, the posterior and anterior fontanels are sunken when palpated. Between ages 4 and 18 months, the posterior fontanel is normally closed, but the anterior fontanel is sunken in hypovolemic infants.

- decreased urine output caused by decreased renal perfusion from renal vasoconstriction
- prolonged capillary refill time caused by increased systemic vascular resistance.

COMPLICATIONS

Possible complications of hypovolemia include:
- shock
- acute renal failure
- death.

Estimating fluid loss

These assessment parameters indicate the severity of fluid loss.

MINIMAL FLUID LOSS
Intravascular volume loss of 10% to 15% is regarded as minimal. Signs and symptoms include:
◆ slight tachycardia
◆ normal supine blood pressure
◆ positive postural vital signs, including a decrease in systolic blood pressure more than 10 mm Hg or an increase in pulse rate more than 20 beats/minute
◆ increased capillary refill time (> 3 seconds)
◆ urine output greater than 30 ml/hour
◆ cool, pale skin on arms and legs
◆ anxiety.

MODERATE FLUID LOSS
Intravascular volume loss of about 25% is regarded as moderate. Signs and symptoms include:
◆ rapid, thready pulse
◆ supine hypotension
◆ cool truncal skin
◆ urine output of 10 to 30 ml/hour
◆ severe thirst
◆ restlessness, confusion, or irritability.

SEVERE FLUID LOSS
Intravascular volume loss of 40% or more is regarded as severe. Signs and symptoms include:
◆ marked tachycardia
◆ marked hypotension
◆ weak or absent peripheral pulses
◆ cold, mottled, or cyanotic skin
◆ urine output less than 10 ml/hour
◆ unconsciousness.

DIAGNOSIS
No single diagnostic finding confirms hypovolemia, but the following test results suggest hypovolemia:
■ increased blood urea nitrogen level (early sign)
■ elevated creatinine level (late sign)
■ increased protein, hemoglobin, and hematocrit (unless caused by hemorrhage, when loss of blood elements causes subnormal values)
■ rising glucose level
■ elevated osmolality (except in hyponatremia, where osmolality is low)
■ electrolyte and arterial blood gas analysis may reflect associated clinical problems caused by underlying cause of hypovolemia or treatment regimen.

If the patient has no underlying renal disorder, typical urinalysis findings include:
■ urine specific gravity greater than 1.03
■ increased urine osmolality
■ urine sodium level less than 50 mEq/L.

TREATMENT
Possible treatments for hypovolemia include:
■ oral fluids (may be adequate in mild hypovolemia if the patient is alert enough to swallow and can tolerate it)
■ parenteral fluids to supplement or replace oral therapy (moderate to severe hypovolemia; choice of parenteral fluid depends on type of fluids lost, severity of hypovolemia, and patient's cardiovascular, electrolyte, and acid-base status)
■ fluid resuscitation by I.V. administration (severe volume depletion; depending on patient's condition, 100 to 500 ml of fluid over 15 minutes to 1 hour; fluid bolus may be given more quickly if needed)
■ blood or blood products (with hemorrhage)
■ antidiarrheal agent as needed
■ antiemetic agent as needed
■ I.V. dopamine (Intropin) or norepinephrine (Levophed) to increase cardiac contractility and renal perfusion (if patient remains symptomatic after fluid replacement)
■ oxygen therapy to ensure sufficient tissue perfusion
■ autotransfusion (for some patients with hypovolemia caused by trauma).

Hypervolemia

The expansion of extracellular fluid (ECF) volume, called *hypervolemia*, may involve the interstitial or intravascular space. Hypervolemia develops when excess sodium and water are retained in about the same proportions. It's always secondary to an increase in total-body sodium content, which causes water retention. Usually the body can compensate and restore fluid balance.

CAUSES

Conditions that increase the risk of sodium and water retention include:
- heart failure
- cirrhosis of the liver
- nephrotic syndrome
- corticosteroid therapy
- low dietary protein intake
- renal failure.

Sources of excessive sodium and water intake include:
- parenteral fluid replacement with normal saline or lactated Ringer's solution
- blood or plasma replacement
- dietary intake of water, sodium chloride, or other salts.

Fluid shift to the ECF compartment may occur after:
- remobilization of fluid after burn treatment
- hypertonic fluids, such as mannitol (Osmitrol) or hypertonic saline solution
- colloidal oncotic fluids such as albumin.

PATHOPHYSIOLOGY

Increased ECF volume causes the following sequence of events:
- circulatory overload
- increased cardiac contractility and mean arterial pressure
- increased capillary hydrostatic pressure
- shift of fluid to the interstitial space
- edema.

Elevated mean arterial pressure inhibits secretion of antidiuretic hormones and aldosterone, which leads to increased urinary elimination of water and sodium. These compensatory mechanisms usually restore normal intravascular volume. If hypervolemia is severe or prolonged or the patient has a history of cardiovascular dysfunction, compensatory mechanisms may fail, and heart failure and pulmonary edema may follow.

SIGNS AND SYMPTOMS

Possible signs and symptoms of hypervolemia include:
- rapid breathing caused by fewer red blood cells per milliliter of blood (dilution causes a compensatory increase in respiratory rate to increase oxygenation)
- dyspnea (labored breathing) caused by increased fluid volume in pleural spaces
- crackles (gurgling or bubbling sounds on auscultation) caused by elevated hydrostatic pressure in pulmonary capillaries
- rapid, bounding pulse caused by increased cardiac contractility (from circulatory overload)
- hypertension (unless heart is failing) caused by circulatory overload (which causes increased mean arterial pressure)
- distended jugular veins caused by increased blood volume and increased preload
- moist skin (compensatory to increase water excretion through perspiration)
- acute weight gain caused by increased volume of total-body fluid from circulatory overload (best indicator of ECF volume excess)
- edema caused by fluid shift from plasma to interstitial spaces (resulting from increased capillary hydrostatic pressure because of increased mean arterial pressure)
- S_3 gallop (abnormal heart sound caused by rapid filling and volume overload of the ventricles during diastole) caused by fluid volume overload.

COMPLICATIONS

Possible complications of hypervolemia include:
- skin breakdown
- acute pulmonary edema with hypoxemia.

DIAGNOSIS

No single diagnostic test confirms the disorder, but the following findings indicate hypervolemia:
- decreased potassium and blood urea nitrogen (BUN) levels caused by hemodilution (increased potassium and BUN levels usually indicate renal failure or impaired renal perfusion)
- decreased hematocrit caused by hemodilution

Interpreting ABG values

This table compares abnormal arterial blood gas (ABG) values and indicates their significance for patient care.

DISORDER	pH	Paco$_2$ (mm Hg)	HCO$_3^-$ (mEq/L)
Normal	*7.35 – 7.45*	*35 – 45 (4.66 – 5.99 kPa)*	*22 – 26*
Respiratory acidosis	< 7.35	> 45 (5.99 kPa)	◆ Acute: may be normal ◆ Chronic: > 26
Respiratory alkalosis	> 7.45	< 35 (4.66 kPa)	◆ Acute: may be normal ◆ Chronic: < 22
Metabolic acidosis	< 7.35	< 35 (4.66 kPa)	< 22
Metabolic alkalosis	> 7.45	> 45 (5.99 kPa)	> 26

■ normal sodium (unless associated sodium imbalance is present)
■ low urine sodium excretion (usually less than 10 mEq/day because an edematous patient is retaining sodium)
■ increased hemodynamic values (including pulmonary artery, pulmonary artery wedge, and central venous pressures).

TREATMENT
Possible treatments for hypervolemia include:
■ restricted sodium and water intake
■ preload reduction agents, such as morphine, furosemide (Lasix), and nitroglycerin (Nitro-Bid), and afterload reduction agents, such as hydralazine (Apresoline) and captopril (Capoten) for pulmonary edema.

CLINICAL ALERT
Carefully monitor I.V. fluid administration rate and patient response, especially in elderly patients or those with impaired cardiac or renal function,

who are particularly vulnerable to acute pulmonary edema.

For severe hypervolemia or renal failure, the patient may undergo renal replacement therapy, such as:
■ hemodialysis or peritoneal dialysis
■ continuous arteriovenous hemofiltration (allows removal of excess fluid from critically ill patients who may not need dialysis; the patient's arterial pressure serves as a natural pump, driving blood through the arterial line)
■ continuous venovenous hemofiltration (similar to arteriovenous hemofiltration, but a mechanical pump is used when mean arterial pressure is less than 60 mm Hg).

Supportive care includes:
■ oxygen administration
■ use of thromboembolic disease support hose to help mobilize edematous fluid
■ bed rest
■ treatment of underlying condition that caused or contributed to hypervolemia.

PATHOPHYSIOLOGIC CHANGES IN ACID-BASE IMBALANCE

Acid-base balance is essential to life. Concepts related to imbalance include acidemia, acidosis, alkalemia, alkalosis, and compensation.

Acidemia

Acidemia is an arterial pH of less than 7.35, which reflects a relative excess of acid in the blood. The hydrogen ion content in extracellular fluid (ECF) increases, and the hydrogen ions move to the intracellular fluid (ICF). To keep the ICF electrically neutral, an equal amount of potassium leaves the cell, creating a relative hyperkalemia.

Acidosis

Acidosis is a systemic increase in hydrogen ion level. If the lungs fail to eliminate carbon dioxide (CO_2) or if volatile (carbonic) or nonvolatile (lactic) acid products of metabolism accumulate, hydrogen ion level rises. Acidosis can also occur if persistent diarrhea causes loss of basic bicarbonate anions or the kidneys fail to reabsorb bicarbonate or secrete hydrogen ions.

Alkalemia

Alkalemia is arterial blood pH greater than 7.45, which reflects a relative excess of base in the blood. In alkalemia, an excess of hydrogen ions in the ICF forces them into the ECF. To keep the ICF electrically neutral, potassium moves from the ECF to the ICF, creating a relative hypokalemia.

Alkalosis

Alkalosis is a bodywide decrease in hydrogen ion level. An excessive loss of CO_2 during hyperventilation, loss of nonvolatile acids during vomiting, or excessive ingestion of base may decrease hydrogen ion level.

Compensation

The lungs and kidneys, along with a number of chemical buffer systems in the intracellular and extracellular compartments, work together to maintain plasma pH in the range of 7.35 to 7.45 (compensation). For a description of acid-base values and compensatory mechanisms, see *Interpreting ABG values*.

BUFFER SYSTEMS

A buffer system consists of a weak acid (that doesn't readily release free hydrogen ions) and a corresponding base such as sodium bicarbonate. These buffers resist or minimize a change in pH when an acid or base is added to the buffered solution. Buffers work in seconds.

The four major buffers or buffer systems are:

■ carbonic acid — bicarbonate system (the most important, works in lungs)
■ hemoglobin-oxyhemoglobin system — (works in red blood cells) hemoglobin binds free hydrogen, blood flows through lungs, hydrogen combines with CO_2
■ other protein buffers (in ECF and ICF)
■ phosphate system (primarily in ICF).

When primary disease processes alter either the acid or base component of the ratio, the lungs or kidneys (whichever isn't affected by the disease process) restore the ratio and normalize pH. Because the body's mechanisms that regulate pH work stepwise over time, the body tolerates gradual changes in pH better than abrupt ones.

COMPENSATION BY THE KIDNEYS

If a respiratory disorder causes acidosis or alkalosis, the kidneys respond by altering their handling of hydrogen and bicarbonate ions to return the pH to normal. Renal compensation begins hours to days after a respiratory alteration in pH. Despite this delay, renal compensation is powerful.
- Acidemia: the kidneys excrete excess hydrogen ions, which may combine with phosphate or ammonia to form titratable acids in the urine. The net effect is to raise the level of bicarbonate ions in the ECF and so restore acid-base balance.
- Alkalemia: the kidneys excrete excess bicarbonate ions, usually with sodium ions. The net effect is to reduce the level of bicarbonate ions in the ECF and restore acid-base balance.

COMPENSATION BY THE LUNGS

If acidosis or alkalosis results from a metabolic or renal disorder, the respiratory system regulates the respiratory rate to return the pH to normal. The partial pressure of arterial carbon dioxide ($PaCO_2$) reflects CO_2 levels proportionate to blood pH. As the level of the gas increases, so does its partial pressure. Within minutes after the slightest change in $PaCO_2$, central chemoreceptors in the medulla that regulate the rate and depth of ventilation detect the change.
- Acidemia increases respiratory rate and depth to eliminate CO_2.
- Alkalemia decreases respiratory rate and depth to retain CO_2.

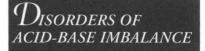

DISORDERS OF ACID-BASE IMBALANCE

Acid-base disturbances can cause respiratory acidosis or alkalosis or metabolic acidosis or alkalosis.

Respiratory acidosis

Respiratory acidosis is an acid-base disturbance characterized by reduced alveolar ventilation. The patient's pulmonary system can't clear enough carbon dioxide (CO_2) from the body. This leads to hypercapnia (partial pressure of arterial carbon dioxide [$PaCO_2$] greater than 45 mm Hg) and acidosis (pH less than 7.35). Respiratory acidosis can be acute (caused by a sudden failure in ventilation) or chronic (in long-term pulmonary disease). Any compromise in the essential components of breathing—ventilation, perfusion, and diffusion—may cause respiratory acidosis.

Prognosis depends on the severity of the underlying disturbance as well as the patient's general clinical condition. The prognosis is least optimistic for a patient with a debilitating disorder.

CAUSES

Factors leading to respiratory acidosis include:
- drugs (opioids, general anesthetics, hypnotics, alcohol, and sedatives—as well as some of the new "designer" drugs, such as MCMA, or "ecstasy"—decrease the sensitivity of the respiratory center)
- central nervous system (CNS) trauma (injury to the medulla may impair ventilatory drive)
- cardiac arrest (acute)
- sleep apnea
- chronic metabolic alkalosis as respiratory compensatory mechanisms try to normalize pH by decreasing alveolar ventilation
- ventilation therapy (use of high-flow oxygen in patients with chronic respiratory disorders suppresses the patient's hypoxic drive to breathe; high positive end-expiratory pressure in the presence of reduced cardiac output may cause hypercapnia caused by large increases in alveolar dead space)

- neuromuscular diseases, such as myasthenia gravis, Guillain-Barré syndrome, and poliomyelitis (respiratory muscles can't respond properly to respiratory drive)
- airway obstruction or parenchymal lung disease (interferes with alveolar ventilation)
- chronic obstructive pulmonary disease (COPD) or asthma
- severe adult respiratory distress syndrome (reduced pulmonary blood flow and poor exchange of CO_2 and oxygen between the lungs and blood)
- chronic bronchitis
- large pneumothorax
- extensive pneumonia
- pulmonary edema.

PATHOPHYSIOLOGY

When pulmonary ventilation decreases, $PaCO_2$ is increased, and the CO_2 level rises in all tissues and fluids, including the medulla and cerebrospinal fluid. Retained CO_2 combines with water to form carbonic acid (H_2CO_3). The carbonic acid dissociates to release free hydrogen and bicarbonate (HCO_3^-) ions. Increased $PaCO_2$ and free hydrogen ions stimulate the medulla to increase respiratory drive and expel CO_2.

As pH falls, 2,3-diphosphoglycerate (2,3-DPG) accumulates in red blood cells, where it alters hemoglobin so that it releases oxygen. This reduced hemoglobin, which is strongly alkaline, picks up hydrogen ions and CO_2 and removes them from the serum.

As respiratory mechanisms fail, rising $PaCO_2$ stimulates the kidneys to retain bicarbonate and sodium ions and excrete hydrogen ions. As a result, more sodium bicarbonate ($NaHCO_3$) is available to buffer free hydrogen ions. Some hydrogen is excreted in the form of ammonium ion (NH_4^+), neutralizing ammonia, an important CNS toxin.

As the hydrogen ion level overwhelms compensatory mechanisms, hydrogen ions move into the cells and potassium ions move out. Without enough oxygen, anaerobic metabolism produces lactic acid. Electrolyte imbalances and acidosis critically depress neurologic and cardiac functions.

SIGNS AND SYMPTOMS

Clinical features vary according to the severity and duration of respiratory acidosis, the underlying disease, and the presence of hypoxemia. Carbon dioxide and hydrogen ions dilate cerebral blood vessels and increase blood flow to the brain, causing cerebral edema and depressing CNS activity.

Possible signs and symptoms affecting the CNS include:
- restlessness or apprehension caused by hypoxemia
- changes in levels of consciousness — such as confusion, somnolence, or coma — caused by hypoxemia
- headaches resulting from cerebral vasodilation
- fine or flapping tremor (asterixis) caused by continued elevation of CO_2 levels
- papilledema caused by increased intracranial pressure as a result of cerebral vasodilation
- depressed reflexes related to elevated CO_2 levels and CNS depression.

Respiratory acidosis may also cause cardiovascular abnormalities, including:
- tachycardia and hypertension caused by sudden onset of hypercapnia and effects of hypoxemia
- atrial and ventricular arrhythmias secondary to development of hyperkalemia
- hypotension with vasodilation (bounding pulses and warm periphery, in severe acidosis).

COMPLICATIONS

Possible complications include:
- profound CNS and cardiovascular deterioration caused by dangerously low blood pH (less than 7.15)
- myocardial depression (leading to shock and cardiac arrest)
- elevated $PaCO_2$ despite optimal treatment (in chronic lung disease).

DIAGNOSIS

The following tests and findings help diagnose respiratory acidosis:
- arterial blood gas (ABG) analysis ($PaCO_2$ greater than 45 mm Hg; pH less than 7.35 to 7.45; and normal HCO_3^- in the acute stage and elevated HCO_3^- in the chronic stage confirm the diagnosis)

- chest X-ray (often shows such causes as heart failure, pneumonia, COPD, and pneumothorax)
- potassium greater than 5 mEq/L
- low chloride level
- urine acidic pH (as the kidneys excrete hydrogen ions to return blood pH to normal)
- drug screening (may confirm suspected drug overdose).

TREATMENT
Effective treatment of respiratory acidosis requires correction of the underlying source of alveolar hypoventilation. Treatment of pulmonary causes of respiratory acidosis includes:

- removal of a foreign body from the airway
- creating an artificial airway through endotracheal intubation or tracheotomy and mechanical ventilation (if the patient can't breathe independently)
- increasing the partial pressure of arterial oxygen to at least 60 mm Hg and blood pH to greater than 7.2 to avoid cardiac arrhythmias
- aerosolized or I.V. bronchodilators to open constricted airways
- antibiotics to treat pneumonia
- chest tubes to correct pneumothorax
- positive end-expiratory pressure to prevent alveolar collapse
- thrombolytic or anticoagulant therapy for massive pulmonary emboli
- bronchoscopy and removal of excessive retained secretions.

Treatment for patients with COPD includes:

- bronchodilators
- oxygen at low flow rates (more oxygen than the person's normal level removes the hypoxic drive, further reducing alveolar ventilation)
- corticosteroids
- gradual reduction in $PaCO_2$ to baseline to provide sufficient chloride and potassium ions to enhance renal excretion of bicarbonate (in chronic respiratory acidosis).

Other treatments include:

- drug therapy for such conditions as myasthenia gravis
- dialysis or charcoal to remove toxic drugs
- correction of metabolic alkalosis

- careful administration of I.V. sodium bicarbonate.

Respiratory alkalosis

Respiratory alkalosis is an acid-base disturbance characterized by a partial pressure of arterial carbon dioxide ($PaCO_2$) less than 35 mm Hg and blood pH greater than 7.45; alveolar hyperventilation is the cause. Hypocapnia (below normal $PaCO_2$) occurs when the lungs eliminate more carbon dioxide (CO_2) than the cells produce.

Respiratory alkalosis is the most common acid-base disturbance in critically ill patients and, when severe, has a poor prognosis.

CAUSES
Causes of respiratory alkalosis fall into two categories:

- pulmonary — severe hypoxemia, pneumonia, interstitial lung disease, pulmonary vascular disease, and acute asthma
- nonpulmonary — anxiety, fever, aspirin toxicity, metabolic acidosis, central nervous system (CNS) disease (inflammation or tumor), sepsis, hepatic failure, and pregnancy.

PATHOPHYSIOLOGY
When pulmonary ventilation increases more than is needed to maintain normal CO_2 levels, excessive amounts of CO_2 are exhaled. The consequent hypocapnia leads to a chemical reduction of carbonic acid, excretion of hydrogen and bicarbonate ions, and a rising serum pH.

In defense against the increasing serum pH, the hydrogen-potassium buffer system pulls hydrogen ions out of the cells and into the blood in exchange for potassium ions. The hydrogen ions entering the blood combine with available bicarbonate ions to form carbonic acid, and the pH falls.

Hypocapnia stimulates the carotid and aortic bodies as well as the medulla, increasing the heart rate (which hypokalemia can further aggravate) but not the blood pressure. At the same time, hypocapnia causes cerebral vasoconstriction and decreased cerebral blood flow. It also overexcites the medulla, pons, and other parts of the autonomic nervous system. When hypocapnia lasts more than 6 hours, the kidneys secrete more bicarbonate and less hydrogen. Full renal adaptation to respiratory alkalosis requires normal volume status and renal function, and it may take several days.

Continued low $PaCO_2$ and the vasoconstriction it causes increases cerebral and peripheral hypoxia. Severe alkalosis inhibits calcium ionization; as calcium ions become unavailable, nerves and muscles become progressively more excitable. Eventually, alkalosis overwhelms the CNS and heart.

SIGNS AND SYMPTOMS

Possible signs and symptoms of respiratory alkalosis include:
■ deep, rapid breathing (possibly more than 40 breaths/minute and much like the Kussmaul's respirations that are typical of diabetic acidosis) usually causing CNS and neuromuscular disturbances (cardinal sign of respiratory alkalosis)
■ light-headedness, dizziness, or agitation caused by decreased cerebral blood flow
■ paresthesias (abnormal sensations such as burning, prickling, or tingling) around the mouth or the extremities caused by hypokalemia
■ carpopedal (wrist and foot, or hands and feet) spasms, twitching (possibly progressing to tetany), and muscle weakness caused by overstimulation of autonomic nervous system from hypocapnia.

COMPLICATIONS

Possible complications of severe respiratory alkalosis include:
■ cardiac arrhythmias that may not respond to conventional treatment as the hemoglobin-oxygen buffer system becomes overwhelmed
■ hypocalcemic tetany, seizures
■ periods of apnea if pH remains high and $PaCO_2$ remains low.

DIAGNOSIS

The following tests and findings indicate respiratory alkalosis:
■ arterial blood gas (ABG) analysis showing $PaCO_2$ less than 35 mm Hg; elevated pH in proportion to decrease in $PaCO_2$ in the acute stage but decreasing toward normal in the chronic stage; normal bicarbonate in acute stage but less than normal in the chronic stage (confirms respiratory alkalosis, rules out respiratory compensation for metabolic acidosis)
■ electrolyte studies (detect metabolic disorders causing compensatory respiratory alkalosis)
■ electrocardiogram findings (may indicate cardiac arrhythmias)
■ low chloride level (in severe respiratory alkalosis)
■ toxicology screening (for salicylate poisoning)
■ urine basic pH (as kidneys excrete bicarbonate to raise blood pH).

TREATMENT

Possible treatments to correct the underlying condition include:
■ removal of ingested toxins, such as salicylates, by inducing emesis or using gastric lavage
■ treatment of fever or sepsis
■ administration of oxygen for acute hypoxemia
■ treatment of CNS disease
■ having patient breathe into a paper bag to increase CO_2 and help relieve anxiety (for hyperventilation caused by severe anxiety)
■ adjustment of tidal volume and minute ventilation in patients on mechanical ventilation to prevent hyperventilation (by monitoring ABG analysis results).

Metabolic acidosis

Metabolic acidosis is an acid-base disorder characterized by excess acid and deficient bicarbonate (HCO_3^-) caused by an underlying nonrespiratory disorder. A primary decrease in plasma HCO_3^- causes pH to fall. Metabolic acidosis can occur with increased production of a nonvolatile acid (such as lactic acid), decreased renal clearance of a nonvolatile acid (as in renal failure), or loss of HCO_3^- (as in chronic diarrhea). Symptoms result from action of compensatory mechanisms in the lungs, kidneys, and cells.

AGE ALERT
Metabolic acidosis is more prevalent among children, who are vulnerable to acid-base imbalance because their metabolic rates are rapid and ratios of water to total-body weight are low.

Severe or untreated metabolic acidosis can be fatal. The prognosis improves with prompt treatment of the underlying cause and rapid reversal of the acidotic state.

CAUSES

Metabolic acidosis usually results from excessive fat metabolism in the absence of usable carbohydrates. This can be caused by diabetic ketoacidosis; chronic alcoholism; malnutrition; or a diet low in carbohydrates and high in fat — all of which produce more ketoacids than the metabolic process can handle. Other causes include:

■ anaerobic carbohydrate metabolism (decreased tissue oxygenation or perfusion — as in cardiac pump failure after myocardial infarction, pulmonary or hepatic disease, shock, or anemia — forces a shift from aerobic to anaerobic metabolism, causing a corresponding increase in lactic acid level)

■ underexcretion of metabolized acids or inability to conserve base caused by renal insufficiency and failure (renal acidosis)

■ diarrhea, intestinal malabsorption, or loss of sodium bicarbonate from the intestines, causing the bicarbonate buffer system to shift to the acidic side (for example, ureteroenterostomy and Crohn's disease can also induce metabolic acidosis)

■ salicylate intoxication (overuse of aspirin); exogenous poisoning; or, less frequently, addisonism (increased excretion of sodium and chloride and retention of potassium)

■ inhibited secretion of acid caused by hypoaldosteronism or the use of potassium-sparing diuretics.

PATHOPHYSIOLOGY

As acid (hydrogen) starts to accumulate in the body, chemical buffers (plasma HCO_3^- and proteins) in the cells and ECF bind the excess hydrogen ions.

Excess hydrogen ions that the buffers can't bind lower the blood pH and stimulate chemoreceptors in the medulla to increase respiration. The consequent fall of $PaCO_2$ frees hydrogen ions to bind with HCO_3^-. Respiratory compensation occurs in minutes but isn't sufficient to correct the acidosis.

Healthy kidneys try to compensate by secreting excess hydrogen ions into the renal tubules. There these ions are buffered by either phosphate or ammonia and excreted into the urine in the form of weak acid. For each hydrogen ion secreted into the renal tubules, the tubules reabsorb and return to the blood one sodium ion and one HCO_3^- ion.

The excess hydrogen ions in extracellular fluid (ECF) passively diffuse into cells. To maintain the balance of charge across the membranes, the cells release potassium ions. Excess hydrogen ions change the normal balance of potassium, sodium, and calcium ions and thereby impair neural excitability.

SIGNS AND SYMPTOMS

In mild acidosis, symptoms of the underlying disease may hide the direct clinical evidence. Signs and symptoms include:

■ headache and lethargy progressing to drowsiness, stupor, and (if condition is severe and untreated) coma and death caused by CNS depression

■ Kussmaul's respirations (as the lungs attempt to compensate by blowing off CO_2), hypotension

■ associated GI distress leading to anorexia, nausea, vomiting, diarrhea, and possibly dehydration

■ warm, flushed skin caused by a pH-sensitive decrease in vascular response to sympathetic stimuli

■ fruity-smelling breath from fat catabolism and excretion of accumulated acetone through the lungs caused by underlying diabetes mellitus.

COMPLICATIONS

Metabolic acidosis depresses the CNS and, if untreated, may lead to:

■ weakness, flaccid paralysis

■ coma

■ ventricular arrhythmias, possibly cardiac arrest.

In the metabolic acidosis of chronic renal failure, HCO_3^- is drawn from bone to buffer hydrogen ions; the results include:

■ growth retardation in children

■ bone disorders such as renal osteodystrophy.

METABOLIC ALKALOSIS ◆ **101**

DIAGNOSIS
The following test results confirm the diagnosis of metabolic acidosis:
■ arterial pH less than 7.35 (as low as 7.10 in severe acidosis)
■ $PaCO_2$ normal or less than 34 mm Hg as respiratory compensatory mechanisms take hold
■ HCO_3^- may be 22 mEq/L.
The following test results support the diagnosis of metabolic acidosis:
■ urine pH less than 4.5 in the absence of renal disease (as the kidneys excrete acid to raise blood pH)
■ potassium level greater than 5.5 mEq/L from chemical buffering
■ glucose level greater than 150 mg/dl
■ serum ketone bodies in diabetes
■ elevated lactic acid level in lactic acidosis
■ anion gap greater than 14 mEq/L in high anion gap metabolic acidosis, lactic acidosis, ketoacidosis, aspirin overdose, alcohol poisoning, renal failure, or other conditions characterized by accumulation of organic acids, sulfates, or phosphates
■ anion gap 12 mEq/L or less in normal anion gap metabolic acidosis from HCO_3^- loss, GI or renal loss, increased acid load (hyperalimentation fluids), rapid I.V. saline solution administration, or other conditions characterized by HCO_3^- loss.

TREATMENT
Treatment to correct the acidosis as quickly as possible by addressing the symptoms and the underlying cause may include:
■ sodium bicarbonate I.V. for severe high anion gap to neutralize blood acidity in patients with pH less than 7.20 and HCO_3^- loss; monitor electrolyte levels, especially potassium level, during sodium bicarbonate therapy (potassium level may fall as pH rises)
■ lactated Ringer's solution I.V. to correct normal anion gap metabolic acidosis and ECF volume deficit
■ evaluation and correction of electrolyte imbalances
■ correction of the underlying cause (for example, in diabetic ketoacidosis, continuous low-dose I.V. insulin infusion)
■ mechanical ventilation to maintain respiratory compensation if needed

■ antibiotic therapy to treat infection
■ dialysis for patients with renal failure or certain drug toxicities
■ antidiarrheals for diarrhea-induced HCO_3^- loss
■ monitoring for secondary changes caused by hypovolemia, such as falling blood pressure (in diabetic acidosis).

Metabolic alkalosis
Metabolic alkalosis occurs when low levels of acid or high bicarbonate (HCO_3^-) cause metabolic, respiratory, and renal responses, producing characteristic symptoms (most notably, hypoventilation). With early diagnosis and prompt treatment, prognosis is good, but untreated metabolic alkalosis may lead to coma and death.

CAUSES
Metabolic alkalosis results from loss of acid, retention of base, or renal mechanisms linked to low potassium and chloride levels.
Causes of critical acid loss include:
■ chronic vomiting
■ nasogastric tube drainage or lavage without adequate electrolyte replacement
■ fistulas
■ use of steroids or certain diuretics (furosemide [Lasix], thiazides, and ethacrynic acid [Edecrin])
■ massive blood transfusions
■ Cushing disease, primary hyperaldosteronism, and Bartter's syndrome (lead to sodium and chloride retention and urinary loss of potassium and hydrogen).
Excessive HCO_3^- retention causing chronic hypercapnia can result from:
■ excessive intake of bicarbonate of soda or other antacids (usually for treatment of gastritis or peptic ulcer)
■ excessive intake of absorbable alkali (as in milk-alkali syndrome, commonly seen in patients with peptic ulcers)
■ excessive amounts of I.V. fluids with high bicarbonate or lactate levels
■ respiratory insufficiency.
Alterations in extracellular electrolyte levels that can cause metabolic alkalosis include:
■ low chloride level (as chloride diffuses out of the cell, hydrogen diffuses into the cell)

■ low potassium level, causing increased hydrogen ion excretion by the kidneys.

PATHOPHYSIOLOGY

Chemical buffers in the extracellular fluid (ECF) and intracellular fluid bind the HCO_3^- that accumulates in the body. Excess unbound HCO_3^- raises blood pH, which depresses chemoreceptors in the medulla, inhibiting respiration and raising partial pressure of arterial carbon dioxide ($PaCO_2$). Carbon dioxide combines with water to form carbonic acid. Low oxygen levels limit respiratory compensation.

When the blood HCO_3^- rises to 28 mEq/L or more, the amount filtered by the renal glomeruli exceeds the reabsorptive capacity of the renal tubules. Excess HCO_3^- is excreted in the urine, and hydrogen ions are retained. To maintain electrochemical balance, sodium ions and water are excreted with the bicarbonate ions.

When hydrogen ion levels in ECF are low, hydrogen ions diffuse passively out of the cells and, to maintain the balance of charge across the cell membrane, extracellular potassium ions move into the cells. As intracellular hydrogen ion levels fall, calcium ionization decreases, and nerve cells become more permeable to sodium ions. As sodium ions move into the cells, they trigger neural impulses, first in the peripheral nervous system and then in the central nervous system.

SIGNS AND SYMPTOMS

Clinical features of metabolic alkalosis result from the body's attempt to correct the acid-base imbalance, primarily through hypoventilation. Signs and symptoms include:

■ irritability, picking at bedclothes (carphology), twitching, and confusion caused by decreased cerebral perfusion

■ nausea, vomiting, and diarrhea (which aggravate alkalosis) caused by continued production of gastric acid

■ cardiovascular abnormalities caused by hypokalemia and hypocalcemia

■ respiratory disturbances (such as cyanosis and apnea) and slow, shallow respirations resulting from hypoventilation as a compensatory mechanism

■ diminished peripheral blood flow during repeated blood pressure checks may provoke carpopedal spasm in the hand (Trousseau's sign, a possible sign of impending tetany) caused by hypocalcemia.

COMPLICATIONS

Uncorrected metabolic alkalosis may progress to:

■ seizures

■ coma.

DIAGNOSIS

Findings that indicate metabolic alkalosis include:

■ blood pH greater than 7.45 and HCO_3^- greater than 26 mEq/L (confirm the diagnosis)

■ $PaCO_2$ greater than 45 mm Hg (indicates attempts at respiratory compensation)

■ low potassium (less than 3.5 mEq/L), calcium (less than 8.9 mg/dl), and chloride (less than 98 mEq/L) levels

■ urine pH about 7

■ alkaline urine after the renal compensatory mechanism begins to excrete bicarbonate

■ electrocardiogram possibly showing low T wave, merging with a P wave, and atrial or sinus tachycardia.

TREATMENT

The goal of treatment is to correct the underlying cause of metabolic alkalosis. Possible treatments include:

■ cautious use of ammonium chloride I.V. (rarely) or hydrochloric acid to restore ECF hydrogen and chloride levels

■ potassium chloride (KCl) and normal saline solution (except in heart failure); usually sufficient to replace losses from gastric drainage

■ discontinuation of diuretics and administration of supplementary KCl (metabolic alkalosis from potent diuretic therapy)

■ oral or I.V. acetazolamide (Diamox; assists renal bicarbonate excretion) to correct metabolic alkalosis without rapid volume expansion (acetazolamide also enhances potassium excretion; therefore, potassium may be given before the drug).

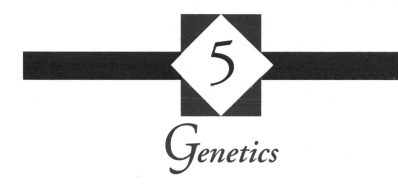

Genetics

Genetics is the study of heredity— the passing of physical, biochemical, and physiologic traits from biological parents to their children. In this transmission, disorders can be transmitted and mistakes or mutations can result in disability or death.

Genetic information is carried in genes, which are strung together on the strands of the deoxyribonucleic acid double helix structure to form chromosomes. Every normal human cell (except reproductive cells) has 46 chromosomes: 22 paired chromosomes called autosomes, and 2 sex chromosomes (a pair of Xs in females and an X and a Y in males). A representation of a person's individual set of chromosomes is called the person's karyotype. (See *Normal human karyotype,* page 104.)

The human genome (the full set of genes in a human) has been under intense study for only about 15 years to determine the structure of each gene in the genome and its location within each of the 23 pairs of chromosomes that make up the set of chromosomes. In June 2000, two teams of scientists completed the "rough draft" of the entire genome sequence. The sequence consists of more than 3.1 billion pairs of chemicals. Decoding the genome will enable scientists to know who is likely to get a specific inherited disease and enable researchers to eradicate many diseases or improve their treatment.

For various reasons, not every gene that might be expressed actually is. Genetic principles are based on studies of thou-

sands of people. Those studies have led to generalities that are usually true, but exceptions occur. Genetics is an inexact science.

GENETIC COMPONENTS

Each of the two strands of deoxyribonucleic acid (DNA) in a chromosome consists of thousands of combinations of four nucleotides— adenine (A), thymine (T), cytosine (C), and guanine (G). Some of our DNA is arranged into genes, which are composed of complementary triplet pairs called codons. The strands are loosely held together by chemical bonds between adenine and thymine or cytosine and guanine— for example, a triplet ACT on one strand is linked to the triplet TGA on the other. The looseness of the bonds allows the strands to separate easily during cell division. (See *DNA duplication: Two double helices from one,* page 105.) The genes carry a code for each trait a person inherits, from blood type to eye color to body shape and myriad other traits.

DNA ultimately controls the formation of essential substances throughout the life of every cell in the body. It does this through the genetic code, the precise sequence of AT and CG pairs on the DNA molecule. Genes not only control heredi-

Normal human karyotype

The illustration represents the arrangement of chromosomes (karyotype) in a normal male.

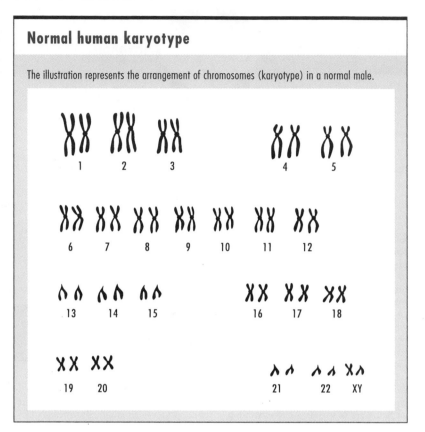

tary traits, transmitted from parents to children, but also cell reproduction and the daily functions of all cells. Genes control cell function by controlling the structures and chemicals that are made within the cell. For example, they control the formation of ribonucleic acid, which in turn controls the formation of specific proteins, most of which are enzymes that assist chemical reactions in the cells.

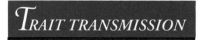

Germ cells, or gametes (ovum and sperm), are one of two classes of cells in the body; each germ cell contains 23 chromosomes (called the *haploid* number)

in its nucleus. All the other cells in the body are somatic cells, which are *diploid*, meaning they contain 23 *pairs* of chromosomes.

When ovum and sperm unite, the corresponding chromosomes pair up so that the fertilized cell and every somatic cell of the new person has 23 pairs of chromosomes in its nucleus.

Germ cells

The body produces germ cells through a type of cell division called meiosis. Meiosis occurs only when the body is creating haploid germ cells from their diploid precursors. Each of the 23 pairs of chromosomes in the diploid cell separates so that when the cell divides, each resulting hap-

DNA duplication: Two double helices from one

The nucleotide, the basic structural unit of deoxyribonucleic acid (DNA), contains a phosphate group, deoxyribose, and a nitrogen base made of adenine (A), thymine (T), cytosine (C), and guanine (G). A DNA molecule's double helix forms from the twisting of nucleotide strands (shown below).

During duplication, a DNA chain separates and new complementary chains form and link to the separated originals (parents). The result is two identical double helices — each containing an original parent strand and the newly formed complementary (daughter) strand.

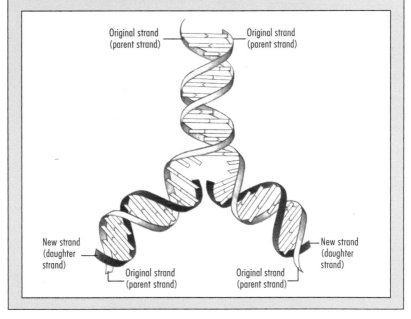

Original strand (parent strand)

Original strand (parent strand)

New strand (daughter strand)

New strand (daughter strand)

Original strand (parent strand)

Original strand (parent strand)

loid germ cell (ovum or sperm) contains one set of 23 chromosomes.

Most of the genes on one chromosome are identical or almost identical to the gene on its mate. (As we discuss later, each chromosome may carry a different version of the same gene.) The location (or locus) of a gene on a chromosome is specific and doesn't vary from person to person. This allows each of the thousands of genes on a strand of deoxyribonucleic acid (DNA) in an ovum to join the corresponding gene in a sperm when the chromosomes pair up at fertilization.

DETERMINING SEX

Only one pair of chromosomes in each cell — pair 23, the sex chromosomes — determines a person's sex. The other 22 numbered chromosome pairs are called *autosomes*. Females have two X chromosomes in pair 23, and males have one X and one Y chromosome in the pair.

Each germ cell (gamete) produced by a male contains either an X or a Y chromosome. When a sperm with an X chromosome fertilizes an ovum, the child will be a girl (two X chromosomes); when a sperm with a Y chromosome fertilizes an ovum, the child will be a boy (one X and one Y

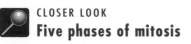

CLOSER LOOK
Five phases of mitosis

In mitosis (used by all cells except gametes), the nuclear contents of a cell reproduce and divide, forming two daughter cells. The five phases of this process are illustrated below.

INTERPHASE
The nucleus and nuclear membrane are well defined and the nucleolus is prominent. Chromosomes (each composed of two chromatids) replicate, each forming a double strand that remains attached at the center of each chromosome by a structure called the centromere; they appear as an indistinguishable matrix within the nucleus. Centrioles appear outside the nucleus.

PROPHASE
The nucleolus disappears and chromosomes become distinct. Halves of each duplicated chromosome (chromatids) remain attached by a centromere. Centrioles move to opposite sides of the cell and radiate spindle fibers.

METAPHASE
Chromosomes line up randomly in the center of the cell between spindles, along the metaphase plate. The centromere of each chromosome replicates.

ANAPHASE
Centromeres move apart, pulling the separate chromosomes to opposite ends of the cell. Each end of the cell now contains 46 chromosomes. The number of chromosomes at each end of the cell equals the original number.

TELOPHASE
A nuclear membrane forms around each end of the cell, and spindle fibers disappear. The cytoplasm compresses and divides the cell in half. Each new cell contains the diploid number (46 in humans) of chromosomes.

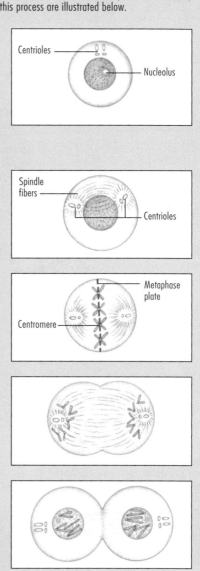

chromosome). Very rare errors in cell division can result in a germ cell that has no sex chromosome or two sex chromosomes. After fertilization, if one of the gametes contains an abnormal number of sex chromosomes, the fertilized ovum may have an XO, XXY, XXX, or XYY in its karyotype and still survive. Most other errors in sex chromosome division are incompatible with life.

Mitosis

The fertilized ovum — now called a *zygote* — undergoes a type of cell division called *mitosis*. Before a cell divides, its chromosomes duplicate. During this process, the double helix of DNA separates into two chains; each chain serves as a template for constructing a new chain. Individual DNA nucleotides are linked into new strands with bases complementary to those in the originals. In this way, two identical double helices are formed, each containing one of the original strands and a newly formed complementary strand. These double helices are duplicates of the original DNA chain.

Mitotic cell division occurs in five phases: an inactive phase called *interphase* and four active phases: *prophase, metaphase, anaphase,* and *telophase.* (See *Five phases of mitosis.*) The result of every mitotic cell division is two new daughter cells, each genetically identical to the original and to each other. Each of the two resulting cells likewise divides, and so on, eventually forming a many-celled human embryo. Thus, each cell in a person's body (except ovum or sperm) contains an identical set of 46 chromosomes that are unique to that person.

TRAIT PREDOMINANCE

Each parent contributes one set of chromosomes (and therefore one set of genes) so that every child has two genes for every locus (location on the chromosome) on the autosomal chromosomes.

Some characteristics, or traits, of the child are determined by one gene that may have many variants, such as eye color. Others, called polygenic traits, require the interaction of one or more genes. In addition, environmental factors may affect how a gene or genes are expressed.

Variations in a particular gene — such as brown, blue, or green eye color — are called alleles. A person who has identical alleles on each chromosome is homozygous for that gene; if the alleles are different, they're said to be heterozygous.

Autosomal inheritance

For unknown reasons, on autosomal chromosomes, one allele may be more influential than the other in determining a specific trait. The more powerful, or *dominant,* gene is more likely to be expressed in the child than the less influential, or *recessive,* gene. Children will express a dominant allele when one or both chromosomes in a pair carry it. A recessive allele won't be expressed unless both chromosomes carry the recessive alleles. For example, a child may receive a gene for brown eyes from one parent and a gene for blue eyes from the other parent. The gene for brown eyes is dominant, and the gene for blue eyes is recessive. Because the dominant gene is more likely to be expressed, the child is more likely to have brown eyes.

Sex-linked inheritance

The X and Y chromosomes aren't literally a pair because the X chromosome is much larger than the Y. The male literally has less genetic material than the female, which means he has only one copy of most genes on the X chromosome. Inheritance of those genes is called *X-linked.* A man will transmit one copy of each X-linked gene to his daughters and none to his sons. A woman will transmit one copy to each daughter or son.

Inheritance of genes on the X chromosomes is different in another way. Some recessive genes on the X chromosomes act like dominants in females. Because of X-inactivation, one recessive allele will be expressed in some somatic cells and another in other somatic cells. The most common example occurs not in people but in cats. Only female cats have calico (tricolor) coat patterns. Hair color in the cat is carried on the X chromosome. Some hair cells in females express the brown allele, others the white, and still others a third color.

Multifactorial inheritance

Environmental factors can affect the expression of some genes; this is called *multifactorial inheritance*. Height is a classic example of a multifactorial trait. Although in general, a child's height will be in a range between the height of the two parents. But nutritional patterns, health care, and other environmental factors also influence development. The better-nourished, healthier children of two short parents may be taller than either. Some diseases have genetic predisposition but multifactorial inheritance; that is, the gene for the disease is expressed only under certain environmental conditions.

Factors that may contribute to multifactorial inheritance include:
- maternal age
- use of drugs, alcohol, or hormones by either parent
- maternal or paternal exposure to radiation
- maternal infection during pregnancy or existing diseases in the mother
- nutritional factors
- general maternal or paternal health
- other factors, including high altitude, maternal smoking, maternal-fetal blood incompatibility, and inadequate prenatal care.

PATHOPHYSIOLOGIC CHANGES

Autosomal, sex-linked, and multifactorial inheritance disorders originate from damage to genes or chromosomes. Some defects arise spontaneously, whereas others may be caused by environmental teratogens.

Gene errors

A permanent change in genetic material is a mutation, which may occur spontaneously or after exposure of a cell to radiation, certain chemicals, or viruses. Mutations can occur anywhere in the genome — the person's entire inventory of genes.

Every cell has built-in defenses against genetic damage. However, if a mutation isn't identified or repaired, it may produce a trait different from the original trait, which is transmitted to children during reproduction. The mutation first causes the cell to produce some abnormal protein that makes the cell differ from its ancestors. Some mutations have no effect, some may change expression of a trait, and others may change the way a cell functions. Some mutations cause serious or deadly defects, such as cancer or congenital anomalies.

AUTOSOMAL DISORDERS

In single-gene disorders, an error occurs at a single gene site on the deoxyribonucleic acid strand. A mistake may occur in the copying and transcribing of a single codon (nucleotide triplet) through additions, deletions, excessive repetitions, or base changes.

Single-gene disorders are inherited in clearly identifiable patterns that are the same as those seen in inheritance of normal traits. Because every person has 22 pairs of autosomes and only 1 pair of sex chromosomes, most hereditary disorders are caused by autosomal defects.

Autosomal dominant transmission usually affects daughters and sons equally. If one parent is affected, each child has a 50% chance of being affected. If both parents are affected (usually a highly unlikely situation), the child has a 25% chance of being disease-free; a 50% chance of having the disorder; and a 25% chance of having two dominant genes for the disorder, a situation that's most likely incompatible with life. An example of this type of inheritance occurs in Marfan syndrome. (See *Autosomal inheritance*.)

Autosomal recessive inheritance also usually affects daughters and sons equally.

Autosomal inheritance

AUTOSOMAL DOMINANT INHERITANCE

The diagram shows the inheritance pattern of an abnormal trait when one parent has recessive normal genes (aa) and the other has a dominant abnormal gene (Aa). Each child has a 50% chance of inheriting A.

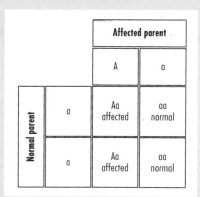

		Affected parent	
		A	a
Normal parent	a	Aa affected	aa normal
	a	Aa affected	aa normal

AUTOSOMAL RECESSIVE INHERITANCE

The diagram shows the inheritance pattern of an abnormal trait when both unaffected parents are heterozygous (Aa) for a recessive abnormal gene (a) on an autosome. As shown, each child has one chance in four (25%) of being affected (aa), a 25% chance of having two normal genes (AA) and no chance of transmittal, and a 50% chance of being a carrier (Aa) who can transmit the gene.

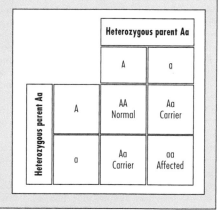

		Heterozygous parent Aa	
		A	a
Heterozygous parent Aa	A	AA Normal	Aa Carrier
	a	Aa Carrier	aa Affected

If both parents are affected, all their children will be affected. If both parents are unaffected but are heterozygous for the trait (carriers of the defective gene), each child has one chance in four of being affected. If only one parent is affected and the other parent isn't a carrier, none of their children will be affected but all will carry the defective gene. If one parent is affected and the other is a carrier, their children will have a 50% chance of being affected. Autosomal recessive disorders may occur when there's no family history of the disease.

SEX-LINKED DISORDERS

Genetic disorders caused by genes located on the sex chromosomes are termed sex-linked disorders. Most sex-linked disorders are passed on the X chromosome, usually as recessive traits. Because males have only one X chromosome, a single X-linked recessive gene can cause disease to be exhibited in a male. Females receive two X chromosomes, so they can be homozygous for a disease allele, homozygous for a normal allele, or heterozygous (a carrier).

Most people who express X-linked recessive traits are males with unaffected parents. In rare cases, the father is affected and the mother is a carrier. All daughters of an affected male will be carriers. Sons of an affected father will be unaffected, and the unaffected sons aren't carriers. Unaffected sons of a carrier mother don't transmit the disorder. Hemophilia is an example of an X-linked inheritance disorder. (See *X-linked inheritance.*)

Characteristics of X-linked dominant inheritance include evidence of the inherited trait in the family history. A person with the abnormal trait must have one affected parent. If the father has an X-linked dominant disorder, all his daughters and none of his sons will be affected. If a mother has an X-linked dominant disorder, each of her children has a 50% chance of being affected.

MULTIFACTORIAL DISORDERS

Most multifactorial disorders result from the effects of several different genes and an environmental component. In polygenic inheritance, each gene has a small additive effect, and the effect of a combination of genetic errors in a person is unpredictable. Multifactorial disorders can result from a less-than-optimum expression of many different genes, not from a specific error.

Some multifactorial disorders are apparent at birth, such as cleft lip, cleft palate, congenital heart disease, anencephaly, clubfoot, and myelomeningocele. Others don't become apparent until later, such as type II diabetes mellitus, hypertension, hyperlipidemia, most autoimmune diseases, and many cancers. Multifactorial disorders that develop in adulthood may be strongly related to environmental factors, not only in incidence but also in the degree of expression.

Teratogens are environmental agents that can harm the developing fetus by causing congenital structural or functional defects. Teratogens may also cause spontaneous miscarriage, complications during labor and delivery, hidden defects in later development (such as cognitive or behavioral problems), or neoplastic transformations. (See *Teratogens and associated disorders,* pages 112 and 113.)

Environmental factors of maternal or paternal origin include the use of chemicals (such as drugs, alcohol, or hormones), exposure to radiation, general health, and age. Maternal factors include infections during pregnancy, existing diseases, nutritional factors, exposure to high altitude, smoking, maternal-fetal blood incompatibility, and poor prenatal care.

The embryonic period — the first 8 weeks after fertilization — is a vulnerable time when specific organ systems are actively differentiating. Exposure to teratogens usually kills the embryo. During the fetal period, organ systems are formed and continue to mature. Exposure during this time can cause intrauterine growth retardation, cognitive abnormalities, or structural defects.

Chromosome defects

Aberrations in chromosome structure or number cause a class of disorders called congenital anomalies, or birth defects. The aberration may be loss, addition, or rearrangement of genetic material. If the remaining genetic material is sufficient to maintain life, an endless variety of clinical manifestations may occur. Most clinically significant chromosome aberrations arise during meiosis. Meiosis is an incredibly complex process that can go wrong in many ways. Potential contributing factors include maternal age, radiation, and use of some therapeutic or recreational drugs.

Translocation, the shifting or moving of chromosomal material, occurs when chromosomes split apart and rejoin in an abnormal arrangement. The cells still have a normal amount of genetic material, so often there are no visible abnormalities. However, the children of parents with translocated chromosomes may have serious genetic defects, such as monosomies or trisomies. Parental age doesn't seem to be a factor in translocation.

ERRORS IN CHROMOSOME NUMBER

During both meiosis and mitosis, chromosomes normally separate in a process called *disjunction.* Failure to separate, called *nondisjunction,* causes an unequal distribution of chromosomes between the two resulting cells. If nondisjunction occurs during mitosis soon after fertilization, it may

X-linked inheritance

X-LINKED RECESSIVE INHERITANCE

The diagram shows the children of a normal parent and a parent with a recessive gene on the X chromosome (shown by an open dot). All daughters of an affected father will be carriers. The son of a carrier mother may inherit a recessive gene on the X chromosome and be affected by the disease. Unaffected sons can't transmit the disorder.

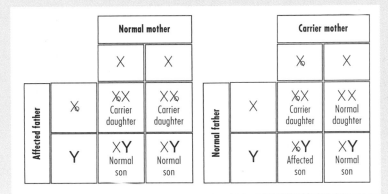

X-LINKED DOMINANT INHERITANCE

This diagram shows the children of a normal parent and a parent with an abnormal, X-linked dominant gene on the X chromosome (shown by the dot on the X). When the father is affected, only his daughters have the abnormal gene. When the mother is affected, both sons and daughters may be affected.

Teratogens and associated disorders

This chart lists common teratogens and their associated disorders.

TERATOGENS	ASSOCIATED DISORDERS
INFECTIONS	
Toxoplasmosis Rubella Cytomegalovirus Herpes simplex Other infections (syphilis, hepatitis B, mumps, gonorrhea, parvovirus, varicella)	◆ Growth deficiency ◆ Mental retardation ◆ Hepatosplenomegaly ◆ Hearing loss ◆ Cardiac and ocular defects ◆ Active infection ◆ Carrier state
MATERNAL DISORDERS	
Diabetes mellitus	◆ Abnormalities of the spine, legs, heart, kidney, or external genitalia
Phenylketonuria	◆ Mental retardation ◆ Microcephaly ◆ Congenital heart defects ◆ Intrauterine growth retardation
Hyperthermia	◆ Intrauterine growth retardation ◆ Central nervous system (CNS) and neural tube defects ◆ Facial defects
DRUGS, CHEMICALS, AND PHYSICAL AGENTS	
Alcohol	◆ Fetal alcohol syndrome ◆ Learning disabilities
Anticonvulsants	◆ Intrauterine growth retardation ◆ Mental deficiency ◆ Facial abnormalities ◆ Cardiac defects ◆ Cleft lip and palate ◆ Malformed ears ◆ Genital defects
Cocaine	◆ Premature delivery ◆ Abruptio placentae ◆ Intracranial hemorrhage ◆ GI and genitourinary (GU) abnormalities

Teratogens and associated disorders *(continued)*

TERATOGENS	ASSOCIATED DISORDERS
DRUGS, CHEMICALS, AND PHYSICAL AGENTS *(continued)*	
Diethylstilbestrol	◆ Clear-cell adenocarcinoma of vagina ◆ Structural and functional defects of female GU tract
Lithium	◆ Congenital heart disease
Methotrexate	◆ Intrauterine growth retardation ◆ Decreased ossification of skull ◆ Prominent eyes ◆ Arm and leg abnormalities ◆ Mild developmental delay
Radiation	◆ Microcephaly ◆ Mental retardation
Tetracycline	◆ Brown staining of decidual teeth ◆ Dental caries ◆ Enamel hypoplasia
Vitamin A derivatives	◆ Facial defects ◆ Cardiac defects ◆ CNS defects ◆ Incomplete development of thymus
Warfarin (Coumadin)	◆ Intrauterine growth retardation ◆ Mental retardation ◆ Seizures ◆ Nasal hypoplasia ◆ Abnormal calcification of axial skeleton

affect all the resulting cells. Gain or loss of chromosomes is usually caused by nondisjunction of autosomes or sex chromosomes during meiosis. The incidence of nondisjunction increases with parental age. (See *Chromosomal disjunction and nondisjunction,* page 114.)

The presence of one chromosome less than the normal number is called *monosomy;* an autosomal monosomy is nonviable. The presence of an extra chromosome is called a *trisomy.* A mixture of both trisomic and normal cells results in mosaicism, which is the presence of two or more cell lines in the same person. The effect of mosaicism depends on the proportion and anatomic location of abnormal cells.

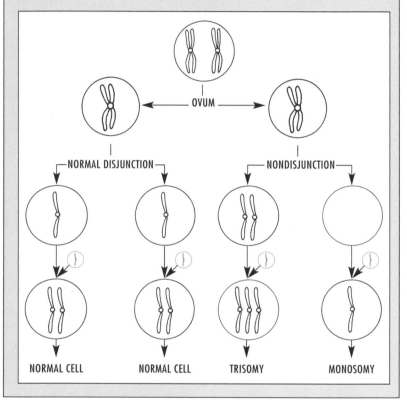

CLOSER LOOK
Chromosomal disjunction and nondisjunction

This illustration shows normal disjunction and nondisjunction of an ovum. In normal disjunction, fertilization with a normal sperm results in a zygote with the correct number of chromosomes. In nondisjunction, the sister chromatids fail to separate; the result is one trisomic cell and one monosomic cell.

OVUM

NORMAL DISJUNCTION

NONDISJUNCTION

NORMAL CELL

NORMAL CELL

TRISOMY

MONOSOMY

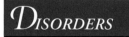

DISORDERS

This section discusses disorders in the context of their pattern of inheritance as well as environmental factors. The alphabetically listed disorders have the following patterns of inheritance:

■ Autosomal recessive: cystic fibrosis, sickle cell anemia, Tay-Sachs disease

■ Autosomal dominant: Marfan syndrome

■ X-linked recessive: fragile X syndrome, hemophilia

■ Polygenic multifactorial: cleft lip and cleft palate, neural tube defects

■ Chromosome number: Down syndrome, Klinefelter syndrome, trisomy 18 syndrome, trisomy 13 syndrome.

Cleft lip and cleft palate

Cleft lip and cleft palate may occur separately or in combination. They originate in the second month of pregnancy if the front and sides of the face and the palatine shelves (embryonic palate structures) fuse imperfectly. Cleft lip with or without cleft palate occurs twice as often in boys as in girls. Cleft palate without cleft lip is more common in girls.

Cleft lip deformities can occur unilaterally, bilaterally, or rarely, in the midline. Only the lip may be involved, or the defect may extend into the upper jaw or nasal cavity. (See *Types of cleft deformities*.)

Incidence is highest in children with a family history of cleft defects. Cleft lip with or without cleft palate occurs in about 1 in 1,000 births among Whites; the incidence is higher among Asians (1.7 in 1,000) and Native Americans (more than 3.6 in 1,000) but lower in Blacks (1 in 2,500).

CAUSES

Causes include:
- chromosomal or Mendelian syndrome (cleft defects are associated with more than 300 syndromes)
- exposure to teratogens during fetal development
- combined genetic and environmental factors.

PATHOPHYSIOLOGY

During the second month of pregnancy, the front and sides of the face and the palatine shelves develop. Because of a chromosomal abnormality, exposure to teratogens, genetic abnormality, or environmental factors, the lip or palate fuses imperfectly.

The deformity may range from a simple notch to a complete cleft. A cleft palate may be partial or complete. A complete cleft includes the soft palate, the bones of the maxilla, and the alveolus on one or both sides of the premaxilla.

A double cleft is the most severe of the deformities. The cleft runs from the soft palate forward to either side of the nose. A double cleft separates the maxilla and premaxilla into freely moving segments. The

Types of cleft deformities

These illustrations show variations of cleft lip and cleft palate.

NOTCH IN THE VERMILLION BORDER (JUNCTION OF THE LIP AND SURROUNDING SKIN)

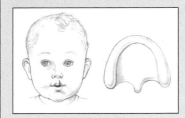

UNILATERAL CLEFT LIP AND PALATE

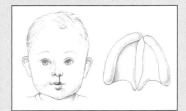

BILATERAL CLEFT LIP AND PALATE

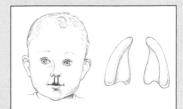

CLEFT PALATE

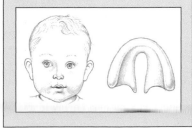

tongue and other muscles can displace the segments, enlarging the cleft.

CLINICAL ALERT
Isolated cleft palate is more commonly associated with other congenital defects than isolated cleft lip with or without cleft palate. The constellation of U-shaped cleft palate, mandibular hypoplasia, and glossoptosis is known as Pierre Robin sequence, or Robin sequence. Robin sequence can occur as an isolated defect or one feature of many different syndromes; therefore, a comprehensive genetic evaluation is suggested for infants with Robin sequence. Because of the mandibular hypoplasia and glossoptosis, careful evaluation and management of the airway are mandatory for infants with Robin sequence.

SIGNS AND SYMPTOMS
Signs and symptoms may include:
■ obvious cleft lip or cleft palate caused by imperfect fusion during embryonic or fetal development
■ feeding difficulties caused by incomplete fusion of the palate.

COMPLICATIONS
Complications may include:
■ malnutrition, because the abnormal lip and palate affect nutritional intake
■ hearing impairment, commonly caused by middle-ear damage or recurrent infections
■ permanent speech disability, even after surgical repair.

DIAGNOSIS
■ Clinical presentation, obvious at birth
■ Prenatal targeted ultrasound

TREATMENT
Correcting cleft lip or palate may involve:
■ surgical correction of cleft lip in the first few days of life to permit sucking, or delayed for 8 to 10 weeks (sometimes as long as 6 to 8 months) to allow the infant to grow and mature—thereby minimizing surgical and anesthesia risks, ruling out associated congenital anomalies, and allowing time for parental bonding
■ orthodontic prosthesis to improve sucking

■ surgical correction of cleft palate at 12 to 18 months, after the infant gains weight and is infection-free
■ speech therapy to correct speech patterns
■ use of a contoured speech bulb attached to the posterior of a denture to occlude the nasopharynx (to help the child develop intelligible speech) when a wide horseshoe defect makes surgery impossible
■ adequate nutrition for normal growth and development
■ use of a large soft nipple with large holes, such as a lamb's nipple, to improve feeding patterns and promote nutrition.

CLINICAL ALERT
Daily use of folic acid before conception decreases the risk of isolated (not associated with another genetic or congenital malformation) cleft lip or palate by up to 25%. Women of childbearing age should be encouraged to take a daily multivitamin containing folic acid until menopause or until they're no longer fertile.

Cystic fibrosis

In cystic fibrosis, dysfunction of the exocrine glands affects multiple organ systems. The disease affects both males and females and is the most common fatal genetic disease in white children.

Cystic fibrosis is accompanied by many complications and now carries an average life expectancy of 32 years. The disorder is characterized by chronic airway infection leading to bronchiectasis, bronchiolectasis, exocrine pancreatic insufficiency, intestinal dysfunction, abnormal sweat gland function, and reproductive dysfunction.

The incidence of cystic fibrosis varies with ethnic origin. It occurs in 1 of 2,000 births among Whites of North America and northern European descent, 1 in 17,000 births among Blacks, and 1 in 90,000 births in the Asian population in Hawaii.

CAUSES
The responsible gene is on chromosome 7q; it encodes a membrane-associated protein called the cystic fibrosis transmembrane regulator (CFTR). The exact function of the CFTR remains unknown, but it appears to help regulate chloride and

sodium transport across epithelial membranes.

Causes of cystic fibrosis include:
- abnormal coding found on as many as 350 CFTR alleles
- autosomal recessive inheritance.

PATHOPHYSIOLOGY

Most cases arise from the mutation that affects the genetic coding for a single amino acid, resulting in a protein (the CFTR) that doesn't function properly. The CFTR resembles other transmembrane transport proteins, but it lacks phenylalanine, an essential amino acid produced by normal genes. This abnormal protein interferes with cAMP-regulated chloride transport and that of other ions by preventing adenosine triphosphate from binding to the protein or by interfering with activation by protein kinase.

The mutation affects volume-absorbing epithelia (in the airways and intestines), salt-absorbing epithelia (in sweat ducts), and volume-secretory epithelia (in the pancreas). Lack of phenylalanine leads to dehydration, increasing the viscosity of mucous gland secretions, leading to obstruction of glandular ducts. Cystic fibrosis has a varying effect on electrolyte and water transport.

SIGNS AND SYMPTOMS

Signs and symptoms may include:
- thick secretions and dehydration caused by ionic imbalance
- chronic airway infections by *Staphylococcus aureus*, *Pseudomonas aeruginosa*, and *Pseudomonas cepacia*, possibly caused by abnormal airway surface fluids and failure of lung defenses
- dyspnea caused by accumulation of thick secretions in bronchioles and alveoli
- paroxysmal cough caused by stimulation of the secretion-removal reflex
- barrel chest, cyanosis, and clubbing of fingers and toes from chronic hypoxia
- crackles on auscultation caused by thick, airway-occluding secretions
- wheezes heard on auscultation caused by constricted airways
- retention of bicarbonate and water caused by the absence of the CFTR chloride channel in the pancreatic ductile epithelia; limits membrane function and leads to retention of pancreatic enzymes, chronic cholecystitis and cholelithiasis, and ultimate destruction of the pancreas
- obstruction of the small and large intestine caused by inhibited secretion of chloride and water and excessive absorption of liquid
- biliary cirrhosis caused by retention of biliary secretions
- fatal shock and arrhythmias caused by hyponatremia and hypochloremia from excessive sodium lost in sweat
- failure to thrive: poor weight gain, poor growth, distended abdomen, thin extremities, and sallow skin with poor turgor caused by malabsorption
- clotting problems, retarded bone growth, and delayed sexual development caused by deficiency of fat-soluble vitamins
- rectal prolapse in infants and children caused by malnutrition and wasting of perirectal supporting tissues
- esophageal varices caused by cirrhosis and portal hypertension.

COMPLICATIONS

Complications may include:
- obstructed glandular ducts (leading to peribronchial thickening) caused by increased viscosity of bronchial, pancreatic, and other mucous-gland secretions
- atelectasis or emphysema caused by respiratory effects
- diabetes, pancreatitis, and hepatic failure caused by effects on the intestines, pancreas, and liver
- malnutrition and malabsorption of fat-soluble vitamins (A, D, E, and K) caused by deficiencies of trypsin, amylase, and lipase (from obstructed pancreatic ducts, preventing the conversion and absorption of fat and protein in the intestinal tract)
- lack of sperm in the semen (azoospermia)
- secondary amenorrhea and increased mucus in the reproductive tracts, blocking the passage of ova.

DIAGNOSIS

The Cystic Fibrosis Foundation has developed certain criteria for a definitive diagnosis:

- Two sweat tests (to detect elevated sodium chloride levels) using a pilocarpine solution (a sweat inducer).
- Presence of an obstructive pulmonary disease, as determined by chest X-ray.
- Confirmed pancreatic insufficiency based on stool sample analysis indicating absence of trypsin or failure to thrive, or a family history of cystic fibrosis.

AGE ALERT
The sweat test may be inaccurate in very young infants because they may not produce enough sweat for a valid test. The test may need to be repeated.

The following test results may support the diagnosis:

- DNA testing can now locate the presence of the Delta F 508 deletion (found in about 70% of patients with cystic fibrosis, although the disease can cause more than 100 other mutations). This testing allows prenatal diagnosis in families with a previously affected child.
- Pulmonary function tests reveal decreased vital capacity, elevated residual volume caused by air entrapments, and decreased forced expiratory volume in 1 second. This test is used if pulmonary exacerbation already exists.
- Liver enzyme tests may reveal hepatic insufficiency.
- Sputum culture reveals organisms that cystic fibrosis patients typically and chronically colonize, such as staphylococcus and pseudomonas.
- Serum albumin measurement helps assess nutritional status.
- Electrolyte analysis assesses hydration status.

TREATMENT

The aim of treatment is to help the child lead as normal a life as possible. The type of treatment depends on the organ system involved. Possible treatments include:

- hypertonic radiocontrast materials delivered by enema to treat acute obstructions caused by meconium ileus
- breathing exercises, postural drainage, and chest percussion to clear pulmonary secretions
- antibiotics to treat lung infection, guided by sputum culture results
- drugs to increase mucus clearance
- inhaled beta-adrenergic agonists to control airway constriction
- pancreatic enzyme replacement to maintain adequate nutrition
- sodium-channel blocker to decrease sodium reabsorption from secretions and improve viscosity
- uridine triphosphate to stimulate chloride secretion by a non-CFTR
- salt supplements to replace electrolytes lost through sweat
- Domase alfa, a genetically engineered pulmonary enzyme, to help liquefy mucus
- recombinant alpha-antitrypsin to counteract excessive proteolytic activity produced during airway inflammation
- gene therapy to introduce normal CFTR into affected epithelial cells
- transplantation of heart or lungs in severe organ failure.

Down syndrome

Down syndrome, or *trisomy 21,* is a spontaneous chromosome abnormality that causes characteristic facial features, other distinctive physical abnormalities, and mental retardation; 60% of affected persons have cardiac defects. Down syndrome occurs in 1 of 650 to 700 of live births. Improved treatment for heart defects, respiratory and other infections, and acute leukemia has significantly increased life expectancy. Fetal and neonatal mortality remain high, usually resulting from complications of associated heart defects.

CAUSES
Causes include:

- advanced parental age (when the mother is age 35 or older at delivery or the father is age 42 or older)
- cumulative effects of environmental factors, such as radiation and viruses.

PATHOPHYSIOLOGY
Nearly all cases of Down syndrome result from trisomy 21 (three copies of chromosome 21). The result is a karyotype of 47

Karyotype of Down syndrome

Each autosome is normally one of a pair. A person with Down syndrome, or trisomy 21, has an extra chromosome 21.

MALE WITH DOWN SYNDROME

chromosomes instead of the usual 46. (See *Karyotype of Down syndrome.*) In 4% of patients, Down syndrome results from an unbalanced translocation or chromosomal rearrangement in which the long arm of chromosome 21 breaks and attaches to another chromosome.

Some affected persons and some asymptomatic parents may have chromosomal mosaicism, a mixture of two cell types, some with the normal 46 and some with 47 (an extra chromosome 21).

SIGNS AND SYMPTOMS

The signs and symptoms manifested by a child with Down syndrome are related to the genetic alteration that affects the growth and development of the fetus while in utero.

CLINICAL ALERT
The physical signs of Down syndrome are apparent at birth. The infant is lethargic and has distinctive craniofacial features.

Other signs and symptoms include:
■ distinctive facial features (low nasal bridge, epicanthic folds, protruding tongue, and low-set ears); small open mouth and disproportionately large tongue
■ single transverse crease on the palm (Simian crease)
■ small white spots on the iris (Brushfield's spots)
■ mental retardation (estimated IQ of 30 to 70)
■ developmental delay from hypotonia and decreased cognitive processing

- congenital heart disease, mainly septal defects and especially of the endocardial cushion
- impaired reflexes because of decreased muscle tone in limbs.

COMPLICATIONS
Possible complications include:
- early death from cardiac complications
- increased susceptibility to leukemia
- premature senile dementia, usually in the fourth decade if the patient survives
- increased susceptibility to acute and chronic infections
- strabismus and cataracts as the child grows
- poorly developed genitalia and delayed puberty (females may menstruate and be fertile; males may be infertile with low testosterone levels and often with undescended testes).

DIAGNOSIS
Diagnostic tests include:
- definitive karyotype
- amniocentesis or chorionic villi sampling for prenatal diagnosis, recommended for pregnant women age 34 and older, even with a negative family history
- prenatal targeted ultrasonography for duodenal obstruction or an atrioventricular canal defect (suggestive of Down syndrome)
- blood tests for reduced alpha-fetoprotein levels (suggestive of Down syndrome).

TREATMENT
Treatment of Down syndrome includes:
- surgery to correct heart defects and other related congenital abnormalities
- antibiotics for recurrent infections
- plastic surgery to correct characteristic facial traits (especially protruding tongue; possibly improving speech, reducing susceptibility to dental caries, and resulting in fewer orthodontic problems)
- early intervention programs and supportive therapies to maximize mental and physical capabilities
- thyroid hormone replacement for hypothyroidism.

Fragile X syndrome

Fragile X is the most common inherited cause of mental retardation. About 85% of males and 50% of females who inherit the fragile X mental retardation 1 (FMR1) mutation will demonstrate clinical features of the syndrome. Postpubescent males with fragile X syndrome often have distinct physical features, behavioral difficulties, and cognitive impairment. Females with fragile X syndrome tend to have more subtle symptoms.

Fragile X syndrome is estimated to occur in about 1 in 1,500 males and 1 in 2,500 females. It has been reported in almost all races and ethnic populations.

CAUSES
Causes may include:
- genetic defect on the X chromosome
- well-defined mutation at a specific location on the FMR1 gene.

PATHOPHYSIOLOGY
Fragile X syndrome is an X-linked condition that doesn't follow a simple X-linked inheritance pattern. The normal sequence of the FMR1 gene was identified at Xq27.3 in 1991. The unique mutation that results in fragile X syndrome consists of an expanding region of a specific triplet of nitrogenous bases: cytosine, guanine, guanine (CGG) within the gene's DNA sequence. Normally, FMR1 contains 6 to 49 sequential copies of the CGG triplet. When the number of CGG triplets expands to the range of 50 to 200 repeats, the region of DNA becomes unstable and is referred to as a premutation. A full mutation consists of more than 200 CGG triplet repeats.

The full mutation typically causes abnormal methylation (methyl groups attach to components of the gene) of FMR1. Methylation inhibits gene transcription and, thus, protein production. The reduced or absent protein product is responsible for the clinical features of fragile X syndrome. About 15% to 20% of males with a full mutation don't have fragile X. This may be because the males have unmethylated portions of mutated FMR1 that can be transcribed for eventual protein production or because the males are mosaic for the FMR1 premutation. It's believed that in asymptomatic mosaic males the cells with a premutation can produce enough protein to compensate for the cells that contain a full mutation and consequently produce no protein.

About 50% of females who inherit a full mutation from their mother have clinical features of fragile X syndrome. This is primarily because of the normal process of random X inactivation. At the time of meiosis, both X chromosomes must be activated. However, shortly after the zygote stage, an X chromosome is inactivated in every cell. Clinically measurable effects of the full FMR1 mutation will be more likely in relevant tissues or organs that have a disproportionate number of cells in which the normal X chromosome has been inactivated.

Males with a premutation don't have fragile X. They're considered unaffected or normal-transmitting males. Because males have only one X chromosome, all daughters of a transmitting male will inherit their father's X chromosome with the premutation. None of the male's sons will inherit the premutation because they inherit their father's Y chromosome rather than the X chromosome.

Females with the premutation don't have fragile X syndrome. However, the premutation can expand into the full mutation range (greater than 200 CGG triplets) when it's transmitted from a premutation carrier mother to her child. This expansion can occur during or after maternal meiosis. Therefore, the following possibilities exist for every child of a mother with a premutation:

■ A daughter receives the mother's X chromosome with the nonmutated FMR1 gene. She won't be affected with fragile X. None of her future children will be at risk for inheriting the syndrome from her.

■ A son receives the mother's X with the nonmutated FMR1 gene. He won't be affected with fragile X. None of his future children will be at risk for inheriting the syndrome from him.

■ A daughter receives the mother's X chromosome with the FMR1 premutation. She will be a carrier like her mother but won't have fragile X syndrome. Her future children will be at risk for inheriting a full mutation from her.

■ A son receives the mother's X with the FMR1 premutation. He won't be affected with fragile X. All of his future daughters but none of his future sons will inherit the premutation from him.

■ A daughter receives the mother's X chromosome with the FMR1 gene whose premutation expanded into a full mutation during or after maternal meiosis. Depending on the outcome of random X inactivation, the daughter may have clinically definable fragile X syndrome. Her future children will be at risk for inheriting the full mutation and, thus, the syndrome from her.

■ A son receives the mother's X chromosome with the FMR1 gene whose premutation has expanded into a full mutation during or after maternal meiosis. In 85% of cases, the son in this situation will have fragile X syndrome. Evidence indicates, however, that the FMR1 gene in the son's gametes may have the CGG triplet repeat within the premutation range, not the full mutation range like his somatic cells. Therefore, his future daughters wouldn't be expected to have fragile X syndrome.

Usually, the FMR1 status of a mother is determined after her son is clinically and later molecularly diagnosed with fragile X syndrome. Health care professionals need to be sensitive to the fact that the mother could find out she is a carrier of a premutation or she has a full mutation. Consequently, not only will she learn her son's diagnosis but she, herself, could be diagnosed with fragile X if she has a full mutation and clinical symptoms.

SIGNS AND SYMPTOMS
Reduced or absent protein production caused by inhibited gene transcription is the underlying pathophysiologic basis the signs and symptoms show. Small children may have relatively few identifiable physical characteristics; behavioral or learning difficulties may be the first indications. Signs and symptoms in affected males include:

■ a prominent jaw and forehead and a head circumference exceeding the 90th percentile

- a long, narrow face with long or large ears that may be posteriorly rotated
- connective tissue abnormalities, including hyperextension of the fingers, a floppy mitral valve (in 80% of adults), and mild to severe pectus excavatum
- unusually large testes, found in most affected males after puberty
- average IQ of 30 to 70
- hyperactivity, speech difficulties, language delay, and autistic-like behaviors, which may be attributed to other disorders such as attention deficit hyperactivity disorder and thus delay the diagnosis.

About 50% of females with the FMR1 full mutation will have symptoms, although their degree of severity and number vary widely among females with fragile X syndrome. Those who are symptomatic typically have a much milder clinical presentation than males because they have an unaffected X chromosome in addition to the one with a FMR1 full mutation. Symptoms in females include:

- some degree of cognitive impairment; most commonly, learning disabilities (math difficulties, language deficits, and attentional problems)
- IQ scores in the mental retardation range
- autistic-like features (rare)
- excessive shyness or social anxiety
- prominent ears and connective tissue manifestations (possibly as significant as in males).

Although males with the FMR1 premutation are asymptomatic, some female carriers of an FMR1 premutation can have associated symptoms. These symptoms include significantly earlier menopause and a low-normal performance IQ.

COMPLICATIONS
Complications of fragile X syndrome may include:

- behavioral or learning difficulties
- cognitive impairment
- connective tissue abnormalities.

DIAGNOSIS
- Identification of clinical symptoms
- Positive genetic test results, preferably DNA analysis of blood or buccal samples

to detect the size of the CGG repeat and the methylation status of FMR1

Before identification of the FMR1 mutation, a special cytogenetic (chromosome) blood test was used to microscopically detect the fragile site on the long arm of the affected X chromosome. It's now common knowledge that a full FMR1 mutation doesn't always result in a cytogenetically detectable fragile site. Therefore, chromosome analysis alone can provide false-negative results. Chromosome analysis still has utility together with FMR1 mutation analysis when genetic evaluation is performed for a male with mental retardation of unknown etiology.

In addition to diagnosing fragile X syndrome, genetic testing can determine whether the mother of a diagnosed individual is a carrier of the FMR1 premutation or has a full mutation. This information can be used for preconceptional genetic counseling by a trained professional and prenatal testing if the woman so chooses. FMR1 mutation analysis also can be subsequently performed on at-risk family members. It should be noted, however, that communication of genetic test results to at-risk family members constitutes a breech of patient confidentiality and privacy unless prior written permission to communicate results has been obtained from the previously tested patients.

TREATMENT
Fragile X syndrome has no known cure. Treatment is aimed at controlling individual symptoms. Most patients are on individualized pharmacotherapy for seizures, mood disorders, aggression, or sleep disorders. Surgery may be needed to repair a defective mitral valve.

Hemophilia

Hemophilia is an X-linked recessive bleeding disorder resulting from a deficiency of specific clotting factors. Hemophilia occurs in 20 of 100,000 male births; the severity and prognosis of bleeding vary with the degree of deficiency, or nonfunction, and the site of bleeding.

Hemophilia A, or classic hemophilia, is a deficiency of clotting factor VIII; it's more common than type B, affecting more than 80% of all persons with hemophilia. Hemophilia B, or Christmas disease, affects 15% of all persons with hemophilia and results from a deficiency of factor IX. There's no relationship between factor VIII and factor IX inherited defects.

CAUSES

Causes include:

- defect in a specific gene on the X chromosome that codes for factor VIII synthesis (hemophilia A)
- more than 300 different base-pair substitutions involving the factor IX gene on the X chromosome (hemophilia B).

PATHOPHYSIOLOGY

Hemophilia is an X-linked recessive genetic disease causing abnormal bleeding because of specific clotting factor malfunction. Factors VIII and IX are components of the intrinsic clotting pathway; factor IX is an essential factor, and factor VIII is a critical cofactor. Factor VIII accelerates the activation of factor X by several thousandfold. Excessive bleeding occurs when these clotting factors are reduced by more than 75%. A deficiency or nonfunction of factor VIII causes hemophilia A, and a deficiency or nonfunction of factor IX causes hemophilia B.

Hemophilia may be severe, moderate, or mild, depending on the degree of activation of clotting factors. Patients with severe disease have no detectable factor VIII or factor IX activity or less than 1% of normal. Moderately afflicted patients have 1% to 4% of normal clotting activity, and mildly afflicted patients have 5% to 25% of normal clotting activity.

A person with hemophilia forms a platelet plug at a bleeding site, but clotting factor deficiency impairs the ability to form a stable fibrin clot. Delayed bleeding is more common than immediate hemorrhage.

SIGNS AND SYMPTOMS

Signs and symptoms may include:

- spontaneous bleeding in severe hemophilia (prolonged or excessive bleeding after circumcision is often the first sign) because of absence of clotting factors

- excessive or continued bleeding or bruising after minor trauma or surgery caused by inability to form a stable fibrin clot because of clotting factor deficiency
- large subcutaneous and deep intramuscular hematomas caused by mild trauma from bleeding into the tissue or muscle
- prolonged bleeding in mild hemophilia after major trauma or surgery, but no spontaneous bleeding after minor trauma
- pain, swelling, and tenderness caused by bleeding into joints (especially weight-bearing joints)
- internal bleeding, commonly manifested as abdominal, chest, or flank pain
- hematuria from bleeding into kidney
- hematemesis or tarry stools from bleeding into the GI tract.

COMPLICATIONS

Complications may include:

- peripheral neuropathy, pain, paresthesia, and muscle atrophy caused by bleeding near peripheral nerves
- ischemia and gangrene caused by impaired blood flow through a major vessel
- decreased tissue perfusion and hypovolemic shock (shown as restlessness, anxiety, confusion, pallor, cool and clammy skin, chest pain, decreased urine output, hypotension, and tachycardia).

DIAGNOSIS

- Specific coagulation factor assays to diagnose the type and severity of hemophilia
- Factor VIII assay of 0% to 30% of normal and prolonged activated partial thromboplastin time (hemophilia A)
- Deficient factor IX and normal factor VIII levels (hemophilia B)
- Normal platelet count and function, bleeding time, and prothrombin time (hemophilia A and B)
- Positive family history, prenatal diagnosis, and carrier testing (although nearly one-third of all patients have no family history)

TREATMENT

Hemophilia isn't curable, but treatment can prevent disabling deformities and prolong life expectancy.

Treatment of hemophilia includes:

Spermatogenic mistake

Fertilization by a sperm with X and Y chromosomes produces an XXY zygote.

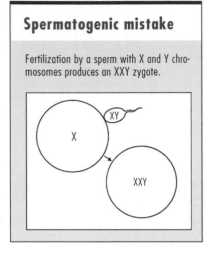

■ cryoprecipitate (for hemophilia A) or lyophilized factor VIII or IX to increase clotting factor levels and to permit normal hemostasis levels
■ factor IX concentrate during bleeding episodes (hemophilia B)
■ aminocaproic acid (Amicar) for oral bleeding (inhibits plasminogen activator substances)
■ prophylactic desmopressin (DDAVP) before dental procedures or minor surgery to release stored von Willebrand's factor and factor VIII (to reduce bleeding)
■ cold compress or ice bag application and elevation of injured part during acute bleeding episode.

 CLINICAL ALERT
To help prevent injury, young children should wear clothing with padded patches on the knees and elbows. Older children should avoid contact sports.

Klinefelter syndrome

Klinefelter syndrome, a relatively common genetic abnormality, results from an extra X chromosome — creating an XXY sex chromosome constitution — and affects only males. It usually becomes apparent at puberty, when the secondary sex characteristics develop. The testicles fail to mature and degenerative testicular changes begin that eventually result in irreversible infertility. Klinefelter syndrome common-

ly causes gynecomastia and is also associated with a tendency toward learning disabilities. Because not all patients with the extra X chromosome will display the same characteristics, the term "XXY male" has come into favor, as opposed to labeling all males with an extra X chromosome as having Klinefelter syndrome. Some of these XXY males may develop Klinefelter syndrome, and some may not.

The XXY chromosome arrangement, probably the most common cause of hypogonadism, appears in about 1 in every 600 males, and may be one of the most common genetic abnormalities.

CAUSES
Causes may include:
■ cells with one extra X chromosome create a 47,XXY complement instead of the normal 46,XY (see *Spermatogenic mistake*)
■ in the rare mosaic form, only some cells contain the extra X chromosomes and others contain the normal XY complement
■ lack of one X chromosome, 45X (see *Turner's syndrome*).

PATHOPHYSIOLOGY
The extra chromosome responsible for Klinefelter syndrome probably results from either meiotic nondisjunction during parental gametogenesis or from mitotic nondisjunction in the zygote. The incidence of meiotic nondisjunction increases with maternal age.

SIGNS AND SYMPTOMS
Klinefelter syndrome may not be apparent until puberty or later in mild cases. Because many of the persons with Klinefelter syndrome are not mentally retarded, behavioral problems in adolescence or infertility may be the only presenting features initially. The signs and symptoms exhibited are the result of the genetic defect involving the extra X chromosome.

The syndrome's characteristic features include:
■ a small penis and prostate gland
■ small testicles
■ sparse facial and abdominal hair
■ feminine distribution of pubic hair (triangular shape)

Turner's syndrome

In Turner's syndrome, one of the X chromosomes (or part of the second X chromosome) may be lost from either the ovum or sperm through nondisjunction or chromosome lag. Mixed aneuploidy may result from mitotic nondisjunction.

This disorder occurs in 1 in 2,500 to 7,000 births; up to 95% of affected fetuses are spontaneously aborted. Maternal age isn't a risk factor in this disorder.

SIGNS AND SYMPTOMS

In utero, the fetus may have a cystic hygroma, seen on ultrasound; however, these may also be seen in fetuses that don't have Turner's syndrome. The mother may have an elevated or low alpha-fetoprotein level.

At birth, 50% of infants with this syndrome measure below the third percentile in length. Many have swollen hands and feet, a wide chest with laterally displaced nipples, and a low hairline that becomes more obvious as they grow. They may have webbing of the neck and coarse, enlarged, prominent ears. Gonadal dysgenesis is seen at birth and typically causes sterility in adult females (unless they have the mosaic form).

Cardiovascular defects, such as bicuspid aortic valve and coarctation of the aorta, occur in 10% to 40% of patients. Short stature (usually under 5′ [1.5 m]) is the most common adult sign.

Most patients have average or slightly below-average intelligence; they commonly exhibit spatial defects, right-left disorientation for extrapersonal space, and defective figure drawing.

DIAGNOSIS AND TREATMENT

Turner's syndrome can be diagnosed by chromosome analysis. Differential diagnosis should rule out mixed gonadal dysgenesis, Noonan syndrome, and other similar disorders.

Treatment should begin in early childhood and may include hormonal therapy (androgens, human growth hormone and, possibly, small doses of estrogen). Later, progesterone and estrogen can induce sexual maturation, but most patients remain sterile.

- sexual dysfunction (impotence, lack of libido)
- in fewer than 50% of patients, gynecomastia
- in the mosaic form, delay of pathologic changes and resulting infertility
- abnormal body build (long legs with short, obese trunk)
- tall stature
- in some individuals, behavioral problems beginning in adolescence
- increased incidence of pulmonary disease and varicose veins.

COMPLICATIONS

Complications may include:
- lack of sperm production and infertility, caused by progressive sclerosis and hyalinization of the seminiferous tubules in the testicles and testicular fibrosis during and after puberty

- learning disabilities and behavioral problems
- osteoporosis
- breast cancer because of the extra X chromosome.

DIAGNOSIS

- A karyotype (chromosome analysis) determined by culturing lymphocytes from the patient's peripheral blood
- Decreased urinary 17-ketosteroid levels
- Increased excretion of follicle-stimulating hormone
- Decreased levels of plasma testosterone after puberty

TREATMENT

Depending on the severity of symptoms, treatment may include:
- mastectomy in patients with persistent gynecomastia

- supplemental testosterone to induce secondary sexual characteristics of puberty
- psychological counseling for body image problems or emotional maladjustment caused by sexual dysfunction.

Marfan syndrome

Marfan syndrome is a rare degenerative, generalized disease of the connective tissue. It results from elastin and collagen defects and causes ocular, skeletal, and cardiovascular anomalies. Death results from cardiovascular complications from early infancy to adulthood. The syndrome occurs in 1 of 20,000 persons, affecting males and females equally.

CAUSES

Causes may include:
- autosomal dominant mutation
- among patients with a negative family history (15% of patients), possibly advanced age of the father.

PATHOPHYSIOLOGY

Marfan syndrome is caused by a mutation in a single allele of a gene located on chromosome 15; the gene codes for fibrillin, a glycoprotein component of connective tissue. These small fibers are abundant in large blood vessels and the suspensory ligaments of the ocular lenses. The effect on connective tissue is varied and includes excessive bone growth, ocular disorders, and cardiac defects.

SIGNS AND SYMPTOMS

Signs and symptoms may include:
- increased height, long extremities, and arachnodactyly (long spiderlike fingers) caused by effects on long bones and joints and excessive bone growth
- defects of sternum (funnel chest or pigeon breast, for example), chest asymmetry, scoliosis, and kyphosis caused by effects on bone
- hypermobile joints caused by effects on connective tissue
- nearsightedness caused by elongated ocular globe
- lens displacement caused by altered connective tissue (the ocular hallmark of the syndrome)
- valvular abnormalities (redundancy of leaflets, stretching of chordae tendineae, and dilation of valvulae annulus) from effects on cardiac connective tissue
- mitral valve prolapse caused by weakened connective tissue
- aortic insufficiency caused by dilation of aortic root and ascending aorta.

COMPLICATIONS

Possible complications include:
- weak joints and ligaments, predisposing to injury
- cataracts caused by lens displacement
- retinal detachments and retinal tears
- severe mitral valve regurgitation caused by mitral valve prolapse
- spontaneous pneumothorax caused by chest wall instability
- inguinal and incisional hernias
- dilation of the dural sac (portion of the dura mater beyond caudal end of the spinal cord).

DIAGNOSIS

- Positive family history in one parent (85% of patients) and typical clinical features
- Presence of lens displacement and aneurysm of the ascending aorta without other symptoms or familial tendency
- Detection of fibrillin defects in cultured skin
- X-rays confirming skeletal abnormalities
- Echocardiogram showing dilation of the aortic root
- DNA analysis of the gene

TREATMENT

Treatment for Marfan syndrome is basically aimed at relieving symptoms and may involve:
- surgical repair of aneurysms to prevent rupture
- surgical correction of ocular deformities to improve vision
- steroid and sex hormone therapy to induce early epiphyseal closure and limit adult height
- beta-adrenergic blockers to delay or prevent aortic dilation
- surgical replacement of aortic valve and mitral valve for extreme dilation

■ mechanical bracing and physical therapy for mild scoliosis if curvature is greater than 20 degrees
■ surgery for scoliosis if curvature is greater than 45 degrees.

Neural tube defects

Neural tube defects (NTDs) are serious congenital anomalies that involve the spine or skull; they result from failure of the neural tube to close at about 28 days after conception. The most common forms of NTDs are spina bifida (50% of cases), anencephaly (40%), and encephalocele (10%). Spina bifida occulta is the most common and least severe spinal cord defect.

The incidence of NTDs varies greatly among countries and by region in the United States. For example, the incidence is significantly higher in the British Isles and low in southern China and Japan. In the United States, North and South Carolina have at least twice the incidence of NTDs as most other parts of the country. These birth defects are also less common in blacks than in whites.

Recent research sponsored by the March of Dimes and others has indicated that the risk of an open NTD may be reduced 50% to 70% among pregnant women who take a daily multivitamin with folic acid. All women of childbearing are urged to take such a vitamin supplement until menopause or the end of childbearing potential. (See *Folic acid supplement recommendations*.)

CAUSES
Causes may include:
■ exposure to a teratogen
■ part of a multiple malformation syndrome (for example, chromosomal abnormalities such as trisomy 18 or 13 syndrome)
■ in isolated birth defects, a combination of genetic and environmental factors (mostly unknown, though possibly a lack of folic acid in the mother's diet).

PATHOPHYSIOLOGY
Neural tube closure normally occurs at 24 days' gestation in the cranial region and

---

Folic acid supplement recommendations

The following recommendations for folic acid supplement dosages have been endorsed by the Centers for Disease Control and Prevention, the U.S. Public Health Service, the March of Dimes Birth Defects Foundation, and the Spina Bifida Association of America, among other groups.

ALL WOMEN OF CHILDBEARING AGE
All women who are capable of becoming pregnant should:
◆ consume 0.4 mg of folic acid daily to reduce their risk of having a child with spina bifida or another neural tube defect (NTD)
◆ continue to consume 0.4 mg of folic acid daily when pregnant until their health care provider prescribes other prenatal vitamins.

WOMEN AT HIGH RISK
Women with a previous pregnancy affected by an NTD should:
◆ receive genetic counseling before their next pregnancy
◆ consume 0.4 mg of folic acid daily
◆ start taking 4 mg of folic acid daily for about 1 month before conception when trying to become pregnant (by taking a separate folic acid supplement, not by increasing multivitamin intake)
◆ continue to take 4 mg of folic acid daily through the first 3 months of pregnancy.

---

continues distally, with closure of the lumbar regions by 28 days.

Spina bifida occulta is characterized by incomplete closure of one or more vertebrae without protrusion of the spinal cord or meninges.

In more severe forms of spina bifida, however, incomplete closure of one or more vertebrae causes protrusion of the spinal contents in an external sac or cystic lesion (spina bifida cystica). Spina bifida cystica has two classifications: myelomeningocele (meningomyelocele) and meningocele. In myelomeningocele, the external sac contains meninges, cerebrospinal fluid (CSF), and a portion of the spinal cord or nerve roots distal to the conus medullaris. When the spinal nerve roots end at the sac, motor and sensory functions below the sac are terminated. In meningocele, less severe than myelomeningocele, the sac contains only meninges and CSF. Meningocele may produce no neurologic symptoms.

In encephalocele, a saclike portion of the meninges and brain protrudes through a defective opening in the skull. Usually, it occurs in the occipital area, but it may also occur in the parietal, nasopharyngeal, or frontal area.

In anencephaly, the most severe form of NTD, the closure defect occurs at the cranial end of the neuroaxis and, as a result, part or the entire top of the skull is missing, severely damaging the brain. Portions of the brain stem and spinal cord may also be missing. No diagnostic or therapeutic efforts are helpful; this condition is invariably fatal.

SIGNS AND SYMPTOMS

Signs and symptoms depend on the type and severity of NTD:

- possibly, a depression or dimple, tuft of hair, soft fatty deposits, port wine nevi, or a combination of these abnormalities on the skin over the spinal defect (spina bifida occulta) caused by incomplete closure
- foot weakness or bowel and bladder disturbances, especially likely during rapid growth phases (spina bifida occulta) related to effect on spinal nerve roots
- saclike structure that protrudes over the spine (myelomeningocele, meningocele) caused by incomplete closure
- depending on the level of the defect, permanent neurologic dysfunction, such as flaccid or spastic paralysis and bowel and bladder incontinence (myelomeningocele) caused by effect on spinal nerve roots.

The child may also exhibit disorders typically associated with NTDs. These disorders include:

- trophic skin disturbances (ulcerations, cyanosis)
- clubfoot
- knee contractures
- hydrocephalus (in about 90% of patients)
- mental retardation
- Arnold-Chiari syndrome (part of the brain protrudes into the spinal canal)
- curvature of the spine.

Clinical effects of encephalocele vary with the degree of tissue involvement and location of the defect. Paralysis and hydrocephalus are common. Infants with this defect have a better chance of survival than anencephalic infants and usually have less paralysis; however, surviving infants are usually severely mentally retarded.

COMPLICATIONS

Complications may include:

- paralysis below the level of the defect
- infection, such as meningitis.

DIAGNOSIS

- Amniocentesis to detect elevated alpha-fetoprotein (AFP) levels in amniotic fluid, which indicates the presence of an open NTD
- Acetylcholinesterase levels (not usually effective for closed NTDs)
- Fetal karyotype to detect chromosomal abnormalities (present in 5% to 7% of NTDs)
- Maternal serum AFP screening in combination with other serum markers, such as human chorionic gonadotropin (HCG), free beta-HCG, or unconjugated estriol (for patients with a lower risk of NTDs and those who will be younger than age 34½ at the time of delivery) to estimate a fetus's risk of NTD as well as possible increased risk for perinatal complications, such as premature rupture of the membranes, abruptio placentae, or fetal death
- Ultrasound when increased risk of open NTD exists, based on family history or abnormal serum screening results (not conclusive for open NTDs or ventral wall defects)

If the NTD isn't diagnosed before birth, other tests are used to make the diagnosis, including:

■ palpation and spinal X-ray for spina bifida occulta

■ myelography to differentiate spina bifida occulta from other spinal abnormalities, especially spinal cord tumors

■ transillumination of the protruding sac to distinguish between myelomeningocele (typically doesn't transilluminate) and meningocele (typically does transilluminate)

■ pinprick examination of the legs and trunk to show the level of sensory and motor involvement in myelomeningocele

■ skull X-rays, cephalic measurements, and computed tomography (CT) scan to reveal associated hydrocephalus.

Other appropriate laboratory tests for patients with myelomeningocele include urinalysis, urine cultures, and tests for renal function starting in the neonatal period and continuing at regular intervals.

In encephalocele, X-rays show a basilar bony skull defect. CT scan and ultrasonography further define the defect.

TREATMENT
Spina bifida occulta usually requires no treatment. Prompt neurosurgical repair and aggressive management may improve the condition of children with some NTDs. However, surgery doesn't reverse neurologic deficits, and serious and permanent disabilities are likely. Fetal surgery has been successful at repairing some open defects, thereby reducing damage. Treatment may include:

■ surgical closure of the protruding sac and continual assessment of growth and development (meningocele)

■ repair of the sac and supportive measures to promote independence and prevent further complications (myelomeningocele)

■ shunt to relieve associated hydrocephalus

■ surgery during infancy to place protruding tissues back into the skull, excise the sac, and correct associated craniofacial abnormalities (encephalocele).

Sickle cell anemia

Sickle cell anemia is a congenital hemolytic anemia resulting from defective hemoglobin molecules. Half the patients with sickle cell anemia die by their early twenties, and few live to middle age.

Sickle cell anemia occurs primarily in persons of African and Mediterranean descent, but it also affects other populations. Although most common among tropical Africans and people of African descent, it also occurs in Puerto Rico, Turkey, India, the Middle East, and the Mediterranean.

CAUSE
■ Mutation of hemoglobin S gene (heterozygous inheritance results in sickle cell trait, usually an asymptomatic condition)

PATHOPHYSIOLOGY
Sickle cell anemia results from substitution of the amino acid valine for glutamic acid in the hemoglobin S gene encoding the beta chain of hemoglobin. Abnormal hemoglobin S, found in the red blood cells (RBCs) of patients, becomes insoluble during hypoxia. As a result, these cells become rigid, rough, and elongated, forming a crescent or sickle shape. (See *Characteristics of sickle cells,* page 130.) The sickling produces hemolysis. The altered cells also pile up in the capillaries and smaller blood vessels, making the blood more viscous. Normal circulation is impaired, causing pain, tissue infarctions, and swelling.

Each patient with sickle cell anemia has a different hypoxic threshold and different factors that trigger a sickle cell crisis. Illness, exposure to cold, stress, acidotic states, or a pathophysiologic process that pulls water out of the sickle cells precipitates a crisis in most patients. (See *Sickle cell crisis*, page 131.) The blockages then cause anoxic changes that lead to further sickling and obstruction.

SIGNS AND SYMPTOMS

CLINICAL ALERT
Symptoms of sickle cell anemia don't develop until after age 6 months because fetal hemoglobin protects infants for the first few months after birth.
Signs and symptoms may include:

Characteristics of sickle cells

Normal red blood cells (RBCs) and sickle cells vary in shape, life span, oxygen-carrying capacity, and the rate at which they're destroyed. These illustrations show normal and sickle cells and lists the major differences.

NORMAL RBCS
◆ 120-day life span
◆ Hemoglobin (Hb) has normal oxygen-carrying capacity
◆ 12 to 14 g/ml of Hb
◆ RBCs destroyed at normal rate

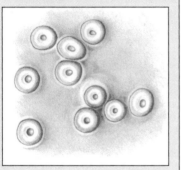

SICKLE CELLS
◆ 30- to 40-day life span
◆ Hb has decreased oxygen-carrying capacity
◆ 6 to 9 g/ml of Hb
◆ RBCs destroyed at accelerated rate

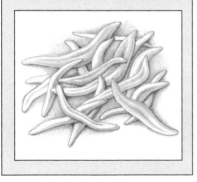

■ tachycardia, cardiomegaly, chronic fatigue, and unexplained dyspnea caused by tissue ischemia
■ hepatomegaly caused by infarction secondary to sluggish blood flow
■ joint swelling caused by aseptic infarction of the bones
■ severe pain in the chest, abdomen, thorax, muscle, or bones (characterizes painful crisis) caused by obstructed blood flow to the area and subsequent ischemia
■ jaundice, dark urine, and low-grade fever caused by blood vessel obstruction by rigid, tangled, sickle cells (leading to tissue anoxia and possibly necrosis)
■ *Streptococcus pneumoniae* sepsis caused by autosplenectomy (splenic damage and scarring in patients with long-term disease).

Suspect any of these crises in a sickle cell anemia patient with pale lips, tongue, palms, or nail beds; lethargy; listlessness; sleepiness; irritability; severe pain; and fever:
■ aplastic crisis (megaloblastic crisis) caused by bone marrow depression (associated with infection, usually viral, and characterized by pallor, lethargy, sleepiness, dyspnea, possible coma, markedly decreased bone marrow activity, and RBC hemolysis)
■ acute sequestration crisis (rare; affects infants ages 8 months to 2 years; may cause lethargy, pallor, and hypovolemic shock) caused by the sudden massive entrapment of cells in spleen and liver
■ hemolytic crisis (rare; usually affects patients who also have glucose-6-phosphate dehydrogenase deficiency; degenerative changes cause liver congestion and enlargement, and chronic jaundice worsens).

COMPLICATIONS
Complications may include:
■ retinopathy, nephropathy, and cerebral vessel occlusion caused by organ infarction
■ hypovolemic shock and death caused by massive entrapment of cells
■ necrosis
■ infection and gangrene.

DIAGNOSIS
■ Positive family history and typical clinical features

CLOSER LOOK
Sickle cell crisis

Infection, exposure to cold, high altitudes, overexertion, or other situations that cause cellular oxygen deprivation may trigger a sickle cell crisis. The deoxygenated, sickle-shaped red blood cells stick to the capillary wall and each other, blocking blood flow and causing cellular hypoxia. The crisis worsens as tissue hypoxia and acidic waste products cause more sickling and cell damage. With each new crisis, organs and tissues are slowly destroyed, especially the spleen and kidneys.

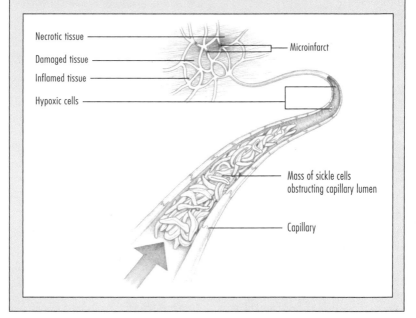

Necrotic tissue
Damaged tissue
Inflamed tissue
Hypoxic cells
Microinfarct
Mass of sickle cells obstructing capillary lumen
Capillary

■ Hemoglobin electrophoresis, showing hemoglobin S
■ Electrophoresis of umbilical cord blood to provide screening for all neonates at risk
■ Stained blood smear showing sickle cells
■ Low RBC counts, elevated white blood cell and platelet counts, decreased erythrocyte sedimentation rate, increased serum iron levels, decreased RBC survival, and reticulocytosis (hemoglobin levels may be low or normal)
■ Lateral chest X-ray showing "Lincoln log" deformity in the vertebrae of many adults and some adolescents

■ Neonatal screening; some states mandate neonate screening for hemoglobin abnormalities, including sickle cell anemia
■ Prenatal and preimplantation diagnosis is available, especially if the mutation in the family is known

TREATMENT
Possible treatments include:
■ packed RBC transfusion to correct hypovolemia (if hemoglobin levels decrease)
■ sedation and analgesics, such as meperidine (Demerol) or morphine, and heat in the form of warm compresses for pain
■ oxygen administration to correct hypoxia

- large amounts of oral or I.V. fluids to correct hypovolemia and prevent dehydration and vessel occlusion
- prophylactic penicillin before age 4 months to prevent infection
- hydroxyurea to reduce painful episodes by increasing the production of fetal hemoglobin, which seems to alleviate symptoms
- iron and folic acid supplements to prevent anemia.

CLINICAL ALERT
Vaccines to prevent illness and anti-infectives, such as low-dose penicillin, should be considered to prevent complications in patients with sickle cell anemia.

Tay-Sachs disease

Tay-Sachs disease, also known as *GM$_2$ gangliosidosis,* is the most common lipid-storage disease.

CLINICAL ALERT
Progressive mental and motor deterioration often causes death before age 5 years. Tay-Sachs disease appears in fewer than 100 infants born each year in the United States.

Tay-Sachs affects persons of Eastern European Jewish (Ashkenazi) ancestry about 100 times more often than the general population, occurring in about 1 in 3,600 live births in this ethnic group. About 1 in 30 Ashkenazi Jews, French Canadians, and American Cajuns are heterozygous carriers. If two such carriers have children, each of their children has a 25% chance of having Tay-Sachs disease.

CAUSE
- Congenital deficiency of the enzyme hexosaminidase A

PATHOPHYSIOLOGY
Tay-Sachs disease is an autosomal recessive disorder in which the enzyme hexosaminidase A is absent or deficient. This enzyme is necessary to metabolize gangliosides, water-soluble glycolipids found primarily in the CNS. Without hexosaminidase A, lipid pigments accumulate and progressively destroy and demyelinate the CNS cells.

SIGNS AND SYMPTOMS
Signs and symptoms of Tay-Sachs disease may include:
- exaggerated Moro reflex (also called *startle reflex*) at birth and apathy (response only to loud sounds) by ages 3 to 6 months caused by demyelination of CNS cells
- inability to sit up, lift the head, or grasp objects; difficulty turning over; progressive vision loss caused by CNS involvement
- deafness, blindness, seizure activity, paralysis, spasticity, and continued neurologic deterioration (by age 18 months) secondary to continued demyelination
- recurrent bronchopneumonia caused by diminished protective reflexes.

COMPLICATIONS
Complications may include:
- blindness
- generalized paralysis
- recurrent bronchopneumonia, usually fatal by age 5.

DIAGNOSIS
- Clinical features
- Serum analysis showing deficient hexosaminidase A
- Amniocentesis or chorionic villus sampling can detect hexosaminidase A deficiency in the fetus

Diagnostic screening is essential for all couples of Ashkenazi Jewish ancestry and for others with a familial history of the disease. A blood test can detect carriers.

TREATMENT
Tay-Sachs disease has no known cure. Supportive treatment for Tay-Sachs disease includes the following measures:
- tube feedings to provide nutritional supplements
- suctioning and postural drainage to maintain a patent airway
- skin care to prevent pressure ulcers in bedridden children
- laxatives to relieve neurogenic constipation.

Trisomy 18 syndrome

Trisomy 18 syndrome (also known as *Edwards' syndrome*) is the second most common multiple malformation syndrome. Most affected infants have full trisomy 18, involving an extra (third) copy of chromosome 18 in each cell, but partial trisomy 18 (with varying phenotypes) and translocation types have also been reported. Most infants with this disorder present with intrauterine growth retardation, congenital heart defects, microcephaly, and other malformations.

Full trisomy 18 syndrome is generally fatal or has an extremely poor prognosis; most trisomic conceptions are spontaneously aborted; 30% to 50% of these infants die within the first 2 months of life and 90% die within the first year. Most surviving patients are profoundly mentally retarded.

Incidence ranges from 1 in 3,000 to 8,000 neonates, with 3 to 4 females affected for every male.

CAUSE
■ Chromosomal abnormality (risk typically increases with maternal age; however, the mean maternal age for this disorder is 32½)

PATHOPHYSIOLOGY
Most cases of trisomy 18 result from spontaneous nondisjunction during meiosis, effecting an extra copy of chromosome 18 in each cell.

SIGNS AND SYMPTOMS
Signs and symptoms of trisomy 18 syndrome include:
■ growth retardation, which begins in utero and remains significant after birth
■ initial hypotonia that may soon give way to hypertonia
■ microcephaly and dolichocephaly
■ micrognathia
■ short and narrow nose with upturned nares
■ unilateral or bilateral cleft lip and palate
■ low-set, slightly pointed ears
■ short neck
■ conspicuous clenched hand with overlapping fingers (commonly seen on ultrasound as well)
■ cystic hygroma

■ choroid plexus cysts (also seen in some normal infants).

COMPLICATIONS
Complications may include:
■ congenital heart defects—such as ventricular septal defect, tetralogy of Fallot, transposition of the great vessels, and coarctation of the aorta (in 80% to 90% of patients)—that may be the cause of death in many infants
■ other congenital anomalies, such as diaphragmatic hernia, various renal defects, omphalocele, neural tube defects, genital and perineal abnormalities (including imperforate anus), and oligohydramnios.

DIAGNOSIS
■ Karyotype, done either prenatally or using peripheral blood or skin fibroblasts after birth (diagnostic)
■ Abnormal results in multiple marker maternal serum screening tests involving different combinations of AFP, HCG, and unconjugated estriol (not diagnostic)
■ Fetal ultrasound revealing varying degrees of abnormalities although many fetuses have few detectable defects

TREATMENT
Treatment is aimed at providing comfort for the infant and emotional support for the parents. Because the infant's sucking reflex is poor, nutrition is maintained using gavage feedings. Teach parents about home care and feeding techniques.

Trisomy 13 syndrome
Trisomy 13 syndrome (also known as *Patau's syndrome*) is the third most common multiple malformation syndrome. Most affected infants have full trisomy 13 at birth; a few have the rare mosaic partial trisomy 13 syndrome (with varying phenotypes) or translocation types. Infants with this disorder typically have brain and facial abnormalities as well as major cardiac, GI, and limb malformations. Full trisomy 13 syndrome is fatal. Many trisomic zygotes are spontaneously aborted; 50% to 70% die within 1 month after birth and 85% by the first year. Only isolated cases of survival beyond 5 years have been re-

ported in full trisomy 13 patients. All survivors have profound mental retardation.

Incidence is estimated to be 1 in 4,000 to 10,000 neonates.

CAUSE
- Chromosomal abnormality (risk increases with advanced maternal age; however, the mean maternal age for this abnormality is 31)

PATHOPHYSIOLOGY
About 75% of all cases result from chromosomal nondisjunction. About 20% result from chromosomal translocation, involving a rearrangement of chromosomes 13 and 14. About 5% of cases are estimated to be mosaics; the clinical effects in these cases may be less severe.

SIGNS AND SYMPTOMS
Signs and symptoms of trisomy 13 syndrome include:
- microcephaly
- varying degrees of holoprosencephaly
- sloping forehead with wide sutures and fontanel
- scalp defect at the vertex
- bilateral cleft lip with associated cleft palate (45%)
- flat and broad nose
- low-set ears and inner ear abnormalities
- polydactyly of the hands and feet
- club feet
- omphaloceles
- neural tube defects
- cystic hygroma
- genital abnormalities
- cystic kidneys
- hydronephrosis
- failure to thrive, seizures, apnea, and feeding difficulties.

COMPLICATIONS
Complications may include:
- congenital heart defects (common), especially hypoplastic left heart, ventricular septal defect, patent ductus arteriosus, or dextroposition, which may significantly contribute to the cause of death
- musculoskeletal abnormalities
- microphthalmos, cataracts, and other eye abnormalities.

DIAGNOSIS
- Karyotype, done either prenatally or on peripheral blood lymphocytes or skin fibroblasts in a neonate or an aborted fetus (diagnostic)
- Abnormal results in multiple marker maternal serum screening tests, involving different combinations of alpha-fetoprotein, human chorionic gonadotropin (HCG) or free beta-HCG in some laboratories, and unconjugated estriol (not diagnostic)
- Ultrasound, which commonly reveals multiple abnormalities in the fetus

TREATMENT
Supportive care is the only treatment for the infant with trisomy 13 syndrome.

Cardiovascular system

The cardiovascular system begins its activity when the fetus is barely 4 weeks old and is the last system to cease activity at the end of life. This body system is so vital that it helps define the presence of life.

The heart, arteries, veins, and lymphatics form the cardiovascular network that serves as the body's transport system. This system brings life-supporting oxygen and nutrients to cells, removes metabolic waste products, and carries hormones from one part of the body to another.

The cardiovascular system, commonly called the *circulatory system,* may be divided into two branches: pulmonary and systemic circulations. In *pulmonary circulation,* blood picks up oxygen and liberates the waste product carbon dioxide. In *systemic circulation* (which includes coronary circulation), blood carries oxygen and nutrients to all active cells and carries waste products to the kidneys, liver, and skin for excretion.

Circulation requires normal heart function, which propels blood through the system by continuous rhythmic contractions. Blood circulates through three types of vessels: arteries, veins, and capillaries. The sturdy, pliable walls of the arteries adjust to the volume of blood leaving the heart. The aorta is the major artery arching out of the left ventricle; its segments and branches ultimately divide into minute, thin-walled (one cell thick) capillaries. Capillaries pass the blood to the veins, which return it to the heart. In the veins, valves prevent blood backflow.

Pathophysiologic manifestations of cardiovascular disease may stem from aneurysm, cardiac shunt, embolus, release of cardiac enzymes and proteins, stenosis, thrombus, and valve incompetence.

Aneurysm

An aneurysm is a localized outpouching or dilation of a weakened arterial wall. This weakness can be the result of either atherosclerotic plaque formation that erodes the vessel wall, or the loss of elastin and collagen in the vessel wall. Congenital abnormalities in the media of the arterial wall, trauma, and infections, such as syphilis, may lead to aneurysm formation. A ruptured aneurysm may cause massive hemorrhage and death.

Several types of aneurysms can occur:
■ A *saccular aneurysm* occurs when increased pressure in the artery pushes out a pouch on one side of the artery, creating a bulge. (See *Types of aortic aneurysms,* page 136.)
■ A *fusiform aneurysm* develops when the arterial wall weakens around its circumference, creating a spindle-shaped aneurysm.
■ A *dissecting aneurysm* occurs when blood is forced between the layers of the arterial wall, causing them to separate and creating a false lumen.

135

CLOSER LOOK
Types of aortic aneurysms

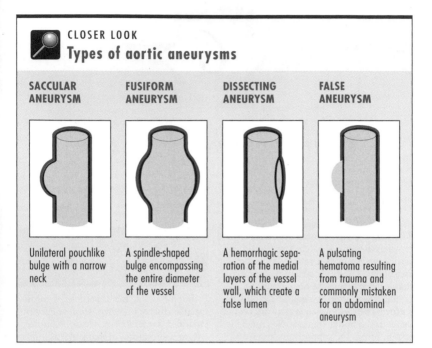

SACCULAR ANEURYSM	FUSIFORM ANEURYSM	DISSECTING ANEURYSM	FALSE ANEURYSM
Unilateral pouchlike bulge with a narrow neck	A spindle-shaped bulge encompassing the entire diameter of the vessel	A hemorrhagic separation of the medial layers of the vessel wall, which create a false lumen	A pulsating hematoma resulting from trauma and commonly mistaken for an abdominal aneurysm

■ A *false aneurysm* develops when a break is present in all layers of the arterial wall and blood leaks out but is contained by surrounding structures, creating a pulsating hematoma.

Common locations of aneurism include:

■ abdominal aortic aneurysm—an abnormal dilation in the arterial wall, usually occurring in the aorta between the renal arteries and iliac branches

■ thoracic aortic aneurysm—an abnormal widening of the ascending, transverse, or descending part of the aorta

■ cerebral aneurysm—a localized dilation of a cerebral artery that may arise at an arterial junction in the circle of Willis, the circular anastomosis formed by the major cerebral arteries at the base of the brain

■ femoral and popliteal aneurysm (sometimes called *peripheral arterial aneurysm*)—the end result of progressive atherosclerotic changes in the walls (medial layer) of these major peripheral arteries.

Cardiac shunt

A cardiac shunt provides communication between the pulmonary and systemic circulations. Before birth, shunts between the right and left sides of the heart and between the aorta and pulmonary artery are a normal part of fetal circulation. After birth, however, the mixing of pulmonary and systemic blood or the movement of blood between the left and right sides of the heart is abnormal. Blood flows through a shunt from an area of high pressure to an area of low pressure or from an area of high resistance to an area of low resistance.

LEFT-TO-RIGHT SHUNT
In a left-to-right shunt, blood flows from the left side of the heart to the right side through an atrial or ventricular defect, or from the aorta to the pulmonary circulation through a patent ductus arteriosus. Because the blood in the left side of the heart is rich in oxygen, a left-to-right shunt delivers oxygenated blood back to the right side of the heart or to the lungs.

Consequently, a left-to-right shunt that occurs as a result of a congenital heart defect is called an *acyanotic defect.*

In a left-to-right shunt, pulmonary blood flow increases as blood is continually recirculated to the lungs, leading to hypertrophy of the pulmonary vessels. The increased amounts of blood circulated from the left side of the heart to the right side can cause right-sided heart failure. Eventually, left-sided heart failure may also occur.

RIGHT-TO-LEFT SHUNT

A right-to-left shunt occurs when blood flows from the right side of the heart to the left side, such as in tetralogy of Fallot, or from the pulmonary artery directly into the systemic circulation through a patent ductus arteriosus. Because blood returning to the right side of the heart and the pulmonary artery is low in oxygen, a right-to-left shunt adds deoxygenated blood to the systemic circulation, causing hypoxia and cyanosis. Congenital defects that involve right-to-left shunts are therefore called *cyanotic defects.* Right-to-left shunt related to poor tissue and organ perfusion commonly causes fatigue, increased respiratory rate, and clubbing of the fingers.

Embolus

An embolus (plural emboli) is a substance that circulates from one location in the body to another through the bloodstream. Although most emboli are blood clots from a thrombus, they may also consist of pieces of tissue, an air bubble, amniotic fluid, fat, bacteria, tumor cells, or a foreign substance.

Emboli that originate in the venous circulation, such as from deep vein thrombosis, travel to the right side of the heart to the pulmonary circulation and eventually lodge in a capillary, causing pulmonary infarction and even death. Most emboli in the arterial system originate from the left side of the heart from such conditions as arrhythmias, valvular heart disease, myocardial infarction, heart failure, or endocarditis. Arterial emboli may lodge in the brain, kidneys, or arms or legs, causing ischemia or infarction.

Release of cardiac enzymes and proteins

Damage to the heart muscle impairs the cell membrane's integrity, and intracellular contents — including cardiac enzymes and proteins — are released and can be measured in the bloodstream. The release of the intracellular contents follows a characteristic pattern of rising and falling values. The released enzymes include creatine kinase, lactate dehydrogenase, and aspartate aminotransferase; the proteins released include troponin T, troponin I, and myoglobin. (See *Release of cardiac enzymes and proteins,* page 138.)

Stenosis

Stenosis is the narrowing of a tubular structure (such as a blood vessel or heart valve). When an artery is stenosed, the tissues and organs perfused by that blood vessel may become ischemic, function abnormally, or die. An occluded vein may result in venous congestion and chronic venous insufficiency.

When a heart valve is stenosed, blood flow through that valve is reduced, causing blood to accumulate in the chamber behind the valve. Pressure in that chamber increases to pump against the resistance of the stenosed valve, causing the heart to work harder, resulting in hypertrophy. Hypertrophy and an increase in workload raise the heart's oxygen demands. A heart with diseased coronary arteries may not be able to sufficiently increase oxygen supply to meet the increased demand.

When stenosis occurs in a valve on the left side of the heart, the increased pressure leads to greater pulmonary venous pressure and pulmonary congestion. As pulmonary vascular resistance rises, right-sided heart failure may occur. Stenosis in a valve on the right side of the heart causes an increase in pressures on the right side of the heart, leading to systemic venous congestion.

Thrombus

A thrombus is a blood clot, consisting of platelets, fibrin, and red and white blood cells, that forms anywhere in the vascular system, such as the arteries, veins, heart chambers, or heart valves.

Release of cardiac enzymes and proteins

Because they're released by damaged tissue, serum proteins and isoenzymes (catalytic proteins that vary in concentration in specific organs) can help identify the compromised organ and assess the extent of damage. After acute myocardial infarction, cardiac enzymes and proteins rise and fall in a characteristic pattern, as shown in the graph below.

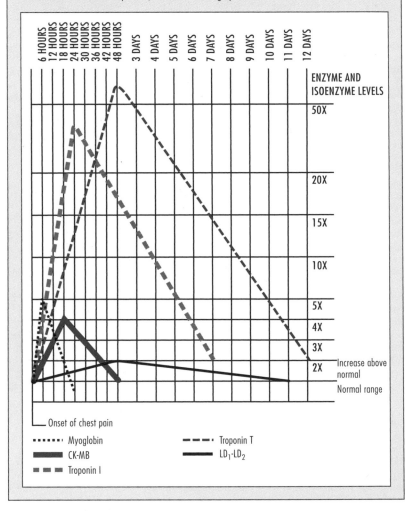

Three conditions, known as *Virchow's triad,* promote thrombus formation: endothelial injury, sluggish blood flow, and increased coagulability. When a blood vessel wall is injured, the endothelial lining attracts platelets and other inflammatory mediators, which may stimulate clot formation. Sluggish or abnormal blood flow also promotes thrombus formation by allowing platelets and clotting factors to accumulate and adhere to the blood vessel walls. Conditions that increase the coagulability of blood also promote clot formation.

The consequences of thrombus formation include occlusion of the blood vessel or the formation of an embolus (if a portion of a thrombus breaks loose and travels through the circulatory system until it lodges in a smaller vessel).

Valve incompetence

Valve incompetence, also called *insufficiency* or *regurgitation,* occurs when valve leaflets don't completely close. Incompetence may affect valves of the veins or heart.

In the veins, valves keep the blood flowing in one direction, toward the heart. When valve leaflets close improperly, blood flows backward and pools behind the valve, causing that valve to weaken and become incompetent. Eventually, the veins become distended, which may result in varicose veins, chronic venous insufficiency, and venous stasis ulcers. Blood clots may form as blood flow becomes sluggish.

In the heart, incompetent valves let blood flow in both directions through the valve, increasing the volume of blood that must be pumped (as well as the heart's workload) and resulting in hypertrophy. As blood volume in the heart increases, the involved heart chambers dilate to accommodate the increased volume. Although incompetence may occur in any heart valve, it's more common in the mitral and aortic valves.

ᴅISORDERS

Arterial occlusive disease

Arterial occlusive disease is the obstruction or narrowing of the lumen of the aorta and its major branches, causing an interruption of blood flow, usually to the legs and feet. This disorder may affect the carotid, vertebral, innominate, subclavian,

mesenteric, and celiac arteries. (See *Possible sites of major artery occlusion,* page 140.)

Arterial occlusive disease is more common in men than in women. The prognosis depends on the occlusion's location, the development of collateral circulation to counteract reduced blood flow and, in acute disease, the time elapsed between occlusion and its removal.

CAUSES

Arterial occlusive disease is a common complication of atherosclerosis. The occlusive mechanism may be endogenous, caused by emboli formation or thrombosis, or exogenous, caused by trauma or fracture. Predisposing factors include smoking; aging; conditions such as hypertension, hyperlipidemia, and diabetes; and a family history of vascular disorders, myocardial infarction, or stroke.

PATHOPHYSIOLOGY

Arterial occlusive disease is usually the result of atherosclerosis, in which fatty, fibrous plaques narrow the lumen of blood vessels. This occlusion can occur acutely or progressively over 20 to 40 years. The most common sites are areas of vessel branching, or bifurcation. The narrowing of the lumina (the channels through the vessels) reduces the blood volume that can flow through them, causing arterial insufficiency to the affected area. Ischemia usually occurs after the vessel lumina have narrowed by at least 50%, reducing blood flow to a level at which it no longer meets the needs of tissue and nerves.

SIGNS AND SYMPTOMS

Signs and symptoms of arterial occlusive disease depend on the site of the occlusion. (See *Types of arterial occlusive disease,* page 141.)

COMPLICATIONS

Complications of arterial occlusive disease may include:
■ severe ischemia and necrosis
■ skin ulceration
■ gangrene, which can lead to limb amputation
■ impaired nail and hair growth

(Text continues on page 142.)

Possible sites of major artery occlusion

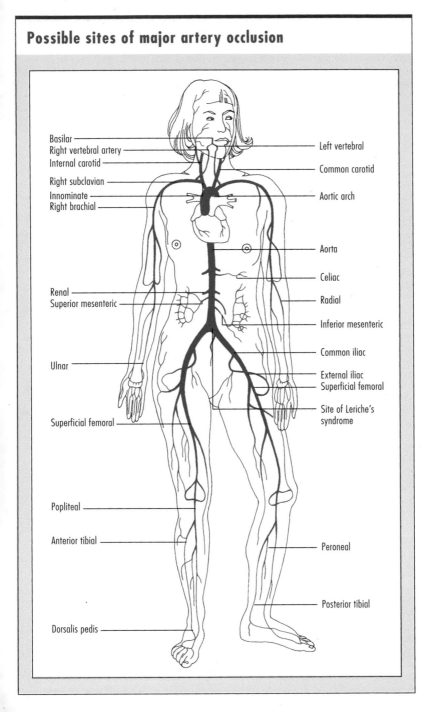

Basilar
Right vertebral artery
Internal carotid

Right subclavian
Innominate
Right brachial

Left vertebral
Common carotid

Aortic arch

Aorta

Celiac

Renal
Superior mesenteric

Radial

Inferior mesenteric

Common iliac

Ulnar

External iliac
Superficial femoral

Site of Leriche's syndrome

Superficial femoral

Popliteal

Anterior tibial

Peroneal

Posterior tibial

Dorsalis pedis

Types of arterial occlusive disease

SITE OF OCCLUSION	SIGNS AND SYMPTOMS
Carotid arterial system ◆ Internal carotids ◆ External carotids	Neurologic dysfunction: transient ischemic attacks (TIAs) caused by reduced cerebral circulation produce unilateral sensory or motor dysfunction (transient monocular blindness, hemiparesis), possible aphasia or dysarthria, confusion, decreased mentation, and headache. These recurrent clinical features usually last 5 to 10 minutes but may last up to 24 hours and may herald a stroke. Absent or decreased pulsation is from reduced blood flow with an auscultatory bruit indicating turbulent blood flow over the affected vessels.
Vertebrobasilar system ◆ Vertebral arteries ◆ Basilar arteries	Neurologic dysfunction: TIAs of brain stem and cerebellum from reduced cerebral circulation produce binocular vision disturbances, vertigo, dysarthria, and "drop attacks" (falling down without loss of consciousness). Less common than carotid TIA.
Innominate ◆ Brachiocephalic artery	Neurologic dysfunction: signs and symptoms as for vertebrobasilar occlusion. Indications of ischemia (claudication) of right arm secondary to reduced or obstructed blood flow; possible bruit indicating turbulent blood flow over right side of neck.
Subclavian artery	Subclavian steal syndrome (characterized by blood backflow from the brain through the vertebral artery on the same side as the occlusion, into the subclavian artery distal to the occlusion); clinical effects of vertebrobasilar occlusion and exercise-induced arm claudication; possible gangrene from prolonged ischemia, usually limited to the digits.
Mesenteric artery ◆ Superior (most commonly affected) ◆ Celiac axis ◆ Inferior	Bowel ischemia, infarct necrosis, and gangrene from obstruction or reduction in blood flow; sudden, acute abdominal pain from ischemia; nausea, vomiting, diarrhea; leukocytosis in response to necrosis; and shock caused by massive intraluminal fluid and plasma loss.
Aortic bifurcation (saddle block occlusion, a medical emergency associated with cardiac embolization)	Sensory and motor deficits (muscle weakness, numbness, paresthesias, paralysis) resulting from effects of reduced blood flow, and signs of ischemia (sudden pain; cold, pale legs with decreased or absent peripheral pulses) in both legs from reduced blood flow.
Iliac artery (Leriche syndrome)	Intermittent claudication of lower back, buttocks, and thighs relieved by rest; absent or reduced femoral or distal pulses caused by complete or partial obstruction of blood flow; possible bruit over femoral arteries related to turbulent blood flow around obstruction; impotence in men because of reduced blood flow to penile tissue.
Femoral and popliteal artery (associated with aneurysm formation)	Intermittent claudication of the calves on exertion; ischemic pain in feet; pretrophic pain (heralds necrosis and ulceration); leg pallor and coolness from reduced blood flow; blanching of feet on elevation caused by gravity's effect of further reducing blood flow; gangrene from prolonged ischemia; no palpable pulses in ankles and feet because of complete obstruction of blood flow.

- stroke or transient ischemic attack
- peripheral or systemic embolism.

DIAGNOSIS

Diagnosis of arterial occlusive disease is usually indicated by patient history and physical examination. The following tests support the diagnosis:

- Arteriography demonstrates the type (thrombus or embolus), location, and degree of obstruction and the collateral circulation. Arteriography is particularly useful in chronic disease or for evaluating candidates for reconstructive surgery.
- Doppler ultrasonography and plethysmography are noninvasive tests that show decreased blood flow distal to the occlusion in acute disease.
- Ophthalmodynamometry helps determine the degree of obstruction in the internal carotid artery by comparing ophthalmic artery pressure to brachial artery pressure on the affected side. More than a 20% difference between pressures suggests insufficiency.
- Electroencephalography and computed tomography scan may be necessary to rule out brain lesions.

TREATMENT

Treatment of arterial occlusive disease depends on the cause, location, and size of the obstruction. For mild chronic disease, supportive measures include smoking cessation, hypertension control, and mild exercise such as walking. For carotid artery occlusion, antiplatelet therapy may begin with ticlopidine or clopidogrel and aspirin. For intermittent claudication of chronic occlusive disease, pentoxifylline and cilostazol may improve blood flow through the capillaries, particularly for patients who are poor candidates for surgery.

Acute arterial occlusive disease typically requires surgery to restore circulation to the affected area, for example:

- *Embolectomy*—A balloon-tipped Fogarty catheter is used to remove thrombotic material from the artery. Embolectomy is used mainly for mesenteric, femoral, or popliteal artery occlusion.
- *Thromboendarterectomy*—Opening of the occluded artery and direct removal of

the obstructing thrombus and the medial layer of the arterial wall; usually performed after angiography and commonly used with autogenous vein or Dacron bypass surgery (femoral-popliteal or aortofemoral).

- *Patch grafting*—The thrombosed arterial segment is removed and replaced with an autogenous vein or Dacron graft.
- *Bypass graft*—Blood flow is diverted through an anastomosed autogenous or Dacron graft past the thrombosed segment.
- *Thrombolytic therapy*—Urokinase, streptokinase, or alteplase causes lysis of clot around or in the plaque.
- *Atherectomy*—Plaque is excised using a drill or slicing mechanism.
- *Balloon angioplasty*—Balloon inflation compresses the obstruction.
- *Laser angioplasty*—Obstruction is excised and vaporized using hot-tip lasers.
- *Stents*—A mesh of wires that stretch and mold to the arterial wall is inserted to prevent reocclusion. This new adjunct follows laser angioplasty or atherectomy.

Combined therapy, which is simply the concomitant use of any of the surgical treatments listed above, may be appropriate. Also, lumbar sympathectomy is a possible adjunct to surgery, depending on the condition of the sympathetic nervous system.

Amputation becomes necessary if arterial reconstructive surgery fails or if gangrene, persistent infection, or intractable pain develops.

Other therapy includes heparin to prevent emboli (for embolic occlusion) and bowel resection after restoration of blood flow (for mesenteric artery occlusion).

Atrial septal defect

In atrial septal defect (ASD), a congenital heart defect involving increased pulmonary blood flow (also called an *acyanotic* congenital heart defect), an opening between the left and right atria allows blood to flow from left to right, resulting in ineffective pumping of the heart, thus increasing the risk of heart failure.

The four types of ASDs are:

- an *ostium secundum defect,* the most common but least serious type, which occurs in the region of the fossa ovalis and, occasionally, extends inferiorly, close to the vena cava
- a *sinus venosus defect* that occurs in the superior-posterior portion of the atrial septum, sometimes extending into the vena cava, and is almost always associated with abnormal drainage of pulmonary veins into the right atrium
- an *ostium primum defect* that occurs in the inferior portion of the septum primum and is usually associated with atrioventricular valve abnormalities (cleft mitral valve) and conduction defects
- a *coronary sinus septal defect,* the least common type, that occurs at the roof of the coronary sinus allowing blood to shunt from the left atrium to the coronary sinus and then into the right atrium.

ASD accounts for about 10% of congenital heart defects and appears almost twice as commonly in females as in males, with a strong familial tendency. Although an ASD is usually a benign defect during infancy and childhood, delayed development of symptoms and complications makes it one of the most common congenital heart defects diagnosed in adults.

The prognosis is excellent in asymptomatic patients and in those with uncomplicated surgical repair, but poor in patients with cyanosis caused by large, untreated defects.

CAUSES

The cause of an ASD is unknown. Ostium primum defects commonly occur in patients with Down syndrome.

PATHOPHYSIOLOGY

In an ASD, blood shunts from the left atrium to the right atrium because the left atrial pressure is normally slightly higher than the right atrial pressure. This pressure difference forces large amounts of blood through a defect. This shunt results in right heart volume overload, affecting the right atrium, right ventricle, and pulmonary arteries. Eventually, the right atrium enlarges, and the right ventricle dilates to accommodate the increased blood volume. If pulmonary artery hypertension develops, increased pulmonary vascular resistance and right ventricular hypertrophy follow. In some adults, irreversible pulmonary artery hypertension causes reversal of the shunt direction, which results in unoxygenated blood entering the systemic circulation, causing cyanosis.

SIGNS AND SYMPTOMS

Signs and symptoms of an ASD include:
- fatigue after exertion from decreased cardiac output from the left ventricle
- early to midsystolic murmur at the second or third left intercostal space, caused by extra blood passing through the pulmonic valve
- low-pitched diastolic murmur at the lower left sternal border, more pronounced on inspiration, resulting from increased tricuspid valve flow in patients with large shunts
- fixed, widely split S_2 caused by delayed closure of the pulmonic valve, resulting from an increased volume of blood
- systolic click or late systolic murmur at the apex, resulting from mitral valve prolapse in older children with an ASD
- clubbing of the fingers (resulting from chronic hypoxia) and cyanosis (resulting from deoxygenated blood entering the systemic circulation), if a right-to-left shunt develops.

AGE ALERT
An infant may be cyanotic because he has a cardiac or pulmonary disorder. Cyanosis that worsens with crying is most likely associated with cardiac causes because crying increases pulmonary resistance to blood flow, resulting in an increased right-to-left shunt. Cyanosis that improves with crying is most likely from pulmonary causes, because deep breathing improves tidal volume.

COMPLICATIONS

Complications of an ASD may include:
- physical underdevelopment
- respiratory infections
- heart failure
- atrial arrhythmias
- mitral valve prolapse.

DIAGNOSIS

A history of increasing fatigue and characteristic physical features suggest an ASD. These tests confirm the diagnosis:

■ Chest X-ray shows an enlarged right atrium and right ventricle, a prominent pulmonary artery, and increased pulmonary vascular markings.

■ Electrocardiography (ECG) results may be normal, but they commonly show right axis deviation, a prolonged PR interval, varying degrees of right bundle branch block, right ventricular hypertrophy, atrial fibrillation (particularly in severe cases after age 30) and, in ostium primum defect, left axis deviation.

■ Echocardiography measures right ventricular enlargement, may locate the defect, and shows volume overload in the right side of the heart. It may reveal right ventricular and pulmonary artery dilation.

■ Two-dimensional echocardiography with color Doppler flow, contrast echocardiography, or both, have supplanted cardiac catheterization as the confirming tests for an ASD. Cardiac catheterization is used if inconsistencies exist in the clinical data or if significant pulmonary hypertension is suspected.

TREATMENT

Treatment for a small ASD may involve inserting an umbrella-like flexible wire mesh using X-ray and ultrasound during cardiac catheterization, instead of open-heart surgery. Open-heart surgical repair may be used for the patient with an uncomplicated ASD with evidence of significant left-to-right shunting. Ideally, this repair is performed when the patient is between ages 2 and 4. Operative treatment shouldn't be performed on a patient with small defects and trivial left-to-right shunts. Because an ASD seldom produces complications in an infant or a toddler, surgery can be delayed until preschool or early school age. A large defect may need immediate surgical closure with sutures or a patch graft.

Buerger's disease

Buerger's disease (sometimes called *thromboangiitis obliterans*) — an inflammatory,

nonatheromatous occlusive condition — impairs circulation to the legs, feet and, occasionally, the hands. Incidence is highest among men of Jewish ancestry, ages 20 to 40, who smoke heavily.

CAUSES

Although the cause of Buerger's disease is unknown, a definite link to smoking has been found, suggesting a hypersensitivity reaction to nicotine.

PATHOPHYSIOLOGY

In Buerger's disease, polymorphonuclear leukocytes infiltrate the walls of small and medium-sized arteries and veins. Thrombus develops in the vascular lumen, eventually occluding and obliterating portions of the small vessels, resulting in decreased blood flow to the feet and legs. This diminished blood flow may produce ulceration and, eventually, gangrene.

SIGNS AND SYMPTOMS

Signs and symptoms of Buerger's disease include:

■ intermittent claudication of the instep that's aggravated by exercise and relieved by rest, resulting from tissue ischemia

■ initially, coldness, cyanosis, and numbness of the feet during exposure to low temperatures, resulting from diminished blood flow; later, redness, heat, and tingling

■ impaired peripheral pulses, diminished blood flow, and migratory superficial thrombophlebitis, caused by inflammatory changes in vessel wall.

COMPLICATIONS

Complications of Buerger's disease may include:

■ ulceration, muscle atrophy, and gangrene caused by impaired blood flow

■ painful fingertip ulcerations if the hands are affected.

DIAGNOSIS

Patient history and physical examination strongly suggest Buerger's disease. Supportive diagnostic tests include:

- Doppler ultrasonography to show diminished circulation in the peripheral vessels
- plethysmography to help detect decreased circulation in the peripheral vessels
- arteriography to locate lesions and rule out atherosclerosis.

TREATMENT

The primary goals of treatment are to relieve symptoms and prevent complications. Such therapy may include:
- an exercise program that uses gravity to fill and drain the blood vessels
- in severe disease, a lumbar sympathectomy to increase blood supply to the skin
- possibly amputation for nonhealing ulcers, intractable pain, or gangrene.

Cardiac arrhythmias

In arrhythmias, abnormal electrical conduction or automaticity changes the heart's rate and rhythm. Arrhythmias vary in severity, from those that are mild, asymptomatic, and require no treatment (such as sinus arrhythmia, in which heart rate increases and decreases with respiration) to catastrophic ventricular fibrillation, which requires immediate resuscitation. Arrhythmias are generally classified according to their origin (ventricular or supraventricular). Their effect on cardiac output and blood pressure, partially influenced by the site of origin, determines their clinical significance.

CAUSES

Common causes of arrhythmias include:
- congenital defects
- myocardial infarction (MI) or ischemia
- organic heart disease
- drug toxicity
- degeneration of the conductive tissue
- connective tissue disorders
- electrolyte imbalances
- cellular hypoxia
- hypertrophy of the heart muscle
- acid-base imbalances
- emotional stress.

However, each arrhythmia may have its own specific causes. (See *Types of cardiac arrhythmias,* pages 146 to 153.)

PATHOPHYSIOLOGY

Arrhythmias may result from enhanced automaticity, reentry, escape beats, or abnormal electrical conduction. (See *Comparing normal and abnormal conduction,* pages 154 and 155.)

SIGNS AND SYMPTOMS

Signs and symptoms of arrhythmias result from reduced cardiac output and altered perfusion to the organs, and may include:
- dyspnea
- hypotension
- dizziness, syncope, and weakness
- chest pain
- cool, clammy skin
- altered level of consciousness
- reduced urinary output.

COMPLICATIONS

Complications of arrhythmias may include:
- sudden cardiac death
- MI
- heart failure
- thromboembolism.

DIAGNOSIS

These tests help identify arrhythmias:
- Electrocardiography detects arrhythmias as well as ischemia and infarction that may result in arrhythmias.
- Laboratory testing may reveal electrolyte abnormalities, acid-base abnormalities, or drug toxicities that may cause arrhythmias.
- Holter monitoring, event monitoring, and loop recording can detect arrhythmias and the effectiveness of drug therapy during a patient's daily activities.
- Exercise testing may detect exercise-induced arrhythmias.
- Electrophysiologic testing identifies the mechanism of an arrhythmia and the location of accessory pathways; it also assesses the effectiveness of antiarrhythmic drugs, radio-frequency ablation, and implantable cardioverter-defibrillators.

TREATMENT

Follow the specific treatment guidelines for each arrhythmia. (See *Types of cardiac arrhythmias,* pages 146 to 153.)

(Text continues on page 152.)

Types of cardiac arrhythmias

This chart reviews many common cardiac arrhythmias and outlines their features, causes, and treatments. Use a normal electrocardiogram strip, if available, to compare normal cardiac rhythm configurations with the rhythm strips below. Characteristics of normal sinus rhythm include:
◆ ventricular and atrial rates of 60 to 100 beats/minute
◆ regular and uniform QRS complexes and P waves
◆ PR interval of 0.12 to 0.20 second
◆ QRS duration < 0.12 second
◆ identical atrial and ventricular rates, with constant PR intervals.

ARRHYTHMIA AND FEATURES

Sinus tachycardia

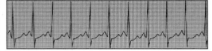

◆ Atrial and ventricular rhythms regular
◆ Rate > 100 beats/minute; rarely,
  > 160 beats/minute
◆ Normal P wave preceding each QRS complex

Sinus bradycardia

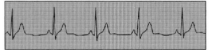

◆ Atrial and ventricular rhythms regular
◆ Rate < 60 beats/minute
◆ Normal P waves preceding each QRS complex

Paroxysmal supraventricular tachycardia

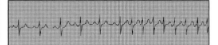

◆ Atrial and ventricular rhythms regular
◆ Heart rate > 160 beats/minute; rarely
  exceeds 250 beats/minute
◆ P waves regular but aberrant; difficult to
  differentiate from preceding T wave
◆ P wave preceding each QRS complex
◆ Sudden onset and termination of arrhythmia

CAUSES	TREATMENT
◆ Normal physiologic response to fever, exercise, anxiety, pain, dehydration; may also accompany shock, left ventricular failure, cardiac tamponade, hyperthyroidism, anemia, hypovolemia, pulmonary embolism, and anterior wall myocardial infarction (MI) ◆ May also occur with atropine, epinephrine, isoproterenol, quinidine, caffeine, alcohol, cocaine, amphetamine, and nicotine use	◆ Correction of underlying cause ◆ Beta-adrenergic blockers or calcium channel blocker
◆ Normal occurrence in well-conditioned heart, as in an athlete ◆ Increased intracranial pressure; increased vagal tone due to straining during defecation, vomiting, intubation, or mechanical ventilation; sick sinus syndrome; hypothyroidism; and inferior wall MI ◆ May also occur with anticholinesterase, beta-adrenergic blocker, digoxin, and morphine use	◆ Correction of underlying cause ◆ For low cardiac output, dizziness, weakness, altered level of consciousness, or low blood pressure: advanced cardiac life support (ACLS) protocol for administration of atropine ◆ Temporary or permanent pacemaker ◆ Dopamine or epinephrine infusion
◆ Intrinsic abnormality of atrioventricular (AV) conduction system ◆ Physical or psychological stress, hypoxia, hypokalemia, cardiomyopathy, congenital heart disease, MI, valvular disease, Wolff-Parkinson-White syndrome, cor pulmonale, hyperthyroidism, and systemic hypertension ◆ Digoxin toxicity; use of caffeine, marijuana, or central nervous system stimulants	◆ If patient is unstable, immediate cardioversion ◆ If patient is stable, vagal stimulation, Valsalva maneuver, and carotid sinus massage ◆ If cardiac function is preserved, treatment priority: calcium channel blocker, beta-adrenergic blocker, digoxin, and cardioversion; then consider procainamide, amiodarone, or sotolol if each preceding treatment is ineffective in rhythm conversion ◆ If the ejection fraction is less than 40% or if the patient is in heart failure, treatment order: digoxin, amiodarone, then diltiazem

(continued)

Types of cardiac arrhythmias *(continued)*

ARRHYTHMIA AND FEATURES

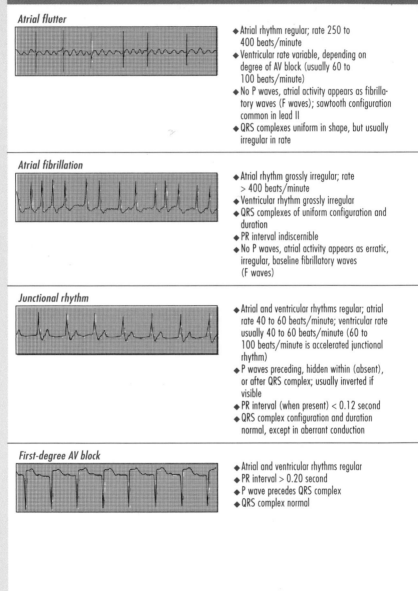

Atrial flutter

- Atrial rhythm regular; rate 250 to 400 beats/minute
- Ventricular rate variable, depending on degree of AV block (usually 60 to 100 beats/minute)
- No P waves, atrial activity appears as fibrillatory waves (F waves); sawtooth configuration common in lead II
- QRS complexes uniform in shape, but usually irregular in rate

Atrial fibrillation

- Atrial rhythm grossly irregular; rate > 400 beats/minute
- Ventricular rhythm grossly irregular
- QRS complexes of uniform configuration and duration
- PR interval indiscernible
- No P waves, atrial activity appears as erratic, irregular, baseline fibrillatory waves (F waves)

Junctional rhythm

- Atrial and ventricular rhythms regular; atrial rate 40 to 60 beats/minute; ventricular rate usually 40 to 60 beats/minute (60 to 100 beats/minute is accelerated junctional rhythm)
- P waves preceding, hidden within (absent), or after QRS complex; usually inverted if visible
- PR interval (when present) < 0.12 second
- QRS complex configuration and duration normal, except in aberrant conduction

First-degree AV block

- Atrial and ventricular rhythms regular
- PR interval > 0.20 second
- P wave precedes QRS complex
- QRS complex normal

CAUSES	TREATMENT
◆ Heart failure, tricuspid or mitral valve disease, pulmonary embolism, cor pulmonale, inferior wall MI, and pericarditis ◆ Digoxin toxicity	◆ If patient is unstable with a ventricular rate > 150 beats/minute, immediate cardioversion ◆ If patient is stable, follow ACLS protocol for cardioversion and drug therapy, which may include calcium channel blockers, beta-adrenergic blockers, or antiarrhythmics ◆ Anticoagulation therapy may also be necessary ◆ Radio-frequency ablation to control rhythm
◆ Heart failure, chronic obstructive pulmonary disease, thyrotoxicosis, constrictive pericarditis, ischemic heart disease, sepsis, pulmonary embolus, rheumatic heart disease, hypertension, mitral stenosis, atrial irritation, or complication of coronary bypass or valve replacement surgery ◆ Nifedipine and digoxin use	◆ If patient is unstable with a ventricular rate > 150 beats/minute, immediate cardioversion ◆ If patient is stable, follow ACLS protocol and drug therapy, which may include calcium channel blockers, beta-adrenergic blockers, or antiarrhythmics ◆ Anticoagulation therapy may also be necessary ◆ In some patients with refractory atrial fibrillation uncontrolled by drugs, radiofrequency catheter ablation
◆ Inferior wall MI or ischemia, hypoxia, vagal stimulation, and sick sinus syndrome ◆ Acute rheumatic fever ◆ Valve surgery ◆ Digoxin toxicity	◆ Correction of underlying cause ◆ Atropine for symptomatic slow rate ◆ Pacemaker insertion if patient doesn't respond to drugs ◆ Discontinuation of digoxin if appropriate
◆ May be seen in healthy persons ◆ Inferior wall MI or ischemia, hypothyroidism, hypokalemia, and hyperkalemia ◆ Digoxin toxicity; use of quinidine, procainamide, beta-adrenergic blockers, calcium channel blockers, or amiodarone	◆ Correction of underlying cause ◆ Possibly atropine if severe symptomatic bradycardia develops ◆ Cautious use of digoxin, calcium channel blockers, and beta-adrenergic blockers

(continued)

Types of cardiac arrhythmias *(continued)*

ARRHYTHMIA AND FEATURES

Second-degree AV block
Mobitz I (Wenckebach)

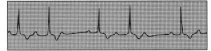

- ◆ Atrial rhythm regular
- ◆ Ventricular rhythm irregular
- ◆ Atrial rate exceeds ventricular rate
- ◆ PR interval progressively, but only slightly, longer with each cycle until QRS complex disappears (dropped beat); PR interval shorter after dropped beat

Second-degree AV block
Mobitz II

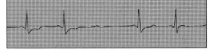

- ◆ Atrial rhythm regular
- ◆ Ventricular rhythm regular or irregular, with varying degree of block
- ◆ P-P interval constant
- ◆ QRS complexes periodically absent

Third-degree AV block
(complete heart block)

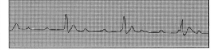

- ◆ Atrial rhythm regular
- ◆ Ventricular rhythm regular and rate slower than atrial rate
- ◆ No relation between P waves and QRS complexes
- ◆ No constant PR interval
- ◆ QRS duration normal (junctional pacemaker) or wide and bizarre (ventricular pacemaker)

Premature ventricular contraction (PVC)

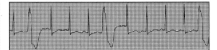

- ◆ Atrial rhythm regular
- ◆ Ventricular rhythm irregular
- ◆ QRS complex premature, usually followed by a complete compensatory pause
- ◆ QRS complex wide and distorted, usually > 0.14 second
- ◆ Premature QRS complexes occurring alone, in pairs, or in threes, alternating with normal beats; focus from one or more sites
- ◆ Ominous when clustered, multifocal, with R wave on T pattern

CAUSES	TREATMENT
◆ Inferior wall MI, cardiac surgery, acute rheumatic fever, and vagal stimulation ◆ Digoxin toxicity; use of propranolol, quinidine, or procainamide	◆ Treatment of underlying cause ◆ Atropine or temporary pacemaker for symptomatic bradycardia ◆ Discontinuation of digoxin if appropriate
◆ Severe coronary artery disease, anterior wall MI, and acute myocarditis ◆ Digoxin toxicity	◆ Temporary or permanent pacemaker ◆ Atropine, dopamine, or epinephrine for symptomatic bradycardia ◆ Discontinuation of digoxin if appropriate
◆ Inferior or anterior wall MI, congenital abnormality, rheumatic fever, hypoxia, postoperative complication of mitral valve replacement, postprocedure complication of radiofrequency ablation in or near AV nodal tissue, Lev's disease (fibrosis and calcification that spreads from cardiac structures to the conductive tissue), and Lenègre's disease (conductive tissue fibrosis) ◆ Digoxin toxicity	◆ Atropine, dopamine, or epinephrine for symptomatic bradycardia ◆ Temporary or permanent pacemaker
◆ Heart failure; old or acute MI, ischemia, or contusion; myocardial irritation by ventricular catheter or a pacemaker; hypercapnia; hypokalemia; hypocalcemia; and hypomagnesemia ◆ Drug toxicity (digoxin, aminophylline, tricyclic antidepressants, beta-adrenergic blockers, isoproterenol, or dopamine) ◆ Caffeine, tobacco, or alcohol use ◆ Psychological stress, anxiety, pain, or exercise	◆ If warranted, procainamide, amiodarone, or lidocaine I.V. ◆ Treatment of underlying cause ◆ Discontinuation of drug causing toxicity ◆ Potassium chloride I.V. if PVC induced by hypokalemia ◆ Magnesium sulfate I.V. if PVC induced by hypomagnesemia

(continued)

Types of cardiac arrhythmias *(continued)*

ARRHYTHMIA AND FEATURES

Ventricular tachycardia

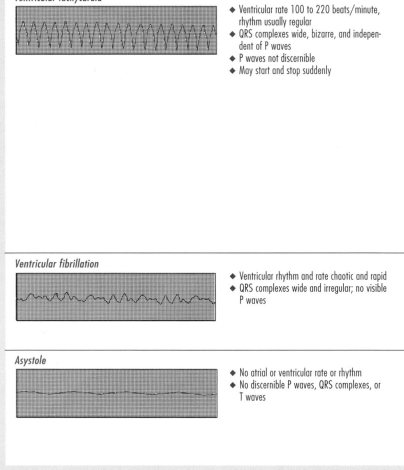

- ◆ Ventricular rate 100 to 220 beats/minute, rhythm usually regular
- ◆ QRS complexes wide, bizarre, and independent of P waves
- ◆ P waves not discernible
- ◆ May start and stop suddenly

Ventricular fibrillation

- ◆ Ventricular rhythm and rate chaotic and rapid
- ◆ QRS complexes wide and irregular; no visible P waves

Asystole

- ◆ No atrial or ventricular rate or rhythm
- ◆ No discernible P waves, QRS complexes, or T waves

Cardiac tamponade

Cardiac tamponade is a rapid, unchecked increase in pressure in the pericardial sac that compresses the heart, impairs diastolic filling, and reduces cardiac output. The pressure increase usually results from blood or fluid accumulation in the pericardial sac. Even a small amount of fluid (50 to 100 ml) can cause a serious tamponade if it accumulates rapidly.

Prognosis depends on the rate of fluid accumulation. If it accumulates rapidly, cardiac tamponade requires emergency lifesaving measures to prevent death. A slow accumulation and increase in pressure, as in pericardial effusion associated

CAUSES	TREATMENT
◆ Myocardial ischemia, MI, or aneurysm; coronary artery disease; rheumatic heart disease; mitral valve prolapse; heart failure; cardiomyopathy; ventricular catheters; hypokalemia; hypercalcemia; hypomagnesemia; and pulmonary embolism ◆ Digoxin, procainamide, epinephrine, or quinidine toxicity ◆ Anxiety	◆ With pulse: If hemodynamically stable with monomorphic QRS complexes, administration of procainamide, sotalol, amiodarone, or lidocaine (follow ACLS protocol); if drugs are ineffective, cardioversion ◆ If polymorphic QRS complexes and normal QT interval, administration of beta-adrenergic blockers, lidocaine, amiodarone, procainamide, or sotalol (follow ACLS protocol); if drug is unsuccessful, cardioversion ◆ If polymorphic QRS and QT interval is prolonged, magnesium I.V., then overdrive pacing if rhythm persists; may also administer isoproterenol, phenytoin, or lidocaine ◆ Pulseless: Initiate CPR; follow ACLS protocol for defibrillation, endotracheal (ET) intubation, and administration of epinephrine or vasopressin, followed by amiodarone or lidocaine and, if ineffective, magnesium sulfate or procainamide ◆ Implantable cardioverter-defibrillator (ICD) if recurrent ventricular tachycardia
◆ Myocardial ischemia, MI, untreated ventricular tachycardia, R-on-T phenomenon, hypokalemia, hyperkalemia, hypercalcemia, hypoxemia, alkalosis, electric shock, and hypothermia ◆ Digoxin, epinephrine, or quinidine toxicity	◆ CPR; follow ACLS protocol for defibrillation, ET intubation, and administration of epinephrine or vasopressin, amiodarone, or lidocaine and, if ineffective, magnesium sulfate or procainamide ◆ ICD if risk for recurrent ventricular fibrillation
◆ Myocardial ischemia, MI, aortic valve disease, heart failure, hypoxia, hypokalemia, severe acidosis, electric shock, ventricular arrhythmia, AV block, pulmonary embolism, heart rupture, cardiac tamponade, hyperkalemia, and electromechanical dissociation ◆ Cocaine overdose	◆ Continue CPR, follow ACLS protocol for ET intubation, transcutaneous pacing, and administration of epinephrine and atropine.

with malignant tumors, may not produce immediate symptoms because the fibrous wall of the pericardial sac can gradually stretch to accommodate as much as 1 to 2 L of fluid.

CAUSES
Cause of cardiac tamponade may include:

■ idiopathic causes (Dressler's syndrome)
■ effusion (from cancer, bacterial infections, tuberculosis and, rarely, acute rheumatic fever)
■ hemorrhage from trauma (such as gunshot or stab wounds to the chest or perforation by a catheter during cardiac or cen-

CLOSER LOOK
Comparing normal and abnormal conduction

NORMAL CARDIAC CONDUCTION
The heart's conduction system, shown below, begins at the sinoatrial (SA) node — the heart's pacemaker. When an impulse leaves the SA node, it travels through the atria along Bachmann's bundle and the internodal pathways to the atrioventricular (AV) node, and then down the bundle of His, along the bundle branches and, finally, down the Purkinje fibers to the ventricles.

ABNORMAL CARDIAC CONDUCTION
Altered automaticity, reentry, or conduction disturbances may cause cardiac arrhythmias.

Altered automaticity
Altered automaticity is the result of partial depolarization, which may increase the intrinsic rate of the SA node or latent pacemakers, or may induce ectopic pacemakers to reach threshold and depolarize.

Automaticity may be altered by drugs, such as epinephrine, atropine, and digoxin, and such conditions as acidosis, alkalosis, hypoxia, myocardial infarction, hypokalemia, and hypocalcemia. Examples of arrhythmias caused by altered automaticity include atrial fibrillation and flutter; supraventricular tachycardia; premature atrial, junctional, and ventricular complexes; ventricular tachycardia and fibrillation; and ac-

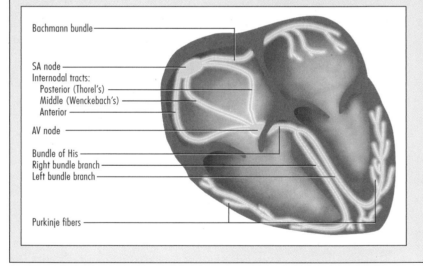

Bachmann bundle

SA node
Internodal tracts:
    Posterior (Thorel's)
    Middle (Wenckebach's)
    Anterior
AV node

Bundle of His
Right bundle branch
Left bundle branch

Purkinje fibers

tral venous catheterization or postcardiac surgery)
■ hemorrhage from nontraumatic causes (such as anticoagulant therapy in patients with pericarditis or rupture of the heart or great vessels)
■ viral or postirradiation pericarditis
■ chronic renal failure requiring dialysis
■ drug reaction from procainamide, hydralazine, minoxidil, isoniazid, penicillin, methysergide maleate, or daunorubicin

■ connective tissue disorders (such as rheumatoid arthritis, systemic lupus erythematosus, rheumatic fever, vasculitis, and scleroderma)
■ acute myocardial infarction.

PATHOPHYSIOLOGY
In cardiac tamponade, the progressive accumulation of fluid in the pericardial sac causes compression of the heart chambers. This compression obstructs blood flow

celerated idioventricular and junctional rhythms.

Reentry

Ischemia or a deformity causes an abnormal circuit to develop within conductive fibers. Although current flow is blocked in one direction within the circuit, the descending impulse can travel in the other direction. By the time the impulse completes the circuit, the previously depolarized tissue within the circuit is no longer refractory to stimulation, allowing reentry of the impulse and repetition of this cycle.

Conditions that increase the likelihood of reentry include hyperkalemia, myocardial ischemia, and the use of certain antiarrhythmic drugs. Reentry may be responsible for such arrhythmias as paroxysmal supraventricular tachycardia; premature atrial, junctional, and ventricular complexes; and ventricular tachycardia.

An alternative reentry mechanism depends on the presence of a congenital accessory pathway linking the atria and the ventricles outside the AV junction (for example, Wolff-Parkinson-White syndrome).

Conduction disturbances

Conduction disturbances occur when impulses are conducted too quickly or too slowly. Causes may include trauma, drug toxicity, myocardial ischemia, myocardial infarction, and electrolyte abnormalities. The AV blocks occur as a result of conduction disturbances.

into the ventricles and reduces the amount of blood that can be pumped out of the heart with each contraction. (See *Understanding cardiac tamponade,* page 156.)

Each time the ventricles contract, more fluid accumulates in the pericardial sac. This further limits the amount of blood that can fill the ventricular chambers — especially the left ventricle — during the next cardiac cycle.

The amount of fluid necessary to cause cardiac tamponade varies greatly; it may be as little as 50 ml when the fluid accumulates rapidly or more than 2 L if the fluid accumulates slowly and the pericardium stretches to adapt.

SIGNS AND SYMPTOMS

Signs and symptoms of cardiac tamponade include:
- elevated central venous pressure (CVP) with jugular vein distention caused by increased jugular venous pressure
- muffled heart sounds caused by fluid in the pericardial sac
- pulsus paradoxus (an inspiratory decrease in systemic blood pressure greater than 15 mm Hg) caused by impaired diastolic filling
- diaphoresis and cool, clammy skin caused by a decrease in cardiac output
- anxiety, restlessness, and syncope caused by a drop in cardiac output
- cyanosis caused by reduced oxygenation of the tissues
- weak, rapid pulse in response to a drop in cardiac output
- cough, dyspnea, orthopnea, and tachypnea caused by lung compression by an expanding pericardial sac and the inability to move blood from the pulmonary vasculature into the compromised left ventricle.

COMPLICATIONS

Reduced cardiac output may be fatal without prompt treatment.

DIAGNOSIS

These tests help confirm cardiac tamponade:
- Chest X-rays show a slightly widened mediastinum and possible cardiomegaly. The cardiac silhouette may have a goblet-shaped appearance.
- Electrocardiography (ECG) may show a low-amplitude QRS complex and electrical alternans, an alternating beat-to-beat change in amplitude of the P wave, QRS complex, and T wave. Generalized ST-segment elevation is noted in all leads. An ECG is used to rule out other cardiac disorders; it also may reveal changes produced by acute pericarditis.

CLOSER LOOK

Understanding cardiac tamponade

The pericardial sac, which surrounds and protects the heart, is composed of several layers. The fibrous pericardium is the tough outermost membrane; the inner membrane, called the serous membrane, consists of the visceral and parietal layers. The visceral layer clings to the heart and is also known as the epicardial layer of the heart. The parietal layer lies between the visceral layer and the fibrous pericardium. The pericardial space, between the visceral and parietal layers, contains 10 to 30 ml of pericardial fluid. This fluid lubricates the layers and minimizes friction when the heart contracts.

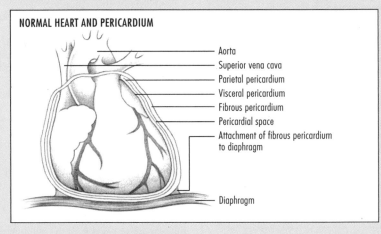

NORMAL HEART AND PERICARDIUM

- Aorta
- Superior vena cava
- Parietal pericardium
- Visceral pericardium
- Fibrous pericardium
- Pericardial space
- Attachment of fibrous pericardium to diaphragm
- Diaphragm

In cardiac tamponade, blood or fluid fills the pericardial space, compressing the heart chambers, increasing intracardiac pressure, and obstructing venous return. As blood flow into the ventricles falls, so does cardiac output. Without prompt treatment, low cardiac output can be fatal.

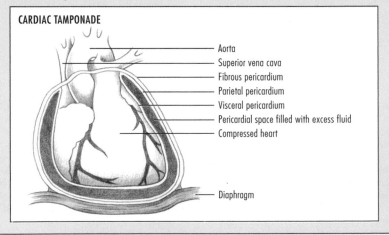

CARDIAC TAMPONADE

- Aorta
- Superior vena cava
- Fibrous pericardium
- Parietal pericardium
- Visceral pericardium
- Pericardial space filled with excess fluid
- Compressed heart
- Diaphragm

- Pulmonary artery catheterization detects increased right atrial pressure, right ventricular diastolic pressure, and CVP.
- Echocardiography may reveal pericardial effusion with signs of right ventricular and atrial compression.

TREATMENT
Correcting cardiac tamponade typically involves:
- supplemental oxygen to improve oxygenation
- continuous ECG and hemodynamic monitoring in an intensive care unit to detect complications and monitor effects of therapy
- pericardiocentesis (needle aspiration of the pericardial cavity) to reduce fluid in the pericardial sac and improve systemic arterial pressure and cardiac output (A catheter may be left in the pericardial space attached to a drainage container to allow for continuous fluid drainage.)
- a pericardial window (surgical creation of an opening) to remove accumulated fluid from the pericardial sac
- pericardiectomy (resection of a portion or all of the pericardium) to allow full communication with the pleura, if repeated pericardiocentesis fails to prevent recurrence
- trial volume loading with crystalloids, such as I.V. normal saline solution, to maintain systolic blood pressure
- inotropic drugs, such as isoproterenol or dopamine, to improve myocardial contractility until fluid in the pericardial sac can be removed
- blood transfusion or a thoracotomy to drain reaccumulating fluid or to repair bleeding sites may be necessary in cases of traumatic injury
- administration of the heparin antagonist protamine sulfate to stop bleeding, in heparin-induced tamponade
- use of vitamin K to stop bleeding, in warfarin-induced tamponade.

Cardiomyopathy

Cardiomyopathy generally applies to disease of the heart muscle fibers, and it occurs in three main forms: dilated, hypertrophic, and restrictive (extremely rare). Cardiomyopathy is the second most common direct cause of sudden death, after coronary artery disease (CAD). About 5 to 8 per 100,000 Americans have *dilated cardiomyopathy,* the most common type. At greatest risk for dilated cardiomyopathy are men and blacks; other risk factors include CAD, hypertension, pregnancy, viral infections, and alcohol or illegal drug use. Because dilated cardiomyopathy usually isn't diagnosed until its advanced stages, the prognosis is usually poor.

There are two types of *hypertrophic cardiomyopathy.* The more common form — nonobstructive hypertrophic cardiomyopathy — is caused by pressure overload hypertension or aortic valve stenosis. The second form, hypertrophic obstructive cardiomyopathy (HOCM), is caused by a genetic abnormality. The course of hypertrophic cardiomyopathy is variable. Some patients progressively deteriorate, whereas others remain stable for years. Almost 50% of all sudden deaths in competitive athletes age 35 or younger are caused by HOCM.

If severe, *restrictive cardiomyopathy* is irreversible.

CAUSES
Most patients with dilated cardiomyopathy have idiopathic, or primary, disease but some dilated cardiomyopathy is caused by another condition. (See *Comparing the cardiomyopathies,* pages 158 to 159.) HOCM is almost always inherited as a non–sex-linked autosomal dominant trait. Restrictive cardiomyopathy results from cardiac muscle fibrosis secondary to infiltration.

PATHOPHYSIOLOGY
Dilated cardiomyopathy results from extensively damaged myocardial muscle fibers. Consequently, contractility in the left ventricle is reduced. As systolic function declines, stroke volume, ejection fraction, and cardiac output fall. As end-diastolic volumes rise, pulmonary congestion may occur. The elevated end-diastolic volume is a compensatory response to preserve stroke volume despite a reduced ejection fraction. The sympathetic nervous system is also stimulated to increase heart rate and contractility. The kidneys are

Comparing the cardiomyopathies

Cardiomyopathies include a variety of structural or functional abnormalities of the ventricles. They're grouped into three main pathophysiologic types — dilated, hypertrophic, and restrictive. These conditions may lead to heart failure by impairing myocardial structure and function.

NORMAL HEART	DILATED CARDIOMYOPATHY
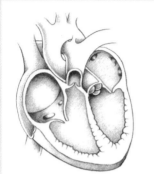	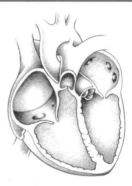
Ventricles	◆ Greatly increased chamber size ◆ Thinning of left ventricular muscle
Atrial chamber size	◆ Increased
Myocardial mass	◆ Increased
Ventricular inflow resistance	◆ Normal
Contractility	◆ Decreased
Possible causes	◆ Viral or bacterial infection ◆ Hypertension ◆ Peripartum syndrome related to toxemia ◆ Ischemic heart disease ◆ Valvular disease ◆ Drug hypersensitivity ◆ Chemotherapy ◆ Cardiotoxic effects of drugs or alcohol

stimulated to retain sodium and water to maintain cardiac output, and vasoconstriction also occurs as the renin-angiotensin system is stimulated. When these compensatory mechanisms can no longer maintain cardiac output, the heart begins to fail. Left ventricular dilation occurs as venous return and systemic vascular resistance rise. Eventually, the atria also dilate as more work is required to pump blood

HYPERTROPHIC CARDIOMYOPATHY	RESTRICTIVE CARDIOMYOPATHY

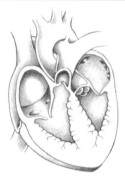 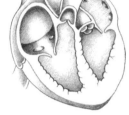

◆ Normal right and decreased left chamber size ◆ Left ventricular hypertrophy ◆ Thickened interventricular septum (hypertrophic obstructive cardiomyopathy [HOCM])	◆ Decreased ventricular chamber size ◆ Left ventricular hypertrophy
◆ Increased on left	◆ Increased
◆ Increased	◆ Normal
◆ Increased	◆ Increased
◆ Increased or decreased	◆ Decreased
◆ Autosomal dominant trait (HOCM) ◆ Hypertension ◆ Obstructive valvular disease ◆ Thyroid disease	◆ Amyloidosis ◆ Sarcoidosis ◆ Hemochromatosis ◆ Infiltrative neoplastic disease

into the full ventricles. Cardiomegaly occurs as a consequence of dilation of the atria and ventricles. Blood pooling in the ventricles increases the risk of emboli.

CLINICAL ALERT
Barth syndrome is a rare genetic disorder that can cause dilated cardiomyopathy in boys. This syndrome may cause skeletal muscle changes, short

stature, neutropenia, and increased susceptibility to bacterial infections. Evidence of dilated cardiomyopathy may appear as early as the first few days or months of life.

Unlike dilated cardiomyopathy, which affects systolic function, hypertrophic cardiomyopathy primarily affects diastolic function. The hypertrophied ventricle becomes stiff, noncompliant, and unable to relax during ventricular filling. Consequently, ventricular filling is reduced and left ventricular filling pressure rises, causing a rise in left atrial and pulmonary venous pressures and leading to venous congestion and dyspnea. Ventricular filling time is further reduced as a compensatory response to tachycardia leading to low cardiac output. If papillary muscles (attached to the atrioventricular valves) become hypertrophied and don't close completely during contraction, mitral insufficiency occurs. The features of HOCM include asymmetrical left ventricular hypertrophy; hypertrophy of the intraventricular septum; rapid, forceful contractions of the left ventricle; impaired relaxation; and obstruction to left ventricular outflow. The forceful ejection of blood draws the anterior leaflet of the mitral valve to the intraventricular septum. This causes early closure of the outflow tract, decreasing ejection fraction. Moreover, intramural coronary arteries are abnormally small and may not be sufficient to supply the hypertrophied muscle with enough blood and oxygen to meet the increased needs of the hyperdynamic muscle.

Restrictive cardiomyopathy is characterized by stiffness of the ventricle caused by left ventricular hypertrophy and endocardial fibrosis and thickening, thus reducing the ability of the ventricle to relax and fill during diastole. Moreover, the rigid myocardium fails to contract completely during systole. As a result, cardiac output falls.

SIGNS AND SYMPTOMS

Clinical manifestations of *dilated cardiomyopathy* may include:
- shortness of breath, orthopnea, dyspnea on exertion, paroxysmal nocturnal dyspnea, fatigue, and a dry cough at night caused by left-sided heart failure
- peripheral edema, hepatomegaly, jugular vein distention, and weight gain caused by right-sided heart failure
- peripheral cyanosis associated with a low cardiac output
- tachycardia as a compensatory response to low cardiac output
- pansystolic murmur associated with mitral and tricuspid insufficiency secondary to cardiomegaly and weak papillary muscles
- S_3 and S_4 gallop rhythms associated with heart failure
- irregular pulse if atrial fibrillation exists
- worsening renal function as decreased cardiac output produces decreased renal perfusion.

Clinical manifestations of *hypertropic cardiomyopathy* may include:
- dyspnea caused by elevated left ventricular filling pressure
- fatigue associated with a reduced cardiac output
- angina caused by the inability of the intramural coronary arteries to supply enough blood to meet the increased oxygen demands of the hypertrophied heart
- peripheral pulse with a characteristic double impulse (pulsus biferiens) caused by powerful left ventricular contractions and rapid ejection of blood during systole
- abrupt arterial pulse resulting from vigorous left ventricular contractions
- irregular pulse if an enlarged atrium causes atrial fibrillation.

Clinical manifestations of HOCM may include:
- systolic ejection murmur along the left sternal border and at the apex caused by mitral insufficiency
- angina caused by the inability of the intramural coronary arteries to supply enough blood to meet the increased oxygen demands of the hypertrophied heart
- syncope resulting from arrhythmias or reduced ventricular filling leading to a reduced cardiac output
- activity intolerance caused by worsening of outflow-tract obstruction from exercise-induced catecholamine release
- abrupt arterial pulse resulting from vigorous left ventricular contractions and early termination of left ventricular ejection

■ irregular pulse if an enlarged atrium causes atrial fibrillation.

Clinical manifestations of *restrictive cardiomyopathy* may include:

■ fatigue, dyspnea, orthopnea, chest pain, edema, liver engorgement, peripheral cyanosis, pallor, and S_3 or S_4 gallop rhythms caused by heart failure

■ systolic murmurs caused by mitral and tricuspid insufficiency.

COMPLICATIONS

Possible complications of cardiomyopathy include:

■ heart failure
■ arrhythmias
■ systemic or pulmonary embolization
■ sudden death.

DIAGNOSIS

These tests help diagnose cardiomyopathy:

■ Echocardiography confirms dilated cardiomyopathy.

■ Chest X-ray may reveal cardiomegaly associated with any of the cardiomyopathies.

■ Cardiac catheterization with possible heart biopsy can be definitive with HOCM.

■ Diagnosis requires elimination of other possible causes of heart failure and arrhythmias. (See *Comparing diagnostic tests in cardiomyopathy,* pages 162 and 163.)

TREATMENT

Management of *dilated cardiomyopathy* may involve:

■ treatment of the underlying cause, if identifiable

■ angiotensin-converting enzyme (ACE) inhibitors, as first-line therapy, to reduce afterload through vasodilation

■ diuretics, taken with ACE inhibitors, to reduce fluid retention

■ digoxin to improve myocardial contractility when ACE inhibitor and diuretic therapy are ineffective

■ hydralazine and isosorbide dinitrate in combination, to produce vasodilation

■ beta-adrenergic blockers for the patient with New York Heart Association (NYHA) class II or III heart failure (see *Classifying heart failure*)

Classifying heart failure

The New York Heart Association classification is a universal gauge of heart failure severity based on physical limitations.

CLASS I: MINIMAL
◆ No limitations
◆ Ordinary physical activity doesn't cause undue fatigue, dyspnea, palpitations, or angina

CLASS II: MILD
◆ Slightly limited physical activity
◆ Comfortable at rest
◆ Ordinary physical activity results in fatigue, palpitations, dyspnea, or angina

CLASS III: MODERATE
◆ Markedly limited physical activity
◆ Comfortable at rest
◆ Less than ordinary activity produces symptoms

CLASS IV: SEVERE
◆ Unable to perform physical activity without discomfort
◆ Angina or symptoms of cardiac inefficiency may develop at rest

---

■ antiarrhythmics, such as amiodarone, used cautiously, to control arrhythmias

■ an implantable cardioverter-defibrillator (ICD) to prevent and treat ventricular arrhythmias (because of the high incidence of sudden death in patients with NYHA class III or IV heart failure)

■ cardioversion to convert atrial fibrillation to sinus rhythm

■ pacemaker insertion to correct arrhythmias

■ a biventricular pacemaker for cardiac resynchronization therapy if symptoms continue despite optimal drug therapy, the patient is classified as NYHA class III or IV heart failure, QRS complex duration is 0.13 second or more, or ejection fraction is 35% or less

Comparing diagnostic tests in cardiomyopathy

Cardiomyopathies include a variety of structural or functional abnormalities of the ventricles. Dilated, hypertrophic, and restrictive cardiomyopathies may lead to heart failure by impairing myocardial structure and function.

DILATED CARDIOMYOPATHY	HYPERTROPHIC CARDIOMYOPATHY
ELECTROCARDIOGRAPHY	
Biventricular hypertrophy, sinus tachycardia, atrial enlargement, atrial and ventricular arrhythmias, bundle branch block, and ST-segment and T-wave abnormalities	Left ventricular hypertrophy, ST-segment and T-wave abnormalities, left anterior hemiblock, Q waves in precordial and inferior leads, ventricular arrhythmias, and, possibly, atrial fibrillation
ECHOCARDIOGRAPHY	
Left ventricular thrombi, global hypokinesia, enlarged atria, left ventricular dilation, and, possibly, valvular abnormalities	Symmetrical thickening of the left ventricular wall and intraventricular septum and left atrial dilation
CHEST X-RAY	
Cardiomegaly, pulmonary congestion, pulmonary venous hypertension, and pleural or pericardial effusions	Cardiomegaly
CARDIAC CATHETERIZATION	
Elevated left atrial and left ventricular end-diastolic pressures, left ventricular enlargement, and mitral and tricuspid incompetence; may identify coronary artery disease as a cause	Elevated ventricular end-diastolic pressure and, possibly, mitral insufficiency, hyperdynamic systolic function, and aortic valve pressure gradient if aortic valve is stenotic
RADIONUCLIDE STUDIES	
Left ventricular dilation and hypokinesis, reduced ejection fraction	Reduced left ventricular volume, increased muscle mass, and ischemia

■ revascularization, such as coronary artery bypass graft surgery, if dilated cardiomyopathy is from ischemia
■ valve repair or replacement, if dilated cardiomyopathy is from valve dysfunction
■ heart transplantation in cases refractory to medical therapy

■ lifestyle modifications, such as smoking cessation; low-fat, low-sodium diet; physical activity; and abstinence from alcohol
■ anticoagulants (controversial) to reduce the risk of emboli.
Management of *hypertrophic cardiomyopathy* may involve:
■ optimal control of hypertension

HYPERTROPHIC OBSTRUCTIVE CARDIOMYOPATHY	RESTRICTIVE CARDIOMYOPATHY
Left ventricular hypertrophy with QRS complexes tallest across mid-precordium, ST segment and T-wave abnormalities, left axis deviation, left atrial abnormality, supraventricular tachycardia, and ventricular tachycardia	Low voltage, hypertrophy, atrioventricular conduction defects, and arrhythmias
Asymmetrical septal hypertrophy; anterior movement of the anterior mitral leaflet during systole, early termination of left ventricular ejection that worsens with dobutamine or nitrate provocation, mitral insufficiency, and atrial dilation	Increased left ventricular muscle mass, normal or reduced left ventricular cavity size, and decreased systolic function; rules out constrictive pericarditis
Normal or mild cardiomegaly	Cardiomegaly, pericardial effusion, and pulmonary congestion
Asymmetrical septal hypertrophy, early termination of systole with decreased ejection fraction, outflow tract pressure gradient increasing from the apex to just below the aortic valve, and mitral insufficiency	Reduced systolic function and myocardial infiltration; increased left ventricular end-diastolic pressure; rules out constrictive pericarditis
Reduced left ventricular volume, increased septal muscle mass, septal ischemia	Left ventricular hypertrophy with restricted ventricular filling and reduced ejection fraction

■ aortic valve replacement if valve is stenotic
■ verapamil or diltiazem to reduce ventricular stiffness and elevated diastolic pressures
■ cardioversion to treat atrial fibrillation

■ anticoagulant therapy to reduce the risk of systemic embolism with atrial fibrillation.

Management of HOCM may involve:
■ beta-adrenergic blockers to slow the heart rate, reduce myocardial oxygen demands, and increase ventricular filling by

relaxing the obstructing muscle, thereby increasing cardiac output
- antiarrhythmic drugs, such as amiodarone, to reduce arrhythmias
- cardioversion to treat atrial fibrillation
- anticoagulant therapy to reduce the risk of systemic embolism with atrial fibrillation
- verapamil or diltiazem to reduce septal stiffness and elevated diastolic pressures
- an ICD to treat ventricular arrhythmias
- ventricular myotomy or myectomy (resection of the hypertrophied septum) to ease outflow tract obstruction and relieve symptoms
- heart transplantation for intractable symptoms
- mitral valve replacement to treat mitral insufficiency (controversial)
- ablation of the atrioventricular node and implantation of a dual-chamber pacemaker (controversial), in the patient with HOCM and ventricular tachycardia, to reduce the outflow gradient by altering the pattern of ventricular contractions.

Management of *restrictive cardiomyopathy* may involve:
- treatment of the underlying cause such as giving deferoxamine to bind iron in restrictive cardiomyopathy caused by hemochromatosis
- although no therapy exists for restricted ventricular filling, digoxin, diuretics, and a restricted sodium diet to ease the symptoms of heart failure
- oral vasodilators to decrease afterload and facilitate ventricular ejection.

Coarctation of the aorta

Coarctation is a narrowing of the aorta, usually just below the left subclavian artery, near the site where the ligamentum arteriosum (the remnant of the ductus arteriosus, a fetal blood vessel) joins the pulmonary artery to the aorta. Coarctation may occur with aortic valve stenosis (usually of a bicuspid aortic valve) and with severe cases of hypoplasia of the aortic arch, patent ductus arteriosus (PDA), and ventricular septal defect (VSD). The obstruction to blood flow results in ineffective pumping by the heart and increases the risk for heart failure.

This acyanotic condition accounts for about 7% of all congenital heart defects in children and is twice as common in boys as in girls. When coarctation of the aorta occurs in girls, it's commonly caused by Turner's syndrome, a chromosomal disorder resulting in ovarian dysgenesis.

The prognosis depends on the severity of associated cardiac anomalies. If corrective surgery is performed before isolated coarctation induces severe systemic hypertension or degenerative changes in the aorta, the prognosis is good.

CAUSES
Although the cause is usually unknown, this defect may be caused by Turner's syndrome.

PATHOPHYSIOLOGY
Coarctation of the aorta may develop as a result of spasm and constriction of the smooth muscle in the ductus arteriosus as it closes. This contractile tissue may extend into the aortic wall, causing narrowing. The obstructive process causes hypertension in the aortic branches above the constriction (arteries that supply the arms, neck, and head) and diminished pressure in the vessel below the constriction.

Restricted blood flow through the narrowed aorta increases the pressure load on the left ventricle and causes dilation of the proximal aorta and ventricular hypertrophy.

As oxygenated blood leaves the left ventricle, a portion travels through the arteries that branch off the aorta proximal to the coarctation. If PDA is present, the rest of the blood travels through the coarctation, mixes with deoxygenated blood from the PDA and travels to the legs. If the PDA is closed, the legs and lower portion of the body must rely solely on the blood that gets through the coarctation.

Untreated, this condition may lead to left-sided heart failure and, rarely, to cerebral hemorrhage and aortic rupture. If VSD accompanies coarctation, blood shunts from left to right, straining the right side of the heart. This situation leads to pulmonary hypertension and, eventually, right-sided heart hypertrophy and failure.

If coarctation is asymptomatic in infancy, it usually remains so throughout adolescence as collateral circulation develops to bypass the narrowed segment.

SIGNS AND SYMPTOMS
Signs and symptoms of this defect may include:
- tachypnea, dyspnea, pulmonary edema, pallor, tachycardia, failure to thrive, cardiomegaly, and hepatomegaly caused by heart failure during an infant's first year of life
- claudication caused by reduced blood flow to the legs
- hypertension in the upper body caused by increased pressure in the arteries proximal to the coarctation
- headache, vertigo, and epistaxis resulting from hypertension
- upper-extremity blood pressure greater than lower-extremity blood pressure because blood flow through the coarctation is greater to the upper body
- pink upper extremities and cyanotic lower extremities because of less oxygenated blood reaching the legs
- absent or diminished femoral pulses caused by restricted blood flow to the lower extremities through the constricted aorta
- normal heart sounds unless a cardiac defect coexists
- chest and arms that are more developed than legs because circulation to the legs is restricted.

COMPLICATIONS
Possible complications of this defect include:
- heart failure
- severe hypertension
- cerebral aneurysms and hemorrhage
- rupture of the aorta
- aortic aneurysm
- infective endocarditis.

DIAGNOSIS
These tests help diagnose coarctation of the aorta:
- Physical examination reveals the cardinal signs — resting systolic hypertension in the upper body, absent or diminished femoral pulses, and a wide pulse pressure.
- Chest X-rays may show left ventricular hypertrophy, heart failure, a wide ascending and descending aorta, and notching of the undersurfaces of the ribs caused by erosion by collateral circulation.
- Electrocardiography may reveal left ventricular hypertrophy.
- Echocardiography may show increased left ventricular muscle thickness, coexisting aortic valve abnormalities, and the coarctation site.
- Cardiac catheterization evaluates collateral circulation and measures pressure in the right and left ventricles and in the ascending and descending aortas (on both sides of the obstruction).
- Aortography locates the site and extent of coarctation.

TREATMENT
Correction of coarctation of the aorta may involve:
- digoxin, diuretics, oxygen, and sedatives in infants with heart failure
- prostaglandin infusion to keep the ductus open
- antibiotic prophylaxis against infective endocarditis before and after surgery
- antihypertensive therapy for children with previous undetected coarctation until surgery is performed
- immediate surgery for the infant with heart failure or hypertension; otherwise, surgery delayed until the preschool years. A flap of the left subclavian artery may be used to reconstruct the aorta. Balloon angioplasty or resection with end-to-end anastomosis or use of a tubular graft may also be performed.

Coronary artery disease
Coronary artery disease (CAD) results from the narrowing of the coronary arteries over time from atherosclerosis. The primary effect of CAD is the loss of oxygen and nutrients to myocardial tissue because of diminished coronary blood flow. The prevalence of CAD is increasing as the population ages. About 11 million people in the United States have CAD; it occurs more commonly in men, whites, and middle-age and elderly people. When patients with CAD receive proper care, prognosis is favorable.

CLOSER LOOK
Atherosclerotic plaque development

The coronary artery walls are made of three layers: intima (the innermost layer, media (the middle layer), and adventitia (the outermost layer).

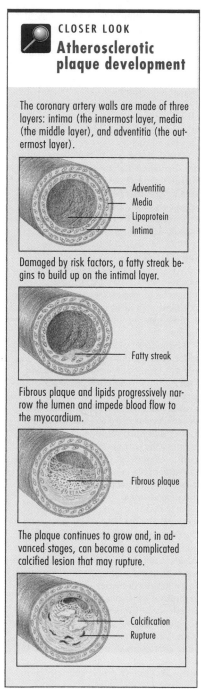

Adventitia
Media
Lipoprotein
Intima

Damaged by risk factors, a fatty streak begins to build up on the intimal layer.

Fatty streak

Fibrous plaque and lipids progressively narrow the lumen and impede blood flow to the myocardium.

Fibrous plaque

The plaque continues to grow and, in advanced stages, can become a complicated calcified lesion that may rupture.

Calcification
Rupture

CAUSES

CAD is commonly caused by atherosclerosis. Less common causes of reduced coronary artery blood flow include:

- dissecting aneurysm
- infectious vasculitis
- syphilis
- congenital defects.

PATHOPHYSIOLOGY

Fatty, fibrous plaques progressively narrow the coronary artery lumina, reducing the volume of blood that can flow through them and leading to myocardial ischemia. (See *Atherosclerotic plaque development*.)

As atherosclerosis progresses, luminal narrowing is accompanied by vascular changes that impair the ability of the diseased vessel to dilate. This causes a precarious balance between myocardial oxygen supply and demand, threatening the myocardium beyond the lesion. When oxygen demand exceeds what the diseased vessel can supply, localized myocardial ischemia results.

Myocardial cells become ischemic within 10 seconds of a coronary artery occlusion. Transient ischemia causes reversible changes at the cellular and tissue levels, depressing myocardial function. Untreated, this can lead to tissue injury or necrosis. Within several minutes, oxygen deprivation forces the myocardium to shift from aerobic to anaerobic metabolism, leading to accumulation of lactic acid and reduction of cellular pH.

The combination of hypoxia, reduced energy availability, and acidosis rapidly impairs left ventricular function. The strength of contractions in the affected myocardial region is reduced as the fibers shorten inadequately, resulting in less force and velocity. Moreover, wall motion is abnormal in the ischemic area, resulting in less blood being ejected from the heart with each contraction. Restoring blood flow through the coronary arteries restores aerobic metabolism and contractility. However, if blood flow isn't restored, myocardial infarction (MI) results.

SIGNS AND SYMPTOMS

Signs and symptoms of CAD may include:

■ angina, the classic sign of CAD, results from a reduced supply of oxygen to the myocardium. It may be described as burning, squeezing, or tightness in the chest that may radiate to the left arm, neck, jaw, or shoulder blade (see *Types of angina*)

 CLINICAL ALERT
Not all patients experience angina in the same way. Some, particularly women and Black and Hispanic patients, may experience no chest discomfort, only dyspnea and fatigue. This is called an anginal equivalent. Patients with diabetes may develop central neuropathies and therefore not experience chest pain; signs of sympathetic stimulation may be their primary angina symptom.

■ nausea and vomiting as a result of reflex stimulation of the vomiting centers by pain

■ cool extremities and pallor caused by sympathetic stimulation

■ diaphoresis from sympathetic stimulation

■ xanthelasma (fat deposits on the eyelids) occurring as a result of hyperlipidemia and atherosclerosis.

CLINICAL ALERT
CAD may produce no symptoms in the older adult because of a decrease in sympathetic response. Dyspnea and fatigue are two key signals of ischemia in an active, older adult.

COMPLICATIONS
Complications of CAD include:
■ arrhythmias
■ MI
■ ischemic cardiomyopathy.

DIAGNOSIS
These tests help diagnose CAD:
■ Electrocardiography may be normal between anginal episodes. During angina, it may show ischemic changes, such as T-wave inversion, ST-segment depression and, possibly, arrhythmias. ST-segment elevation suggests either MI or Prinzmetal's angina.

■ Ultra-fast computerized tomography scan may be used to identify calcium deposits in coronary arteries. Calcium scoring correlates with the degree of CAD.

Types of angina

There are four types of angina:
◆ *Stable angina:* pain is predictable in frequency and duration and is relieved by rest and nitroglycerin.
◆ *Unstable angina:* pain increases in frequency and duration and is more easily induced; it indicates a worsening of coronary artery disease that may progress to myocardial infarction.
◆ *Prinzmetal's* or *variant angina:* pain is caused by spasm of the coronary arteries; it may occur spontaneously and may not be related to physical exercise or emotional stress.
◆ *Microvascular angina:* impairment of vasodilator reserve causes anginalike chest pain in a person with normal coronary arteries.

■ Stress testing may be performed to detect ST-segment changes during exercise or pharmacologic stress, indicating ischemia, and to determine a safe exercise prescription.

■ Coronary angiography reveals the location and degree of coronary artery stenosis or obstruction, collateral circulation, and the condition of the artery beyond the narrowing.

■ Intravascular ultrasound may be used to further define coronary anatomy and luminal narrowing.

■ Myocardial perfusion imaging with thallium-201 may be performed during treadmill exercise to detect ischemic areas of the myocardium; these areas appear as "cold spots," which normalize during rest, indicating viable tissue.

■ Stress echocardiography may show abnormal wall motion in ischemic areas.

■ Rest perfusion imaging with sestamibi can be used to rule out myocardial ischemia in the patient with a chest pain syndrome that isn't clearly cardiac in nature.

TREATMENT

Treatment of CAD may involve:

■ nitrates, such as nitroglycerin (given sublingually, orally, transdermally, or topically in ointment form), isosorbide dinitrate (given sublingually or orally), or isosorbide mononitrate (given orally) to reduce myocardial oxygen consumption

■ beta-adrenergic blockers to reduce the heart's workload and oxygen demands by reducing heart rate and peripheral resistance to blood flow

■ calcium channel blockers to prevent coronary artery spasm

■ antiplatelet drugs to minimize platelet aggregation and the risk of coronary occlusion

■ antilipemic drugs to reduce serum cholesterol or triglyceride levels

■ antihypertensive drugs to control hypertension

■ estrogen replacement therapy to reduce the risk of CAD in postmenopausal women

■ coronary artery bypass graft (CABG) surgery to restore blood flow by bypassing an occluded artery using another vessel

■ "key-hole" or minimally invasive surgery, an alternative to traditional CABG surgery, using fiber-optic cameras inserted through small cuts in the chest, to correct blockages in one or two accessible arteries

■ angioplasty, to relieve occlusion in patients with partial occlusion and without calcification

■ laser angioplasty to correct occlusion by vaporizing fatty deposits

■ rotational atherectomy to remove arterial plaque with a high-speed burr

■ stent placement in a reopened artery to hold the artery open

■ drug-eluting stent placement, currently under clinical trials, to hold a reopened artery open and to minimize the risk of in-stent restenosis.

■ lifestyle modifications to reduce further progression of CAD; these include smoking cessation, regular exercise, stress management, maintaining an ideal body weight, and following a low-fat, low-sodium diet.

Endocarditis

Endocarditis (also known as *infective* or *bacterial endocarditis*) is an infection of the endocardium, heart valves, or cardiac prosthesis resulting from bacterial or fungal invasion.

Untreated endocarditis is usually fatal but, with proper treatment, 70% of patients recover. The prognosis is worst when endocarditis causes severe valvular damage, leading to insufficiency and heart failure, or when it involves a prosthetic valve.

CAUSES

Most cases of endocarditis occur in patients:

■ who are I.V. drug abusers

■ with prosthetic heart valves

■ with mitral valve prolapse (especially male patients with a systolic murmur)

■ with rheumatic heart disease.

Other predisposing conditions include coarctation of the aorta; tetralogy of Fallot; subaortic and valvular aortic stenosis; ventricular septal defects; pulmonary stenosis; Marfan syndrome; degenerative heart disease, especially calcific aortic stenosis; and, rarely, a syphilitic aortic valve. However, some patients with endocarditis have no underlying heart disease.

Infecting organisms differ among these groups. In patients with native valve endocarditis who aren't I.V. drug abusers, causative organisms usually include (in order of frequency) streptococci, especially *Streptococcus viridans;* staphylococci; or enterococci. Although other bacteria occasionally cause the disorder, fungal causes are rare in this group. The mitral valve is involved most commonly, followed by the aortic valve.

In patients who are I.V. drug users, *Staphylococcus aureus* is the most common infecting organism. Less commonly, streptococci, enterococci, gram-negative bacilli, or fungi cause the disorder. The tricuspid valve is involved most commonly, followed by the aortic valve and then the mitral valve.

In patients with prosthetic valve endocarditis, early cases (those that develop within 60 days of valve insertion) are usually caused by staphylococcal infection.

However, gram-negative aerobic organisms, fungi, streptococci, enterococci, or diphtheroids may also cause the disorder. The course is usually fulminant and is associated with a high mortality rate. Late cases (occurring after 60 days) show signs and symptoms similar to native valve endocarditis.

PATHOPHYSIOLOGY

In endocarditis, bacteremia — even transient bacteremia following dental or urogenital procedures — introduces the pathogen into the bloodstream. This infection causes fibrin and platelets to aggregate on the valve tissue and engulf circulating bacteria or fungi that flourish and form friable wartlike vegetative growths on the heart valves, the endocardial lining of a heart chamber, or the epithelium of a blood vessel. (See *Degenerative changes in endocarditis*.) Such growths may cover the valve surfaces, causing ulceration and necrosis; they may also extend to the chordae tendineae, leading to rupture and subsequent valvular insufficiency. Ultimately, they may embolize to the spleen, kidneys, central nervous system, and lungs.

SIGNS AND SYMPTOMS

Early clinical features of endocarditis are usually nonspecific and include malaise, weakness, fatigue, weight loss, anorexia, arthralgia, night sweats, chills, valvular insufficiency and, in 90% of patients, an intermittent fever that may recur for weeks. These features are typically related to the infectious process. A more acute onset is associated with organisms of high pathogenicity such as *Staphylococcus aureus*. Endocarditis commonly causes a loud, regurgitant murmur typical of the underlying heart lesion from the vegetative growths on the valve. A suddenly changing murmur or the discovery of a new murmur in the presence of fever is a classic physical sign of endocarditis.

In about 30% of patients, embolization from growing lesions or diseased valvular tissue may produce:
- *splenic infarction* — pain in the left upper quadrant, radiating to the left shoulder, and abdominal rigidity

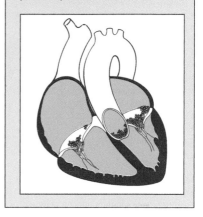

Degenerative changes in endocarditis

This illustration shows typical growths on the endocardium produced by fibrin and platelet deposits on infection sites.

- *renal infarction* — hematuria, pyuria, flank pain, and decreased urine output
- *cerebral infarction* — hemiparesis, aphasia, or other neurologic deficits
- *pulmonary infarction* (most common in right-sided endocarditis, which commonly occurs among I.V. drug users and after cardiac surgery) — cough, pleuritic pain, pleural friction rub, dyspnea, and hemoptysis
- *peripheral vascular occlusion* — numbness and tingling in an arm, leg, finger, or toe or signs of impending peripheral gangrene.

Other signs may include splenomegaly; petechiae of the skin (especially common on the upper anterior trunk) and buccal, pharyngeal, or conjunctival mucosa caused by small emboli lodging in the small vessels; and splinter hemorrhages under the nails secondary to bleeding in the small vessels of the nail beds from emboli lodging there.

Rarely, endocarditis produces Osler's nodes (tender, raised, subcutaneous lesions on the fingers or toes), Roth's spots (hemorrhagic areas with white centers on the retina from emboli in the nerve fiber layer of the eye), and Janeway lesions (purplish macules on the palms or soles from emboli).

COMPLICATIONS

Complications of endocarditis may include:

- heart failure
- death
- aortic root abscesses
- myocardial abscesses
- pericarditis
- cardiac arrhythmia
- meningitis
- cerebral emboli
- brain abscesses
- septic pulmonary infarcts
- arthritis
- glomerulonephritis
- acute renal failure.

DIAGNOSIS

Three or more blood cultures in a 24- to 48-hour period (each from a separate venipuncture) identify the causative organism in up to 90% of patients. Blood cultures should be drawn from three different sites, with 1 hour between each venipuncture.

The remaining 10% of patients may have negative blood cultures, possibly suggesting fungal infection or infections that are difficult to diagnose such as *Haemophilus parainfluenzae.*

Other abnormal but nonspecific laboratory test results may include:
- normal or elevated white blood cell count
- abnormal histiocytes (macrophages)
- elevated erythrocyte sedimentation rate
- normocytic, normochromic anemia (in 70% to 90% of patients)
- proteinuria and microscopic hematuria (in about 50% of patients)
- positive serum rheumatoid factor (in about one-half of all patients after endocarditis is present for 3 to 6 weeks)
- valvular damage, identified by echocardiography — particularly transesophageal
- atrial fibrillation and other arrhythmias that accompany valvular disease, identified by electrocardiography.

TREATMENT

The goal of treatment is to eradicate the infecting organism. First-line therapy is usually a combination of penicillin and an aminoglycoside, usually gentamicin. Antimicrobial therapy should start promptly and continue over 4 to 6 weeks. Selection of an antibiotic is based on identification of the infecting organism and on sensitivity studies. While results are pending, or if blood cultures are negative, empiric antimicrobial therapy is based on the likely infecting organism.

Supportive treatment includes bed rest, aspirin for fever and aches, and sufficient fluid intake. Severe valvular damage, especially aortic or mitral insufficiency, may require corrective surgery if refractory heart failure develops or in cases requiring that an infected prosthetic valve be replaced.

Heart failure

A syndrome rather than a disease, heart failure occurs when the heart can't pump enough blood to meet the body's metabolic needs. Heart failure results in intravascular and interstitial volume overload and poor tissue perfusion. An individual with heart failure experiences reduced exercise tolerance, a reduced quality of life, and a shortened life span.

Although the most common cause of heart failure is coronary artery disease, it also occurs in infants, children, and adults with congenital and acquired heart defects. The incidence of heart failure increases with age. About 1% of people older than age 50 experience heart failure; it occurs in 10% of people older than age 80. About 700,000 Americans die of heart failure each year. Mortality from heart failure is greater for males, blacks, and elderly people.

Although advances in diagnostic and therapeutic techniques have greatly improved the outlook for patients with heart failure, the prognosis still depends on the underlying cause and its response to treatment.

Causes of heart failure

The causes of heart failure may be divided into four general categories. The chart below highlights some of the disorders associated with each underlying cause.

CAUSE	EXAMPLES
Abnormal cardiac muscle function	◆ Myocardial infarction ◆ Cardiomyopathy
Abnormal left ventricular volume	◆ Valvular insufficiency ◆ High-output states: – Chronic anemia – Arteriovenous fistula – Thyrotoxicosis – Pregnancy – Septicemia – Beriberi – Infusion of a large volume of I.V. fluids in a short period
Abnormal left ventricular pressure	◆ Hypertension ◆ Pulmonary hypertension ◆ Chronic obstructive pulmonary disease ◆ Aortic or pulmonic valve stenosis
Abnormal left ventricular filling	◆ Mitral valve stenosis ◆ Tricuspid valve stenosis ◆ Atrial myxoma ◆ Constrictive pericarditis ◆ Atrial fibrillation ◆ Impaired ventricular relaxation: – Hypertension – Myocardial hibernation – Myocardial stunning

CAUSES

Causes of heart failure may be divided into four general categories. (See *Causes of heart failure.*)

PATHOPHYSIOLOGY

Heart failure may be classified according to the side of the heart affected (left- or right-sided heart failure) or by the cardiac cycle involved (systolic or diastolic dysfunction).

Left-sided heart failure. Left-sided heart failure occurs as a result of ineffective left ventricular contractile function. As the pumping ability of the left ventricle fails, cardiac output falls. Blood is no longer effectively pumped out into the body; it backs up into the left atrium and then into the lungs, causing pulmonary congestion, dyspnea, and activity intolerance. If the condition persists, pulmonary edema and right-sided heart failure may result. Common causes include left ventricular infarction, hypertension, and aortic and mitral valve stenosis.

Right-sided heart failure. Right-sided heart failure results from ineffective right ventricular contractile function. Consequently, blood isn't pumped effectively through the right ventricle to the lungs, causing blood to back up into the right atrium and the peripheral circulation. The patient gains weight and develops peripheral edema and engorgement of the kidney and other organs. It may be caused by an acute right ventricular infarction, pulmonary hypertension, or a pulmonary embolus. However, the most common cause is profound backward blood flow from left-sided heart failure.

Systolic dysfunction. Systolic dysfunction occurs when the left ventricle can't pump enough blood out to the systemic circulation during systole and the ejection fraction falls. Consequently, blood backs up into the pulmonary circulation and pressure increases in the pulmonary venous system. Cardiac output falls; weakness, fatigue, and shortness of breath may occur. Causes of systolic dysfunction include myocardial infarction and dilated cardiomyopathy.

Diastolic dysfunction. Diastolic dysfunction occurs when the ability of the left ventricle to relax and fill during diastole is reduced and the stroke volume falls. Therefore, higher volumes are needed in the ventricles to maintain cardiac output. Consequently, pulmonary congestion and peripheral edema develop. Diastolic dysfunction may occur as a result of left ventricular hypertrophy, hypertension, or restrictive cardiomyopathy. This type of heart failure is less common than systolic dysfunction, and its treatment isn't as clear.

All causes of heart failure eventually lead to reduced cardiac output, which triggers compensatory mechanisms, such as increased sympathetic activity, activation of the renin-angiotensin-aldosterone system, ventricular dilation, and hypertrophy. These mechanisms improve cardiac output at the expense of increased ventricular work.

Increased sympathetic activity—a response to decreased cardiac output and blood pressure—enhances peripheral vascular resistance, contractility, heart rate, and venous return. Signs of increased sympathetic activity, such as cool extremities and clamminess, may indicate impending heart failure.

Increased sympathetic activity also restricts blood flow to the kidneys, causing them to secrete renin which, in turn, converts angiotensinogen to angiotensin I, which then becomes angiotensin II—a potent vasoconstrictor. Angiotensin causes the adrenal cortex to release aldosterone, leading to sodium and water retention and an increase in circulating blood volume. This renal mechanism is initially helpful; however, if it persists unchecked, it can aggravate heart failure as the heart struggles to pump against the increased volume.

In ventricular dilation, an increase in end-diastolic ventricular volume (preload) causes increased stroke work and stroke volume during contraction, stretching cardiac muscle fibers so that the ventricle can accept the increased intravascular volume. Eventually, the muscle becomes stretched beyond optimum limits and contractility declines.

In ventricular hypertrophy, an increase in ventricular muscle mass allows the heart to pump against increased resistance to the outflow of blood, improving cardiac output. However, this increased muscle mass also increases myocardial oxygen requirements. An increase in the ventricular diastolic pressure necessary to fill the enlarged ventricle may compromise diastolic coronary blood flow, limiting the oxygen supply to the ventricle and causing ischemia and impaired muscle contractility.

In heart failure, counterregulatory substances—prostaglandins and atrial natriuretic factor—are produced in an attempt to reduce the negative effects of volume overload and vasoconstriction caused by the compensatory mechanisms.

The kidneys release the prostaglandins prostacyclin and prostaglandin E_2, which are potent vasodilators. These vasodilators also act to reduce volume overload produced by the renin-angiotensin-aldosterone system by inhibiting sodium and water reabsorption by the kidneys.

Atrial natriuretic factor is a hormone secreted mainly by the atria in response to stimulation of the stretch receptors in the atria caused by excess fluid volume. B-type natriuretic factor is secreted by the ventricles because of fluid volume overload. These natriuretic factors work to counteract the negative effects of sympathetic nervous system stimulation and the renin-angiotensin-aldosterone system by producing vasodilation and diuresis.

SIGNS AND SYMPTOMS

Early clinical manifestations of left-sided heart failure include:
- dyspnea caused by pulmonary congestion
- orthopnea as blood is redistributed from the legs to the central circulation when the patient lies down at night
- paroxysmal nocturnal dyspnea caused by the reabsorption of interstitial fluid when the patient is lying down and reduced sympathetic stimulation during sleep
- fatigue associated with reduced oxygenation and an inability to increase cardiac output in response to physical activity
- nonproductive cough associated with pulmonary congestion.

Later clinical manifestations of left-sided heart failure may include:
- crackles from pulmonary congestion
- hemoptysis (spitting of blood derived from the lungs) resulting from bleeding veins in the bronchial system caused by venous distention
- point of maximal impulse displaced toward the left anterior axillary line caused by left ventricular hypertrophy
- tachycardia from sympathetic stimulation
- S_3 caused by rapid ventricular filling
- S_4 resulting from atrial contraction against a noncompliant ventricle
- cool, pale skin resulting from peripheral vasoconstriction
- restlessness and confusion from reduced cardiac output.

Clinical manifestations of right-sided heart failure include:
- elevated jugular vein distention from venous congestion
- positive hepatojugular reflux and hepatomegaly secondary to venous congestion
- right upper quadrant pain caused by liver engorgement

- anorexia, fullness, and nausea, which may be from congestion of the liver and intestines
- nocturia as fluid is redistributed at night and reabsorbed
- weight gain caused by sodium and water retention
- edema associated with fluid volume excess
- ascites or anasarca caused by fluid retention.

COMPLICATIONS

Acute complications of heart failure include:
- pulmonary edema
- acute renal failure
- arrhythmias.

Chronic complications include:
- activity intolerance
- renal impairment
- cardiac cachexia
- metabolic impairment
- thromboembolism.

DIAGNOSIS

These tests help diagnose heart failure:
- Chest X-rays show increased pulmonary vascular markings, interstitial edema, or pleural effusion and cardiomegaly.
- Electrocardiography may indicate hypertrophy, ischemic changes, or infarction and may also reveal tachycardia and extrasystoles.
- Laboratory testing may reveal abnormal liver function tests and elevated blood urea nitrogen and creatinine levels. Prothrombin time may be prolonged as congestion impairs the liver's ability to synthesize procoagulants.
- Brain natriuretic peptide assay, a blood test, may show elevated levels. Along with such clinical signs as edematous ankles, elevated brain natriuretic peptide levels strongly indicate heart failure.
- Echocardiography may reveal left ventricular hypertrophy, dilation, and abnormal contractility.
- Pulmonary artery monitoring typically demonstrates elevated pulmonary artery and pulmonary artery wedge pressures, left ventricular end-diastolic pressure in left-sided heart failure, and elevated right atrial

pressure or central venous pressure in right-sided heart failure.

■ Radionuclide ventriculography may reveal an ejection fraction less than 40%; in diastolic dysfunction, the ejection fraction may be normal.

TREATMENT

Management of heart failure may involve:

■ treatment of the underlying cause, if known

■ angiotensin-converting enzyme (ACE) inhibitors for patients with left ventricle dysfunction to reduce production of angiotensin II, resulting in preload and afterload reduction

 AGE ALERT
An elderly patient may require lower doses of ACE inhibitors because of impaired renal clearance. Monitor the patient for severe hypotension, signifying a toxic effect.

■ digoxin for the patient with heart failure caused by left ventricular systolic dysfunction to increase myocardial contractility, improve cardiac output, reduce the volume of the ventricle, and decrease ventricular stretch

■ diuretics to reduce fluid volume overload and venous return

■ beta-adrenergic blockers in the patient with New York Heart Association (NYHA) class II or III heart failure caused by left ventricular systolic dysfunction to prevent remodeling (see *Classifying heart failure,* page 161)

■ inotropic therapy with dobutamine or milrinone for acute treatment of heart failure exacerbation

■ chronic or chronic intermittent inotropic therapy to augment ventricular contractility to avoid exacerbations of heart failure in the patient with NYHA class IV heart failure

■ nesiritide, a human B-type natriuretic peptide, to augment diuresis and to decrease afterload in acute management of heart failure exacerbation

■ diuretics, nitrates, morphine, and oxygen to treat pulmonary edema

■ lifestyle modifications (to reduce symptoms of heart failure), such as weight loss (if obese), limited sodium (2 g/day) and alcohol intake, reduced fat intake, smoking cessation, stress reduction, and development of an exercise program (Heart failure is no longer a contraindication to exercise and cardiac rehabilitation.)

■ coronary artery bypass surgery or angioplasty for heart failure caused by coronary artery disease

■ heart transplantation in the patient receiving aggressive medical treatment, but still experiencing limitations or repeated hospitalizations

■ other surgery or invasive procedures may be recommended for the patient with severe limitations or repeated hospitalizations, despite maximal medical therapy. Some procedures are controversial and may include cardiomyoplasty, insertion of an intra-aortic balloon pump, use of a mechanical ventricular assist device, and implanting an internal cardioverter-defibrillator.

 AGE ALERT
Heart failure in children occurs mainly as a result of congenital heart defects. Therefore, treatment guidelines are directed toward the specific cause.

Hypertension

Hypertension, an elevation in diastolic or systolic blood pressure, occurs as two major types: essential (primary) hypertension, the most common, and secondary hypertension, which results from renal disease or another identifiable cause. Malignant hypertension is a severe, fulminant form of hypertension common to both types. Hypertension is a major cause of stroke, cardiac disease, and renal failure.

Hypertension affects 15% to 20% of adults in the United States. The risk of hypertension increases with age and is higher in Blacks than Whites and in those with less education and lower income. Men have a higher incidence of hypertension in young and early middle adulthood; thereafter, women have a higher incidence.

Essential hypertension usually begins insidiously as a benign disease, slowly progressing to a malignant state. If untreated, even mild cases can cause major complications and death. Carefully managed treatment, which may include lifestyle modifications and drug therapy, improves the prognosis. Untreated, essential hypertension carries a high mortality rate. Severely elevated blood pressure (hypertensive crisis) may be fatal.

CAUSES

Risk factors for *essential hypertension* include:
- family history
- advancing age
- sleep apnea

AGE ALERT
Elderly people may have isolated systolic hypertension, in which just the systolic blood pressure is elevated, because atherosclerosis causes a loss of elasticity in large arteries. Previously, it was believed that isolated systolic hypertension was a normal part of the aging process and shouldn't be treated. Results of the Systolic Hypertension in the Elderly Program, however, found that treating isolated systolic hypertension with antihypertensive drugs lowered the incidence of stroke, coronary artery disease (CAD), and left-sided heart failure.

- race (most common in blacks)

CLINICAL ALERT
Blacks are at an increased risk for primary hypertension when predisposition to low plasma renin levels diminishes the ability to excrete excess sodium. Hypertension develops at an earlier age and is more severe in Blacks than in Whites.

- obesity
- tobacco use
- high intake of sodium
- high intake of saturated fat
- excessive alcohol consumption
- sedentary lifestyle
- stress
- excess renin
- mineral deficiencies (calcium, potassium, and magnesium)
- diabetes mellitus.

Causes of *secondary hypertension* include:
- coarctation of the aorta
- renal artery stenosis and parenchymal disease
- brain tumor, quadriplegia, and head injury

- pheochromocytoma, Cushing's syndrome, hyperaldosteronism, or thyroid, pituitary, or parathyroid dysfunction
- hormonal contraceptives, cocaine, epoetin alfa, sympathetic stimulants, monoamine oxidase inhibitors taken with tyramine, estrogen replacement therapy, and nonsteroidal anti-inflammatory drugs
- pregnancy-induced hypertension (PIH)
- excessive alcohol consumption.

PATHOPHYSIOLOGY

Arterial blood pressure is a product of total peripheral resistance and cardiac output. Cardiac output is increased by conditions that increase heart rate, stroke volume, or both. Peripheral resistance is increased by factors that increase blood viscosity or reduce the lumen size of vessels, especially the arterioles.

Several theories help to explain the development of hypertension, including:
- changes in the arteriolar bed, causing increased peripheral vascular resistance
- abnormally increased tone in the sympathetic nervous system that originates in the vasomotor system centers, causing increased peripheral vascular resistance
- increased blood volume resulting from renal or hormonal dysfunction
- an increase in arteriolar thickening caused by genetic factors, leading to increased peripheral vascular resistance
- abnormal renin release, resulting in the formation of angiotensin II, which constricts the arteriole and increases blood volume. (See *Understanding blood pressure regulation,* page 176.)

Prolonged hypertension increases the heart's workload as resistance to left ventricular ejection increases. To increase contractile force, the left ventricle hypertrophies, raising the heart's oxygen demands and workload. Cardiac dilation and failure may occur when hypertrophy can no longer maintain sufficient cardiac output. Because hypertension promotes coronary atherosclerosis, the heart may be further compromised by reduced blood flow to the myocardium, resulting in angina or myocardial infarction (MI). Hypertension also causes vascular damage, leading to accelerated atherosclerosis and target organ damage, such as retinal injury, renal fail-

Understanding blood pressure regulation

Hypertension may result from a disturbance in one of these intrinsic mechanisms.

RENIN-ANGIOTENSIN SYSTEM
The renin-angiotensin system acts to increase blood pressure through these mechanisms:
◆ sodium depletion, reduced blood pressure, and dehydration stimulate renin release
◆ renin reacts with angiotensin, a liver enzyme, and converts it to angiotensin I, which increases preload and afterload
◆ angiotensin I converts to angiotensin II in the lungs; angiotensin II is a potent vasoconstrictor that targets the arterioles
◆ angiotensin II works to increase preload and afterload by stimulating the adrenal cortex to secrete aldosterone; this increases blood volume by conserving sodium and water.

AUTOREGULATION
Several intrinsic mechanisms work to change an artery's diameter to maintain tissue and organ perfusion despite fluctuations in systemic blood pressure. These mechanisms include stress relaxation and capillary fluid shifts:

◆ in stress relaxation, blood vessels gradually dilate when blood pressure increases to reduce peripheral resistance
◆ in capillary fluid shift, plasma moves between vessels and extravascular spaces to maintain intravascular volume.

SYMPATHETIC NERVOUS SYSTEM
When blood pressure drops, baroreceptors in the aortic arch and carotid sinuses decrease their inhibition of the medulla's vasomotor center. The consequent increases in sympathetic stimulation of the heart by norepinephrine increases cardiac output by strengthening the contractile force, raising the heart rate, and augmenting peripheral resistance by vasoconstriction. Stress can also stimulate the sympathetic nervous system to increase cardiac output and peripheral vascular resistance.

ANTIDIURETIC HORMONE
The release of antidiuretic hormone can regulate hypotension by increasing reabsorption of water by the kidney. With reabsorption, blood plasma volume increases, thus raising blood pressure.

ure, stroke, and aortic aneurysm and dissection.

The pathophysiology of secondary hypertension is related to the underlying disease. For example:
■ The most common cause of secondary hypertension is chronic renal disease. Insult to the kidney from chronic glomerulonephritis or renal artery stenosis interferes with sodium excretion, the renin-angiotensin-aldosterone system, or renal perfusion, causing blood pressure to increase.
■ In Cushing's syndrome, increased cortisol levels raise blood pressure by increasing renal sodium retention, angiotensin II levels, and vascular response to norepinephrine.
■ In primary aldosteronism, increased intravascular volume, altered sodium con-

centrations in vessel walls, or very high aldosterone levels cause vasoconstriction and increased resistance.
■ Pheochromocytoma is a chromaffin cell tumor of the adrenal medulla that secretes epinephrine and norepinephrine. Epinephrine increases cardiac contractility and rate, whereas norepinephrine increases peripheral vascular resistance.

SIGNS AND SYMPTOMS
Although hypertension commonly produces no symptoms, these signs and symptoms may occur:
■ elevated blood pressure readings on at least two consecutive occasions after initial screening, caused by pathophysiologic changes in blood vessels

AGE ALERT
Because many older adults have a wide auscultatory gap — the pause between the first Korotkoff's sound and the next sound — failure to pump the blood pressure cuff up high enough can lead to missing the first beat and underestimating systolic blood pressure. To avoid missing the first Korotkoff's sound, palpate the radial artery and inflate the cuff to a point about 20 mm beyond which the pulse beat disappears.

■ occipital headache (may worsen on rising in the morning as a result of increased intracranial pressure) resulting from vascular changes; nausea and vomiting may also occur
■ epistaxis possibly caused by vascular involvement
■ bruits (which may be heard over the abdominal aorta or carotid, renal, and femoral arteries) caused by stenosis or aneurysm
■ dizziness, confusion, and fatigue caused by decreased tissue perfusion caused by vasoconstriction of blood vessels
■ blurry vision as a result of retinal damage
■ nocturia caused by an increase in blood flow to the kidneys and an increase in glomerular filtration
■ edema caused by increased capillary pressure.

If secondary hypertension exists, other signs and symptoms may be related to the cause. For example, Cushing's syndrome may cause truncal obesity and purple striae, whereas patients with pheochromocytoma may develop headache, nausea, vomiting, palpitations, pallor, and profuse perspiration.

COMPLICATIONS
Complications of hypertension include:
■ hypertensive crisis, peripheral arterial disease, dissecting aortic aneurysm, CAD, angina, MI, heart failure, arrhythmias, and sudden death (see *What happens in hypertensive crisis,* page 178)
■ transient ischemic attacks, stroke, retinopathy, and hypertensive encephalopathy
■ renal failure.

DIAGNOSIS
These tests help diagnose hypertension:
■ Serial blood pressure measurements may be useful. (See *Classifying blood pressure readings,* page 179.)
■ Urinalysis may show protein, casts, red blood cells, or white blood cells, suggesting renal disease; presence of catecholamines associated with pheochromocytoma; or glucose, suggesting diabetes.
■ Laboratory testing may reveal elevated blood urea nitrogen and serum creatinine levels suggestive of renal disease, or hypokalemia indicating adrenal dysfunction (primary hyperaldosteronism).
■ Complete blood count may reveal other causes of hypertension, such as polycythemia or anemia.
■ Excretory urography may reveal renal atrophy, indicating chronic renal disease. One kidney smaller than the other suggests unilateral renal disease.
■ Electrocardiogram may show left ventricular hypertrophy or ischemia.
■ Chest X-rays may show cardiomegaly.
■ Echocardiography may reveal left ventricular hypertrophy.

TREATMENT
The Seventh Report of the Joint National Committee on Prevention, Detection, Evaluation, and Treatment of High Blood Pressure of the National Institutes of Health, National Heart, Lung, and Blood Institute recommends:
■ Lifestyle modification including weight reduction, use of a Dietary Approaches to Stop Hypertension (DASH) diet (involves consumption of a diet rich in fruits, vegetables, and lowfat dairy products with a reduced content of saturated and total fat), reduction of dietary sodium intake, physical activity (regular aerobic activity such as brisk walking), and moderation of alcohol intake.
■ Pharmacologic therapy initially with thiazide diuretics for patients with a systolic blood pressure ranging from 140 to 159 mm Hg and a diastolic blood pressure ranging from 90 to 99 mm Hg. Other agents, such as angiotensin-converting enzyme (ACE) inhibitors, angiotensin receptor blockers, beta-adrenergic blockers, and calcium channel blockers may be used

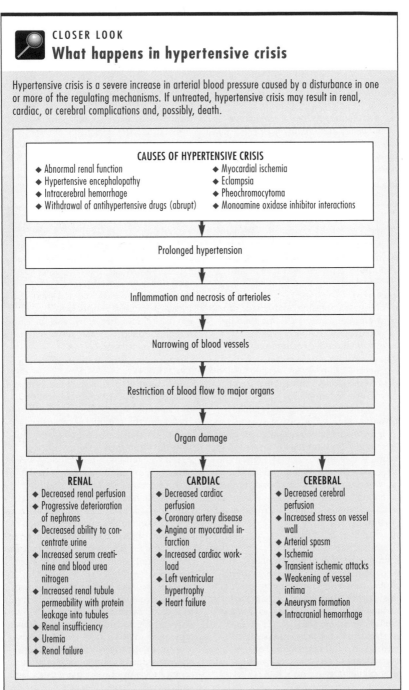

CLOSER LOOK

What happens in hypertensive crisis

Hypertensive crisis is a severe increase in arterial blood pressure caused by a disturbance in one or more of the regulating mechanisms. If untreated, hypertensive crisis may result in renal, cardiac, or cerebral complications and, possibly, death.

CAUSES OF HYPERTENSIVE CRISIS

- ◆ Abnormal renal function
- ◆ Hypertensive encephalopathy
- ◆ Intracerebral hemorrhage
- ◆ Withdrawal of antihypertensive drugs (abrupt)

- ◆ Myocardial ischemia
- ◆ Eclampsia
- ◆ Pheochromocytoma
- ◆ Monoamine oxidase inhibitor interactions

Prolonged hypertension

Inflammation and necrosis of arterioles

Narrowing of blood vessels

Restriction of blood flow to major organs

Organ damage

RENAL
- ◆ Decreased renal perfusion
- ◆ Progressive deterioration of nephrons
- ◆ Decreased ability to concentrate urine
- ◆ Increased serum creatinine and blood urea nitrogen
- ◆ Increased renal tubule permeability with protein leakage into tubules
- ◆ Renal insufficiency
- ◆ Uremia
- ◆ Renal failure

CARDIAC
- ◆ Decreased cardiac perfusion
- ◆ Coronary artery disease
- ◆ Angina or myocardial infarction
- ◆ Increased cardiac workload
- ◆ Left ventricular hypertrophy
- ◆ Heart failure

CEREBRAL
- ◆ Decreased cerebral perfusion
- ◆ Increased stress on vessel wall
- ◆ Arterial spasm
- ◆ Ischemia
- ◆ Transient ischemic attacks
- ◆ Weakening of vessel intima
- ◆ Aneurysm formation
- ◆ Intracranial hemorrhage

Classifying blood pressure readings

In 2003, the National Institutes of Health issued a revised method of classifying blood pressure. The updated categories are highlighted below. A new category of prehypertension has been added; stages 2 and 3, previously identified, have been combined.

The revised categories are based on the average of two or more readings taken on separate visits after an initial screening. The categories apply to adults age 18 and older who aren't taking antihypertensive medication, who don't have a short-term serious illness, and who don't have other conditions such as diabetes or kidney disease.

(If the systolic and diastolic pressures fall into different categories, use the higher of the two pressures to classify the reading. For example, a reading of 160/92 mm Hg should be classified as stage 2.)

In addition to classifying stages of hypertension based on average blood pressure readings, clinicians should also note target organ disease and additional risk factors. For example, a patient with diabetes, heart failure, and a blood pressure reading of 144/98 mm Hg would be classified as "stage 1 hypertension with compelling indications (heart failure and diabetes)." This additional information is important to obtain a true picture of the patient's cardiovascular health.

CATEGORY	SYSTOLIC	DIASTOLIC
Normal	< 120 mm Hg AND	< 80 mm Hg
Prehypertension	120 to 139 mm Hg OR	80 to 89 mm Hg
Stage 1 hypertension	140 to 159 mm Hg OR	90 to 99 mm Hg
Stage 2 hypertension	≤ 160 mm Hg	≥ 100

instead or in combination with thiazide diuretics.

■ Pharmacologic therapy with a two-drug combination for patients with blood pressure greater than 160/100 mm Hg. Usually, a thiazide diuretic in combination with ACE inhibitors, angiotensin receptor blockers, beta-adrenergic blockers, and calcium channel blockers.

■ Pharmacologic therapy with multidrug therapy for patients with hypertension and other underlying disorders such as heart failure, history of previous MI, diabetes, chronic renal disease, or history of stroke.

■ Dosage adjustments based on the patient's response to drug therapy, to achieve a target goal; for patients with diabetes or chronic renal disease, the target blood pressure to achieve is 130/80 mm Hg.

Treatment of secondary hypertension focuses on correcting the underlying cause and controlling hypertensive effects.

Typically, hypertensive emergencies require parenteral administration of a vasodilator or an adrenergic inhibitor or oral administration of a selected drug, such as nifedipine, captopril, clonidine, or labetalol, to rapidly reduce blood pressure. The goal is to reduce mean arterial blood pressure first by no more than 25% (within minutes to hours), then to 160/110 mm Hg within 2 hours while avoiding excessive decreases in blood pressure that can precipitate renal, cerebral, or myocardial ischemia.

Examples of hypertensive emergencies include hypertensive encephalopathy, intracranial hemorrhage, acute left-sided heart failure with pulmonary edema, and dissecting aortic aneurysm. Hypertensive emergencies are also associated with eclampsia or severe PIH, unstable angina, and acute MI.

Hypertension without accompanying symptoms or target-organ disease seldom requires emergency drug therapy.

Myocardial infarction

In myocardial infarction (MI) — also known as a *heart attack* — reduced blood flow through one of the coronary arteries results in myocardial ischemia and necrosis. In cardiovascular disease, death usually results from cardiac damage or complications of MI — the leading cause of death in the United States and Western Europe. Each year, about 900,000 people in the United States experience MI. Mortality is high when treatment is delayed, and almost one-half of sudden deaths from MI occur before hospitalization, within 1 hour of the onset of symptoms. The prognosis improves if vigorous treatment begins immediately.

CAUSES

Predisposing risk factors for MI include:
- family history of MI
- gender (men and postmenopausal women are more susceptible to MI than premenopausal women, although the incidence is increasing among women, especially those who smoke and take hormonal contraceptives)
- hypertension
- smoking
- elevated triglyceride, total cholesterol, and low-density lipoprotein levels
- obesity
- excessive intake of saturated fats
- sedentary lifestyle
- aging
- stress or type A personality
- drug use, especially cocaine and amphetamines.

PATHOPHYSIOLOGY

MI results from occlusion of one or more of the coronary arteries. Occlusion can stem from atherosclerosis, thrombosis, platelet aggregation, or coronary artery stenosis or spasm. If coronary artery occlusion causes prolonged ischemia, lasting longer than 30 to 45 minutes, irreversible myocardial cell damage and muscle death occur. The site of the MI depends on the vessels involved. Occlusion of the circumflex branch of the left coronary artery causes a lateral wall infarction; occlusion of the anterior descending branch of the left coronary artery, an anterior wall infarction. True posterior or inferior wall infarctions generally result from occlusion of the right coronary artery or one of its branches.

Right ventricular infarctions can also result from right coronary artery occlusion, can accompany inferior infarctions, and may cause right-sided heart failure. In Q-wave (transmural) MI, tissue damage extends through all myocardial layers; in non-Q-wave (subendocardial) MI, damage occurs only in the innermost and, possibly, middle layers.

All infarcts have a central area of necrosis or infarction surrounded by an area of potentially viable hypoxic injury. This zone may be salvaged if circulation is restored or it may progress to necrosis. The zone of injury, in turn, is surrounded by an area of viable ischemic tissue. (See *Zones of myocardial infarction*.) Although ischemia begins immediately, the size of the infarct can be limited if circulation is restored within 6 hours.

Several changes occur after MI. Cardiac enzymes and proteins are released by the infarcted myocardial cells, which are used in the diagnosis of an MI. Within 24 hours, the infarcted muscle becomes edematous and cyanotic. During the next several days, leukocytes infiltrate the necrotic area and begin to remove necrotic cells, thinning the ventricular wall. Scar formation begins by the third week after MI, and by the sixth week, scar tissue is well established.

Zones of myocardial infarction

Myocardial infarction has a central area of necrosis surrounded by a zone of injury that may recover if revascularization occurs. This zone of injury is surrounded by an outer ring of reversible ischemia. Characteristic electrocardiographic changes are associated with each zone. A disruption at any point in the menstrual cycle can produce amenorrhea, as illustrated in the flow chart below.

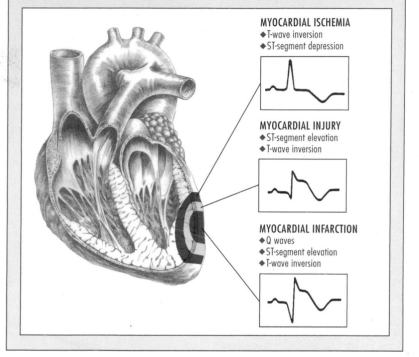

MYOCARDIAL ISCHEMIA
◆ T-wave inversion
◆ ST-segment depression

MYOCARDIAL INJURY
◆ ST-segment elevation
◆ T-wave inversion

MYOCARDIAL INFARCTION
◆ Q waves
◆ ST-segment elevation
◆ T-wave inversion

The scar tissue that forms on the necrotic area inhibits contractility. When this occurs, the compensatory mechanisms (vascular constriction, increased heart rate, and renal retention of sodium and water) try to maintain cardiac output. Ventricular dilation may also occur in a process called *remodeling*. Functionally, an MI may cause reduced contractility with abnormal wall motion, altered left ventricular compliance, reduced stroke volume, reduced ejection fraction, and elevated left ventricular end-diastolic pressure.

SIGNS AND SYMPTOMS

Signs and symptoms of MI may include:
■ persistent, crushing substernal chest pain that may radiate to the left arm, jaw, neck, or shoulder blades caused by reduced oxygen supply to the myocardial cells; it may be described as heavy, squeezing, or crushing

AGE ALERT
Many older adults don't have chest pain with MI, but experience atypical symptoms, such as fatigue, dyspnea, falls, tingling of the extremities, nau-

Pinpointing myocardial infarction

Depending on the location, ischemia or infarction causes changes in specific electrocardiographic leads.

TYPES OF MYOCARDIAL INFARCTION	LEADS
Inferior	II, III, aV$_F$
Anterior	V$_3$, V$_4$
Septal	V$_1$, V$_2$
Lateral	I, aV$_L$, V$_5$, V$_6$
Anterolateral	I, aV$_L$, V$_3$ to V$_6$
Posterior	V$_1$ or V$_2$
Right ventricular	V$_{1R}$ to V$_{4R}$

sea, vomiting, weakness, syncope, and confusion.
■ cool extremities, perspiration, anxiety, and restlessness from the release of catecholamines
■ blood pressure and pulse initially elevated as a result of sympathetic nervous system activation (If cardiac output is reduced, blood pressure may fall. Bradycardia may be associated with conduction disturbances, particularly with damage to the inferior wall of the left ventricle.)
■ fatigue and weakness caused by reduced perfusion to skeletal muscles
■ nausea and vomiting as a result of reflex stimulation of vomiting centers by pain fibers or from vasovagal reflexes
■ shortness of breath and crackles reflecting heart failure
■ low-grade temperature in the days after acute MI caused by the inflammatory response

■ jugular vein distention reflecting right ventricular dysfunction and pulmonary congestion
■ S$_3$ and S$_4$ reflecting ventricular dysfunction
■ loud holosystolic murmur in apex, possibly caused by papillary muscle rupture
■ reduced urine output secondary to reduced renal perfusion and increased aldosterone and antidiuretic hormone.

COMPLICATIONS
Complications of MI include:
■ arrhythmias
■ cardiogenic shock
■ heart failure causing pulmonary edema
■ pericarditis
■ rupture of the atrial or ventricular septum, ventricular wall, or valves
■ mural thrombi causing cerebral or pulmonary emboli
■ ventricular aneurysms
■ myocardial rupture
■ extensions of the original infarction.

DIAGNOSIS
These tests help diagnose an MI:
■ Serial 12-lead electrocardiogram (ECG) may reveal characteristic changes, such as serial ST-segment depression in non-Q-wave MI (a more limited area of damage insufficient to cause changes in the pattern of ventricular depolarization) and ST-segment elevation in Q-wave MI (a larger area of damage, which causes permanent change in the pattern of ventricular depolarization). An ECG can also identify the location of MI, arrhythmias, hypertrophy, and pericarditis. (See *Pinpointing myocardial infarction.*)
■ Serial cardiac enzymes and proteins may show a characteristic rise and fall, specifically CK-MB, the proteins troponin T and I, and myoglobin to confirm the diagnosis of MI. (See *Release of cardiac enzymes and proteins,* page 138.)
■ Laboratory testing may reveal elevated white blood cell count, C-reactive protein level, and erythrocyte sedimentation rate caused by inflammation; and increased glucose levels following the release of catecholamines.

■ Echocardiography may show ventricular wall motion abnormalities and may detect septal or papillary muscle rupture.

■ Chest X-rays may show left-sided heart failure or cardiomegaly caused by ventricular dilation.

■ Nuclear imaging scanning using sestamibi, thallium-201, and technetium-99m can be used to identify areas of infarction and viable muscle cells.

■ Cardiac catheterization may be used to identify the involved coronary artery as well as to provide information on ventricular function and pressures and volumes within the heart.

TREATMENT

Treatment of an MI typically involves following the treatment guidelines recommended by the American College of Cardiology/American Heart Association (ACC/AHA) Task Force on Practice Guidelines. These include:

■ assessment of the patient with chest pain in the emergency department within 10 minutes of symptom onset because at least 50% of deaths take place within 1 hour of the onset of symptoms (Moreover, thrombolytic therapy is most effective when started within the first 3 hours after the onset of symptoms.)

■ oxygen by nasal cannula for 2 to 3 hours to increase blood oxygenation (see *Treating myocardial infarction,* pages 184 and 185)

■ nitroglycerin sublingually or I.V. to relieve chest pain, unless systolic blood pressure is less than 90 mm Hg or heart rate is less than 50 or greater than 100 beats/minute

■ morphine or meperidine for analgesia because pain stimulates the sympathetic nervous system, leading to an increase in heart rate and vasoconstriction

■ aspirin every day indefinitely, to inhibit platelet aggregation

■ continuous cardiac monitoring to detect arrhythmias and ischemia

■ I.V. fibrinolytic therapy for the patient with chest pain of at least 30 minutes' duration who reaches the hospital within 12 hours of the onset of symptoms (unless contraindications exist) and whose ECG shows new left bundle-branch block (LBBB) or ST-segment elevation of at least 1 to 2 mm in two or more ECG leads (However, reperfusion therapy is most beneficial within 3 hours after symptoms start.)

■ I.V. heparin for the patient who has received fibrinolytic therapy to increase the chances of patency in the affected coronary artery

■ percutaneous transluminal coronary angioplasty (PTCA), which is superior to fibrinolytic therapy if it can be performed in a timely manner in a facility with personnel skilled in the procedure

■ glycoprotein IIb/IIIa receptor blocking agents, which strongly inhibit platelet aggregation (They're indicated as adjunct therapy with PTCA in acute ST-segment elevation MI and as primary therapy in non-ST-segment elevation MI; use with fibrinolytic agents controversial.)

■ limitation of physical activity for the first 12 hours to reduce cardiac workload, thereby limiting the area of necrosis

■ keeping atropine, amiodarone, transcutaneous pacing patches or a transvenous pacemaker, a defibrillator, and epinephrine readily available to treat arrhythmias (The ACC/AHA doesn't recommend the prophylactic use of antiarrhythmic drugs during first 24 hours.)

■ I.V. nitroglycerin for 24 to 48 hours in the patient without hypotension, bradycardia, or excessive tachycardia to reduce afterload and preload and relieve chest pain

■ early I.V. beta-adrenergic blockers to the patient with an evolving acute MI followed by oral therapy, as long as there are no contraindications, to reduce heart rate and myocardial contractile force, thereby reducing myocardial oxygen requirements

■ angiotensin-converting enzyme inhibitors in the patient with an evolving MI with ST-segment elevation or LBBB, but without hypotension or other contraindications, to reduce afterload and preload and prevent remodeling

■ magnesium sulfate for 24 hours to correct hypomagnesemia, if needed

■ angiography and possible percutaneous or surgical revascularization for the patien

DISRUPTING DISEASE
Treating myocardial infarction

This chart shows how treatments can be applied to myocardial infarction at various stages of its development.

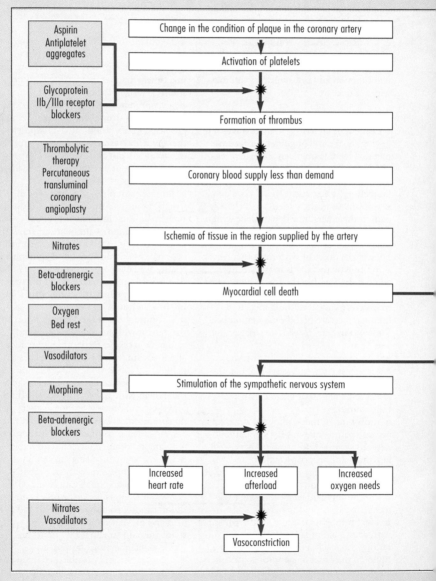

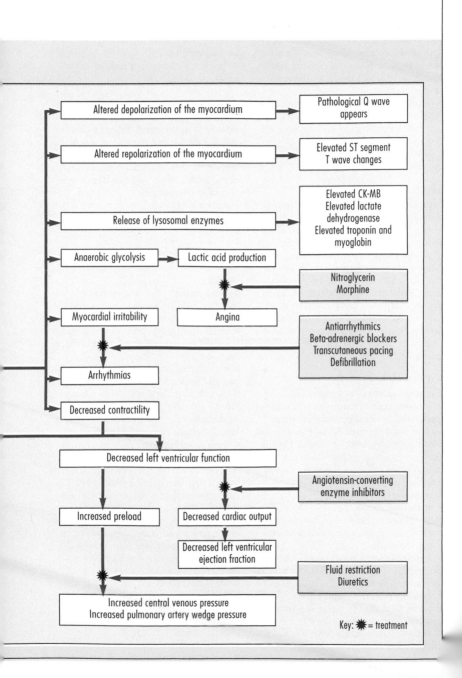

with spontaneous or provoked myocardial ischemia following an acute MI
- exercise testing before discharge to determine the adequacy of medical therapy and to obtain baseline information for an appropriate exercise prescription (It can also determine functional capacity and stratify the patient's risk of a subsequent cardiac event.)
- cardiac risk modification program of weight control; a low-fat, low-cholesterol diet; smoking cessation; and regular exercise to reduce cardiac risk
- lipid-lowering agents, as indicated by the fasting lipid profile.

Myocarditis

Myocarditis is focal or diffuse inflammation of the cardiac muscle (myocardium). It may be acute or chronic and can occur at any age. In many cases, myocarditis fails to produce specific cardiovascular symptoms or electrocardiogram (ECG) abnormalities, and recovery is usually spontaneous without residual defects. Occasionally, myocarditis is complicated by heart failure; in some cases, it leads to cardiomyopathy. Rarely, it can produce fulminant fatal heart failure caused by diffuse myocarditis.

CAUSES

Common causes of myocarditis include:
- viral infections (most common cause in the United States and western Europe), such as coxsackievirus A and B strains and, possibly, poliomyelitis, influenza, Epstein-Barr virus, human immunodeficiency virus, cytomegalovirus, measles, mumps, rubeola, rubella, and adenoviruses and echoviruses
- bacterial infections, such as diphtheria, tuberculosis, typhoid fever, tetanus, and staphylococcal, pneumococcal, and gonococcal infections
- hypersensitive immune reactions, including acute rheumatic fever and postcardiotomy syndrome
- radiation therapy — large doses of radiation to the chest in treating lung or breast cancer
- toxins (such as lead, chemicals, and cocaine) and chronic alcoholism
- parasitic infections, especially South American trypanosomiasis (Chagas' disease) in infants and immunosuppressed adults; also, toxoplasmosis
- fungal infections, including candidiasis and aspergillosis
- helminthic infections such as trichinosis.

PATHOPHYSIOLOGY

Damage to the myocardium occurs when an infectious organism triggers an autoimmune, cellular, and humoral reaction. The resulting inflammation may lead to hypertrophy, fibrosis, and inflammatory changes of the myocardium and conduction system. The heart muscle weakens and contractility is reduced. The heart muscle becomes flabby and dilated and pinpoint hemorrhages may develop.

SIGNS AND SYMPTOMS

Signs and symptoms of myocarditis may include:
- nonspecific symptoms, such as fatigue, dyspnea, palpitations, and fever caused by systemic infection
- mild, continuous pressure or soreness in the chest (occasionally), related to inflammation
- tachycardia from a compensatory sympathetic response
- S_3 and S_4 gallops as a result of heart failure
- murmur of mitral insufficiency may be heard, if papillary muscles involved
- pericardial friction rub, if pericarditis exists
- if myofibril degeneration occurs, it may lead to right-sided and left-sided heart failure, with cardiomegaly, jugular vein distention, dyspnea, edema, pulmonary congestion, persistent fever with resting or exertional tachycardia disproportionate to the degree of fever, and supraventricular and ventricular arrhythmias.

COMPLICATIONS

Complications of myocarditis include:
- recurrence of myocarditis
- chronic valvulitis (when it results from rheumatic fever)
- dilated cardiomyopathy
- arrhythmias and sudden death

- heart failure
- pericarditis
- ruptured myocardial aneurysm
- thromboembolism.

DIAGNOSIS

History reveals recent febrile upper respiratory infection. These tests help confirm the diagnosis of myocarditis:

- Laboratory testing may reveal elevated levels of creatine kinase (CK), CK-MB, troponin I, troponin T, aspartate aminotransferase, and lactate dehydrogenase. Also, inflammation and infection can cause elevated white blood cell count and erythrocyte sedimentation rate.
- Antibody titers may be elevated such as antistreptolysin-O titer in rheumatic fever.
- ECG may reveal diffuse ST-segment and T-wave abnormalities, conduction defects (prolonged PR interval, bundle branch block, or complete heart block), supraventricular arrhythmias, and ventricular extrasystoles.
- Chest X-rays may show an enlarged heart and pulmonary vascular congestion.
- Echocardiography may demonstrate some degree of left ventricular dysfunction.
- Radionuclide scanning may identify inflammatory and necrotic changes characteristic of myocarditis.
- Laboratory cultures of stool, throat, and body fluids may identify bacterial or viral causes of infection.
- Endomyocardial biopsy may confirm the diagnosis. A negative biopsy result doesn't exclude the diagnosis.

TREATMENT

Correction of myocarditis may involve:

- antibiotics to treat bacterial infections
- antipyretics to reduce fever and decrease stress on the heart
- bed rest to reduce oxygen demands and the heart's workload
- restricted activity to minimize myocardial oxygen consumption, supplemental oxygen therapy, sodium restriction and diuretics to decrease fluid retention, angiotensin-converting enzyme inhibitors, and digoxin to increase myocardial contractility for patients with heart failure

CLINICAL ALERT
Administer digoxin cautiously because some patients may show a paradoxical sensitivity even to small doses.

- antiarrhythmic drugs, such as quinidine or procainamide, to treat arrhythmias

CLINICAL ALERT
Use antiarrhythmic drugs cautiously because these drugs may depress myocardial contractility. A temporary pacemaker may be inserted if complete atrioventricular block occurs.

- anticoagulation to prevent thromboembolism
- corticosteroids and immunosuppressants, although controversial, to combat life-threatening complications such as intractable heart failure
- nonsteroidal anti-inflammatory drugs are contraindicated during the acute phase (first 2 weeks) because they increase myocardial damage
- cardiac assist devices or transplantation as a last resort in severe cases that resist treatment.

Patent ductus arteriosus

The ductus arteriosus is a fetal blood vessel that connects the pulmonary artery to the descending aorta, just distal to the left subclavian artery. Normally, the ductus closes within days to weeks after birth. In patent ductus arteriosus (PDA), the lumen of the ductus remains open after birth. This creates a left-to-right shunt of blood from the aorta to the pulmonary artery and results in recirculation of arterial blood through the lungs. Thus, it's considered a congenital heart defect associated with increased pulmonary blood flow. Initially, PDA may produce no clinical effects, but over time it can precipitate pulmonary vascular disease, causing symptoms to appear by age 40. PDA affects twice as many females as males and is the most common acyanotic congenital heart defect found in adults.

The prognosis is good if the shunt is small or surgical repair is effective. Otherwise, PDA may advance to intractable heart failure, which may be fatal.

CAUSES

PDA is associated with:

■ premature birth, probably as a result of abnormalities in oxygenation or the relaxant action of prostaglandin E, which prevents ductal spasm and contracture necessary for closure

■ rubella syndrome
■ coarctation of the aorta
■ ventricular septal defect
■ pulmonary and aortic stenosis
■ living at high altitudes.

PATHOPHYSIOLOGY

The ductus arteriosus normally closes as prostaglandin levels from the placenta fall and oxygen levels rise. This process should begin as soon as the neonate takes its first breath, but may take as long as 3 months in some children.

In PDA, relative resistances in pulmonary and systemic vasculature and the size of the ductus determine the quantity of blood that's shunted from left to right. Because of increased aortic pressure, oxygenated blood is shunted from the aorta through the ductus arteriosus to the pulmonary artery. The blood returns to the left side of the heart and is pumped out to the aorta once more.

The left atrium and left ventricle must accommodate the increased pulmonary venous return, increasing filling pressure and workload on the left side of the heart and causing left ventricular hypertrophy and possibly heart failure. In the final stages of untreated PDA, the left-to-right shunt leads to chronic pulmonary artery hypertension that becomes fixed and unreactive. This causes the shunt to reverse so that unoxygenated blood enters systemic circulation, causing cyanosis.

SIGNS AND SYMPTOMS

Signs and symptoms of PDA may include:

■ respiratory distress with signs of heart failure in infants, especially those who are premature, from the tremendous volume of blood shunted to the lungs through a patent ductus and the increased workload on the left side of the heart

■ classic machinery murmur (Gibson murmur), a continuous murmur heard throughout systole and diastole in older children and adults from shunting of blood from the aorta to the pulmonary artery throughout systole and diastole (It's best heard at the base of the heart, at the second left intercostal space under the left clavicle. The murmur may obscure S_2. However, in a right-to-left shunt, this murmur may be absent.)

■ thrill palpated at the left sternal border caused by the shunting of blood from the aorta to the pulmonary artery

■ prominent left ventricular impulse from left ventricular hypertrophy

■ bounding peripheral pulses (Corrigan's pulse) caused by the high-flow state

■ widened pulse pressure because of an elevated systolic blood pressure and, primarily, a drop in diastolic blood pressure as blood is shunted through the PDA, thus reducing peripheral resistance

■ slow motor development caused by heart failure

■ failure to thrive as a result of heart failure

■ fatigue and dyspnea on exertion, which may develop in adults with undetected PDA.

COMPLICATIONS

Possible complications of PDA may include:

■ infective endocarditis
■ heart failure
■ recurrent pneumonia.

DIAGNOSIS

These tests help diagnose PDA:

■ Chest X-rays may show increased pulmonary vascular markings, prominent pulmonary arteries, and enlargement of the left ventricle and aorta.

■ Electrocardiogram may be normal or may indicate left atrial or ventricular hypertrophy and, in pulmonary vascular disease, biventricular hypertrophy.

■ Echocardiography detects and estimates the size of a PDA. It also reveals an enlarged left atrium and left ventricle, or right ventricular hypertrophy from pulmonary vascular disease.

■ Cardiac catheterization shows higher pulmonary arterial oxygen content than right ventricular content because of the influx of aortic blood. Increased pulmonary artery pressure indicates a large shunt or, if it exceeds systemic arterial pressure, severe pulmonary vascular disease. Cardiac catheterization allows for the calculation of blood volume crossing the ductus, and can rule out associated cardiac defects. Injection of a contrast agent can conclusively demonstrate PDA.

TREATMENT
Correction of PDA may involve:
- surgery to ligate the ductus if medical management can't control heart failure (Asymptomatic infants with PDA don't require immediate treatment. If symptoms are mild, surgical ligation of the PDA is usually delayed until age 1.)
- indomethacin (a prostaglandin inhibitor) to induce ductus spasm and closure in premature infants
- prophylactic antibiotics to protect against infective endocarditis
- treatment of heart failure with fluid restriction, diuretics, and digoxin
- other therapy, including cardiac catheterization, to deposit a plug or umbrella in the ductus to stop shunting.

Pericarditis
Pericarditis is an inflammation of the pericardium — the fibroserous sac that envelops, supports, and protects the heart. It occurs in acute and chronic forms. Acute pericarditis can be fibrinous or effusive, with purulent, serous, or hemorrhagic exudate. Chronic constrictive pericarditis is characterized by dense fibrous pericardial thickening. The prognosis depends on the underlying cause, but is generally good in acute pericarditis, unless constriction occurs.

CAUSES
Common causes of pericarditis include:
- bacterial, fungal, or viral infection (infectious pericarditis)
- neoplasms (primary, or metastases from lungs, breasts, or other organs)
- high-dose radiation to the chest
- uremia
- hypersensitivity or autoimmune disease, such as acute rheumatic fever (most common cause of pericarditis in children), systemic lupus erythematosus, and rheumatoid arthritis
- previous cardiac injury, such as myocardial infarction (Dressler's syndrome), trauma, or surgery (postcardiotomy syndrome), that leaves the pericardium intact but causes blood to leak into the pericardial cavity
- drugs, such as hydralazine or procainamide
- idiopathic factors (most common in acute pericarditis)
- aortic aneurysm with pericardial leakage (less common)
- myxedema with cholesterol deposits in the pericardium (less common).

PATHOPHYSIOLOGY
Pericardial tissue damaged by bacteria or other substances results in the release of chemical mediators of inflammation (prostaglandins, histamines, bradykinins, and serotonin) into the surrounding tissue, thereby initiating the inflammatory process. Friction occurs as the inflamed pericardial layers rub against each other. Histamines and other chemical mediators dilate vessels and increase vessel permeability. Vessel walls then leak fluids and protein (including fibrinogen) into tissues, causing extracellular edema. Macrophages already present in the tissue begin to phagocytize the invading bacteria and are joined by neutrophils and monocytes. After several days, the area fills with an exudate composed of necrotic tissue and dead and dying bacteria, neutrophils, and macrophages. Eventually, the contents of the cavity autolyze and are gradually reabsorbed into healthy tissue.

A pericardial effusion develops if fluid accumulates in the pericardial cavity. Cardiac tamponade results when fluid accumulates rapidly in the pericardial space, compressing the heart and preventing it from filling during diastole and resulting in a drop in cardiac output. (See "Cardiac tamponade," page 152.)

Chronic constrictive pericarditis develops if the pericardium becomes thick and stiff from chronic or recurrent pericarditis, encasing the heart in a stiff shell and preventing it from properly filling during diastole. This causes an increase in left- and right-sided filling pressures, leading to a drop in stroke volume and cardiac output.

SIGNS AND SYMPTOMS

Signs and symptoms of pericarditis may include:

■ pericardial friction rub caused by the roughened pericardial membranes rubbing against one another (Although rub may be heard intermittently, it's best heard when the patient leans forward and exhales.)

■ sharp and typically sudden pain, usually starting over the sternum and radiating to the neck (especially the left trapezius ridge), shoulders, back, and arms caused by inflammation and irritation of the pericardial membranes (pain is usually pleuritic, increasing with deep inspiration and decreasing when the patient sits up and leans forward, pulling the heart away from the diaphragmatic pleurae of the lungs)

■ shallow, rapid respirations to reduce pleuritic pain

■ mild fever caused by the inflammatory process

■ dyspnea, orthopnea, and tachycardia as well as other signs of heart failure may occur as fluid builds up in the pericardial space, causing pericardial effusion, a major complication of acute pericarditis

■ muffled and distant heart sounds from fluid buildup

■ pallor, clammy skin, hypotension, pulsus paradoxus, neck vein distention and, eventually, cardiovascular collapse may occur with the rapid fluid accumulation of cardiac tamponade

■ fluid retention, ascites, hepatomegaly, jugular vein distention, and other signs of chronic right-sided heart failure may occur with chronic constrictive pericarditis as the systemic venous pressure gradually increases

■ pericardial knock in early diastole along the left sternal border produced by restricted ventricular filling

■ Kussmaul's sign, increased jugular venous distention on inspiration, caused by restricted right-sided filling.

COMPLICATIONS

Pericardial effusion is the major complication of acute pericarditis. If fluid accumulates rapidly, cardiac tamponade may oc-

cur. If the pericardium doesn't heal properly after an acute episode, scarring around the heart may occur, leading to impaired diastolic filling of the ventricles.

DIAGNOSIS

These tests help diagnose pericarditis:

■ Electrocardiography may reveal diffuse ST-segment elevation in the limb leads and most precordial leads that reflects the inflammatory process. Downsloping PR segments and upright T waves are present in most leads. QRS segments may be diminished when pericardial effusion exists. Arrhythmias, such as atrial fibrillation and sinus arrhythmias, may occur. In chronic constrictive pericarditis, there may be low-voltage QRS complexes, T-wave inversion or flattening, and P mitrale (wide P waves) in leads I, II, and V_6.

■ Laboratory testing may reveal an elevated erythrocyte sedimentation rate as a result of the inflammatory process or a normal or elevated white blood cell count, especially in infectious pericarditis; blood urea nitrogen may detect uremia as a cause of pericarditis.

■ Blood cultures may identify an infectious cause.

■ Antistreptolysin-O titers may be positive if pericarditis is caused by rheumatic fever.

■ Purified protein derivative skin test may be positive if pericarditis is caused by tuberculosis.

■ Echocardiography may show an echo-free space between the ventricular wall and the pericardium and reduced pumping action of the heart.

■ Chest X-rays may be normal with acute pericarditis. The cardiac silhouette may be enlarged with a water bottle shape caused by fluid accumulation if pleural effusion is present.

TREATMENT

Correcting pericarditis typically involves:

■ bed rest as long as fever and pain persist, to reduce metabolic needs

■ treatment of the underlying cause, if it can be identified

■ nonsteroidal anti-inflammatory drugs (NSAIDs), such as aspirin and indo-

methacin, to relieve pain and reduce inflammation
- corticosteroids, if NSAIDs are ineffective and no infection exists (Corticosteroids must be administered cautiously because episodes may recur when therapy is discontinued.)
- antibacterial, antifungal, or antiviral therapy if an infectious cause is suspected
- pericardiocentesis to remove excess fluid from the pericardial space
- partial pericardectomy, for recurrent pericarditis, to create a window that allows fluid to drain into the pleural space
- total pericardectomy, for constrictive pericarditis, to permit adequate filling and contraction of the heart
- idiopathic pericarditis may be benign and self-limiting.

Raynaud's disease

Raynaud's disease is one of several primary arteriospastic disorders characterized by episodic vasospasm in the small peripheral arteries and arterioles, precipitated by exposure to cold or stress. This condition occurs bilaterally and usually affects the hands or, less commonly, the feet. Raynaud's disease is most prevalent in females, particularly between puberty and age 40. It's a benign condition, requiring no specific treatment and causing no serious sequelae.

Raynaud's phenomenon, however, a condition usually associated with several connective disorders — such as scleroderma, systemic lupus erythematosus (SLE), or polymyositis — has a progressive course, leading to ischemia, gangrene, and amputation. Distinguishing between the two disorders is difficult because some patients who experience mild symptoms of Raynaud's disease for several years may later develop overt connective tissue disease, especially scleroderma.

CAUSES
Although family history is a risk factor, the cause of this disorder is unknown.

Raynaud's phenomenon may develop as a result of:
- connective tissue disorders, such as scleroderma, rheumatoid arthritis, SLE, or polymyositis

- pulmonary hypertension
- thoracic outlet syndrome
- arterio-occlusive disease
- myxedema
- trauma
- serum sickness
- exposure to heavy metals
- previous damage from cold exposure
- long-term exposure to cold, vibrating machinery (such as operating a jackhammer), or pressure to the fingertips (such as in typists and pianists).

PATHOPHYSIOLOGY
Although the cause is unknown, several theories account for reduced digital blood flow, including:
- intrinsic vascular wall hyperactivity to cold
- increased vasomotor tone from sympathetic stimulation
- antigen-antibody immune response (the most likely theory because abnormal immunologic test results accompany Raynaud's phenomenon).

SIGNS AND SYMPTOMS
Signs and symptoms of Raynaud's disease may include:
- blanching of the fingers bilaterally after exposure to cold or stress as vasoconstriction or vasospasm reduces blood flow (This is followed by cyanosis caused by increased oxygen extraction resulting from sluggish blood flow. As the spasm resolves, the fingers turn red as blood rushes back into the arterioles.)
- cold and numbness, possibly occurring during the vasoconstrictive phase because of ischemia
- throbbing, aching pain, swelling, and tingling, possibly occurring during the hyperemic phase
- trophic changes, such as sclerodactyly, ulcerations, or chronic paronychia, possibly occurring as a result of ischemia in long-standing disease.

COMPLICATIONS
Cutaneous gangrene may occur as a result of prolonged ischemia, necessitating amputation of one or more digits (although extremely rare).

DIAGNOSIS

These tests help diagnose Raynaud's disease:

▪ Clinical criteria include skin color changes induced by cold or stress; bilateral involvement; absence of gangrene or, if present, minimal cutaneous gangrene; normal arterial pulses; and patient history of symptoms for at least 2 years.

▪ Antinuclear antibody (ANA) titer is used to identify autoimmune disease as an underlying cause of Raynaud's phenomenon; further tests must be performed if ANA titer is abnormal.

▪ Arteriography rules out arterial occlusive disease.

▪ Doppler ultrasonography may show reduced blood flow if symptoms result from arterial occlusive disease.

TREATMENT

Treatment of this disorder typically involves:

▪ teaching the patient to avoid triggers, such as cold and mechanical or chemical injury

▪ encouraging the patient to stop smoking and avoid decongestants and caffeine to reduce vasoconstriction

▪ keeping fingers and toes warm to reduce vasoconstriction

▪ calcium channel blockers, such as nifedipine, diltiazem, and nicardipine, to produce vasodilation and prevent vasospasm

▪ adrenergic blockers, such as phenoxybenzamine or reserpine, which may improve blood flow to fingers or toes

▪ biofeedback and relaxation exercises to reduce stress and improve circulation

▪ sympathectomy to prevent ischemic ulcers by promoting vasodilation (necessary in less than 25% of patients)

▪ amputation, if ischemia causes ulceration and gangrene.

Rheumatic fever and rheumatic heart disease

A systemic inflammatory disease of childhood, acute rheumatic fever develops after infection of the upper respiratory tract with group A beta-hemolytic streptococci. It mainly involves the heart, joints, central nervous system, skin, and subcutaneous tissues and commonly recurs. Rheumatic heart disease refers to the cardiac manifestations of rheumatic fever and includes pancarditis (myocarditis, pericarditis, and endocarditis) during the early acute phase and chronic valvular disease later. Cardiac involvement develops in up to 50% of patients.

Worldwide, 15 to 20 million new cases of rheumatic fever are reported each year. The disease typically occurs during cool, damp weather in the winter and early spring. In the United States, it's most common in the North.

Rheumatic fever tends to run in families, lending support to the existence of genetic predisposition. Environmental factors also seem to be significant in the development of the disorder. For example, in lower socioeconomic groups, the incidence is highest in children between ages 5 and 15, probably because of malnutrition and crowded living conditions.

Patients without carditis or with mild carditis have a good long-term prognosis. Severe pancarditis occasionally produces fatal heart failure during the acute phase. Of patients who survive this complication, about 20% die within 10 years. Antibiotic therapy has greatly reduced the mortality of rheumatic heart disease. Since 1950, the number of deaths in the United States from this disease had decreased by almost 75%.

CAUSES

Rheumatic fever is caused by group A beta-hemolytic streptococcal pharyngitis.

PATHOPHYSIOLOGY

Rheumatic fever appears to be a hypersensitivity reaction to group A beta-hemolytic streptococcal infection. Because very few persons (3%) with streptococcal infections contract rheumatic fever, altered host resistance must be involved in its development or recurrence. The antigens of group A streptococci bind to receptors in the heart, muscle, brain, and synovial joints, causing an autoimmune response. Because of a similarity between the antigens of the streptococcus bacteria and the antigens of the body's own cells, antibodies may attack healthy body cells by mistake.

Carditis may affect the endocardium, myocardium, or pericardium during the early acute phase. Later, the heart valves may be damaged, causing chronic valvular disease.

Pericarditis produces a serofibrinous effusion. Myocarditis produces characteristic lesions called Aschoff's bodies (fibrin deposits surrounded by necrosis) in the interstitial tissue of the heart as well as cellular swelling and fragmentation of interstitial collagen. These lesions lead to progressively fibrotic nodule and interstitial scar formation.

Endocarditis causes valve leaflet swelling, erosion along the lines of leaflet closure, and blood, platelet, and fibrin deposits, which form beadlike growths. Eventually, the valve leaflets become scarred, lose their elasticity, and begin to adhere to each other. Endocarditis strikes the mitral valve most commonly in females and the aortic valve in males. In both sexes, it occasionally affects the tricuspid valve and, rarely, the pulmonic valve.

SIGNS AND SYMPTOMS

The classic symptoms of rheumatic fever and rheumatic heart disease include:
- polyarthritis or migratory joint pain, caused by inflammation, occurring in most patients (Swelling, redness, and signs of effusion usually accompany such pain, which most commonly affects the knees, ankles, elbows, and hips.)
- erythema marginatum, a nonpruritic, macular, transient rash on the trunk or inner aspects of the upper arms or thighs, that gives rise to red lesions with blanched centers
- subcutaneous nodules — firm, movable, and nontender, about 3 mm to 2 cm in diameter, usually near tendons or bony prominences of joints, especially the elbows, knuckles, wrists, and knees secondary to inflammation (They commonly accompany carditis and may last a few days to several weeks.)
- chorea — rapid jerky movements — possibly developing up to 6 months after the original streptococcal infection. (Mild chorea may produce hyperirritability, a deterioration in handwriting, or inability to

concentrate. Severe chorea causes purposeless, nonrepetitive, involuntary muscle spasms; poor muscle coordination; and weakness.)

Other signs and symptoms of rheumatic fever and rheumatic heart disease include:
- a streptococcal infection a few days to 6 weeks earlier, occurring in 95% of those with rheumatic fever
- temperature of at least 100.4° F (38° C) from infection and inflammation
- a new mitral or aortic heart murmur, or a worsening murmur in a person with a preexisting murmur caused by carditis
- pericardial friction rub caused by inflamed pericardial membranes rubbing against one another, if pericarditis exists
- chest pain, typically pleuritic, from inflammation and irritation of the pericardial membranes (Pain may increase with deep inspiration and decrease when the patient sits up and leans forward, pulling the heart away from the diaphragmatic pleurae of the lungs.)
- dyspnea, tachypnea, nonproductive cough, bibasilar crackles, and edema from heart failure in severe rheumatic carditis.

COMPLICATIONS

Possible complications of rheumatic fever and rheumatic heart disease include:
- destruction of the mitral and aortic valves
- pancarditis (pericarditis, myocarditis, and endocarditis)
- heart failure.

DIAGNOSIS

These tests help diagnose rheumatic fever and rheumatic heart disease:
- Jones criteria revealing either two major criteria, or one major criterion and two minor criteria, plus evidence of a previous group A streptococcal infection, are necessary for diagnosis. (See *Jones criteria for diagnosing rheumatic fever,* page 194.)
- Laboratory testing may reveal an elevated white blood cell count and elevated erythrocyte sedimentation rate during the acute phase.
- Hemoglobin and hematocrit may show slight anemia from suppressed erythropoiesis during inflammation.

Jones criteria for diagnosing rheumatic fever

The Jones criteria are used to standardize the diagnosis of rheumatic fever. Diagnosis requires that the patient be identified with either two major criteria, or one major criterion and two minor criteria, plus evidence of a previous streptococcal infection.

MAJOR CRITERIA
◆ Carditis
◆ Migratory polyarthritis
◆ Sydenham chorea
◆ Subcutaneous nodules
◆ Erythema marginatum

MINOR CRITERIA
◆ Fever
◆ Arthralgia
◆ Elevated acute phase reactants
◆ Prolonged PR interval

■ C-reactive protein level may be abnormal, especially during the acute phase.
■ Cardiac enzyme levels may be increased in severe carditis.
■ Antistreptolysin-O titer may be elevated in 95% of patients within 2 months of onset.
■ Throat cultures may continue to show the presence of group A beta-hemolytic streptococci; however, these usually occur in small numbers.
■ Electrocardiogram may show changes that aren't diagnostic, but the PR interval is prolonged in 20% of patients.
■ Chest X-rays may show normal heart size or cardiomegaly, pericardial effusion, or heart failure.
■ Echocardiography can detect valvular damage and pericardial effusion and can measure chamber size and provide information on ventricular function.
■ Cardiac catheterization provides information on valvular damage and left ventricular function.

TREATMENT
Treatment of these disorders typically involves:
■ prompt treatment of all group A beta-hemolytic streptococcal pharyngitis with oral penicillin V or I.M. penicillin G benzathine, or erythromycin for patients with penicillin hypersensitivity
■ salicylates to relieve fever and pain and minimize joint swelling
■ corticosteroids if the patient has carditis or if salicylates fail to relieve pain and inflammation
■ strict bed rest for about 5 weeks for the patient with active carditis to reduce cardiac demands
■ bed rest, sodium restriction, angiotensin-converting enzyme inhibitors, digoxin, and diuretics to treat heart failure
■ corrective surgery, such as commissurotomy (separation of adherent, thickened valve leaflets of the mitral valve), valvuloplasty (inflation of a balloon within a valve), or valve replacement (with a prosthetic valve) for severe mitral or aortic valvular dysfunction that causes persistent heart failure
■ secondary prevention of rheumatic fever, which begins after the acute phase subsides with monthly I.M. injections of penicillin G benzathine or daily doses of oral penicillin V or sulfadiazine (Treatment usually continues for at least 5 years or until age 21, whichever is longer.)
■ prophylactic antibiotics for dental work and other invasive or surgical procedures to prevent endocarditis.

Shock
Shock isn't a disease, but rather a clinical syndrome leading to reduced tissue and organ perfusion and, eventually, organ dysfunction and failure. Shock can be classified into three major categories based on the precipitating factors: distributive (neurogenic, septic, and anaphylactic), cardiogenic, and hypovolemic shock. Even with treatment, shock has a high mortality rate after the body's compensatory mechanisms fail. (See *Types of shock.*)

Types of shock

DISTRIBUTIVE SHOCK

In distributive shock, vasodilation causes a state of hypovolemia.

◆ *Neurogenic shock.* A loss of sympathetic vasoconstrictor tone in the vascular smooth muscle and reduced autonomic function lead to widespread arterial and venous vasodilation. Venous return is reduced as blood pools in the venous system, leading to a drop in cardiac output and hypotension.

◆ *Septic shock.* An immune response is triggered when bacteria release endotoxins. In response, macrophages secrete tumor necrosis factor (TNF) and interleukins. These mediators, in turn, are responsible for an increased release of platelet-activating factor (PAF), prostaglandins, leukotrienes, thromboxane A_2, kinins, and complement. The consequences are vasodilation and vasoconstriction, increased capillary permeability, reduced systemic vascular resistance, microemboli, and an elevated cardiac output. Endotoxins also stimulate the release of histamine, further increasing capillary permeability. Moreover, myocardial depressant factor, TNF, PAF, and other factors depress myocardial function. Cardiac output falls, resulting in multisystem organ failure.

◆ *Anaphylactic shock.* Triggered by an allergic reaction, anaphylactic shock occurs when a person is exposed to an antigen to which he has already been sensitized. Exposure results in the production of specific immunoglobulin (Ig) E antibodies by plasma cells that bind to membrane receptors on mast cells and basophils. On reexposure, the antigen binds to IgE antibodies or cross-linked IgE receptors, triggering the release of powerful chemical mediators from mast cells. IgG or IgM enters into the reaction and activates the release of complement factors. At the same time, the chemical mediators bradykinin and leukotrienes induce vascular collapse by stimulating contraction of certain groups of smooth muscles and by increasing vascular permeability, leading to decreased peripheral resistance and plasma leakage into the extravascular tissues, thereby reducing blood volume and causing hypotension, hypovolemic shock, and cardiac dysfunction. Bronchospasm and laryngeal edema also occur.

CARDIOGENIC SHOCK

In cardiogenic shock, the left ventricle can't maintain an adequate cardiac output. Compensatory mechanisms increase heart rate, strengthen myocardial contractions, promote sodium and water retention, and cause selective vasoconstriction. However, these mechanisms increase myocardial workload and oxygen consumption, which reduces the heart's ability to pump blood, especially if the patient has myocardial ischemia. Consequently, blood backs up, resulting in pulmonary edema. Eventually, cardiac output falls and multisystem organ failure develops as the compensatory mechanisms fail to maintain perfusion.

HYPOVOLEMIC SHOCK

When fluid is lost from the intravascular space through external losses or the shift of fluid from the vessels to the interstitial or intracellular spaces, venous return to the heart is reduced. This reduction in preload decreases ventricular filling, leading to a drop in stroke volume. Then, cardiac output falls, causing reduced perfusion of the tissues and organs.

CAUSES

Causes of neurogenic shock may include:
- spinal anesthesia
- vasomotor center depression
- severe pain
- medications
- hypoglycemia.

Causes of septic shock may include:
- gram-negative bacteria (most common cause)
- gram-positive bacteria
- viruses, fungi, *Rickettsiae*, parasites, yeast, protozoa, or mycobacteria.

AGE ALERT
The immature immune system of neonates and infants and the weakened immune system of older adults, commonly accompanied by chronic illness, make these populations more susceptible to septic shock.

Causes of anaphylactic shock may include:
- medications, vaccines
- venom
- foods
- contrast media
- ABO-incompatible blood.

Causes of cardiogenic shock may include:
- myocardial infarction (MI) (most common cause)
- heart failure
- cardiomyopathy
- arrhythmias
- obstruction
- pericardial tamponade
- tension pneumothorax
- pulmonary embolism.

Causes of hypovolemic shock may include:
- blood loss (most common cause)
- GI fluid loss
- burns
- renal loss (diabetic ketoacidosis, diabetes insipidus, adrenal insufficiency)
- fluid shifts
- ascites
- peritonitis
- hemothorax.

PATHOPHYSIOLOGY
There are three basic stages common to each type of shock: compensatory, progressive, and irreversible, or refractory, stages.

Compensatory stage. When arterial pressure and tissue perfusion are reduced, compensatory mechanisms are activated to maintain perfusion to the heart and brain. As the baroreceptors in the carotid sinus and aortic arch sense a decrease in blood pressure, epinephrine and norepinephrine are secreted to increase peripheral resistance, blood pressure, and myocardial contractility. Reduced blood flow to the kidney activates the renin-angiotensin-al-

dosterone system, causing vasoconstriction and sodium and water retention, leading to increased blood volume and venous return. As a result of these compensatory mechanisms, cardiac output and tissue perfusion are maintained.

Progressive stage. The progressive stage of shock begins as compensatory mechanisms fail to maintain cardiac output. Tissues become hypoxic because of poor perfusion. As cells switch to anaerobic metabolism, lactic acid builds up, producing metabolic acidosis. This acidotic state depresses myocardial function. Tissue hypoxia also promotes the release of endothelial mediators, which produce vasodilation and endothelial abnormalities, leading to venous pooling and increased capillary permeability. Sluggish blood flow increases the risk of disseminated intravascular coagulation (DIC).

Irreversible (refractory) stage. As the shock syndrome progresses, permanent organ damage occurs as compensatory mechanisms can no longer maintain cardiac output. Reduced perfusion damages cell membranes, lysosomal enzymes are released, and energy stores are depleted, possibly leading to cell death. As cells use anaerobic metabolism, lactic acid accumulates, increasing capillary permeability and the movement of fluid out of the vascular space. This loss of intravascular fluid further contributes to hypotension. Perfusion to the coronary arteries is reduced, causing myocardial depression and a further reduction in cardiac output. Eventually, circulatory and respiratory failure occur. Death is inevitable.

SIGNS AND SYMPTOMS
In the compensatory stage of shock, signs and symptoms may include:
- tachycardia and bounding pulse from sympathetic stimulation
- restlessness and irritability related to cerebral hypoxia
- tachypnea to compensate for hypoxia
- reduced urinary output resulting from vasoconstriction

- cool, pale skin from vasoconstriction; warm, dry skin in septic shock from vasodilation.

In the progressive stage of shock, signs and symptoms may include:
- hypotension as compensatory mechanisms begin to fail
- narrowed pulse pressure associated with reduced stroke volume; weak, rapid, thready pulse caused by decreased cardiac output; shallow respirations as the patient weakens; reduced urinary output as poor renal perfusion continues
- cold, clammy skin caused by vasoconstriction
- cyanosis related to hypoxia.

CLINICAL ALERT
Hypotension, an altered level of consciousness, and hyperventilation may be the only signs of septic shock in infants and elderly people.

In the irreversible stage, clinical findings may include:
- unconsciousness and absent reflexes caused by reduced cerebral perfusion, acid-base imbalance, or electrolyte abnormalities
- rapidly falling blood pressure as decompensation occurs
- weak pulse caused by reduced cardiac output
- slow, shallow, or Cheyne-Stokes respirations following from respiratory center depression
- anuria related to renal failure.

COMPLICATIONS
Possible complications of shock include:
- acute respiratory distress syndrome
- acute tubular necrosis
- DIC
- cerebral hypoxia
- death.

DIAGNOSIS
These tests help diagnose shock:
- Hematocrit may be reduced in hemorrhage or elevated in other types of shock caused by hypovolemia.
- Blood, urine, and sputum cultures may identify the organism responsible for septic shock.
- Coagulation studies may detect coagulopathy from DIC.

- Laboratory testing may reveal increased white blood cell count and erythrocyte sedimentation rate from injury and inflammation; elevated blood urea nitrogen and creatinine levels from reduced renal perfusion; lactate level may be increased because of anaerobic metabolism; and glucose level may be elevated in early stages of shock as the liver releases glycogen stores in response to sympathetic stimulation.
- Cardiac enzymes and proteins may be elevated, indicating MI as a cause of cardiogenic shock.
- Arterial blood gas analysis may reveal respiratory alkalosis in early shock associated with tachypnea, respiratory acidosis in later stages associated with respiratory depression, and metabolic acidosis in later stages resulting from anaerobic metabolism.
- Urine specific gravity may be high in response to effects of antidiuretic hormone.
- Chest X-rays may be normal in early stages; pulmonary congestion may be seen in later stages.
- Hemodynamic monitoring may reveal characteristic patterns of intracardiac pressures and cardiac output, which are used to guide fluid and drug management. (See *Putting hemodynamic monitoring to use,* page 198.)
- Electrocardiography determines the heart rate and detects arrhythmias, ischemic changes, and MI.
- Echocardiography determines left ventricular function and reveals valvular abnormalities.

TREATMENT
Correction of shock typically involves:
- identification and treatment of the underlying cause, if possible
- maintaining a patent airway; preparing for intubation and mechanical ventilation if the patient develops respiratory distress
- supplemental oxygen to increase oxygenation
- continuous cardiac monitoring to detect changes in heart rate and rhythm; administration of antiarrhythmics, as necessary
- initiating and maintaining at least two I.V. lines with large-gauge needles for fluid and drug administration

Putting hemodynamic monitoring to use

Hemodynamic monitoring provides information on intracardiac pressures and cardiac output. To understand intracardiac pressures, picture the cardiovascular system as a continuous loop with constantly changing pressure gradients that keep the blood moving.

RIGHT ATRIAL PRESSURE (RAP), OR CENTRAL VENOUS PRESSURE (CVP)

The RAP reflects right atrial, or right heart, function and end-diastolic pressure.
◆ Normal: 1 to 6 mm Hg (1.34 to 8 cm H_2O). (To convert mm Hg to cm H_2O, multiply mm Hg by 1.34)
◆ Elevated value suggests: right ventricular (RV) failure, volume overload, tricuspid valve stenosis or regurgitation, constrictive pericarditis, pulmonary hypertension, cardiac tamponade, or RV infarction.
◆ Low value suggests: reduced circulating blood volume.

RV PRESSURE

RV systolic pressure normally equals pulmonary artery systolic pressure, RV end-diastolic pressure, which equals RAP, reflects RV function.
◆ Normal: systolic, 15 to 25 mm Hg; diastolic, 0 to 8 mm Hg.
◆ Elevated value suggests: mitral stenosis or insufficiency, pulmonary disease, hypoxemia, constrictive pericarditis, chronic heart failure, atrial and ventricular septal defects, and patent ductus arteriosus.

PULMONARY ARTERY PRESSURE

Pulmonary artery systolic pressure reflects RV function and pulmonary circulation pressures. Pulmonary artery diastolic pressure reflects left ventricular (LV) pressures, specifically LV end-diastolic pressure.

◆ Normal: systolic, 15 to 25 mm Hg; diastolic, 8 to 15 mm Hg; mean, 10 to 20 mm Hg.
◆ Elevated value suggests: LV failure, increased pulmonary blood flow (left or right shunting, as in atrial or ventricular septal defects), mitral stenosis or insufficiency, and in any condition causing increased pulmonary arteriolar resistance.

PULMONARY ARTERY WEDGE PRESSURE (PAWP)

PAWP reflects left atrial and LV pressures unless the patient has mitral stenosis. Changes in PAWP reflect changes in LV filling pressure. The heart momentarily relaxes during diastole as it fills with blood from the pulmonary veins; this permits the pulmonary vasculature, left atrium, and left ventricle to act as a single chamber.
◆ Normal: mean pressure, 6 to 12 mm Hg.
◆ Elevated value suggests: LV failure, mitral stenosis or insufficiency, and pericardial tamponade.
◆ Low value suggests: hypovolemia.

LEFT ATRIAL PRESSURE

This value reflects LV end-diastolic pressure in patients without mitral valve disease.
◆ Normal: 6 to 12 mm Hg.

CARDIAC OUTPUT

Cardiac output is the amount of blood ejected by the heart each minute.
◆ Normal: 4 to 8 L; varies with a patient's weight, height, and body surface area. Adjusting the cardiac output to the patient's size yields a measurement called the cardiac index.

■ I.V. fluids, crystalloids, colloids, or blood products, as necessary, to maintain intravascular volume.
   Additional therapy for hypovolemic shock may include:

■ pneumatic antishock garment, which may be applied to control internal and external hemorrhage by direct pressure
■ fluids, such as normal saline or lactated Ringer's solution, initially, to restore filling pressures

packed red blood cells in hemorrhagic shock to restore blood loss and improve the blood's oxygen-carrying capacity.

Additional measures for cardiogenic shock may include:

- inotropic drugs, such as dopamine, dobutamine, inamrinone, and epinephrine, to increase heart contractility and cardiac output
- vasodilators, such as nitroglycerin or nitroprusside, given with a vasopressor to reduce the left ventricle's workload
- diuretics to reduce preload, if the patient has fluid volume overload
- intra-aortic balloon pump (IABP) therapy to reduce the work of the left ventricle by decreasing systemic vascular resistance (Diastolic pressure is increased, resulting in improved coronary artery perfusion.)
- thrombolytic therapy or coronary artery revascularization to restore coronary artery blood flow, if cardiogenic shock is caused by acute MI
- emergency surgery to repair papillary muscle rupture or ventricular septal defect, if either is the cause of cardiogenic shock
- ventricular assist device to assist the pumping action of the heart when IABP and drug therapy fail
- heart transplantation, which may be considered when other medical and surgical therapeutic measures fail.

Correction of septic shock may also include:

- antibiotic therapy to eradicate the causative organism
- inotropic and vasopressor drugs, such as dopamine, dobutamine, and norepinephrine, to improve perfusion and maintain blood pressure
- although still investigational, monoclonal antibodies to tumor necrosis factor, endotoxin, and interleukin-1, to counteract septic shock mediators.

Additional therapy for neurogenic shock may include:

- vasopressor drugs to raise blood pressure by vasoconstriction
- fluid replacement to maintain blood pressure and cardiac output.

Tetralogy of Fallot

Tetralogy of Fallot is a combination of four cardiac defects: ventricular septal defect (VSD), right ventricular outflow tract obstruction (pulmonic stenosis), right ventricular hypertrophy, and dextroposition of the aorta, with overriding of the VSD. It's considered a congenital heart defect associated with decreased pulmonary blood flow. Blood shunts from right to left through the VSD, allowing unoxygenated blood to mix with oxygenated blood resulting in cyanosis. This cyanotic heart defect sometimes coexists with other congenital, acyanotic, heart defects, such as patent ductus arteriosus or atrial septal defect. It accounts for about 10% of all congenital defects and occurs equally in males and females. Before surgical advances made correction possible, about one-third of affected children died in infancy.

CAUSES
The cause of tetralogy of Fallot is unknown, but may be associated with:
- fetal alcohol syndrome
- thalidomide use during pregnancy.

PATHOPHYSIOLOGY
In tetralogy of Fallot, unoxygenated venous blood returning to the right side of the heart may pass through the VSD to the left ventricle, bypassing the lungs, or it may enter the pulmonary artery, depending on the extent of the pulmonic stenosis. Rather than originating from the left ventricle, the aorta overrides both ventricles.

The VSD usually lies in the outflow tract of the right ventricle and is generally large enough to permit equalization of right and left ventricular pressures. However, the ratio of systemic vascular resistance to pulmonic stenosis affects the direction and magnitude of shunt flow across the VSD. Severe obstruction of right ventricular outflow produces a right-to-left shunt, causing decreased systemic arterial oxygen saturation, cyanosis, reduced pulmonary blood flow, and hypoplasia of the entire pulmonary vasculature. Right ventricular hypertrophy develops in response to the extra force needed to push blood into the stenotic pulmonary artery. Milder forms of pulmonic stenosis result in a left-to-right shunt or no shunt at all.

SIGNS AND SYMPTOMS

Signs and symptoms of tetralogy of Fallot may include:
- cyanosis, the hallmark of tetralogy of Fallot, caused by a right-to-left shunt
- cyanotic or "blue" spells (Tet spells), characterized by dyspnea; deep, sighing respirations; bradycardia; fainting; seizures; and loss of consciousness following exercise, crying, straining, infection, or fever (It may result from reduced oxygen to the brain because of increased right-to-left shunting, possibly caused by spasm of the right ventricular outflow tract, increased systemic venous return, or decreased systemic arterial resistance.)
- clubbing, diminished exercise tolerance, increasing dyspnea on exertion, growth retardation, and eating difficulties in older children from poor oxygenation
- squatting with shortness of breath to reduce venous return of unoxygenated blood from the legs and to increase systemic arterial resistance
- loud systolic murmur best heard along the left sternal border, which may diminish or obscure the pulmonic component of S_2
- continuous murmur of the ductus in a patient with a large patent ductus, which may obscure systolic murmur
- thrill at the left sternal border caused by abnormal blood flow through the heart
- obvious right ventricular impulse and prominent inferior sternum associated with right ventricular hypertrophy.

COMPLICATIONS

Possible complications of tetralogy of Fallot include:
- pulmonary thrombosis
- venous thrombosis
- cerebral embolism
- infective endocarditis
- risk of spontaneous abortion, premature birth, and low-birth-weight neonates born to women with tetralogy of Fallot.

DIAGNOSIS

These tests help diagnose tetralogy of Fallot:
- Chest X-rays may demonstrate decreased pulmonary vascular marking (depending on the severity of the pulmonary obstruction), an enlarged right ventricle, and a boot-shaped cardiac silhouette.
- Electrocardiogram shows right ventricular hypertrophy, right axis deviation and, possibly, right atrial hypertrophy.
- Echocardiography identifies septal overriding of the aorta, the VSD, and pulmonic stenosis and detects the hypertrophied walls of the right ventricle.
- Laboratory testing reveals diminished oxygen saturation and polycythemia (hematocrit may be more than 60%) if the cyanosis is severe and long-standing, predisposing the patient to thrombosis.
- Cardiac catheterization confirms the diagnosis by providing visualization of pulmonic stenosis, the VSD, and the overriding aorta and ruling out other cyanotic heart defects. This test also measures the degree of oxygen saturation in aortic blood.

TREATMENT

Tetralogy of Fallot may be managed by the following measures:
- a knee-chest position and administration of oxygen and morphine to improve oxygenation
- palliative surgery with a Blalock-Taussig procedure, which joins the subclavian artery to the pulmonary artery to enhance blood flow to the lungs to reduce hypoxia
- prophylactic antibiotics to prevent infective endocarditis or cerebral abscesses
- phlebotomy to reduce polycythemia
- corrective surgery to relieve pulmonic stenosis and close the VSD, directing left ventricular outflow to the aorta.

Transposition of the great arteries

Transposition of the great arteries is a congenital heart defect associated with mixed blood flow (previously called *cyanotic congenital heart defect*) in which the great arteries are reversed such that the aorta arises from the right ventricle and the pulmonary artery from the left ventricle, producing two noncommunicating circulatory systems (pulmonic and systemic). Transposition accounts for about 5% of all congenital heart defects and commonly coexists with other congenital heart defects, such as ventricular septal defect (VSD), VSD with pulmonic stenosis, atrial septal defect (ASD), and patent ductus arteriosus (PDA). It affects two to three times more males than females.

CAUSES
The cause of this disorder is unknown.

PATHOPHYSIOLOGY
Transposition of the great arteries results from faulty embryonic development. Oxygenated blood returning to the left side of the heart is carried back to the lungs by a transposed pulmonary artery. Unoxygenated blood returning to the right side of the heart is carried to the systemic circulation by a transposed aorta.

Communication between the pulmonic and systemic circulations is necessary for survival. In infants with isolated transposition, blood mixes only at the patent foramen ovale and at the PDA, resulting in slight mixing of unoxygenated systemic blood and oxygenated pulmonary blood. In infants with concurrent cardiac defects, greater mixing of blood occurs.

SIGNS AND SYMPTOMS
Signs and symptoms of this defect may include:
- cyanosis and tachypnea that worsens with crying within the first few hours after birth, when no other heart defects exist that allow mixing of systemic and pulmonary blood (Cyanosis may be minimized with associated defects, such as ASD, VSD, or PDA.)
- gallop rhythm, tachycardia, dyspnea, hepatomegaly, and cardiomegaly within days to weeks from heart failure
- loud S_2 because the anteriorly transposed aorta is directly behind the sternum
- murmurs of ASD, VSD, or PDA
- diminished exercise tolerance, fatigability, and finger clubbing from reduced oxygenation.

COMPLICATIONS
Transposition of the great arteries may be complicated by:
- heart failure

- infective endocarditis.

DIAGNOSIS
These tests help diagnose transposition of the great arteries:
- Chest X-rays are normal in the first days after birth. Within days to weeks, right atrial and right ventricular enlargement characteristically cause the heart to appear oblong. X-ray may also show increased pulmonary vascular markings, except when pulmonic stenosis exists.
- Electrocardiogram typically reveals right axis deviation and right ventricular hypertrophy, but may be normal in a neonate.
- Echocardiography demonstrates the reversed position of the aorta and pulmonary artery and records echoes from both semilunar valves simultaneously because of aortic valve displacement. It also detects other cardiac defects.
- Cardiac catheterization reveals decreased oxygen saturation in left ventricular blood and aortic blood; increased right atrial, right ventricular, and pulmonary artery oxygen saturation; and right ventricular systolic pressure equal to systemic pressure. Dye injection reveals the transposed vessels and the presence of other cardiac defects.
- Arterial blood gas analysis indicates hypoxia and secondary metabolic acidosis.

TREATMENT
Treatment of this disorder may involve:
- prostaglandin infusion to keep the ductus arteriosus patent until surgical correction
- atrial balloon septostomy (Rashkind procedure) during cardiac catheterization, if needed as a palliative measure until surgery can be performed (It enlarges the patent foramen ovale and thereby improves oxygenation and alleviates hypoxia by allowing greater mixing of blood from the pulmonary and systemic circulations.)
- digoxin and diuretics after atrial balloon septostomy to lessen heart failure until the infant is ready to withstand corrective surgery (usually between birth and age 1)
- surgery to correct transposition, although the procedure depends on the physiology of the defect.

Valvular heart disease

In valvular heart disease, three types of mechanical disruption can occur: stenosis, or narrowing, of the valve opening; incomplete closure of the valve; or valve prolapse.

CAUSES

The causes of valvular heart disease are varied and are different for each type of valve disorder. Valvular disorders in children and adolescents most commonly occur as a result of congenital heart defects. In adults, rheumatic heart disease is a common cause. (See *Types of valvular heart disease,* pages 204 to 207.)

PATHOPHYSIOLOGY

Pathophysiology of valvular heart disease varies according to the valve and the disorder.

Mitral insufficiency. An abnormality of the mitral leaflets, mitral annulus, chordae tendineae, papillary muscles, left atrium, or left ventricle can lead to mitral insufficiency. Blood from the left ventricle flows back into the left atrium during systole, causing the atrium to enlarge to accommodate the backflow. As a result, the left ventricle also dilates to accommodate the increased blood volume from the atrium and to compensate for diminishing cardiac output. Ventricular hypertrophy and increased end-diastolic pressure result in increased pulmonary artery pressure, eventually leading to left-sided and right-sided heart failure.

Mitral stenosis. Narrowing of the valve by valvular abnormalities, fibrosis, or calcification obstructs blood flow from the left atrium to the left ventricle. Consequently, left atrial volume and pressure rise and the chamber dilates. Greater resistance to blood flow causes pulmonary hypertension, right ventricular hypertrophy, and right-sided heart failure. Also, inadequate filling of the left ventricle produces low cardiac output.

Aortic insufficiency. Blood flows back into the left ventricle during diastole, causing fluid overload in the ventricle, which dilates and hypertrophies. The excess volume causes fluid overload in the left atrium and, finally, the pulmonary system. Left-sided heart failure and pulmonary edema eventually result.

Aortic stenosis. Increased left ventricular pressure tries to overcome the resistance of the narrowed valvular opening. The added workload increases the demand for oxygen, and diminished cardiac output causes poor coronary artery perfusion, ischemia of the left ventricle, and left-sided heart failure.

Pulmonic stenosis. Obstructed right ventricular outflow causes right ventricular hypertrophy, eventually resulting in right-sided heart failure.

SIGNS AND SYMPTOMS

The clinical manifestations vary according to the type of valvular defects. (See *Types of valvular heart disease,* pages 204 to 207, for specific clinical features of each valve disorder.)

COMPLICATIONS

Possible complications of valvular heart disease include:
- heart failure
- pulmonary edema
- thromboembolism
- endocarditis
- arrhythmias.

DIAGNOSIS

Diagnosis of valvular heart disease can be made through cardiac catheterization, chest X-rays, echocardiography, or electrocardiography. (See *Types of valvular heart disease,* pages 204 to 207.)

TREATMENT

Correcting this disorder typically involves:
- digoxin, a low-sodium diet, diuretics, vasodilators, and especially angiotensin-converting enzyme inhibitors to treat left-sided heart failure
- oxygen in acute situations, to increase oxygenation
- anticoagulants to prevent thrombus formation around diseased or replaced valves

- prophylactic antibiotics before and after surgery or dental care to prevent endocarditis
- nitroglycerin to relieve angina in conditions such as aortic stenosis
- beta-adrenergic blockers or digoxin to slow the ventricular rate in atrial fibrillation or atrial flutter
- cardioversion to convert atrial fibrillation to sinus rhythm
- open or closed commissurotomy to separate thick or adherent mitral valve leaflets
- balloon valvuloplasty to enlarge the orifice of a stenotic mitral, aortic, or pulmonic valve
- annuloplasty or valvuloplasty to reconstruct or repair the valve in mitral insufficiency
- valve replacement with a prosthetic valve for mitral and aortic valve disease.

Varicose veins

Varicose veins are dilated, tortuous veins, engorged with blood and resulting from improper venous valve function. They can be primary, originating in the superficial veins, or secondary, occurring in the deep veins.

Primary varicose veins tend to be familial and affect both legs; they're twice as common in females as in males. They account for about 90% of varicose veins; about 10% to 20% of people in the United States have primary varicose veins. Usually, secondary varicose veins occur in one leg. Both types are more common in middle adulthood.

Without treatment, varicose veins continue to enlarge. Although there's no cure, certain measures, such as walking and using compression stockings, can reduce symptoms. Surgery may remove varicose veins, but the condition can occur subsequently in other veins.

CAUSES

Primary varicose veins can result from:
- congenital weakness of the valves or venous wall
- conditions that produce prolonged venous stasis or increased intra-abdominal pressure, such as pregnancy, obesity, constipation, or wearing tight clothes

- occupations that necessitate standing for an extended period.

Secondary varicose veins can result from:
- deep vein thrombosis
- venous malformation
- arteriovenous fistulas
- trauma to the venous system
- occlusion.

PATHOPHYSIOLOGY

Veins are thin-walled, distensible vessels with valves that keep blood flowing in one direction. Any condition that weakens, destroys, or distends these valves allows blood backflow to the previous valve. If a valve can't hold the pooling blood, it can become incompetent, allowing even more blood to flow backward. As the volume of venous blood builds, pressure in the vein increases and the vein becomes distended. As the veins are stretched, their walls weaken and they lose their elasticity. As the veins enlarge, they become lumpy and tortuous. As hydrostatic pressure increases, plasma is forced out of the veins and into the surrounding tissues, resulting in edema.

People who stand for prolonged periods may also develop venous pooling because there's no muscular contraction in the legs to force blood back up to the heart. If the valves in the veins are too weak to hold the pooling blood, they begin to leak, allowing blood to flow backward.

SIGNS AND SYMPTOMS

Signs and symptoms of varicose veins may include:
- dilated, tortuous, purplish, ropelike veins, particularly in the calves, caused by venous pooling
- edema of the calves and ankles from deep vein incompetence
- leg heaviness that worsens in the evening and in warm weather; caused by venous pooling
- dull aching in the legs after prolonged standing or walking, which may be caused by tissue breakdown
- aching during menses as a result of increased fluid retention.

(Text continues on page 206.)

Types of valvular heart disease

CAUSES AND INCIDENCE	CLINICAL FINDINGS
Mitral stenosis ◆ Results from rheumatic fever (most common cause) or endocarditis ◆ Most common in females ◆ May be associated with other congenital anomalies	◆ Dyspnea on exertion, paroxysmal nocturnal dyspnea, orthopnea, weakness, fatigue, and palpitations ◆ Peripheral edema, jugular vein distention, ascites, and hepatomegaly (right ventricular failure) ◆ Crackles, atrial fibrillation, and signs of systemic emboli ◆ Auscultation revealing a loud S_1 or opening snap and a diastolic murmur at the apex
Mitral insufficiency ◆ Results from rheumatic fever, hypertrophic obstructive cardiomyopathy, mitral valve prolapse, myocardial infarction, severe left ventricular dilation or failure, or ruptured chordae tendineae ◆ Associated with other congenital anomalies such as transposition of the great arteries ◆ Rare in children without other congenital anomalies	◆ Orthopnea, dyspnea, fatigue, angina, and palpitations ◆ Peripheral edema, jugular vein distention, and hepatomegaly (right-sided heart failure) ◆ Tachycardia, crackles, and pulmonary edema ◆ Auscultation revealing a holosystolic murmur at apex, a possible split S_2, and an S_3
Aortic insufficiency ◆ Results from rheumatic fever, syphilis, hypertension, or endocarditis or may be idiopathic ◆ Associated with Marfan syndrome ◆ Most common in males ◆ Associated with ventricular septal defect, even after surgical closure	◆ Dyspnea, cough, fatigue, palpitations, angina, and syncope ◆ Pulmonary congestion, left-sided heart failure, and "pulsating" nail beds (Quincke sign) ◆ Rapidly rising and collapsing pulses (pulsus biferiens), cardiac arrhythmias, and widened pulse pressure ◆ Auscultation revealing an S_3 and a diastolic blowing murmur at left sternal border ◆ Palpation and visualization of apical impulse in chronic disease
Aortic stenosis ◆ Results from congenital aortic bicuspid valve (associated with coarctation of the aorta), congenital stenosis of valve cusps, rheumatic fever, or atherosclerosis in elderly persons ◆ Most common in males	◆ Dyspnea on exertion, paroxysmal nocturnal dyspnea, fatigue, syncope, angina, and palpitations ◆ Pulmonary congestion and left-sided heart failure ◆ Diminished carotid pulses, decreased cardiac output, and cardiac arrhythmias; may have pulsus alternans ◆ Auscultation revealing systolic murmur heard at base or in carotids and, possibly, an S_4

DIAGNOSTIC MEASURES

- *Cardiac catheterization:* diastolic pressure gradient across valve; elevated left atrial and pulmonary artery wedge pressures (PAWP) > 15 mm Hg with severe pulmonary hypertension; elevated right-sided heart pressure with decreased cardiac output; and abnormal contraction of the left ventricle
- *Chest X-rays:* left atrial and ventricular enlargement, enlarged pulmonary arteries, and mitral valve calcification
- *Echocardiography:* thickened mitral valve leaflets and left atrial enlargement
- *Electrocardiography (ECG):* left atrial hypertrophy, atrial fibrillation, right ventricular hypertrophy, and right axis deviation

- *Cardiac catheterization:* mitral regurgitation with increased left ventricular end-diastolic volume and pressure, increased atrial pressure and PAWP, and decreased cardiac output
- *Chest X-rays:* left atrial and ventricular enlargement and pulmonary venous congestion
- *Echocardiography:* abnormal valve leaflet motion and left atrial enlargement
- *ECG:* may show left atrial and ventricular hypertrophy, sinus tachycardia, and atrial fibrillation

- *Cardiac catheterization:* reduction in arterial diastolic pressures, aortic regurgitation, other valvular abnormalities, and increased left ventricular end-diastolic pressure
- *Chest X-rays:* left ventricular enlargement and pulmonary venous congestion
- *Echocardiography:* left ventricular enlargement, alterations in mitral valve movement (indirect indication of aortic valve disease), and mitral thickening
- *ECG:* sinus tachycardia, left ventricular hypertrophy, and left atrial hypertrophy in severe disease

- *Cardiac catheterization:* pressure gradient across valve (indicating obstruction) and increased left ventricular end-diastolic pressures
- *Chest X-rays:* valvular calcification, left ventricular enlargement, and pulmonary vein congestion
- *Echocardiography:* thickened aortic valve and left ventricular wall, possibly coexistent with mitral valve stenosis
- *ECG:* left ventricular hypertrophy

(continued)

Types of valvular heart disease *(continued)*

CAUSES AND INCIDENCE	CLINICAL FINDINGS
Pulmonic stenosis ◆ Results from congenital stenosis of valve cusp or rheumatic heart disease (uncommon) ◆ Associated with tetralogy of Fallot	◆ Asymptomatic or symptomatic with dyspnea on exertion, fatigue, chest pain, and syncope ◆ May cause jugular vein distention or right-sided heart failure ◆ Auscultation revealing a systolic murmur at the left sternal border and a split S_2 with a delayed or absent pulmonic component

COMPLICATIONS

Possible complications of varicose veins include:

- blood clots secondary to venous stasis
- venous stasis ulcers
- chronic venous insufficiency.

AGE ALERT
As a person ages, veins dilate and stretch, increasing susceptibility to varicose veins and chronic venous insufficiency. Because the skin is very friable and can easily break down, ulcers caused by chronic venous insufficiency in an older adult may take longer to heal.

DIAGNOSIS

These tests help diagnose varicose veins:

- A manual compression test detects a palpable impulse when the vein is firmly occluded at least 8″ (20 cm) above the point of palpation, indicating incompetent valves in the vein.
- Trendelenburg's test (retrograde filling test) detects incompetent deep and superficial vein valves.
- Photoplethysmography characterizes venous blood flow by noting changes in the skin's circulation.
- Doppler ultrasonography detects the presence or absence of venous backflow in deep or superficial veins.
- Venous outflow and reflux plethysmography detects deep venous occlusion; this test is invasive and not routinely used.
- Ascending and descending venography demonstrates venous occlusion and patterns of collateral flow.

TREATMENT

Correction of varicose veins typically involves:

- treatment of the underlying cause, such as an abdominal tumor or obesity, if possible
- antiembolism stockings or elastic bandages to counteract swelling by supporting the veins and improving circulation
- a regular exercise program to promote muscular contraction to force blood through the veins and reduce venous pooling
- injection of a sclerosing agent into small- to medium-sized varicosities
- surgical stripping and ligation of severe varicose veins
- phlebectomy, removing the varicose vein through small incisions in the skin, which may be performed in an outpatient setting.

Additional treatment measures include:

- discouraging the patient from wearing constrictive clothing that interferes with venous return
- encouraging the obese patient to lose weight to reduce increased intra-abdominal pressure
- telling the patient to elevate her legs above her heart whenever possible to promote venous return
- instructing the patient to avoid prolonged standing or sitting because these actions enhance venous pooling.

DIAGNOSTIC MEASURES

◆ *Cardiac catheterization:* increased right ventricular pressure, decreased pulmonary artery pressure, and abnormal valve orifice
◆ *ECG:* may show right ventricular hypertrophy, right axis deviation, right atrial hypertrophy, and atrial fibrillation

Ventricular septal defect

In a ventricular septal defect (VSD), the most common congenital cardiac defect associated with increased pulmonary blood flow (previously classified as an acyanotic congenital heart disorder), an opening in the septum between the ventricles allows blood to shunt between the left and right ventricles. This process results in ineffective pumping of the heart and increases the risk of heart failure.

VSDs account for up to 30% of all congenital heart defects. The prognosis is good for defects that close spontaneously or are correctable surgically, but poor for untreated defects, which are sometimes fatal in children by age 1, usually from secondary complications.

CAUSES

A VSD may be associated with these conditions:
■ fetal alcohol syndrome
■ Down syndrome and other autosomal trisomies
■ renal anomalies
■ patent ductus arteriosus and coarctation of the aorta
■ prematurity.

PATHOPHYSIOLOGY

In infants with a VSD, the ventricular septum fails to close completely by eight weeks' gestation. VSDs are located in the membranous or muscular portion of the ventricular septum and vary in size. Some defects close spontaneously; in other defects, the septum is entirely absent, creating a single ventricle. Small VSDs are likely to close spontaneously. Large VSDs should be surgically repaired before pulmonary vascular disease occurs or while it's still reversible.

A VSD isn't readily apparent at birth because right and left pressures are about equal and pulmonary artery resistance is elevated. Alveoli aren't yet completely opened, so blood doesn't shunt through the defect. As the pulmonary vasculature gradually relaxes, between 4 and 8 weeks after birth, right ventricular pressure decreases, allowing blood to shunt from the left to the right ventricle. Initially, large VSD shunts cause left atrial and left ventricular hypertrophy. Later, an uncorrected VSD causes right ventricular hypertrophy from increasing pulmonary resistance. Eventually, right- and left-sided heart failure and cyanosis (from reversal of the shunt direction) occur. Fixed pulmonary hypertension may occur much later in life with right-to-left shunting (Eisenmenger syndrome), causing cyanosis and clubbing of the nail beds.

SIGNS AND SYMPTOMS

Signs and symptoms of a VSD may include:
■ thin, small infants who gain weight slowly when a large VSD is present secondary to heart failure
■ a loud, harsh, widely transmitted systolic murmur heard best along the left sternal border at the third or fourth inter-

costal space, caused by abnormal blood flow through the VSD

■ a palpable thrill caused by turbulent blood flow between the ventricles through a small VSD

■ loud, widely split pulmonic component of S_2 caused by increased pressure gradient across the VSD

■ displacement of point of maximal impulse to the left caused by hypertrophy of the heart

▲ **AGE ALERT**
Typically, in infants, the apical impulse is palpated over the fourth intercostal space, just to the left of the mid-clavicular line. In children older than age 7, it's palpated over the fifth intercostal space. When the heart is enlarged, the apical beat is displaced to the left or downward.

■ prominent anterior chest secondary to cardiac hypertrophy

■ liver, heart, and spleen enlargement because of systemic congestion

■ feeding difficulties associated with heart failure

■ diaphoresis, tachycardia, and rapid, grunting respirations resulting from heart failure

■ cyanosis and finger clubbing if right-to-left shunting occurs later in life as a result of pulmonary hypertension.

COMPLICATIONS
Complications of a VSD may include:

■ pulmonary hypertension

■ infective endocarditis

■ pneumonia

■ heart failure

■ Eisenmenger's syndrome

he aortic valve is

DIAGNOSIS
These tests help diagnose a VSD:

■ Chest X-rays appear normal in small defects. In large VSDs, the X-ray may show cardiomegaly, left atrial and left ventricular enlargement, and prominent vascular markings.

■ Electrocardiogram may be normal with small VSDs, whereas in large VSDs it may show left and right ventricular

hypertrophy, suggestive of pulmonary hypertension.

■ Echocardiography can detect a VSD in the septum, estimate the size of the left-to-right shunt, suggest pulmonary hypertension, and identify associated lesions and complications.

■ Cardiac catheterization determines the size and exact location of the VSD and the extent of pulmonary hypertension; it also detects associated defects. It calculates the degree of shunting by comparing the blood oxygen saturation in each ventricle. The oxygen saturation of the right ventricle is greater than normal because oxygenated blood is shunted from the left to the right ventricle.

TREATMENT
Correction of a VSD may involve:

■ early surgical correction for a large VSD, usually performed using a patch graft, before heart failure and irreversible pulmonary vascular disease develop

■ placement of a permanent pacemaker, which may be necessary after VSD repair if complete heart block develops from interference with the bundle of His during surgery

■ surgical closure of small defects using sutures (They may not be surgically repaired if the patient has normal pulmonary artery pressure and a small shunt.)

■ pulmonary artery banding to normalize pressures and flow distal to the band and to prevent pulmonary vascular disease if the child has other defects and will benefit from delaying surgery

■ digoxin, sodium restriction, and diuretics before surgery to prevent heart failure

■ prophylactic antibiotics before and after surgery to prevent infective endocarditis.

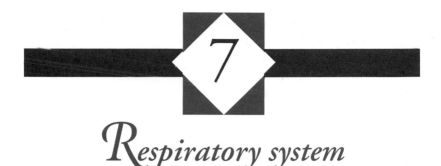

Respiratory system

The respiratory system's major function is gas exchange, in which air enters the body on inhalation (inspiration); travels throughout the respiratory passages, exchanging oxygen for carbon dioxide at the tissue level; and expels carbon dioxide on exhalation (expiration).

The upper airway — composed of the nose, mouth, pharynx, and larynx — allows airflow into the lungs. This area is responsible for warming, humidifying, and filtering the air, thereby protecting the lower airway from foreign matter.

The lower airway consists of the trachea, mainstem bronchi, secondary bronchi, bronchioles, and terminal bronchioles. These structures are anatomic dead spaces and function only as passageways for moving air into and out of the lungs. Distal to each terminal bronchiole is the acinus, which consists of respiratory bronchioles, alveolar ducts, and alveolar sacs. The bronchioles and ducts function as conduits, and the alveoli are the chief units of gas exchange. These final subdivisions of the bronchial tree make up the lobules — the functional units of the lungs. (See *Structure of the lobule,* page 210.)

In addition to warming, humidifying, and filtering inspired air, the lower airway protects the lungs with several defense mechanisms. Clearance mechanisms include the cough reflex and mucociliary system. The mucociliary system produces mucus, trapping foreign particles. Foreign matter is then swept by specialized finger-like projections called cilia to the upper airway for expectoration. A breakdown in the epithelium of the lungs or the mucociliary system can cause the defense mechanisms to malfunction, and pollutants and irritants then enter and inflame the lungs. The lower airway also provides immunologic protection and initiates pulmonary injury responses.

The external component of respiration (ventilation or breathing) delivers inspired air to the lower respiratory tract and alveoli. Contraction and relaxation of the respiratory muscles moves air into and out of the lungs.

Normal expiration is passive; the inspiratory muscles cease to contract, and the elastic recoil of the lungs and the chest wall causes them to contract again. These actions raise the pressure within the lungs to above atmospheric pressure, moving air from the lungs to the atmosphere.

An adult lung contains an estimated 300 million alveoli; each alveolus is supplied by many capillaries. To reach the capillary lumen, oxygen must cross the alveolar capillary membrane.

The pulmonary alveoli promote gas exchange by diffusion — the passage of gas molecules through respiratory membranes. In diffusion, oxygen passes to the blood, and carbon dioxide, a byproduct of cellular metabolism, passes out of the blood and is channeled away.

Circulating blood delivers oxygen to the cells of the body for metabolism and transports metabolic wastes and carbon

CLOSER LOOK
Structure of the lobule

Each lobule contains terminal bronchioles and the acinus. The acinus consists of respiratory bronchioles and the alveolar sacs.

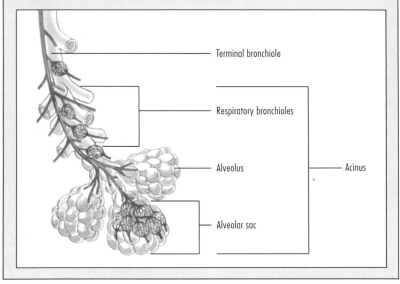

- Terminal bronchiole
- Respiratory bronchioles
- Alveolus
- Alveolar sac
- Acinus

dioxide from the tissues back to the lungs. When oxygenated arterial blood reaches tissue capillaries, the oxygen diffuses from the blood into the cells because of an oxygen tension gradient. The amount of oxygen available to cells depends on the concentration of hemoglobin (the principal carrier of oxygen) in the blood, the regional blood flow, the arterial oxygen content, and cardiac output.

Because circulation is continuous, carbon dioxide doesn't normally accumulate in tissues. Carbon dioxide produced during cellular respiration diffuses from tissues to regional capillaries and is transported by the systemic venous circulation. When carbon dioxide reaches the alveolar capillaries, it diffuses into the alveoli, where the partial pressure of carbon dioxide ($PaCO_2$) is lower. Carbon dioxide is removed from the alveoli during exhalation.

For effective gas exchange, ventilation and perfusion at the alveolar level must match closely. (See *Understanding ventilation and perfusion.*) The ratio of ventilation to perfusion is called the $\dot{V}/\dot{Q}$ ratio. A $\dot{V}/\dot{Q}$ mismatch can result from ventilation-perfusion dysfunction or altered lung mechanics.

The amount of air carrying oxygen that reaches the lungs depends on lung volume and capacity, compliance, and resistance to airflow. Changes in compliance can occur in either the lung or the chest wall. Destruction of the lung's elastic fibers, which occurs in acute respiratory distress syndrome, decreases lung compliance. The lungs become stiff, making breathing difficult. The alveolar capillary membrane may also be affected, causing hypoxia. Chest wall compliance is affected by disorders causing thoracic deformity, muscle spasm, and abdominal distention.

CLOSER LOOK
Understanding ventilation and perfusion

Effective gas exchange depends on the relationship between ventilation and perfusion, expressed as the $\dot{V}/\dot{Q}$ ratio. The illustrations below show what happens when the $\dot{V}/\dot{Q}$ ratio is normal and abnormal.

NORMAL VENTILATION AND PERFUSION

When the $\dot{V}/\dot{Q}$ ratio is matched, unoxygenated blood from the venous system returns to the right ventricle through the pulmonary artery to the lungs, carrying carbon dioxide. The arteries branch into the alveolar capillaries, where gas exchange occurs.

INADEQUATE PERFUSION (DEAD-SPACE VENTILATION)

When the $\dot{V}/\dot{Q}$ ratio is high, ventilation is normal, but alveolar perfusion is reduced or absent (illustrated by the perfusion blockage). This results from a perfusion defect, such as pulmonary embolism or a disorder that decreases cardiac output.

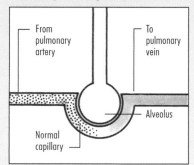

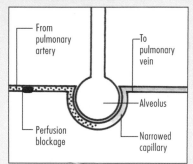

INADEQUATE VENTILATION (SHUNT)

When the $\dot{V}/\dot{Q}$ ratio is low, pulmonary circulation is adequate, but oxygen is inadequate for normal diffusion (illustrated by the ventilation blockage). A portion of the blood flowing through the pulmonary vessels doesn't become oxygenated.

INADEQUATE VENTILATION AND PERFUSION (SILENT UNIT)

The silent unit indicates an absence of ventilation and perfusion to the lung area (illustrated by blockages in perfusion and ventilation). The silent unit may try to compensate for this $\dot{V}/\dot{Q}$ imbalance by delivering blood flow to better-ventilated lung areas.

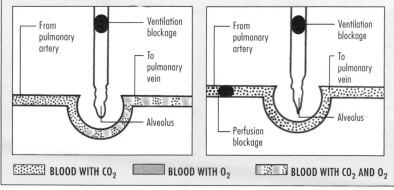

Respiration is also controlled neurologically by the lateral medulla oblongata of the brain stem. Impulses travel down the phrenic nerves to the diaphragm and then down the intercostal nerves to the intercostal muscles between the ribs. The rate and depth of respiration are controlled similarly.

Apneustic and pneumotaxic centers in the pons of the midbrain influence the pattern of breathing. Stimulation of the lower pontine apneustic center (by trauma, tumor, or stroke) produces forceful inspiratory gasps alternating with weak expiration. This pattern doesn't occur if the vagi are intact. The apneustic center continually excites the medullary inspiratory center and thus facilitates inspiration. Signals from the pneumotaxic center and afferent impulses from the vagus nerve inhibit the apneustic center and "turn off" inspiration.

In addition, chemoreceptors respond to the hydrogen ion concentration of arterial blood (pH), $PaCO_2$, and the partial pressure of arterial oxygen (PaO_2). Central chemoreceptors respond indirectly to arterial blood by sensing changes in the pH of the cerebrospinal fluid (CSF). $PaCO_2$ also helps regulate ventilation by impacting the pH of CSF. If $PaCO_2$ is high, the respiratory rate increases; if $PaCO_2$ is low, the respiratory rate decreases. Information from peripheral chemoreceptors in the carotid and aortic bodies also responds to decreased PaO_2 and pH. Either of these changes results in increased respiratory drive within minutes.

PATHOPHYSIOLOGIC CHANGES

Pathophysiologic manifestations of respiratory disease may stem from atelectasis, bronchiectasis, cyanosis, and hypoxemia.

Atelectasis
Atelectasis occurs when the alveolar sacs or entire lung segments expand incompletely, producing a partial or complete lung collapse. This phenomenon removes certain regions of the lung from gas exchange, allowing unoxygenated blood to pass unchanged through these regions and resulting in hypoxia. Atelectasis may be chronic or acute, and commonly occurs in patients undergoing upper abdominal or thoracic surgery. There are two major causes of collapse from atelectasis: absorptional atelectasis, secondary to bronchial or bronchiolar obstruction, and compression atelectasis.

ABSORPTION ATELECTASIS
Bronchial occlusion, which prevents air from entering the alveoli distal to the obstruction, can cause absorption atelectasis — the air present in the alveoli is absorbed gradually into the bloodstream and eventually the alveoli collapse. This may result from intrinsic or extrinsic bronchial obstruction. The most frequent intrinsic cause is retained secretions or exudate forming mucus plugs. Disorders, such as cystic fibrosis, chronic bronchitis, or pneumonia, increase the risk of absorption atelectasis. Extrinsic bronchial atelectasis usually results from occlusion caused by foreign bodies, bronchogenic carcinoma, and scar tissue.

Impaired production of surfactant can also cause absorption atelectasis. Increasing surface tension of the alveolus from reduced surfactant leads to collapse.

COMPRESSION ATELECTASIS
Compression atelectasis results from external compression, which drives the air out and causes the lung to collapse. This may result from upper abdominal surgical incisions, rib fractures, pleuritic chest pain, tight chest dressings, and obesity (which elevates the diaphragm and reduces tidal volume). These situations inhibit full lung expansion or make deep breathing painful, thus resulting in this disorder.

Bronchiectasis
Bronchiectasis is marked by chronic abnormal dilation of the bronchi and destruction of the bronchial walls and can occur throughout the tracheobronchial tree. It may also be confined to a single

segment or lobe. This disorder is usually bilateral in nature and involves the basilar segments of the lower lobes.

There are three forms of bronchiectasis: cylindrical, fusiform (varicose), and saccular (cystic). (See *Forms of bronchiectasis*.) It results from conditions associated with repeated damage to bronchial walls with abnormal mucociliary clearance, which causes a breakdown of supporting tissue adjacent to the airways. (See *Causes of bronchiectasis*, page 214.)

In patients with bronchiectasis, sputum stagnates in the dilated bronchi and leads to secondary infection, characterized by inflammation and leukocytic accumulations. Additional debris collects within and occludes the bronchi. Increasing pressure from the retained secretions induces mucosal injury.

Cyanosis

Cyanosis is a bluish discoloration of the skin and mucous membranes. In most populations, it's readily detectable by a visible blue tinge on the nail beds and lips. Central cyanosis indicates decreased oxygen saturation of hemoglobin in arterial blood, which is best observed in the buccal mucous membranes and the lips. Peripheral cyanosis is a slowed blood circulation of the fingers and toes that's best visualized by examining the nail bed area.

CULTURAL DIVERSITY
In patients with black or dark complexions, cyanosis may not be evident in the lip area or the nail beds. A better indicator in these individuals is to assess the membranes of the oral mucosa (buccal mucous membranes) and of the conjunctivae of the eyes.

Cyanosis is caused by desaturation with oxygen or reduced hemoglobin amounts. It develops when 5 g of hemoglobin is desaturated, even if hemoglobin counts are adequate or reduced. Conditions that result in cyanosis include decreased arterial oxygenation (indicated by low PaO_2), pulmonary or cardiac right-to-left shunts, decreased cardiac output, anxiety, and a cold environment.

A person who isn't cyanotic doesn't necessarily have adequate oxygenation. Inade-

---

Forms of bronchiectasis

The three types of bronchiectasis are cylindrical, fusiform (varicose), and saccular (cystic). In cylindrical bronchiectasis, bronchioles are usually symmetrically dilated, whereas in fusiform bronchiectasis, bronchioles are deformed. In saccular bronchiectasis, large bronchi become enlarged and balloonlike.

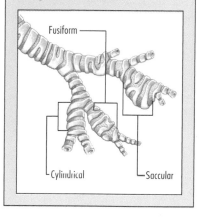

---

quate tissue oxygenation occurs in severe anemia, resulting in inadequate hemoglobin concentration. It also occurs in carbon monoxide poisoning, in which hemoglobin binds to carbon monoxide instead of to oxygen. Although assessment doesn't reveal cyanosis, oxygenation is inadequate.

Another patient may appear cyanotic even though oxygenation is adequate — as in polycythemia, an abnormal increase in the red blood cell count. Because the hemoglobin count is increased and oxygenation occurs at a normal rate, the patient may still present with cyanosis.

Cyanosis as a presenting condition must be interpreted in relation to the patient's underlying pathophysiology. Diagnosis of inadequate oxygenation may be confirmed by analyzing arterial blood gases and measuring PaO_2.

Causes of bronchiectasis

Bronchiectasis results from conditions associated with repeated damage to bronchial walls and with abnormal mucociliary clearance, leading to a breakdown in the supporting tissue adjacent to the airways. Such conditions include:
◆ cystic fibrosis
◆ immune disorders (for example, agammaglobulinemia)
◆ recurrent bacterial respiratory tract infections that were inadequately treated (for example, tuberculosis)
◆ complications of measles, pneumonia, pertussis, or influenza
◆ obstruction (from a foreign body, tumor, or stenosis) with recurrent infection
◆ inhalation of corrosive gas or repeated aspiration of gastric juices into the lungs
◆ congenital anomalies, such as bronchomalacia, congenital bronchiectasis, and Kartagener syndrome (bronchiectasis, sinusitis, and dextrocardia)
◆ rare disorders such as immotile cilia syndrome.

Hypoxemia

Hypoxemia is reduced oxygenation of the arterial blood, evidenced by reduced PaO_2 of arterial blood gases. It's caused by respiratory alterations, whereas hypoxia is diminished tissue oxygenation at the cellular level that may be caused by conditions affecting other body systems that are unrelated to alterations of pulmonary function. Low cardiac output or cyanide poisoning can result in hypoxia, in addition to alterations in respiration. Hypoxia can occur anywhere in the body. If hypoxia occurs in the blood, it's termed hypoxemia. Hypoxemia can lead to tissue hypoxia.

Hypoxemia can be caused by decreased oxygen content of inspired gas, hypoventilation, diffusion abnormalities, abnormal V/Q ratios, and pulmonary right-to-left shunts. The physiologic mechanism for each cause of hypoxemia is variable. (See *Major causes of hypoxemia*.)

DISORDERS

Respiratory disorders can be acute or chronic. The disorders described here include examples from each type.

Acute respiratory distress syndrome

Acute respiratory distress syndrome (ARDS) is a form of pulmonary edema that can quickly lead to acute respiratory failure. Also known as *shock lung, stiff lung, white lung, wet lung,* or *Da Nang lung,* ARDS may follow direct or indirect injury to the lung. However, its diagnosis is difficult, and death can occur within 48 hours of onset if not promptly diagnosed and treated. A differential diagnosis needs to rule out cardiogenic pulmonary edema, pulmonary vasculitis, and diffuse pulmonary hemorrhage. Patients who recover may have little or no permanent lung damage.

CAUSES
Common causes of ARDS include:
■ injury to the lung from trauma (most common cause) such as airway contusion
■ trauma-related factors, such as fat emboli, sepsis, shock, pulmonary contusions, and multiple transfusions, which increase the likelihood that microemboli will develop
■ anaphylaxis
■ aspiration of gastric contents
■ diffuse pneumonia, especially viral pneumonia
■ drug overdose, such as of heroin, aspirin, or ethchlorvynol
■ idiosyncratic drug reaction to ampicillin or hydrochlorothiazide
■ inhalation of noxious gases, such as nitrous oxide, ammonia, or chlorine
■ near drowning
■ oxygen toxicity
■ sepsis
■ coronary artery bypass grafting
■ hemodialysis
■ leukemia
■ acute miliary tuberculosis
■ pancreatitis
■ thrombotic thrombocytopenic purpura

Bacterial infections

Bacteria are simple one-celled microorganisms with a cell wall that protects them from many of the human body's defense mechanisms. Although they lack a nucleus, bacteria possess all the other mechanisms they need to survive and rapidly reproduce.

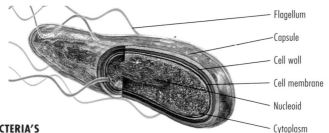

Flagellum
Capsule
Cell wall
Cell membrane
Nucleoid
Cytoplasm

BACTERIA'S DAMAGING WAYS

Bacteria may enter the body through various routes, but once inside the body, bacteria can multiply sufficiently to cause infection. The infection may be caused directly by the bacteria or by the toxins they produce.

1. Some bacteria damage the tissue by adhering to and invading tissue cells. Other bacteria produce toxins that alter the chemical reactions occurring in the cell. As a result, cellular function is disrupted or the cell dies.

2. Some bacterial toxins may cause clotting in the small vessels. As a result, the tissues normally supplied by these vessels become deprived of oxygen, leading to tissue ischemia and damage.

3. Bacteria also may cause fluid to leak from the blood vessel. Toxins produced may damage the walls of small blood vessels, allowing fluid to leak out into the surrounding tissue. Subsequently, fluid is lost, leading to decreased blood pressure and cardiac output.

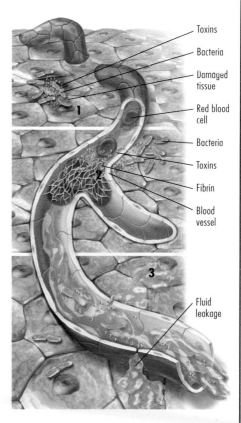

Toxins
Bacteria
Damaged tissue
Red blood cell
Bacteria
Toxins
Fibrin
Blood vessel
Fluid leakage

Viral infections

A virus is a subcellular organism made up of ribonucleic acid (RNA) and deoxyribonucleic acid (DNA) covered with proteins. Viruses are obligate intracellular parasites; that is, they can't grow or reproduce apart from living cells. Instead, they invade a host cell and stimulate it to participate in the formation of additional virus particles.

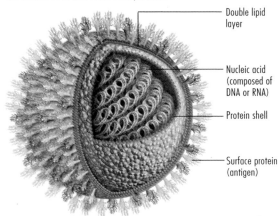

Double lipid layer

Nucleic acid (composed of DNA or RNA)

Protein shell

Surface protein (antigen)

VIRAL STRUCTURE
Generally, a virus has a core of nucleic acid, composed of DNA or RNA, depending on the type of virus. The nucleic acid is enclosed in one or two protein shells. Surface proteins, called *antigens,* cover the outer shell.

VIRAL INFECTION OF A CELL

A virus can't process nutrients or replicate without a host cell. Viruses invade host cells by attaching to a specific molecule on the cell surface, which acts as a receptor. After attachment, a multistep entry process delivers the viral nucleic acid, which contains the genes, into the cytoplasm or the nucleus of the host cell. Once released, the viral genes dictate the synthesis of viral proteins and the replication of its genome, followed by assembly and release of the new virus particles. Cell destruction is required for release of some viruses, but not of others, which "bud" through the plasma membrane.

To invade a cell:
1. The surface proteins on the virus attach to specific receptor sites on the host cell's outer membrane.
2. After attaching to the membrane, part or all of the virus penetrates into the host cell.
3. Depending on the specific virus, the nucleic acid of the virus (RNA or DNA) is released into the host cell's cytoplasm or nucleus. Then the viral genes direct the production of proteins and nucleic acids, the components of the new virus particles.
4. The host cell may burst, releasing the viruses to infect other cells. However, not all viruses destroy the cells as they leave. Some viruses form buds from the host cell's membrane and are released.

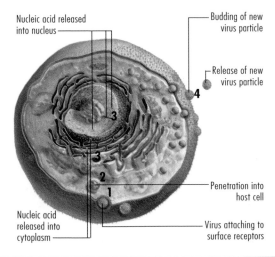

Nucleic acid released into nucleus

Budding of new virus particle

Release of new virus particle

Penetration into host cell

Virus attaching to surface receptors

Nucleic acid released into cytoplasm

VIRAL ENTRY AND SPREAD

To cause infection, the virus must enter the host. This can occur at these sites:

- ◆ conjunctiva
- ◆ mouth or oropharynx (GI tract)
- ◆ skin
- ◆ respiratory tract
- ◆ genitourinary tract.

Once inside the body, some viruses are confined to the site of initial infection and spread only locally, whereas other viruses spread widely. In the body, viruses may spread through the blood or through the peripheral nervous system.

VIRAL SPREAD THROUGH THE BLOOD

Viremia refers to the presence of a virus in the bloodstream. The most common source is a virus that replicates in the regional lymph nodes and is transported by the thoracic duct into the circulation. Blood-borne viruses either circulate freely in the plasma or are cell-associated. Cell-associated viremia means that the virus replicates in cells found in the circulation, particularly B or T lymphocytes or monocytes, or red blood cells. The latter, however, is very rare.

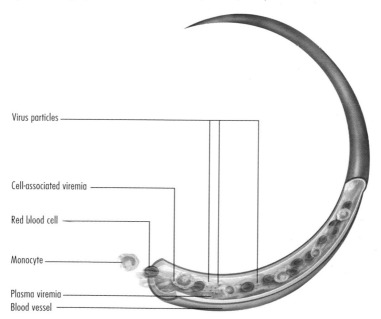

Virus particles

Cell-associated viremia

Red blood cell

Monocyte

Plasma viremia
Blood vessel

VIRAL SPREAD THROUGH THE PERIPHERAL NERVOUS SYSTEM

A virus may be transmitted within the axon of peripheral nerve fibers through neural spread. The neural pathway plays an essential role in the spread of some viruses, although neural spread is a less common method of spreading than viremia is. Neurotropic viruses are usually confined to the peripheral and central nervous systems and replicate in relatively few peripheral tissues.

Cancer

Cancer is a condition characterized by the rapid growth of abnormal (malignant) cells, which invade nearby tissues and may metastasize to other areas of the body.

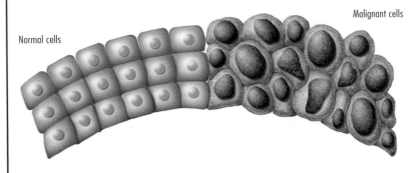

Malignant cells

Normal cells

Cancer cells divide and replicate rapidly; they tend to be aggressive and out of control. In contrast, cells forming a benign tumor multiply slowly and remain localized. Benign tumor cells resemble cells of the original tissue, and the tumor is seldom-life threatening.

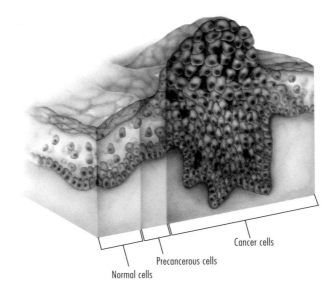

Cancer cells

Precancerous cells

Normal cells

CANCER STAGING

The diagnosis of cancer is determined by a biopsy, a microscopic evaluation of sampled tissue. Determining the extent of spread of the malignant cells is called staging. Although many different systems exist, typically a four-stage system is used.

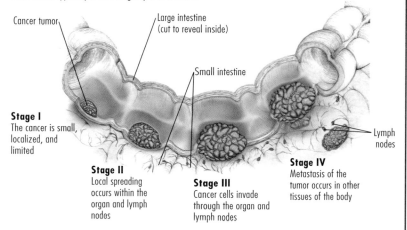

Cancer tumor

Large intestine
(cut to reveal inside)

Small intestine

Stage I
The cancer is small, localized, and limited

Lymph nodes

Stage II
Local spreading occurs within the organ and lymph nodes

Stage III
Cancer cells invade through the organ and lymph nodes

Stage IV
Metastasis of the tumor occurs in other tissues of the body

CANCER SPREAD

Cancer cells may invade nearby tissues or metastasize to other organs. There are three ways in which cancer cells may spread to other tissues:

◆ Through the blood: cancer cells may travel through the blood vessels, often to the liver and the lungs.
◆ Through the lymphatic system: the lymphatic system plays a key role in the immune system by helping to fight conditions as minor as colds or as serious as cancer. Cancer cells may move through the network of channels, from the tissues to the lymph nodes, to the circulatory system, and eventually to other organs.
◆ Through seeding: Cancer may penetrate an organ, moving into a nearby body cavity such as the chest or abdominal area and spread throughout the area.

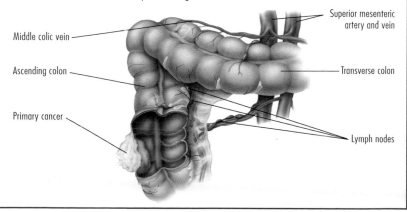

Middle colic vein

Superior mesenteric artery and vein

Ascending colon

Transverse colon

Primary cancer

Lymph nodes

Asthma

Characterized by increased airflow resistance, asthma is a chronic reactive airway disorder that causes episodic airway obstruction. Such obstruction results from bronchospasms, increased mucus secretion, and mucosal edema.

In asthma, bronchial linings overreact to various stimuli, causing episodic smooth muscle spasms that severely constrict the airways. Immunoglobulin (Ig) E antibodies, attached to histamine-containing mast cells and receptors on cell membranes, initiate intrinsic asthma attacks. When exposed to an antigen such as pollen, the IgE antibody combines with the antigen.

On subsequent exposure to the antigen, mast cells degranulate and release mediators. Mast cells in the lung interstitium are stimulated to release histamine and leukotrienes. Histamine attaches to receptor sites in the larger bronchi, where it causes swelling in smooth muscles. Mucous membranes become inflamed, irritated, and swollen.

Leukotrienes attach to receptor sites in the smaller bronchi and cause local swelling of the smooth muscle. Leukotrienes also cause prostaglandins to travel through the bloodstream to the lungs, where they enhance histamine's effect. Histamine stimulates the mucous membranes to secrete excessive mucus, further narrowing the bronchial lumen. Goblet cells secrete viscous mucus that's difficult to cough up. Mucosal edema and thickened secretions further block the airways.

On inhalation, the narrowed bronchial lumen can still expand slightly, allowing air to reach the alveoli. On exhalation, increased intrathoracic pressure closes the bronchial lumen completely. Air enters but can't escape. Thus air is trapped in the alveoli.

Mucus fills the lung bases, inhibiting alveolar ventilation. Blood is shunted to alveoli in other lung parts but still can't compensate for diminished ventilation.

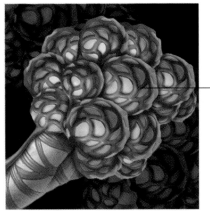

— Air trapped in alveoli

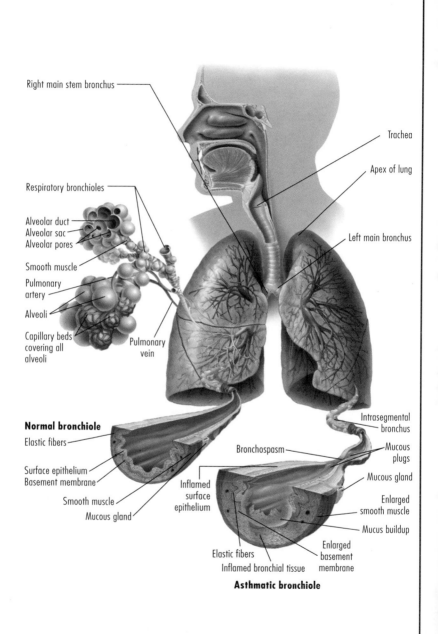

Right main stem bronchus

Trachea

Apex of lung

Respiratory bronchioles

Alveolar duct
Alveolar sac
Alveolar pores

Smooth muscle

Pulmonary
artery

Alveoli

Capillary beds
covering all
alveoli

Pulmonary
vein

Left main bronchus

Normal bronchiole

Elastic fibers

Surface epithelium
Basement membrane

Smooth muscle

Mucous gland

Bronchospasm

Inflamed
surface
epithelium

Intrasegmental
bronchus

Mucous
plugs

Mucous gland

Enlarged
smooth muscle

Mucus buildup

Elastic fibers
Inflamed bronchial tissue

Enlarged
basement
membrane

Asthmatic bronchiole

Chronic bronchitis

Chronic bronchitis is inflammation of the bronchi, caused by irritants or infection. A form of chronic obstructive pulmonary disease (COPD), bronchitis may be classified as acute or chronic. In chronic bronchitis, hypersecretion of mucus and chronic productive cough last for 3 months of the year and occur for at least 2 consecutive years. The distinguishing characteristic of bronchitis is airflow obstruction.

Chronic bronchitis occurs when irritants are inhaled for a prolonged time. The irritants inflame the tracheobronchial tree, leading to increased mucus production and a narrowed or blocked airway. As the inflammation continues, changes in the cells lining the respiratory tract result in resistance of the small airways and severe ventilation-perfusion ($\dot{V}/\dot{Q}$) imbalance, which decreases arterial oxygenation.

Healthy bronchi

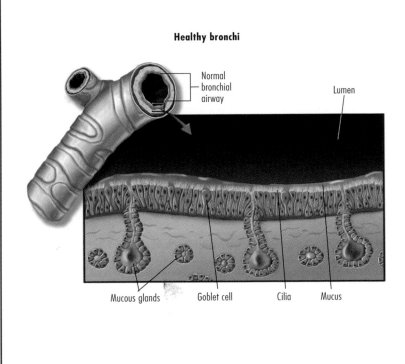

Normal bronchial airway

Lumen

Mucous glands

Goblet cell

Cilia

Mucus

Chronic bronchitis results in hypertrophy and hyperplasia of the mucous glands, increased goblet cells, ciliary damage, squamous metaplasia of the columnar epithelium, and chronic leukocytic and lymphocytic infiltration of bronchial walls. Hypersecretion of the goblet cells blocks the free movement of the cilia, which normally sweep dust, irritants, and mucus away from the airways. With mucus and debris accumulating in the airway, the defenses are altered, and the individual is prone to respiratory tract infections.

Additional effects include widespread inflammation, airway narrowing, and mucus within the airways. Bronchial walls become inflamed and thickened from edema and accumulation of inflammatory cells, and the effects of smooth muscle bronchospasm further narrow the lumen. At first, only large bronchi are involved, but eventually all airways are affected. Airways become obstructed and closure occurs, especially on expiration. The gas is then trapped in the distal portion of the lung. Hypoventilation occurs, leading to a $\dot{V}/\dot{Q}$ mismatch and resultant hypoxemia.

Chronic bronchitis

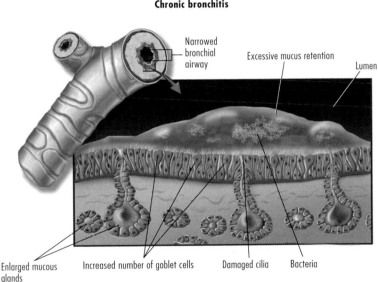

Narrowed bronchial airway

Excessive mucus retention

Lumen

Enlarged mucous glands

Increased number of goblet cells

Damaged cilia

Bacteria

Pulmonary edema

Pulmonary edema is an accumulation of fluid in the extravascular spaces of the lungs. It's a common complication of cardiac disorders and may be a chronic condition or an acute condition that develops quickly and rapidly becomes fatal.

Normal alveoli

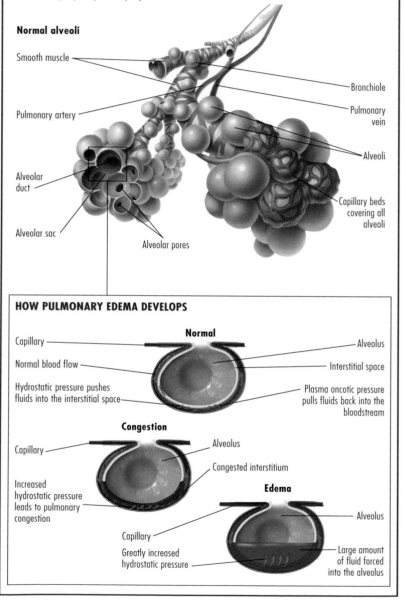

- Smooth muscle
- Pulmonary artery
- Alveolar duct
- Alveolar sac
- Alveolar pores
- Bronchiole
- Pulmonary vein
- Alveoli
- Capillary beds covering all alveoli

HOW PULMONARY EDEMA DEVELOPS

Normal
- Capillary
- Normal blood flow
- Hydrostatic pressure pushes fluids into the interstitial space
- Alveolus
- Interstitial space
- Plasma oncotic pressure pulls fluids back into the bloodstream

Congestion
- Capillary
- Increased hydrostatic pressure leads to pulmonary congestion
- Alveolus
- Congested interstitium

Edema
- Capillary
- Greatly increased hydrostatic pressure
- Alveolus
- Large amount of fluid forced into the alveolus

Severe acute respiratory syndrome

Severe acute respiratory syndrome (SARS) is a severe respiratory tract infection caused by a virus. This virus, identified as a coronavirus, is named SARS-associated coronavirus (SARS-CoV).

SARS-CoV is a ribonucleic acid virus that's believed to be spread by droplets created during coughing and sneezing. There's also some belief that the virus can be spread by contact with objects contaminated with respiratory secretions or stool. After exposure, individuals often develop symptoms within 3 to 7 days. Although it produces symptoms similar to many other respiratory illnesses, the virus causes a severe, rapidly spreading pneumonia that destroys the alveoli.

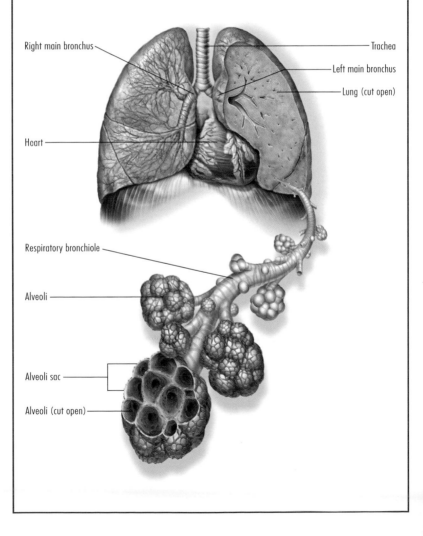

Coronary artery disease

Coronary artery disease (CAD) results as atherosclerotic plaque fills the lumens of the coronary arteries and obstructs blood flow. The primary effect of CAD is a diminished supply of oxygen and nutrients to the myocardial tissue.

PROGRESSION OF CAD IN ATHEROSCLEROSIS

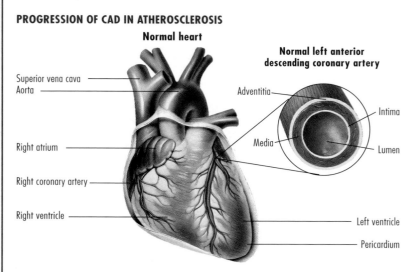

Normal heart

Normal left anterior descending coronary artery

Superior vena cava
Aorta
Right atrium
Right coronary artery
Right ventricle

Adventitia
Media
Intima
Lumen

Left ventricle
Pericardium

NARROW ARTERY LEADS TO ISCHEMIA

The narrowing of a coronary artery reduces blood flow (ischemia). The result is oxygen starvation of heart tissue, which causes symptoms of chest pain and tightness, called angina. Ischemia may be present without anatomical changes to the myocardium.

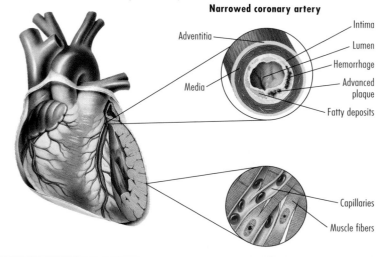

Narrowed coronary artery

Adventitia
Media
Intima
Lumen
Hemorrhage
Advanced plaque
Fatty deposits

Capillaries
Muscle fibers

BLOCKED ARTERY LEADS TO MYOCARDIAL INFARCTION

Sudden insufficient blood supply is commonly caused by ruptured plaque and thrombus formation that occludes the artery lumen. This produces an area of necrosis in the heart muscle, which results in a myocardial infarction (MI).

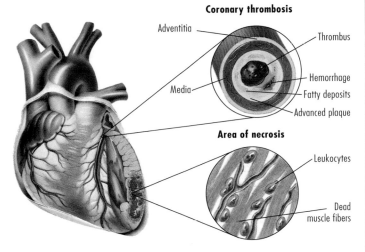

Coronary thrombosis

Adventitia — Thrombus

Media — Hemorrhage

Fatty deposits

Advanced plaque

Area of necrosis

Leukocytes

Dead muscle fibers

RECOVERY THROUGH COLLATERAL BLOOD SUPPLY

Collateral (accessory) blood supply from adjacent vessels travels to the region affected by the MI to provide fresh blood.

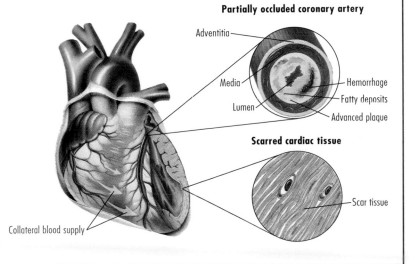

Partially occluded coronary artery

Adventitia

Media — Hemorrhage

Fatty deposits

Lumen

Advanced plaque

Scarred cardiac tissue

Scar tissue

Collateral blood supply

Seizure disorder

Seizure disorder, or epilepsy, is a condition of the brain characterized by susceptibility to recurrent seizures (paroxysmal events associated with abnormal electrical discharges of neurons in the brain). Primary seizure disorder is idiopathic, without apparent structural changes in the brain. Secondary seizure disorder, characterized by structural changes or metabolic alterations of the neuronal membranes, causes increased automaticity.

The brain's ability to turn electrical impulses "on" and "off" lets it control messages and work effectively. In people with seizure disorder, this fine balance is upset and the brain is unable to limit the spread of electrical activity.

HOW A SEIZURE OCCURS

Some neurons in the brain may depolarize easily or be hyperexcitable; this epileptogenic focus fires more readily than normal when stimulated. In these neurons, the membrane potential at rest is less negative or inhibitory connections are missing, possibly as a result of decreased gamma-aminobutyric acid activity or localized shifts in electrolytes.

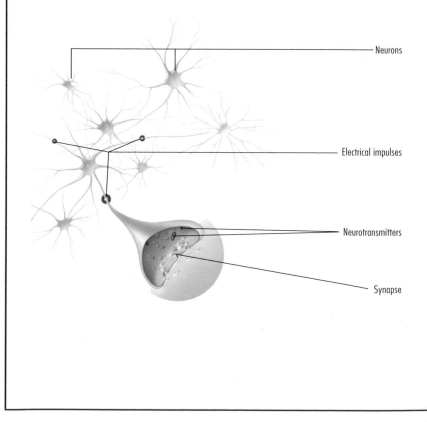

Neurons

Electrical impulses

Neurotransmitters

Synapse

On stimulation, the epileptogenic focus fires and spreads electrical current toward the synapse and to the surrounding cells. These cells fire in turn and the impulse cascades to one side of the brain (a partial seizure), both sides of the brain (a generalized seizure), or cortical, subcortical, and brain stem areas. The brain's metabolic demand for oxygen increases dramatically during a seizure. If this demand isn't met, hypoxia and brain damage ensue. Firing of inhibitory neurons causes the excitatory neurons to slow their firing and eventually stop. If this inhibitory action doesn't occur, the result is status epilepticus: one seizure occurring right after another; without treatment the anoxia is fatal.

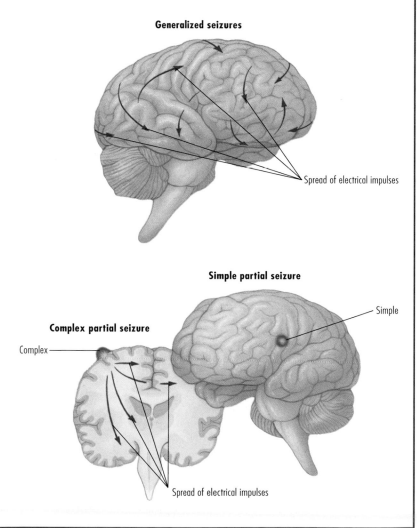

Generalized seizures

Spread of electrical impulses

Simple partial seizure

Simple

Complex partial seizure

Complex

Spread of electrical impulses

Hypercholesterolemia

Cholesterol is a lipid whose nucleus is synthesized from fatty acids. It's insoluble in plasma. Therefore, it must be carried in the blood by specialized fat-carrying proteins called lipoproteins.

Lipoproteins are classified by their density. There are five types of lipoproteins: chylomicrons, very-low-density lipoproteins (VLDLs), intermediate-density lipoproteins (IDLs), low-density lipoproteins (LDLs), and high-density lipoproteins (HDLs). Cholesterol is transported in the bloodstream primarily by LDLs.

Lipoprotein

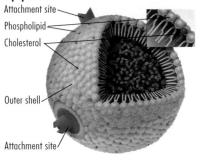

Attachment site
Phospholipid
Cholesterol

Outer shell

Attachment site

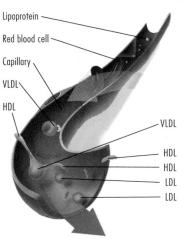

Lipoprotein
Red blood cell
Capillary
VLDL
HDL

VLDL
HDL
HDL
LDL
LDL

Lipoproteins act as shuttles for fat in the bloodstream. VLDLs travel through the blood stream and attach to the lining of the capillaries. Here, the fatty core, cholesterol, is drawn out. IDLs, smaller lipoproteins, remain in the bloodstream and shed tiny disklike particles of HDL. LDLs remain in the blood and travel back to the liver to be removed by specific receptors on the liver cell. However, if the level of cholesterol in the bloodstream is high, fewer receptors are available on the surface of the liver cell for lipoprotein attachment, thereby interfering with the removal of LDLs.

CONSEQUENCES OF HYPERCHOLESTEROLEMIA

Hypercholesterolemia is associated with development of atherosclerosis and heart disease. When the levels of cholesterol in the blood stream are normal, the arterial walls remain smooth and slippery. However, when the cholesterol levels are high, excess cholesterol concentrates in the walls of the arteries, leading to a reduction, and ultimately a blockage, of blood flow.

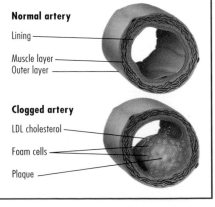

Normal artery

Lining
Muscle layer
Outer layer

Clogged artery

LDL cholesterol
Foam cells
Plaque

Major causes of hypoxemia

This chart lists the major causes of hypoxemia and contributing factors.

MAJOR CAUSE	CONTRIBUTING FACTORS
Decrease in inspired oxygen	High altitudes, inhaling poorly oxygenated gases, or breathing in an enclosed space
Hypoventilation	Respiratory center inappropriately stimulated (such as by oversedation, overdosage, or neurologic damage), chronic obstructive pulmonary disease
Alveolar capillary diffusion abnormality	Emphysema, conditions resulting in fibrosis, or pulmonary edema
Ventilation-perfusion mismatch	Asthma, chronic bronchitis, or pneumonia
Shunting	Acute respiratory distress syndrome, idiopathic respiratory distress syndrome of the newborn, or atelectasis

- uremia
- venous air embolism.

PATHOPHYSIOLOGY

Injury in ARDS involves the alveolar and pulmonary capillary epithelium. A cascade of cellular and biochemical changes is triggered by the specific causative agent. When initiated, this injury triggers neutrophils, macrophages, monocytes, and lymphocytes to produce various cytokines. The cytokines promote cellular activation, chemotaxis, and adhesion. The activated cells produce inflammatory mediators, including oxidants, proteases, kinins, growth factors, and neuropeptides, which initiate the complement cascade, intravascular coagulation, and fibrinolysis.

These cellular triggers result in increased vascular permeability to proteins, affecting the hydrostatic pressure gradient of the capillary. Elevated capillary pressure — such as resulting from insults of fluid overload or cardiac dysfunction in sepsis — greatly increases interstitial and alveolar edema, which is evident in dependent lung areas and can be visualized as whitened areas on chest X-rays. Alveolar closing pressure then exceeds pulmonary pressures, and alveolar closure and collapse begin.

In ARDS, fluid accumulation in the lung interstitium, the alveolar spaces, and the small airways causes the lungs to stiffen, thus impairing ventilation and reducing oxygenation of the pulmonary capillary blood. The resulting injury reduces normal blood flow to the lungs. Damage can occur directly — as in aspiration of gastric contents and inhalation of noxious gases — or indirectly — from chemical mediators released in response to systemic disease.

Platelets begin to aggregate and release substances, such as serotonin, bradykinin, and histamine, which attract and activate neutrophils. These substances inflame and damage the alveolar membrane and later increase capillary permeability. In the early stages of ARDS, signs and symptoms may be undetectable.

Additional chemotactic factors released include endotoxins (such as those present in septic states), tumor necrosis factor, and interleukin-1. The activated neutrophils release several inflammatory mediators and platelet aggravating factors that damage the alveolar capillary membrane and increase capillary permeability.

Histamines and other inflammatory substances increase capillary permeability, allowing fluids to move into the interstitial space. Consequently, the patient experiences tachypnea, dyspnea, and tachycardia. As capillary permeability increases, proteins, blood cells, and more fluid leak out, increasing interstitial osmotic pressure and causing pulmonary edema. Tachycardia, dyspnea, and cyanosis may occur. Hypoxia (usually unresponsive to increasing fraction of inspired oxygen), decreased pulmonary compliance, crackles, and rhonchi develop. The resulting pulmonary edema and hemorrhage significantly reduce lung compliance and impair alveolar ventilation.

The fluid in the alveoli and decreased blood flow damage surfactant in the alveoli. This reduces the ability of alveolar cells to produce more surfactant. Without surfactant, alveoli and bronchioles fill with fluid or collapse, gas exchange is impaired, and the lungs are much less compliant. Ventilation of the alveoli is further decreased. The burden of ventilation and gas exchange shifts to uninvolved areas of the lung, and pulmonary blood flow is shunted from right to left. The work of breathing is increased, and the patient may develop thick frothy sputum and marked hypoxemia with increasing respiratory distress.

Mediators released by neutrophils and macrophages also cause varying degrees of pulmonary vasoconstriction, resulting in pulmonary hypertension. The result of these changes is a ventilation-perfusion mismatch. Although the patient responds with an increased respiratory rate, sufficient oxygen can't cross the alveolar capillary membrane. Carbon dioxide continues to cross easily and is lost with every exhalation. As oxygen and carbon dioxide levels in the blood decrease, the patient develops increasing tachypnea, hypoxemia, and hypocapnia (low partial pressure of arterial carbon dioxide [$PaCO_2$]).

Pulmonary edema worsens, and hyaline membranes form. Inflammation leads to fibrosis, which further impedes gas exchange. Fibrosis progressively obliterates alveoli, respiratory bronchioles, and the interstitium. Functional residual capacity decreases, and shunting becomes more serious. Hypoxemia leads to metabolic acidosis. At this stage, the patient develops increasing $PaCO_2$, decreasing pH and partial pressure of arterial oxygen (PaO_2), decreasing bicarbonate (HCO_3^-) levels, and mental confusion. (See *Looking at acute respiratory distress syndrome.*)

The end result is respiratory failure. Systemically, neutrophils and inflammatory mediators cause generalized endothelial damage and increased capillary permeability throughout the body. Multisystem organ dysfunction syndrome (MODS) occurs as the cascade of mediators affects each system. Death may occur from the influence of ARDS and MODS.

SIGNS AND SYMPTOMS

Signs and symptoms of ARDS include:
- rapid, shallow breathing and dyspnea, which occur hours to days after the initial injury in response to decreasing oxygen levels in the blood
- increased rate of ventilation from hypoxemia and its effects on the pneumotaxic center
- intercostal and suprasternal retractions from the increased effort required to expand the stiff lung
- crackles and rhonchi, which are audible and result from fluid accumulation in the lungs
- restlessness, apprehension, and mental sluggishness, which occur as the result of hypoxic brain cells
- motor dysfunction, which occurs as hypoxia progresses
- tachycardia, which signals the heart's effort to deliver more oxygen to the cells and vital organs
- respiratory acidosis, which occurs as carbon dioxide accumulates in the blood and oxygen levels decrease
- metabolic acidosis, which eventually results from failure of compensatory mechanisms.

COMPLICATIONS

Possible complications of ARDS include:
- hypotension
- decreased urine output
- metabolic acidosis
- respiratory acidosis

CLOSER LOOK
Looking at acute respiratory distress syndrome

These Illustrations show the process and progress of acute respiratory distress syndrome.

In phase 1, injury reduces normal blood flow to the lungs. Platelets aggregate and release histamine (H), serotonin (S), and bradykinin (B).

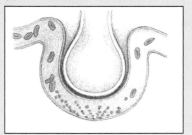

In phase 4, decreased blood flow and fluids in the alveoli damage surfactant and impair the cell's ability to produce more. The alveoli then collapse, thus impairing gas exchange.

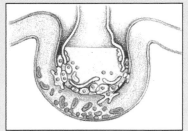

In phase 2, the released substances inflame and damage the alveolar capillary membrane, increasing capillary permeability. Fluids then shift into the interstitial space.

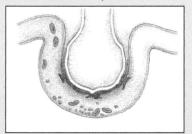

In phase 5, oxygenation is impaired, but carbon dioxide (CO_2) easily crosses the alveolar capillary membrane and is expired. Blood oxygen (O_2) and CO_2 levels are low.

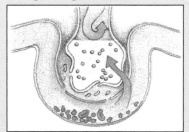

In phase 3, capillary permeability increases and proteins and fluids leak out, increasing interstitial osmotic pressure and causing pulmonary edema.

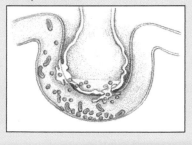

In phase 6, pulmonary edema worsens and inflammation leads to fibrosis. Gas exchange is further impeded.

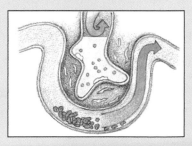

- MODS
- ventricular fibrillation
- ventricular standstill.

DIAGNOSIS

These tests help diagnose ARDS:

- Arterial blood gas (ABG) analysis with the patient breathing room air initially reveals a reduced PaO_2 (less than 60 mm Hg) and a decreased $PaCO_2$ (less than 35 mm Hg). Hypoxemia, despite increased supplemental oxygen, is the hallmark of ARDS; the resulting blood pH reflects respiratory alkalosis. As ARDS worsens, ABG values show respiratory acidosis evident by an increasing $PaCO_2$ (more than 45 mm Hg), metabolic acidosis evident by a decreasing HCO_3^- less than 22 mEq/L, and a declining PaO_2 despite oxygen therapy.
- Pulmonary artery catheterization helps identify the cause of pulmonary edema (cardiac versus noncardiac) by measuring pulmonary artery wedge pressure; allows collection of pulmonary artery blood, which shows decreased oxygen saturation, reflecting tissue hypoxia; measures pulmonary artery pressure; measures cardiac output by thermodilution techniques; and provides information to allow calculation of the percentages of blood shunted through the lungs.
- Serial chest X-rays in early stages show bilateral infiltrates; in later stages, lung fields with a ground-glass appearance and "whiteouts" of both lung fields (with irreversible hypoxemia) may be observed. To differentiate ARDS from heart failure, note that the normal cardiac silhouette appears diffuse; bilateral infiltrates tend to be more peripheral and patchy, as opposed to the usual perihilar "bat wing" appearance of cardiogenic pulmonary edema; and there are fewer pleural effusions.
- Sputum analysis, including Gram stain and culture and sensitivity, identifies causative organisms.
- Blood cultures identify infectious organisms.
- Toxicology testing screens for drug ingestion.
- Serum amylase rules out pancreatitis.

TREATMENT

Treatment is focused on correcting the causes of ARDS and preventing progression of hypoxemia and respiratory acidosis; it may involve:

- administration of humidified oxygen by a tight-fitting mask, which allows for the use of continuous positive airway pressure
- for hypoxemia that doesn't respond adequately to the above measures, ventilatory support with intubation, volume ventilation, and positive end-expiratory pressure
- pressure-controlled inverse ratio ventilation to reverse the conventional inspiration-to-expiration ratio and minimize the risk of trauma (Mechanical breaths are pressure-limited to prevent increased damage to the alveoli.)
- permissive hypercapnia to limit peak inspiratory pressure (Although carbon dioxide removal is compromised, treatment isn't given for subsequent changes in blood hydrogen and oxygen concentration.)
- sedatives, opioids, or neuromuscular blockers such as pancuronium bromide, which may be given during mechanical ventilation to minimize restlessness, oxygen consumption, and carbon dioxide production and to facilitate ventilation
- sodium bicarbonate, which may reverse severe metabolic acidosis
- I.V. fluid administration to maintain blood pressure by treating hypovolemia
- vasopressors to maintain blood pressure
- antimicrobial drugs to treat nonviral infections
- diuretics to reduce interstitial and pulmonary edema
- correction of electrolyte and acid-base imbalances to maintain cellular integrity, particularly the sodium-potassium pump
- fluid restriction to prevent increase of interstitial and alveolar edema.

Acute respiratory failure

When the lungs can't adequately maintain arterial oxygenation or eliminate carbon dioxide, acute respiratory failure (ARF) results, which can lead to tissue hypoxia. In patients with essentially normal lung tissue, ARF usually means partial pressure of arterial carbon dioxide ($PaCO_2$) above 50 mm Hg and partial pressure of arterial oxygen (PaO_2) below 50 mm Hg. These limits, however, don't apply to patients with chronic obstructive pulmonary disease (COPD), who often have a consistently high $PaCO_2$ and low PaO_2. In patients with COPD, only acute deterioration in arterial blood gas (ABG) values, with corresponding clinical deterioration, indicates ARF.

CAUSES

Conditions that can result in alveolar hypoventilation, ventilation-perfusion ($\dot{V}/\dot{Q}$) mismatch, or right-to-left shunting can lead to respiratory failure; these include:

- COPD
- bronchitis
- pneumonia
- bronchospasm
- ventilatory failure
- pneumothorax
- atelectasis
- cor pulmonale
- pulmonary edema
- pulmonary emboli
- central nervous system (CNS) disease
- CNS depression — head trauma or injudicious use of sedatives, opioids, tranquilizers, or oxygen.

PATHOPHYSIOLOGY

Respiratory failure results from impaired gas exchange. Conditions associated with alveolar hypoventilation, $\dot{V}/\dot{Q}$ mismatch, and intrapulmonary (right-to-left) shunting can cause ARF if left untreated.

Decreased oxygen saturation may result from alveolar hypoventilation, in which chronic airway obstruction reduces alveolar minute ventilation. PaO_2 levels fall and $PaCO_2$ levels rise, resulting in hypoxemia.

Hypoventilation can occur with a decrease in the rate or duration of inspiratory signal from the respiratory center, such as with CNS conditions or trauma or CNS-depressant drugs. Neuromuscular diseases, such as poliomyelitis or amyotrophic lateral sclerosis, can result in alveolar hypoventilation if the condition affects normal contraction of the respiratory muscles. The most common cause of alveolar hypoventilation is airway obstruction, commonly seen with COPD (emphysema or bronchitis).

The most common cause of hypoxemia — $\dot{V}/\dot{Q}$ imbalance — occurs when such conditions as pulmonary embolism or acute respiratory distress syndrome interrupt normal gas exchange in a specific lung region. Too little ventilation with normal blood flow or too little blood flow with normal ventilation may cause the imbalance, resulting in decreased PaO_2 levels and, thus, hypoxemia.

Decreased fraction of inspired oxygen is also a cause of respiratory failure, although it's uncommon. Hypoxemia results from inspired air that doesn't contain adequate oxygen to establish an adequate gradient for diffusion into the blood — for example, at high altitudes or in confined spaces.

The hypoxemia and hypercapnia characteristics of respiratory failure stimulate strong compensatory responses by all of the body systems, including the respiratory, cardiovascular, and central nervous systems. In response to hypoxemia, for example, the sympathetic nervous system triggers vasoconstriction, increases peripheral resistance, and increases the heart rate. Untreated $\dot{V}/\dot{Q}$ imbalances can lead to right-to-left shunting in which blood passes from the heart's right side to its left without being oxygenated.

Tissue hypoxemia occurs, resulting in anaerobic metabolism and lactic acidosis. Respiratory acidosis occurs from hypercapnia. Heart rate increases, stroke volume increases, and heart failure may occur. Cyanosis occurs because of increased amounts of unoxygenated blood. Hypoxia of the kidneys results in the release of erythropoietin from renal cells, which causes the bone marrow to increase red blood cell production — an attempt by the body to increase the blood's oxygen-carrying capacity.

The body responds to hypercapnia with cerebral depression, hypotension, circulatory failure, and increased heart rate and cardiac output. Hypoxemia, hypercapnia, or both causes the brain's respiratory control center first to increase respiratory depth (tidal volume) and then to increase the respiratory rate. As respiratory failure worsens, intercostal, supraclavicular, and suprasternal retractions may also occur.

SIGNS AND SYMPTOMS

Specific symptoms vary with the underlying cause of ARF, but may include these systems:

■ *Respiratory*—Rate may be increased, decreased, or normal, depending on the cause; respirations may be shallow, deep, or alternate between the two; air hunger may occur. Cyanosis may or may not be present, depending on the hemoglobin level and arterial oxygenation. Auscultation of the chest may reveal crackles, rhonchi, wheezing, or diminished breath sounds secondary to possible airway obstruction and subsequent hypoventilation.

■ *CNS*—When hypoxemia and hypercapnia occur, a person may show restlessness, confusion, loss of concentration, irritability, tremulousness, diminished tendon reflexes, papilledema, and coma.

■ *Cardiovascular*—Tachycardia, with increased cardiac output and mildly elevated blood pressure as a result of adrenal release of catecholamine, occurs early in response to low PaO_2. With myocardial hypoxia, arrhythmias may develop. Pulmonary hypertension, resulting from pulmonary capillary vasoconstriction, may cause increased pressures on the right side of the heart, distended jugular veins, an enlarged liver, and peripheral edema.

COMPLICATIONS

Complications of ARF may include:
■ tissue hypoxia
■ metabolic acidosis
■ cardiac arrest.

DIAGNOSIS

These tests help identify ARF:

■ ABG analysis indicates respiratory failure by deteriorating values and a pH below 7.35. Patients with COPD may have a lower than normal pH compared with previous levels.

■ Chest X-rays identify pulmonary diseases or such conditions as emphysema, atelectasis, lesions, pneumothorax, infiltrates, and effusions.

■ Electrocardiography can demonstrate ventricular arrhythmias (indicating myo-

cardial hypoxia) or right ventricular hypertrophy (indicating cor pulmonale).

■ Pulse oximetry reveals decreasing arterial oxygen saturation.

■ White blood cell count detects the underlying infection.

■ Abnormally low hemoglobin level and hematocrit signal blood loss, which indicates decreased oxygen-carrying capacity.

■ Hypokalemia may result from compensatory hyperventilation, the body's attempt to correct acidosis.

■ Hypochloremia usually occurs in metabolic alkalosis.

■ Blood cultures may identify pathogens.

■ Pulmonary artery catheterization helps to distinguish pulmonary and cardiovascular causes of ARF and monitors hemodynamic pressures.

TREATMENT

Correcting ARF typically involves:
■ oxygen therapy to promote oxygenation and raise PaO_2
■ mechanical ventilation with an endotracheal or a tracheostomy tube, if needed, to provide adequate oxygenation and reverse acidosis
■ high-frequency ventilation, if treatment is ineffective for the patient, to force the airways open, promoting oxygenation and preventing alveoli collapse
■ antibiotics to treat infection
■ bronchodilators to maintain airway patency
■ corticosteroids to decrease inflammation
■ fluid restrictions in cor pulmonale to reduce volume and cardiac workload
■ positive inotropic agents to increase cardiac output
■ vasopressors to maintain blood pressure
■ diuretics to reduce edema and fluid overload
■ patient's deep breathing with pursed lips (if patient isn't intubated and mechanically ventilated) to help keep airway patent.

Asbestosis

Considered a form of pneumoconiosis, asbestosis is characterized by diffuse interstitial pulmonary fibrosis. Prolonged exposure to airborne particles causes pleural plaques and tumors of the pleura and peritoneum. Asbestosis can develop 15 to 20 years after regular exposure to asbestos has ended. It's a potent co-carcinogen and increases the smoker's risk of lung cancer. An asbestos worker who smokes is 90 times more likely to develop lung cancer as a smoker who has never worked with asbestos.

CAUSES

Common causes of asbestosis include:
- prolonged inhalation of asbestos fibers; people at high risk include workers in the mining, milling, construction, fireproofing, and textile industries
- exposure to asbestos used in paints, plastics, and brake and clutch linings
- family members of asbestos workers who may be exposed to stray fibers from the worker's clothing
- exposure to fibrous asbestos dust in deteriorating buildings or in waste piles from asbestos plants.

PATHOPHYSIOLOGY

Asbestosis occurs when lung spaces become filled with asbestos fibers. The inhaled asbestos fibers (50 microns or more in length and 0.5 microns or less in diameter) travel down the airway and penetrate respiratory bronchioles and alveolar walls. Coughing attempts to expel the foreign matter. Mucus production and goblet cells are stimulated to protect the airway from the debris and aid in expectoration. Fibers then become encased in a brown, iron-rich proteinlike sheath in sputum or lung tissue, called asbestosis bodies. Chronic irritation by the fibers continues to affect the lower bronchioles and alveoli. The foreign material and inflammation swell the airways, and fibrosis develops in response to the chronic irritation. Interstitial fibrosis may develop in lower lung zones, affecting lung parenchyma and the pleurae. Raised hyaline plaques may form in the parietal pleura, the diaphragm, and the pleura adjacent to the pericardium. Hypoxia develops as more alveoli and lower airways are affected.

SIGNS AND SYMPTOMS

Signs and symptoms of asbestosis may include:
- dyspnea on exertion as a result of increased mucus production and airway narrowing
- dyspnea at rest with extensive fibrosis
- severe, nonproductive cough in nonsmokers or productive cough in smokers from chronic irritation of bronchial tree and mucus production
- clubbed fingers from chronic hypoxia
- chest pain (commonly pleuritic) from pleural irritation
- recurrent respiratory tract infections as pulmonary defense mechanisms begin to fail
- pleural friction rub from fibrosis
- crackles on auscultation attributed to air moving through thickened sputum
- decreased lung inflation from lung stiffness
- recurrent pleural effusions from fibrosis
- decreased forced expiratory volume from diminished alveoli
- decreased vital capacity from fibrotic changes.

COMPLICATIONS

Possible complications of asbestosis include:
- pulmonary fibrosis from progression of asbestosis
- respiratory failure
- pulmonary hypertension
- cor pulmonale.

DIAGNOSIS

These tests help identify asbestosis:
- Chest X-rays may show fine, irregular, linear, and diffuse infiltrates. Extensive fibrosis is revealed by a honeycomb or ground-glass appearance. Chest X-rays may also show pleural thickening and calcification, bilateral obliteration of the costophrenic angles and, in later stages, an enlarged heart with a classic "shaggy" border.
- Pulmonary function tests may identify decreased vital capacity, forced vital capacity (FVC), and total lung capacity; decreased or normal forced expiratory volume in 1 second (FEV_1); a normal ratio, or FEV_1 to FVC; and reduced diffusing

capacity for carbon monoxide when fibrosis destroys alveolar walls and thickens the alveolar capillary membrane.

■ Arterial blood gas analysis may reveal decreased partial pressure of arterial oxygen and partial pressure of arterial carbon dioxide ($PaCO_2$) from hyperventilation.

TREATMENT

Asbestosis can't be cured. The goal of treatment is to relieve symptoms and control complications; treatment may involve:

■ chest physiotherapy (controlled coughing and postural drainage with chest percussion and vibration) to help relieve respiratory signs and symptoms and manage hypoxia and cor pulmonale

■ aerosol therapy to liquefy mucus

■ inhaled mucolytics to liquefy and mobilize secretions

■ increased fluid intake to 3 L daily

■ antibiotics to treat respiratory tract infections

■ oxygen administration to relieve hypoxia

■ possibly diuretics to decrease edema, digoxin to enhance cardiac output, and salt restriction to prevent fluid retention for patients with cor pulmonale.

Asthma

Asthma is a chronic inflammatory airway disorder characterized by airflow obstruction and airway hyperresponsiveness to a multiplicity of stimuli. This widespread but variable airflow obstruction is caused by bronchospasm, edema of the airway mucosa, and increased mucus production with plugging and airway remodeling. It's a type of chronic obstructive pulmonary disease (COPD), a long-term pulmonary disease characterized by increased airflow resistance; other types of COPD include chronic bronchitis and emphysema.

 AGE ALERT
Although asthma strikes at any age, about 50% of patients are younger than age 10; twice as many boys as girls are affected in this age-group. One-third of patients develop asthma between ages 10 and 30, and the incidence is the same in both sexes in this age-group. About one-third of all patients share the disease

with at least one immediate family member.

Asthma may result from sensitivity to extrinsic or intrinsic allergens. Extrinsic, or atopic, asthma begins in childhood; typically, patients are sensitive to specific external allergens.

AGE ALERT
Extrinsic asthma is commonly accompanied by other hereditary allergies, such as eczema and allergic rhinitis, in children.

Intrinsic, or nonatopic, patients with asthma react to internal, nonallergenic factors; external substances can't be implicated in patients with intrinsic asthma. Most episodes occur after a severe respiratory tract infection, especially in adults. However, many patients with asthma, especially children, have intrinsic and extrinsic asthma.

A significant number of adults acquire an allergic form of asthma or exacerbation of existing asthma from exposure to agents in the workplace. Irritants, such as chemicals in flour, acid anhydrides, toluene diisocyanates, screw flies, river flies, and excreta of dust mites in carpet, have been identified as agents that trigger asthma.

CAUSES

Extrinsic allergens include:

■ pollen

■ animal dander

■ house dust or mold

■ kapok or feather pillows

■ food additives containing sulfites

■ other sensitizing substances.

Intrinsic allergens include:

■ irritants

■ emotional stress

■ fatigue

■ endocrine changes

■ temperature variations

■ humidity variations

■ exposure to noxious fumes

■ anxiety

■ coughing or laughing

■ genetic factors (see below).

PATHOPHYSIOLOGY

There are two genetic influences identified with asthma, namely the ability of an individual to develop asthma (atopy) and the

CLOSER LOOK
Pathophysiology of asthma

In asthma, hyperresponsiveness of the airways and bronchospasms occur. These illustrations show the progression of an asthma attack.

◆ Histamine (H) attaches to receptor sites in larger bronchi, causing swelling of the smooth muscles.

◆ Leukotrienes (L) attach to receptor sites in the smaller bronchi and cause swelling of smooth muscle there. Leukotrienes also cause prostaglandins to travel through the bloodstream to the lungs, where they enhance histamine's effects.

◆ Histamine stimulates the mucous membranes to secrete excessive mucus, further narrowing the bronchial lumen. On inhalation, the narrowed bronchial lumen can still expand slightly; however, on exhalation, the increased intrathoracic pressure closes the bronchial lumen completely.

◆ Mucus fills lung bases, inhibiting alveolar ventilation. Blood is shunted to alveoli in other parts of the lungs, but it still can't compensate for diminished ventilation.

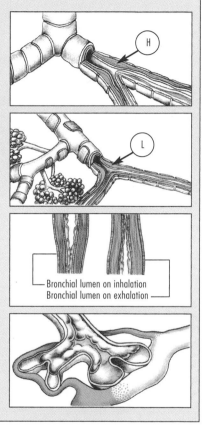

Bronchial lumen on inhalation
Bronchial lumen on exhalation

tendency to develop hyperresponsiveness of the airways independent of atopy. A locus of chromosome 11 associated with atopy contains an abnormal gene that encodes a part of the immunoglobulin (Ig) E receptor. Environmental factors interact with inherited factors to cause asthmatic reactions with associated bronchospasms.

In asthma, bronchial linings overreact to various stimuli, causing episodic smooth muscle spasms that severely constrict the airways. (See *Pathophysiology of asthma*.) IgE antibodies, attached to histamine-containing mast cells and receptors on cell membranes, initiate intrinsic asthma attacks. When exposed to an antigen, such as pollen, the IgE antibody combines with the antigen.

On subsequent exposure to the antigen, mast cells degranulate and release mediators. Mast cells in the lung interstitium are stimulated to release histamine and leuko-

CLOSER LOOK
Looking at a bronchiole in asthma

Asthma is characterized by bronchospasms, increased mucus secretion, and mucosal edema, which contribute to airway narrowing and obstruction. Shown here is a normal bronchiole in cross section and an obstructed bronchiole, as it occurs in asthma.

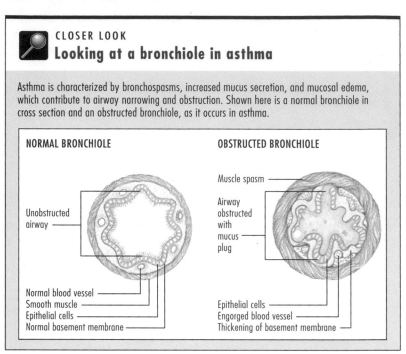

NORMAL BRONCHIOLE

Unobstructed airway

Normal blood vessel
Smooth muscle
Epithelial cells
Normal basement membrane

OBSTRUCTED BRONCHIOLE

Muscle spasm

Airway obstructed with mucus plug

Epithelial cells
Engorged blood vessel
Thickening of basement membrane

trienes. Histamine attaches to receptor sites in the larger bronchi, where it causes swelling in smooth muscles. Mucous membranes become inflamed, irritated, and swollen. The patient may experience dyspnea, prolonged expiration, and an increased respiratory rate.

Leukotrienes attach to receptor sites in the smaller bronchi and cause local swelling of the smooth muscle. Leukotrienes also cause prostaglandins to travel through the bloodstream to the lungs, where they enhance histamine's effect. A wheeze may be audible during coughing—the higher the pitch, the narrower the bronchial lumen. Histamine stimulates the mucous membranes to secrete excessive mucus, further narrowing the bronchial lumen. Goblet cells secrete viscous mucus that's difficult to cough up, resulting in coughing, rhonchi, increased-pitch wheezing, and increased respiratory distress. Mucosal edema and thickened secretions further block the airways. (See *Looking at a bronchiole in asthma.*)

On inhalation, the narrowed bronchial lumen can still expand slightly, allowing air to reach the alveoli. On exhalation, increased intrathoracic pressure closes the bronchial lumen completely. Air enters but can't escape. The patient develops a barrel chest and hyperresonance to percussion.

Mucus fills the lung bases, inhibiting alveolar ventilation. Blood is shunted to alveoli in other lung parts but still can't compensate for diminished ventilation.

Hyperventilation is triggered by lung receptors to increase lung volume because of trapped air and obstructions. Intrapleural and alveolar gas pressures rise, causing a decreased perfusion of alveoli. Increased alveolar gas pressure, decreased ventilation, and decreased perfusion result in uneven ventilation-perfusion ratios and mismatching within different lung segments.

Hypoxia triggers hyperventilation by respiratory center stimulation, which in turn decreases partial pressure of arterial carbon dioxide ($PaCO_2$) and increases pH, resulting in a respiratory alkalosis. As the airway obstruction increases in severity, more alveoli are affected. Ventilation and perfusion remain inadequate, and carbon dioxide retention develops. Respiratory acidosis results, and respiratory failure occurs.

If status asthmaticus occurs, hypoxia worsens and expiratory flows and volumes decrease even further. If treatment isn't initiated, the patient begins to tire out. (See *Averting an asthma attack.*) Acidosis develops as arterial carbon dioxide increases. The situation becomes life-threatening when air becomes audible upon auscultation (a silent chest) and $PaCO_2$ rises to more than 70 mm Hg.

SIGNS AND SYMPTOMS

Extrinsic asthma is usually accompanied by signs and symptoms of atopy (type I IgE-mediated allergy), such as eczema and allergic rhinitis. It commonly follows a severe respiratory tract infection, especially in adults.

An acute asthma attack begins dramatically, with simultaneous onset of severe multiple symptoms, or insidiously, with gradually increasing respiratory distress. Asthma that occurs with cyanosis, confusion, and lethargy indicates the onset of life-threatening status asthmaticus and respiratory failure.

Signs and symptoms of asthma include:
■ sudden dyspnea, wheezing, and tightness in the chest from bronchoconstriction
■ coughing that produces thick, clear, or yellow sputum resulting from excess mucus production
■ tachypnea, along with use of accessory respiratory muscles because of increasing air trapping and respiratory distress
■ rapid pulse resulting from increased workload of the heart because of the effects of hypoxemia and hyperinflation on the pulmonary vasculature
■ hyperresonant lung fields from air trapping
■ diminished breath sounds from obstruction and air trapping.

In 1997, the National Heart, Lung, and Blood Institute of the National Institutes of Health identified four levels of asthma severity based on the frequency of symp-

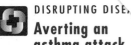

DISRUPTING DISEASE

Averting an asthma attack

This flowchart shows pathophysiologic changes that occur with asthma. Treatments and interventions show where the physiologic cascade would be altered to stop an asthma attack.

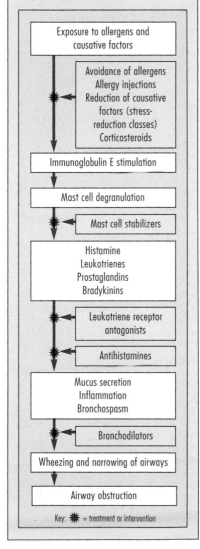

Exposure to allergens and causative factors

Avoidance of allergens
Allergy injections
Reduction of causative factors (stress-reduction classes)
Corticosteroids

Immunoglobulin E stimulation

Mast cell degranulation

Mast cell stabilizers

Histamine
Leukotrienes
Prostaglandins
Bradykinins

Leukotriene receptor antagonists

Antihistamines

Mucus secretion
Inflammation
Bronchospasm

Bronchodilators

Wheezing and narrowing of airways

Airway obstruction

Key: ✳ = treatment or intervention

...is and exacerbations, effects on activity ...el, and lung function study results: mild ...itermittent, mild persistent, moderate persistent, and severe persistent.

Findings for mild intermittent asthma include:

- symptoms occurring fewer than two times per week
- asymptomatic patient with normal peak expiratory flow (PEF) between exacerbations
- brief exacerbations (from a few hours to a few days) varying in intensity
- nighttime symptoms occurring fewer than two times per month
- lung function studies showing FEV_1 or PEF more than 80% of normal values; PEF may vary by less than 20%.

Findings for mild persistent asthma include:

- symptoms occurring more than two times per week, but less than once per day; exacerbations may affect activity
- nighttime symptoms occurring more than two times per month
- lung function studies showing FEV_1 or PEF more than 80% of normal values; PEF may vary by 20% to 30%.

Findings for moderate persistent asthma include:

- symptoms occurring daily
- exacerbations occurring more than two times per week and may last for days; exacerbations affect activity
- bronchodilator therapy used daily
- nighttime symptoms occurring more than once per week
- lung function studies showing FEV_1 or PEF 60% to 80% of normal values; PEF may vary by more than 30%.

Findings for severe persistent asthma include:

- symptoms occurring on a continuous basis
- exacerbations occurring frequently and limit physical activity
- nighttime symptoms occurring frequently
- lung function studies showing FEV_1 or PEF less than 60% of normal values; PEF may vary by more than 30%.

COMPLICATIONS
Possible complications of asthma include:

- status asthmaticus
- respiratory failure.

DIAGNOSIS
These tests help diagnose asthma:

- Pulmonary function tests reveal signs of airway obstructive disease, low-normal or decreased vital capacity, and increased total lung and residual capacities. Pulmonary function may be normal between attacks. Partial pressure of arterial oxygen (PaO_2) and $PaCO_2$ are usually decreased, except in severe asthma, when $PaCO_2$ may be normal or increased, indicating severe bronchial obstruction.
- Serum IgE levels may increase from an allergic reaction.
- Sputum analysis may indicate the presence of Curschmann's spirals (casts of airways), Charcot-Leyden crystals, and eosinophils.
- Complete blood count with differential reveals an increased eosinophil count.
- Chest X-rays can be used to diagnose or monitor the progress of asthma and may show hyperinflation with areas of atelectasis.
- Arterial blood gas (ABG) analysis detects hypoxemia (decreased PaO_2; decreased, normal, or increasing $PaCO_2$) and guides treatment.
- Skin testing may identify specific allergens. Results read in 1 or 2 days detect an early reaction; after 4 or 5 days, a late reaction.
- Bronchial challenge testing evaluates the clinical significance of allergens identified by skin testing.
- Electrocardiography shows sinus tachycardia during an attack; a severe attack may show signs of cor pulmonale (right axis deviation, peaked P wave) that resolve after the attack.

TREATMENT
Treatment for asthma is typically based on the severity of disease. Managing asthma usually involves:

- prevention, by identifying and avoiding precipitating factors, such as environmental allergens or irritants, which is the best treatment
- desensitization to specific antigens—helpful if the stimuli can't be removed en-

tirely—which decreases the severity of attacks of asthma with future exposure
■ bronchodilators—including the methylxanthines (theophylline and aminophylline) and the beta$_2$-adrenergic agonists (albuterol and terbutaline)—to decrease bronchoconstriction, reduce bronchial airway edema, and increase pulmonary ventilation
■ corticosteroids (such as hydrocortisone sodium succinate, prednisone, methylprednisolone, and beclomethasone) for their anti-inflammatory and immunosuppressive effects, which decrease inflammation and edema of the airways
■ mast cell stabilizers (cromolyn sodium and nedocromil sodium), effective in patients with atopic asthma who have seasonal disease (When given prophylactically, they block the acute obstructive effects of antigen exposure by inhibiting the degranulation of mast cells, thereby preventing the release of chemical mediators responsible for anaphylaxis.)
■ leukotriene modifiers, such as zileuton, and leukotriene receptor antagonists (LTRAs), such as montelukast and zafirlukast, inhibit the potent bronchoconstriction and inflammatory effects of the cysteinyl leukotrienes. LTRAs can be used as adjunctive therapy to avoid high-dose inhaled corticosteroids. Although this class of medications doesn't replace inhaled corticosteroids as first-line anti-inflammatory treatment, it can be used successfully in cases where poor compliance with inhaled corticosteroid use is suspected.
■ anticholinergic bronchodilators, such as ipratropium, which block acetylcholine, another chemical mediator
■ low-flow humidified oxygen, which may be needed to treat dyspnea, cyanosis, and hypoxemia (However, the amount delivered should maintain PaO$_2$ between 65 and 85 mm Hg, as determined by ABG analysis.)
■ mechanical ventilation—necessary if the patient's condition doesn't respond to initial ventilatory support and drugs, or if the patient develops respiratory failure
■ relaxation exercises, such as yoga, to help increase circulation and to help a patient recover from an asthma attack.

Chronic bronchitis

Chronic bronchitis is inflammation of the bronchi caused by irritants or infection. A form of chronic obstructive pulmonary disease (COPD), bronchitis may be classified as acute or chronic. In chronic bronchitis, hypersecretion of mucus and chronic productive cough last for 3 months of the year and occur for at least 2 consecutive years. The distinguishing characteristic of bronchitis is airflow obstruction.

 CLINICAL ALERT
COPD is more prevalent in an urban versus rural environment, and is also related to occupational factors (mineral or organic dusts).

AGE ALERT
Children of parents who smoke are at higher risk for respiratory tract infection, which can lead to chronic bronchitis.

CAUSES
Common causes of chronic bronchitis include:
■ exposure to irritants
■ cigarette smoking
■ genetic predisposition
■ exposure to organic or inorganic dusts
■ exposure to noxious gases
■ respiratory tract infection.

PATHOPHYSIOLOGY
Chronic bronchitis occurs when irritants are inhaled for a prolonged time. The irritants inflame the tracheobronchial tree, leading to increased mucus production and a narrowed or blocked airway. As the inflammation continues, changes in the cells lining the respiratory tract result in resistance of the small airways and severe ventilation-perfusion (V/Q) imbalance, which decreases arterial oxygenation.

Chronic bronchitis results in hypertrophy and hyperplasia of the mucous glands, increased goblet cells, ciliary damage, squamous metaplasia of the columnar epithelium, and chronic leukocytic and lymphocytic infiltration of bronchial walls. (See *Changes in chronic bronchitis,* page 228.) Hypersecretion of the goblet cells blocks the free movement of the cilia, which normally sweep dust, irritants, and mucus away from the airways. With mu-

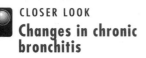

CLOSER LOOK
Changes in chronic bronchitis

In chronic bronchitis, irritants inflame the tracheobronchial tree over time, leading to increased mucus production and a narrowed or blocked airway. As the inflammation continues, goblet and epithelial cells hypertrophy. Because the natural defense mechanisms are blocked, the airways accumulate debris in the respiratory tract. The illllustrations show these changes.

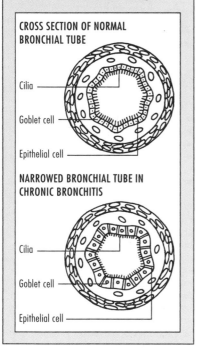

CROSS SECTION OF NORMAL BRONCHIAL TUBE

Cilia

Goblet cell

Epithelial cell

NARROWED BRONCHIAL TUBE IN CHRONIC BRONCHITIS

Cilia

Goblet cell

Epithelial cell

chospasm further narrow the lumen. Initially, only large bronchi are involved but, eventually, all airways are affected. Airways become obstructed and closure occurs, especially on expiration. The gas is then trapped in the distal portion of the lung. Hypoventilation occurs, leading to a V̇/Q̇ mismatch and resultant hypoxemia.

Hypoxemia and hypercapnia occur as a result of hypoventilation. Pulmonary vascular resistance (PVR) increases as inflammatory and compensatory vasoconstriction in hypoventilated areas narrows the pulmonary arteries. Increased PVR leads to increased afterload of the right ventricle. With repeated inflammatory episodes, scarring of the airways occurs, and permanent structural changes develop. Respiratory infections can trigger acute exacerbations, and respiratory failure can occur.

Patients with chronic bronchitis have a diminished respiratory drive. The resulting chronic hypoxia causes the kidneys to produce erythropoietin, which stimulates excessive red blood cell production and leads to polycythemia. Although hemoglobin levels are high, the amount of reduced (not fully oxygenated) hemoglobin in contact with oxygen is low; therefore, cyanosis occurs.

SIGNS AND SYMPTOMS
Signs and symptoms of chronic bronchitis may include:
■ copious gray, white, or yellow sputum from hypersecretion of goblet cells
■ productive cough to expectorate mucus produced by the lungs
■ dyspnea from airflow obstruction to the lower tracheobronchial tree
■ cyanosis related to diminished oxygenation and cellular hypoxia; reduced oxygen is supplied to the tissues
■ use of accessory muscles for breathing from compensated attempts to supply the cells with increased oxygen
■ tachypnea from hypoxia
■ pedal edema from right-sided heart failure
■ jugular vein distention from right-sided heart failure
■ weight gain from edema
■ wheezing from air moving through narrowed respiratory passages

cus and debris accumulating in the airway, the defenses are altered, and the individual is prone to respiratory tract infections.

Additional effects include widespread inflammation, airway narrowing, and mucus within the airways. Bronchial walls become inflamed and thickened from edema and accumulation of inflammatory cells, and the effects of smooth muscle bron-

- prolonged expiratory time from the body's attempt to keep airways patent
- rhonchi from air moving through narrow, mucus-filled passages
- pulmonary hypertension caused by involvement of small pulmonary arteries, from inflammation in the bronchial walls and spasms of pulmonary blood vessels from hypoxia.

COMPLICATIONS

Possible complications of chronic bronchitis include:
- recurrent respiratory tract infections
- cor pulmonale (right ventricular hypertrophy with right-sided heart failure) from increased right ventricular end-diastolic pressure
- pulmonary hypertension
- heart failure, resulting in increased venous pressure, liver engorgement, and dependent edema
- acute respiratory failure.

DIAGNOSIS

These tests help diagnose chronic bronchitis:
- Chest X-rays may show hyperinflation and increased bronchovascular markings.
- Pulmonary function studies indicate increased residual volume, decreased vital capacity and forced expiratory flow, and normal static compliance and diffusing capacity.
- Arterial blood gas analysis reveals decreased partial pressure of arterial oxygen and normal or increased partial pressure of arterial carbon dioxide.
- Sputum analysis may reveal many microorganisms and neutrophils.
- Electrocardiography may show atrial arrhythmias; peaked P waves in leads II, III, and aV$_F$; and, occasionally, right ventricular hypertrophy.

TREATMENT

Correcting chronic bronchitis typically involves:
- avoidance of air pollutants (most effective)
- smoking cessation and avoidance of second-hand smoke
- antibiotics to treat recurring infections

- bronchodilators to relieve bronchospasms and facilitate mucociliary clearance
- adequate hydration to liquefy secretions
- chest physiotherapy to mobilize secretions
- ultrasonic or mechanical nebulizers to loosen and mobilize secretions
- corticosteroids to combat inflammation
- diuretics to reduce edema
- oxygen to treat hypoxia.

Chronic obstructive pulmonary disease

Chronic obstructive pulmonary disease (COPD), also called *chronic obstructive lung disease,* results from emphysema, chronic bronchitis, asthma, or a combination of these disorders. Usually, more than one of these underlying conditions coexist; bronchitis and emphysema often occur together. (See "Asthma," page 222; "Chronic bronchitis," page 227; and "Emphysema," page 233, for a review of these conditions.)

COPD is the most common lung disease and affects an estimated 17 million people in the United States; the incidence is increasing. The disease doesn't always produce symptoms and may cause only minimal disability. However, COPD worsens with time.

CAUSES

Common causes of COPD may include:
- cigarette smoking
- recurrent or chronic respiratory tract infections
- air pollution
- allergies
- familial and hereditary factors such as an alpha$_1$-antitrypsin deficiency.

PATHOPHYSIOLOGY

Smoking, one of the major causes of COPD, impairs ciliary action and macrophage function and causes inflammation in the airways, increased mucus production, destruction of alveolar septa, and peribronchiolar fibrosis. Early inflammatory changes may reverse if the patient stops smoking before lung disease becomes extensive.

The mucus plugs and narrowed airways cause air trapping, as in chronic bronchitis

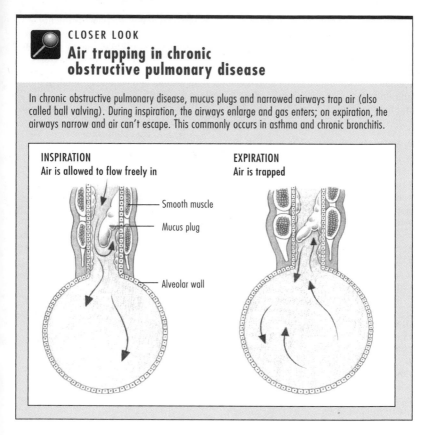

CLOSER LOOK
Air trapping in chronic obstructive pulmonary disease

In chronic obstructive pulmonary disease, mucus plugs and narrowed airways trap air (also called ball valving). During inspiration, the airways enlarge and gas enters; on expiration, the airways narrow and air can't escape. This commonly occurs in asthma and chronic bronchitis.

INSPIRATION
Air is allowed to flow freely in

EXPIRATION
Air is trapped

Smooth muscle

Mucus plug

Alveolar wall

and emphysema. Hyperinflation occurs to the alveoli on expiration. On inspiration, airways enlarge, allowing air to pass beyond the obstruction; on expiration, airways narrow and gas flow is prevented. Air trapping (also called *ball valving*) occurs commonly in asthma and chronic bronchitis. (See *Air trapping in chronic obstructive pulmonary disease.*)

SIGNS AND SYMPTOMS
Signs and symptoms of COPD may include:
■ reduced ability to perform exercises or do strenuous work because of diminished pulmonary reserve
■ productive cough from stimulation of the reflex by mucus
■ dyspnea on minimal exertion from narrowed airways and air trapping

■ frequent respiratory tract infections from impaired ciliary action and macrophage function
■ intermittent or continuous hypoxemia from impaired gas flow
■ grossly abnormal results on pulmonary function studies from effects of air trapping, inflammation, destruction of alveolar septa and peribronchial fibrosis
■ thoracic deformities resulting from chronic air trapping and increased work of breathing.

COMPLICATIONS
Possible complications of COPD include:
■ overwhelming disability
■ cor pulmonale
■ severe respiratory failure
■ death.

DIAGNOSIS

These tests help diagnose COPD:

- Arterial blood gas analysis determines oxygen need by indicating the degree of hypoxia and helps avoid carbon dioxide narcosis.
- Chest X-rays support the underlying diagnosis.
- Pulmonary function studies support the diagnosis of the underlying condition.
- Electrocardiography may show arrhythmias consistent with hypoxemia.

TREATMENT

Managing COPD typically involves:

- bronchodilators to alleviate bronchospasms and enhance mucociliary clearance of secretions
- effective coughing to remove secretions
- postural drainage to help mobilize secretions
- chest physiotherapy to mobilize secretions
- low oxygen concentrations as needed (High flow rates of oxygen can lead to narcosis.)

CLINICAL ALERT

The patient with COPD rarely requires more than 3 L/minute to maintain adequate oxygenation. Higher flow rates can further increase partial pressure of arterial oxygen, but the patient whose ventilatory drive is largely based on hypoxemia commonly develops markedly increased partial pressure of arterial carbon dioxide tensions. In this patient, chemoreceptors in the brain are relatively insensitive to the increase in carbon dioxide. Thus, excessive oxygen therapy may eliminate the hypoxic respiratory drive, causing confusion and drowsiness, signs of carbon dioxide narcosis.

- antibiotics to allow treatment of respiratory tract infections
- smoking cessation
- increased fluid intake to thin the mucus
- use of a humidifier to thin secretions.

Cor pulmonale

Cor pulmonale (also called *right-sided heart failure*) is a condition in which hypertrophy and dilation of the right ventricle develop because of disease affecting the structure or function of the lungs or their vasculature. It can occur at the end stage of various chronic disorders of the lungs, pulmonary vessels, chest wall, and respiratory control center. Cor pulmonale doesn't occur with disorders stemming from congenital heart disease or with those affecting the left side of the heart.

About 85% of patients with cor pulmonale also have chronic obstructive pulmonary disease (COPD), and about 25% of patients with bronchial COPD eventually develop cor pulmonale. The disorder is most common in smokers and in middle-age and elderly males; however, its incidence in females is increasing. Because cor pulmonale occurs late in the course of the individual's underlying condition and with other irreversible diseases, the prognosis is poor.

AGE ALERT

In children, cor pulmonale may be a complication of cystic fibrosis, hemosiderosis, upper airway obstruction, scleroderma, extensive bronchiectasis, neuromuscular diseases that affect respiratory muscles, or abnormalities of the respiratory control area.

CAUSES

Common causes of cor pulmonale include:

- disorders that affect the pulmonary parenchyma
- COPD
- bronchial asthma
- primary pulmonary hypertension
- vasculitis
- pulmonary emboli
- external vascular obstruction resulting from a tumor or aneurysm
- kyphoscoliosis
- pectus excavatum (funnel chest)
- muscular dystrophy
- poliomyelitis
- obesity
- high altitude.

PATHOPHYSIOLOGY

In cor pulmonale, pulmonary hypertension increases the heart's workload. To compensate, the right ventricle hypertrophies to force blood through the lungs. As long as the heart can compensate for the increased pulmonary vascular resistance,

CLOSER LOOK

Cor pulmonale: An overview

Although pulmonary restrictive disorders (such as fibrosis or obesity), obstructive disorders (such as bronchitis), or primary vascular disorders (such as recurrent pulmonary emboli) may cause cor pulmonale, these disorders share this common pathway.

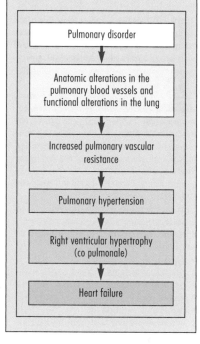

Pulmonary disorder

↓

Anatomic alterations in the pulmonary blood vessels and functional alterations in the lung

↓

Increased pulmonary vascular resistance

↓

Pulmonary hypertension

↓

Right ventricular hypertrophy (co pulmonale)

↓

Heart failure

signs and symptoms reflect only the underlying disorder.

Severity of right ventricular enlargement in cor pulmonale is from increased afterload. An occluded vessel impairs the heart's ability to generate enough pressure. Pulmonary hypertension results from the increased blood flow needed to oxygenate the tissues.

In response to hypoxia, the bone marrow produces more red blood cells (RBCs), causing polycythemia. The blood's viscosity increases, which further aggravates pulmonary hypertension. This increases the right ventricle's workload, causing heart failure. (See *Cor pulmonale: An overview*.)

In COPD, increased airway obstruction makes airflow worse. The resulting hypoxia and hypercarbia can have vasodilatory effects on systemic arterioles. However, hypoxia increases pulmonary vasoconstriction. The liver becomes palpable and tender because it's engorged and displaced downward by the low diaphragm. Hepatojugular reflux may occur.

Compensatory mechanisms begin to fail, and larger amounts of blood remain in the right ventricle at the end of diastole, causing ventricular dilation. Increasing intrathoracic pressures impede venous return and raise jugular venous pressure. Peripheral edema can occur, and right ventricular hypertrophy increases progressively. The main pulmonary arteries enlarge, pulmonary hypertension increases, and heart failure occurs.

SIGNS AND SYMPTOMS

Patients in the early stages of cor pulmonale may present with:
- a chronic productive cough to clear secretions from the lungs
- exertional dyspnea from hypoxia
- wheezing respirations as airways narrow
- fatigue and weakness from hypoxemia.

Patients with progressive cor pulmonale may present with:
- dyspnea at rest from hypoxemia
- tachypnea from decreased oxygenation to the tissues
- orthopnea from pulmonary edema
- dependent edema from right-sided heart failure
- distended jugular veins from pulmonary hypertension
- enlarged, tender liver related to polycythemia and decreased cardiac output
- hepatojugular reflux (distention of the jugular vein induced by pressing over the liver) from right-sided heart failure
- right upper quadrant discomfort from liver involvement
- tachycardia from decreased cardiac output and increasing hypoxia
- weakened pulses from decreased cardiac output

■ pansystolic murmur at the lower left sternal border with tricuspid insufficiency, which increases in intensity when the patient inhales.

COMPLICATIONS

Possible complications of cor pulmonale include:

■ right- and left-sided heart failure as the heart hypertrophies in an attempt to circulate the blood

■ hepatomegaly

■ edema

■ ascites

■ pleural effusions

■ thromboembolism from polycythemia.

DIAGNOSIS

These tests help diagnose cor pulmonale:

■ Pulmonary artery catheterization shows increased right ventricular and pulmonary artery pressures, resulting from increased pulmonary vascular resistance. Right ventricular systolic and pulmonary artery systolic pressures are more than 30 mm Hg, and pulmonary artery diastolic pressure is more than 15 mm Hg.

■ Echocardiography demonstrates right ventricular enlargement.

■ Angiography shows right ventricular enlargement.

■ Chest X-rays reveal large central pulmonary arteries and right ventricular enlargement.

■ Arterial blood gas analysis detects decreased partial pressure of arterial oxygen (usually less than 70 mm Hg and rarely more than 90 mm Hg).

■ Electrocardiography shows arrhythmias, such as premature atrial and ventricular contractions and atrial fibrillation during severe hypoxia, and also right bundle branch block, right axis deviation, prominent P waves, and an inverted T wave in right precordial leads.

■ Pulmonary function tests reflect underlying pulmonary disease.

■ Magnetic resonance imaging measures the right ventricular mass, wall thickness, and ejection fraction.

■ Cardiac catheterization measures pulmonary vascular pressures.

■ Laboratory testing may reveal hematocrit typically over 50%; serum hepatic tests may show an elevated level of aspartate aminotransferase levels with hepatic congestion and decreased liver function, and serum bilirubin levels may be elevated if liver dysfunction and hepatomegaly exist.

TREATMENT

Treatment of cor pulmonale has three aims: reducing hypoxemia and pulmonary vasoconstriction, increasing exercise tolerance, and correcting the underlying condition when possible. Treatment may involve:

■ bed rest to reduce myocardial oxygen demands

■ digoxin to increase the strength of contraction of the myocardium

■ antibiotics to treat an underlying respiratory tract infection

■ a potent pulmonary artery vasodilator, such as diazoxide, nitroprusside, hydralazine, angiotensin-converting enzyme inhibitors, calcium channel blockers or prostaglandins, to reduce primary pulmonary hypertension

■ continuous administration of low concentrations of oxygen to decrease pulmonary hypertension, polycythemia, and tachypnea

■ mechanical ventilation to reduce the workload of breathing in acute disease

■ a low-sodium diet with restricted fluid to reduce edema

■ phlebotomy to decrease excess RBC mass that occurs with polycythemia

■ small doses of heparin to decrease the risk of thromboembolism

■ tracheotomy, which may be required if the patient has an upper airway obstruction

■ corticosteroids to treat vasculitis or an underlying autoimmune disorder.

Emphysema

Emphysema, a form of chronic obstructive pulmonary disease, is the abnormal, permanent enlargement of the acini accompanied by destruction of alveolar walls. Obstruction results from tissue changes rather than mucus production, which occurs with asthma and chronic bronchitis. The distinguishing characteristic of em-

CLOSER LOOK
A look at abnormal alveoli

In the patient with emphysema, recurrent pulmonary inflammation damages and eventually destroys the alveolar walls, creating large air spaces. The damaged alveoli can't recoil normally after expanding; therefore, bronchioles collapse on expiration, trapping air in the lungs and causing overdistension. As the alveolar walls are destroyed, the lungs become enlarged, and the total lung capacity and residual volume then increase. Shown here are changes that occur during emphysema.

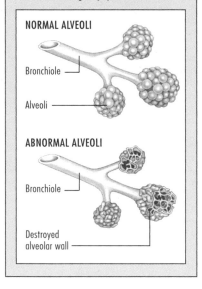

NORMAL ALVEOLI

Bronchiole

Alveoli

ABNORMAL ALVEOLI

Bronchiole

Destroyed alveolar wall

CAUSES
Emphysema is usually caused by:
- alpha₁-antitrypsin (AAT) deficiency
- cigarette smoking.

PATHOPHYSIOLOGY
Primary emphysema has been linked to an inherited deficiency of the enzyme AAT, a major component of alpha₁-globulin. AAT inhibits the activation of several proteolytic enzymes; deficiency of this enzyme is an autosomal recessive trait that predisposes an individual to develop emphysema because proteolysis in lung tissues isn't inhibited. Homozygous individuals have up to an 80% chance of developing lung disease; people who smoke have a greater chance of developing emphysema. Patients who develop emphysema before or during their early 40s and those who are nonsmokers are believed to have an AAT deficiency.

In emphysema, recurrent inflammation is associated with the release of proteolytic enzymes from lung cells. This causes irreversible enlargement of the air spaces distal to the terminal bronchioles. Enlargement of air spaces destroys the alveolar walls, which results in a breakdown of elasticity and loss of fibrous and muscle tissue, thus making the lungs less compliant.

In normal breathing, the air moves into and out of the lungs to meet metabolic needs. A change in airway size compromises the lungs' ability to circulate sufficient air. In patients with emphysema, recurrent pulmonary inflammation damages and eventually destroys the alveolar walls, creating large air spaces. (See *A look at abnormal alveoli*.)

The alveolar septa are initially destroyed, eliminating a portion of the capillary bed and increasing air volume in the acinus. This breakdown leaves the alveoli unable to recoil normally after expanding and results in bronchiolar collapse on expiration. The damaged or destroyed alveolar walls can't support the airways to keep them open. (See *Air trapping in emphysema*.) The amount of air that can be expired passively is diminished, thus trapping air in the lungs and leading to overdistension. Hyperinflation of the alveoli produces bullae (air spaces) adjacent to

physema is airflow limitation caused by lack of elastic recoil in the lungs.

Emphysema appears to be more prevalent in males than in females; about 65% of patients with well-defined emphysema are men and 35% are women.

AGE ALERT
Aging is a risk factor for emphysema. Senile emphysema results from degenerative changes; stretching occurs without destruction in the smooth muscle. Connective tissue usually isn't affected.

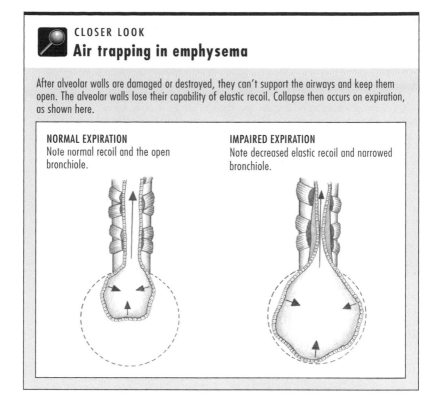

CLOSER LOOK
Air trapping in emphysema

After alveolar walls are damaged or destroyed, they can't support the airways and keep them open. The alveolar walls lose their capability of elastic recoil. Collapse then occurs on expiration, as shown here.

NORMAL EXPIRATION
Note normal recoil and the open bronchiole.

IMPAIRED EXPIRATION
Note decreased elastic recoil and narrowed bronchiole.

the pleura (blebs). Septal destruction also decreases airway calibration. Part of each inspiration is trapped because of increased residual volume and decreased calibration. Septal destruction may affect only the respiratory bronchioles and alveolar ducts, leaving alveolar sacs intact (centriacinar emphysema), or it can involve the entire acinus (panacinar emphysema), with damage more random and involving the lower lobes of the lungs.

AGE ALERT
Panacinar emphysema tends to occur in elderly people with an AAT deficiency, whereas centriacinar emphysema occurs in smokers with chronic bronchitis.

Associated pulmonary capillary destruction usually allows a patient with severe emphysema to match ventilation to perfusion. This process prevents the development of cyanosis. The lungs are usually enlarged; therefore, the total lung capacity and residual volume increase.

SIGNS AND SYMPTOMS
Signs and symptoms of emphysema may include:
■ tachypnea related to decreased oxygenation
■ dyspnea on exertion, commonly the initial symptom from changes in airway size
■ barrel-shaped chest from the lungs overdistending and overinflating
■ prolonged expiration and grunting, which occur because the accessory muscles are used for inspiration and abdominal muscles are used for expiration
■ decreased breath sounds caused by air-trapping in the alveoli and alveolar wall destruction
■ clubbed fingers and toes related to chronic hypoxic changes

- decreased tactile fremitus on palpation as air moves through poorly functioning alveoli
- decreased chest expansion from hypoventilation
- hyperresonance on chest percussion from overinflated air spaces
- crackles and wheezing on inspiration as bronchioles collapse.

COMPLICATIONS
Possible complications of emphysema include:
- right ventricular hypertrophy (cor pulmonale)
- respiratory failure
- recurrent respiratory tract infections
- spontaneous pneumothorax.

 CLINICAL ALERT
Be aware that alveolar blebs and bullae may rupture, leading to spontaneous pneumothorax, requiring immediate intervention. Sudden, sharp pleuritic pain exacerbated by chest movement, breathing, or coughing is highly suggestive of this condition.

DIAGNOSIS
These tests help diagnose emphysema:
- Chest X-rays in advanced disease may show a flattened diaphragm, reduced vascular markings at the lung periphery, overaeration of the lungs, vertical heart, enlarged anteroposterior chest diameter, and a large retrosternal air space.
- Pulmonary function tests indicate increased residual volume and total lung capacity, reduced diffusing capacity, and increased inspiratory flow.
- Arterial blood gas analysis usually reveals reduced partial pressure of arterial oxygen and a normal partial pressure of arterial carbon dioxide until late in the disease process.
- Electrocardiography may show tall, symmetrical P waves in leads II, III, and aV_F; a vertical QRS axis and signs of right ventricular hypertrophy are seen late in the disease.
- Complete blood count usually reveals an increased hemoglobin level late in the disease when the patient has persistent, severe hypoxia.

TREATMENT
Correcting emphysema typically involves:
- avoiding smoking to preserve remaining alveoli
- avoiding air pollution to preserve remaining alveoli
- bronchodilators, such as beta-adrenergic blockers, albuterol, and ipratropium bromide, to reverse bronchospasms and promote mucociliary clearance
- antibiotics to treat respiratory tract infections
- pneumovax to prevent pneumococcal pneumonia
- adequate hydration to liquefy and mobilize secretions
- chest physiotherapy to mobilize secretions
- oxygen therapy at low settings to correct hypoxia
- flu vaccine to prevent influenza
- mucolytics to thin secretions and aid in mucus expectoration
- aerosolized or systemic corticosteroids
- transtracheal catheterization to enable the patient to receive oxygen therapy at home
- lung volume reduction surgery for selected patients. (Nonfunctional parts of the lung [tissue filled with disease providing little ventilation or perfusion] are surgically removed; removal allows more functional lung tissue to expand and the diaphragm to return to its normally elevated position.)

Pleural effusion and empyema

Pleural effusion is excess fluid in the pleural space. Normally, this space contains a small amount of extracellular fluid that lubricates the pleural surfaces. Increased production or inadequate removal of this fluid results in pleural effusion. Empyema is the accumulation of pus and necrotic tissue in the pleural space. Blood (hemothorax) and chyle (chylothorax) may also collect in this space.

CAUSES
Transudative pleural effusions frequently result from heart failure, hepatic disease with ascites, peritoneal dialysis, hypoalbuminemia, and disorders resulting in overexpanded intravascular volume.

Exudative pleural effusions occur with tuberculosis (TB), subphrenic abscess, pancreatitis, bacterial or fungal pneumonitis or empyema, malignancy, pulmonary embolism with or without infarction, collagen disease (lupus erythematosus [LE] and rheumatoid arthritis), myxedema, and chest trauma.

Empyema may result from idiopathic infection or may be related to pneumonitis, carcinoma, perforation, or esophageal rupture.

PATHOPHYSIOLOGY

The balance of osmotic and hydrostatic pressures in parietal pleural capillaries normally results in fluid movement into the pleural space. Balanced pressures in visceral pleural capillaries promote reabsorption of this fluid. Excessive hydrostatic pressure or decreased osmotic pressure can cause excess fluid to pass across intact capillaries. The result is a transudative pleural effusion, an ultrafiltrate of plasma containing low concentrations of protein.

Exudative pleural effusions result when capillaries exhibit increased permeability with or without changes in hydrostatic and colloid osmotic pressures, allowing protein-rich fluid to leak into the pleural space.

Empyema is usually associated with an infection in the pleural space, which results from an extension of an infection of nearby structures.

SIGNS AND SYMPTOMS

Signs and symptoms of pleural effusion may include:
- dyspnea
- pleuritic chest pain
- other clinical features, depending on the cause of the effusion
- fever and malaise in patients with empyema.

COMPLICATIONS

Complications of pleural effusion may include:
- impaired ventilation
- pleurisy.
  Complications of empyema may include:
- pleurisy

- pericarditis
- septicemia.

DIAGNOSIS

Auscultation of the chest reveals decreased breath sounds; percussion detects dullness over the effused area, which doesn't change with breathing. Chest X-ray shows radiopaque fluid in dependent regions. However, diagnosis also requires other tests to distinguish transudative from exudative effusions and to help pinpoint the underlying disorder.

The most useful test is thoracentesis, in which analysis of aspirated pleural fluid shows:
- transudative effusions — lactate dehydrogenase (LD) levels less than 200 IU and protein levels less than 3 g/dl
- exudative effusions — ratio of protein in pleural fluid to serum of 0.5 or more, LD in pleural fluid of 200 IU or more, and ratio of LD in pleural fluid to LD in serum of 0.6 or more
- empyema — acute inflammatory white blood cells and microorganisms
- empyema or exudative effusion occurring with rheumatoid arthritis — extremely decreased pleural fluid glucose levels.

In addition, if a pleural effusion results from esophageal rupture or pancreatitis, fluid amylase levels are usually higher than serum levels. Aspirated fluid may be tested for LE cells, antinuclear antibodies, and neoplastic cells. It may also be analyzed for color and consistency; acid-fast bacillus, fungal, and bacterial cultures; and triglycerides (in chylothorax). Cell analysis shows leukocytosis in empyema. A negative tuberculin skin test strongly rules against TB as the cause. In exudative pleural effusions in which thoracentesis isn't definitive, pleural biopsy may be done. It's particularly useful for confirming TB or malignancy.

TREATMENT

Treatment depends on the amount of fluid present and may include:
- thoracentesis to remove fluid or careful monitoring of the patient's own reabsorption of the fluid (symptomatic effusion)
- drainage to prevent fibrothorax formation (hemothorax)

■ insertion of a chest tube to drain the fluid (Because pleural effusions associated with lung cancer typically reaccumulate quickly, a sclerosing agent, such as talc, may be injected through the tube to cause adhesions between the parietal and visceral pleura, thereby obliterating the potential space for fluid to recollect.)

■ oxygen administration for associated hypoxia.

Treatment of empyema requires:

■ insertion of one or more chest tubes after thoracentesis, to allow drainage of purulent material, and possibly decortication (surgical removal of the thick coating over the lung) or rib resection to allow open drainage and lung expansion

■ parenteral antibiotics

■ oxygen administration for associated hypoxia.

Pneumothorax

Pneumothorax is an accumulation of air in the pleural cavity that leads to partial or complete lung collapse. When the air between the visceral and parietal pleurae collects and accumulates, increasing tension in the pleural cavity can cause the lung to progressively collapse. Air is trapped in the intrapleural space and determines the degree of lung collapse. Venous return to the heart may be impeded to cause a life-threatening condition called *tension pneumothorax.*

The most common types of pneumothorax are open, closed, and tension.

CAUSES

Common causes of open pneumothorax include:

■ penetrating chest injury (gunshot or stab wound)

■ insertion of a central venous catheter

■ chest surgery

■ transbronchial biopsy

■ thoracentesis or closed pleural biopsy.

Causes of closed pneumothorax include:

■ blunt chest trauma

■ air leakage from ruptured blebs

■ rupture resulting from barotrauma caused by high intrathoracic pressures during mechanical ventilation

■ tubercular or cancerous lesions that erode into the pleural space

■ interstitial lung disease such as eosinophilic granuloma.

Tension pneumothorax may be caused by:

■ penetrating chest wound treated with an air-tight dressing

■ fractured ribs

■ mechanical ventilation

■ high-level positive end-expiratory pressure that causes alveolar blebs to rupture

■ chest tube occlusion or malfunction.

PATHOPHYSIOLOGY

A rupture in the visceral or parietal pleura and chest wall causes air to accumulate and separate the visceral and parietal pleurae. Negative pressure is destroyed, and the elastic recoil forces are affected. The lung recoils by collapsing toward the hilus.

Open pneumothorax (also called a *sucking chest wound* or *communicating pneumothorax*) results when atmospheric air (positive pressure) flows directly into the pleural cavity (negative pressure). As the air pressure in the pleural cavity becomes positive, the lung collapses on the affected side, resulting in decreased total lung capacity, vital capacity, and lung compliance. Ventilation-perfusion imbalances lead to hypoxia.

Closed pneumothorax occurs when air enters the pleural space from within the lung, causing increased pleural pressure, which prevents lung expansion during normal inspiration. Spontaneous pneumothorax is another type of closed pneumothorax.

AGE ALERT
Spontaneous pneumothorax is common in older patients with chronic pulmonary disease, but it may also occur in healthy, tall, young adults.

Both types of closed pneumothorax can result in a collapsed lung with hypoxia and decreased total lung capacity, vital capacity, and lung compliance. The range of lung collapse is between 5% and 95%.

Tension pneumothorax results when air in the pleural space is under higher pressure than air in the adjacent lung. The air enters the pleural space from the site of pleural rupture, which acts as a one-way valve. Air is allowed to enter into the pleural space on inspiration, but can't escape as the rupture site closes on expiration. More air enters on inspiration, and air pressure begins to exceed barometric pressure. Increasing air pressure pushes against the recoiled lung, causing compression atelectasis. Air also presses against the mediastinum, compressing and displacing the heart and great vessels. The air can't escape, and the accumulating pressure causes the lung to collapse. As air continues to accumulate and intrapleural pressures increase, the mediastinum shifts away from the affected side and decreases venous return. This forces the heart, trachea, esophagus, and great vessels to the unaffected side, compressing the heart and the contralateral lung. Without immediate treatment, this emergency can rapidly become fatal. (See *Understanding tension pneumothorax.*)

SIGNS AND SYMPTOMS

Signs and symptoms of pneumothorax may include:

■ sudden, sharp pleuritic pain exacerbated by chest movement, breathing, and coughing secondary to increased tension in pleural cavity

■ asymmetrical chest wall movement from lung collapse

■ shortness of breath from hypoxia

■ cyanosis from hypoxia

■ decreased vocal fremitus related to lung collapse

■ absent breath sounds on the affected side from lung collapse

■ chest rigidity on the affected side from decreased expansion

■ tachycardia from hypoxia

■ crackling beneath the skin on palpation (subcutaneous emphysema), which is from air leaking into the tissues.

Tension pneumothorax produces the most severe respiratory symptoms, including:

■ decreased cardiac output related to mediastinal shift and decreased venous return

■ hypotension from decreased cardiac output

■ compensatory tachycardia

■ tachypnea from hypoxia

CLOSER LOOK
Understanding tension pneumothorax

In tension pneumothorax, air accumulates intrapleurally and can't escape. As intrapleural pressure increases, the ipsilateral lung is affected and also collapses.

On inspiration, the mediastinum shifts toward the unaffected lung, impairing ventilation.

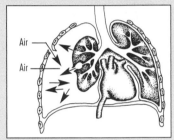

On expiration, the mediastinal shift distorts the vena cava and reduces venous return.

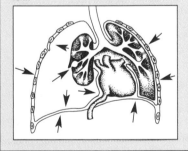

■ lung collapse from air or blood in the intrapleural space

■ mediastinal shift from increasing tension

■ tracheal deviation to the opposite side from mediastinal shift

■ distended jugular veins from intrapleural pressure, mediastinal shift, and increased cardiovascular pressure

■ pallor related to decreased cardiac output

- anxiety related to hypoxia
- weak and rapid pulse from decreased cardiac output.

COMPLICATIONS
Possible complications of pneumothorax include:
- decreased cardiac output
- hypoxemia
- cardiac arrest.

DIAGNOSIS
These tests help diagnose pneumothorax:
- Chest X-rays confirm the diagnosis by revealing air in the pleural space and, possibly, a mediastinal shift.
- Arterial blood gas analysis may reveal hypoxemia, possibly with respiratory acidosis and hypercapnia. Partial pressure of arterial oxygen levels may decrease at first, but typically return to normal within 24 hours.

TREATMENT
Treatment depends on the type of pneumothorax.

Spontaneous pneumothorax with less than 30% of lung collapse, no signs of increased pleural pressure, and no dyspnea or indications of physiologic compromise, may be corrected with:
- bed rest to conserve energy and reduce oxygenation demands
- monitoring of blood pressure and pulse for early detection of physiologic compromise
- monitoring of respiratory rate to detect early signs of respiratory compromise
- oxygen administration to enhance oxygenation and improve hypoxia
- aspiration of air with a large-bore needle attached to a syringe to restore negative pressure within the pleural space.

Correction of pneumothorax with more than 30% of lung collapse may include:
- thoracostomy tube placed in the second or third intercostal space in the midclavicular line with connection to underwaterseal and low-pressure suction to try to reexpand the lung by restoring negative intrapleural pressure
- if recurrent spontaneous pneumothorax, thoracotomy and pleurectomy may be performed, which causes the lung to adhere to the parietal pleura.

Open (traumatic) pneumothorax may be corrected with:
- chest tube drainage to reexpand the lung
- surgical repair of the lung.

Correction of tension pneumothorax typically involves:
- immediate treatment with large-bore needle insertion into the pleural space through the second intercostal space to reexpand the lung
- insertion of a thoracostomy tube
- analgesics to promote comfort and encourage deep breathing and coughing.

Pulmonary edema

Pulmonary edema is an accumulation of fluid in the extravascular spaces of the lungs. It's a common complication of cardiac disorders and may occur as a chronic condition or may develop quickly and rapidly become fatal.

CAUSES
Pulmonary edema is caused by left-sided heart failure due to:
- arteriosclerosis
- cardiomyopathy
- hypertension
- valvular heart disease.

Factors that predispose the patient to pulmonary edema include:
- barbiturate or opiate poisoning
- cardiac failure
- excess infusion of I.V. fluids or overly rapid infusion
- impaired pulmonary lymphatic drainage (from Hodgkin's disease or obliterative lymphangitis after radiation)
- inhalation of irritating gases
- mitral stenosis and left atrial myxoma (which impairs left atrial emptying)
- pneumonia
- pulmonary veno-occlusive disease.

PATHOPHYSIOLOGY
Normally, pulmonary capillary hydrostatic pressure, capillary oncotic pressure, capillary permeability, and lymphatic drainage are in balance. When this balance changes or the lymphatic drainage system is obstructed, fluid infiltrates into the lung and

CLOSER LOOK
Understanding pulmonary edema

In pulmonary edema, diminished function of the left ventricle causes blood to back up into pulmonary veins and capillaries. The increasing capillary hydrostatic pressure pushes fluid into the interstitial spaces and alveoli. These illustrations show a normal alveolus and an alveolus affected by pulmonary edema.

NORMAL ALVEOLUS

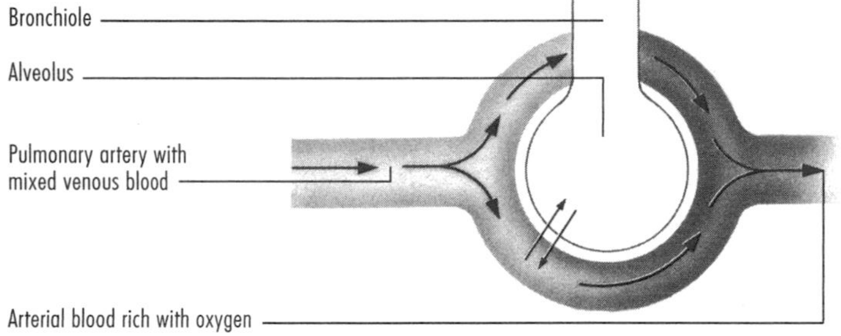

Bronchiole

Alveolus

Pulmonary artery with mixed venous blood

Arterial blood rich with oxygen

ALVEOLUS IN PULMONARY EDEMA

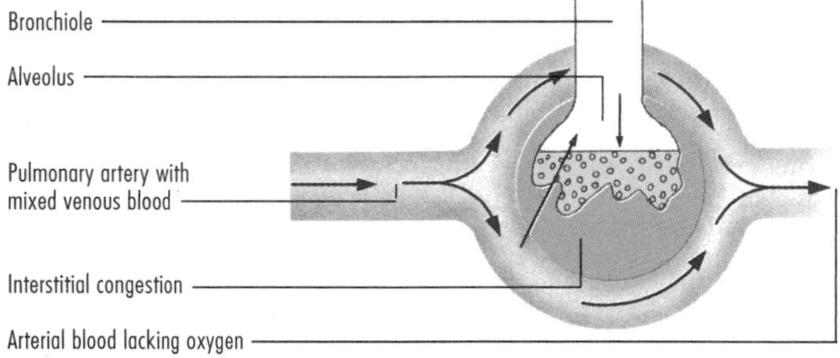

Bronchiole

Alveolus

Pulmonary artery with mixed venous blood

Interstitial congestion

Arterial blood lacking oxygen

pulmonary edema results. If pulmonary capillary hydrostatic pressure increases, the compromised left ventricle requires increased filling pressures to maintain adequate cardiac output. These pressures are transmitted to the left atrium, pulmonary veins, and pulmonary capillary bed, forcing fluids and solutes from the intravascular compartment into the interstitium of the lungs. As the interstitium overloads

with fluid, fluid floods the peripheral alveoli and impairs gas exchange.

If colloid osmotic pressure decreases, the hydrostatic force that regulates intravascular fluids (the natural pulling force) is lost because there's no opposition. Fluid flows freely into the interstitium and alveoli, impairing gas exchange and leading to pulmonary edema. (See *Understanding pulmonary edema*.)

A blockage of the lymph vessels can result from compression by edema or tumor fibrotic tissue and by increased systemic venous pressure. Hydrostatic pressure in the large pulmonary veins increases, the pulmonary lymphatic system can't drain correctly into the pulmonary veins, and excess fluid moves into the interstitial space. Pulmonary edema then results from fluid accumulation.

Capillary injury, such as occurs in acute respiratory distress syndrome (ARDS) or with inhalation of toxic gases, increases capillary permeability. The injury causes plasma proteins and water to leak out of the capillary and move into the interstitium, increasing the interstitial oncotic pressure, which is normally low. As interstitial oncotic pressure begins to equal capillary oncotic pressure, the water begins to move out of the capillary and into the lungs, resulting in pulmonary edema.

SIGNS AND SYMPTOMS
Signs and symptoms of early states of pulmonary edema may include:
- dyspnea on exertion caused by hypoxia
- paroxysmal nocturnal dyspnea caused by decreased lung expansion from alveolar flooding
- orthopnea from decreased ability of the diaphragm to expand
- cough caused by stimulation of cough reflex by excessive fluid
- mild tachypnea from hypoxia
- increased blood pressure from increased pulmonary pressures and decreased oxygenation
- dependent crackles as air moves through fluid in the lungs
- jugular vein distention from decreased cardiac output and increased pulmonary vascular resistance
- tachycardia from hypoxia.

Signs and symptoms of later stages of pulmonary edema may include:
- labored, rapid respiration from hypoxia
- more diffuse crackles as air moves through fluid in the lungs
- cough, producing frothy, bloody sputum
- increased tachycardia from hypoxemia
- arrhythmias from hypoxic myocardium

- cold, clammy skin from peripheral vasoconstriction
- diaphoresis from decreased cardiac output and shock
- cyanosis from hypoxia
- decreased blood pressure from decreased cardiac output and shock
- thready pulse from decreased cardiac output and shock.

COMPLICATIONS
Possible complications of pulmonary edema include:
- respiratory failure
- respiratory acidosis
- cardiac arrest.

DIAGNOSIS
These tests help diagnose pulmonary edema:
- Arterial blood gas analysis usually reveals hypoxia with variable partial pressure of arterial carbon dioxide, depending on the patient's degree of fatigue. Respiratory acidosis may occur.
- Chest X-rays show diffuse haziness of the lung fields and, usually, cardiomegaly and pleural effusion.
- Pulse oximetry may reveal decreasing arterial oxygen saturation levels.
- Pulmonary artery catheterization identifies left-sided heart failure and helps rule out ARDS.
- Electrocardiography may show previous or current myocardial infarction.

TREATMENT
Treatment measures for pulmonary edema are designed to reduce extravascular fluid, to improve gas exchange and myocardial function and, if possible, to correct underlying conditions. Correcting this disorder typically involves:
- high concentrations of oxygen administered by nasal cannula to enhance gas exchange and improve oxygenation
- assisted ventilation to improve oxygen delivery to the tissues and promote acid-base balance
- diuretics, such as furosemide and bumetanide, to increase urination, which helps mobilize extravascular fluid

- positive inotropic agents, such as digoxin and inamrinone, to enhance contractility in myocardial dysfunction
- pressor agents to enhance contractility and promote vasoconstriction in peripheral vessels
- antiarrhythmics for arrhythmias related to decreased cardiac output
- arterial vasodilators, such as nitroprusside, to decrease peripheral vascular resistance, preload, and afterload
- morphine to reduce anxiety and dyspnea and to dilate the systemic venous bed, promoting blood flow from pulmonary circulation to the periphery.

Pulmonary embolism

The most common pulmonary complication in a hospitalized patient, pulmonary embolism is an obstruction of the pulmonary arterial bed by a dislodged thrombus, heart valve growths, or a foreign substance. It strikes an estimated 6 million adults each year in the United States, resulting in 100,000 deaths. Although pulmonary infarction that results from embolism may be so mild as to be asymptomatic, massive embolism (more than 50% obstruction of pulmonary arterial circulation) and the accompanying infarction can be rapidly fatal.

CAUSES
Pulmonary embolism generally results from dislodged thrombi originating in the leg veins or pelvis. More than one-half of such thrombi arise in the deep veins of the legs. Other less common sources of thrombi are the pelvic veins, renal veins, hepatic vein, right side of the heart, and upper extremities.

Predisposing factors for pulmonary embolism include long-term immobility, chronic pulmonary disease, heart failure or atrial fibrillation, thrombophlebitis, polycythemia vera, thrombocytosis, autoimmune hemolytic anemia, sickle cell disease, varicose veins, recent surgery, advanced age, lower-extremity fractures or surgery, burns, obesity, vascular injury, cancer, I.V. drug abuse, or hormonal contraceptives.

PATHOPHYSIOLOGY
Thrombus formation results directly from vascular wall damage, venostasis, or hypercoagulability of the blood. Trauma, clot dissolution, sudden muscle spasm, intravascular pressure changes, or a change in peripheral blood flow can cause the thrombus to loosen or fragment. Then the thrombus — now called an *embolus* — floats to the heart's right side and enters the lung through the pulmonary artery. There, the embolus may dissolve, continue to fragment, or grow.

By occluding the pulmonary artery, the embolus prevents alveoli from producing enough surfactant to maintain alveolar integrity. As a result, alveoli collapse and atelectasis develops. If the embolus enlarges, it may clog most or all of the pulmonary vessels and cause death.

Rarely, the emboli contain air, fat, bacteria, amniotic fluid, talc (from drugs intended for oral administration, which are injected intravenously by addicts), or tumor cells.

SIGNS AND SYMPTOMS
Total occlusion of the main pulmonary artery is rapidly fatal; smaller or fragmented emboli produce symptoms that vary with the size, number, and location:
- dyspnea (usually the first symptom), which may be accompanied by anginal or pleuritic chest pain from pulmonary infarction
- tachycardia related to hypoxemia
- productive cough (sputum may be blood-tinged) related to mucus production from obstruction from embolus
- pleural effusion related to changes in intrapulmonary pressures secondary to embolus.

Less common signs include massive hemoptysis, splinting of the chest, leg edema and, with a large embolus, cyanosis, syncope, and distended jugular veins.

In addition, pulmonary embolism may cause pleural friction rub and signs of circulatory collapse (weak, rapid pulse and hypotension) and of hypoxia (restlessness and anxiety).

COMPLICATIONS

Complications of pulmonary embolism may include:

- pulmonary infarction
- acute respiratory failure
- acute cor pulmonale
- death.

DIAGNOSIS

The patient history should reveal predisposing conditions for pulmonary embolism. A triad of deep vein thrombosis (DVT) formation is stasis, endothelial injury, and hypercoagulability. Risk factors include long car or plane trips, cancer, pregnancy, hypercoagulability, previous DVTs, and pulmonary emboli.

These tests support the diagnosis of pulmonary embolism:

- Chest X-ray helps to rule out other pulmonary diseases; areas of atelectasis, elevated diaphragm and pleural effusion, prominent pulmonary artery and, occasionally, the characteristic wedge-shaped infiltrate suggestive of pulmonary infarction, or focal oligemia of blood vessels, are apparent.
- Lung scan shows perfusion defects in areas beyond occluded vessels; however, it doesn't rule out microemboli.
- Pulmonary angiography is the most definitive test, but requires a skilled angiographer and radiologic equipment; it also poses some risk to the patient. Its use depends on the uncertainty of the diagnosis and the need to avoid unnecessary anticoagulant therapy in a high-risk patient.
- Electrocardiography (ECG) is inconclusive, but helps distinguish pulmonary embolism from myocardial infarction. In extensive embolism, the ECG may show right axis deviation; right bundle-branch block; tall, peaked P waves; depression of ST segments and T-wave inversions (indicative of right-sided heart strain); and supraventricular tachyarrhythmias. A pattern sometimes observed is S_1, Q_3, and T_3 (S wave in lead I, Q wave in lead III, and inverted T wave in lead III).
- Auscultation occasionally reveals a right ventricular S_3 gallop and increased intensity of a pulmonic component of S_2. Also, crackles and a pleural rub may be heard at the embolism site.

- Arterial blood gas measurements showing decreased partial pressure of arterial carbon dioxide and partial pressure of arterial oxygen are characteristic, but don't always occur.
- If pleural effusion is present, thoracentesis may rule out empyema, which indicates pneumonia.

TREATMENT

Treatment is designed to maintain adequate cardiovascular and pulmonary function during resolution of the obstruction and to prevent embolus recurrence. Because most emboli resolve within 10 to 14 days, treatment consists of:

- oxygen therapy, as needed
- anticoagulation with heparin to inhibit new thrombus formation; heparin therapy is monitored by daily coagulation studies (partial thromboplastin time)
- fibrinolytic therapy with urokinase, streptokinase, or alteplase for patients with massive pulmonary embolism and shock to enhance fibrinolysis of the pulmonary emboli and remaining thrombi
- vasopressors for emboli that cause hypotension
- antibiotics for septic emboli, not anticoagulants, and evaluation for the infection's source, particularly endocarditis
- surgery, such as vena caval ligation, plication, or insertion of a device (umbrella filter) to filter blood returning to the heart and lungs, for patients who can't take anticoagulants (because of recent surgery or blood dyscrasia), or who have recurrent emboli during anticoagulant therapy.

Pulmonary hypertension

Pulmonary hypertension occurs when pulmonary artery pressure (PAP) rises above normal for reasons other than aging or altitude. No definitive set of values is used to diagnose pulmonary hypertension, but the National Institutes of Health requires a mean PAP of 25 mm Hg or more. Primary or idiopathic pulmonary hypertension is characterized by increased PAP and increased pulmonary vascular resistance. This form is most common in women ages 20 to 40 and is usually fatal within 3 to 4 years.

CLINICAL ALERT
Mortality is highest in pregnant women.

Secondary pulmonary hypertension results from existing cardiac or pulmonary disease or both. The prognosis in secondary pulmonary hypertension depends on the severity of the underlying disorder.

The patient may have no signs or symptoms of the disorder until lung damage becomes severe. In fact, it may not be diagnosed until an autopsy is performed.

CAUSES

Causes of primary pulmonary hypertension are unknown, but may include:
- hereditary factors
- altered immune mechanisms.

Secondary pulmonary hypertension results from hypoxemia caused by various conditions, including:
- alveolar hypoventilation resulting from:
  - chronic obstructive pulmonary disease
  - sarcoidosis
  - diffuse interstitial pneumonia
  - malignant metastasis
  - scleroderma
  - obesity
  - kyphoscoliosis
- vascular obstruction resulting from:
  - pulmonary embolism
  - vasculitis
  - left atrial myxoma
  - idiopathic veno-occlusive disease
  - fibrosing mediastinitis
  - mediastinal neoplasm
- primary cardiac disease resulting from:
  - patent ductus arteriosus (PDA)
  - atrial septal defect
  - ventricular septal defect (VSD).

Conditions causing acquired cardiac disease include:
- rheumatic valvular disease
- mitral stenosis.

PATHOPHYSIOLOGY

In primary pulmonary hypertension, the smooth muscle in the pulmonary artery wall hypertrophies for no reason, narrowing the small pulmonary artery (arterioles) or obliterating it completely. Fibrous lesions also form around the vessels, impairing distensibility and increasing vascular resistance. Pressures in the left ventricle,

which receives blood from the lungs, remain normal. However, the increased pressures generated in the lungs are transmitted to the right ventricle, which supplies the pulmonary artery. Eventually, the right ventricle fails (cor pulmonale). Although oxygenation isn't severely affected initially, hypoxia and cyanosis eventually occur. Death results from cor pulmonale.

Alveolar hypoventilation can result from diseases caused by alveolar destruction or from disorders that prevent the chest wall from expanding sufficiently to allow air into the alveoli. The resulting decreased ventilation increases pulmonary vascular resistance. Hypoxemia resulting from this ventilation-perfusion mismatch also causes vasoconstriction, further increasing vascular resistance and resulting in pulmonary hypertension.

Coronary artery disease or mitral valvular disease causing increased left ventricular filling pressures may cause secondary pulmonary hypertension. VSD and PDA cause secondary pulmonary hypertension by increasing blood flow through the pulmonary circulation through left-to-right shunting. Pulmonary emboli and chronic destruction of alveolar walls, as in emphysema, cause secondary pulmonary hypertension by obliterating or obstructing the pulmonary vascular bed. Secondary pulmonary hypertension can also occur by vasoconstriction of the vascular bed, such as through hypoxemia, acidosis, or both. Conditions resulting in vascular obstruction can also cause pulmonary hypertension because blood isn't allowed to flow appropriately through the vessels.

Secondary pulmonary hypertension can be reversed if the disorder is resolved. If hypertension persists, hypertrophy occurs in the medial smooth muscle layer of the arterioles. The larger arteries stiffen, and hypertension progresses. Pulmonary pressures begin to equal systemic blood pressure, causing right ventricular hypertrophy and eventually cor pulmonale.

Primary cardiac diseases may be congenital or acquired. Congenital defects cause a left-to-right shunt, rerouting blood through the lungs twice and causing pulmonary hypertension. Acquired cardiac diseases, such as rheumatic valvular disease and mitral stenosis, result in left-sided heart failure that diminishes the flow of oxygenated blood from the lungs. This increases pulmonary vascular resistance and right ventricular pressure.

SIGNS AND SYMPTOMS

Signs and symptoms of pulmonary hypertension may include:

- increasing dyspnea on exertion from left-sided heart failure
- fatigue and weakness from diminished tissue oxygenation
- syncope from diminished oxygenation to brain cells
- difficulty breathing from left-sided heart failure
- shortness of breath from left-sided heart failure
- pain with breathing from lactic acid buildup in the tissues
- ascites from right ventricular failure
- jugular vein distention from right-sided heart failure
- restlessness and agitation from hypoxia
- decreased level of consciousness, confusion, and memory loss because of hypoxia
- decreased diaphragmatic excursion and respiration because of hypoventilation
- possible displacement of point of maximal impulse beyond the midclavicular line from fluid accumulation
- peripheral edema from right-sided heart failure
- easily palpable right ventricular lift from altered cardiac output and pulmonary hypertension
- palpable and tender liver from pulmonary hypertension
- tachycardia from hypoxia
- systolic ejection murmur from pulmonary hypertension and altered cardiac output
- split S_2, S_3, and S_4 from pulmonary hypertension and altered cardiac output
- decreased breath sounds from fluid accumulation in the lungs
- loud, tubular breath sounds from fluid accumulation in the lungs.

COMPLICATIONS

Possible complications of pulmonary hypertension include:

- cor pulmonale
- cardiac failure
- cardiac arrest.

DIAGNOSIS

These tests help diagnose pulmonary hypertension:

- Arterial blood gas analysis reveals hypoxemia.
- Electrocardiography in right ventricular hypertrophy shows right axis deviation and tall or peaked P waves in inferior leads.
- Cardiac catheterization reveals pulmonary systolic pressure above 30 mm Hg. It may also show an increased pulmonary artery wedge pressure (PAWP) if the underlying cause is left atrial myxoma, mitral stenosis, or left-sided heart failure; otherwise, PAWP is normal.
- Pulmonary angiography detects filling defects in pulmonary vasculature such as those that develop with pulmonary emboli.
- Pulmonary function tests may show decreased flow rates and increased residual volume in underlying obstructive disease; in underlying restrictive disease, they may show reduced total lung capacity.
- Radionuclide imaging detects abnormalities in right and left ventricular functioning.
- Open lung biopsy may determine the type of disorder.
- Echocardiography allows the assessment of ventricular wall motion and possible valvular dysfunction. It can also demonstrate right ventricular enlargement, abnormal septal configuration consistent with right ventricular pressure overload, and reduction in left ventricular cavity size.
- Perfusion lung scanning may produce normal or abnormal results, with multiple patchy and diffuse filling defects that don't suggest pulmonary embolism.

TREATMENT

Managing pulmonary hypertension typically involves:

- oxygen therapy to correct hypoxemia and resulting increased pulmonary vascular resistance
- fluid restriction in right-sided heart failure to decrease the heart's workload

- digoxin to increase cardiac output
- diuretics to decrease intravascular volume and extravascular fluid accumulation
- vasodilators to reduce myocardial workload and oxygen consumption
- calcium channel blockers to reduce myocardial workload and oxygen consumption
- bronchodilators to relax smooth muscles and increase airway patency
- beta-adrenergic blockers to improve oxygenation
- treatment of the underlying cause to correct pulmonary edema
- heart-lung transplant in severe cases.

Respiratory distress syndrome of the newborn

Respiratory distress syndrome (RDS), also known as *hyaline membrane disease,* is the most common cause of neonatal death; in the United States alone, it kills about 40,000 neonates every year.

AGE ALERT
RDS occurs most exclusively in neonates born before 37 weeks' gestation; it occurs in about 60% of those born before 28 weeks' gestation.

RDS of the newborn is marked by widespread alveolar collapse. Occurring mainly in premature neonates and in sudden infant death syndrome, it strikes apparently healthy neonates. It's most common in neonates of mothers who have diabetes and in those delivered by cesarean birth, or it may occur suddenly after antepartum hemorrhage.

In RDS of the newborn, premature neonates develop a widespread alveolar collapse from surfactant deficiency. If untreated, the syndrome causes death within 72 hours of birth in up to 14% of neonates weighing less than 5.5 lb (2,500 g). Aggressive management and mechanical ventilation can improve the prognosis, although some surviving neonates are left with bronchopulmonary dysplasia. Mild cases of the syndrome subside after about 3 days.

CAUSES
Common causes of RDS of the newborn include:

- lack of surfactant
- premature birth.

PATHOPHYSIOLOGY
Surfactant, a lipoprotein present in alveoli and respiratory bronchioles, helps to lower surface tension, maintain alveolar patency, and prevent alveolar collapse, particularly at the end of expiration.

Although the neonatal airways are developed by 27 weeks' gestation, the intercostal muscles are weak and the alveoli and capillary blood supply are immature. Surfactant deficiency causes a higher surface tension. The alveoli aren't able to maintain patency and begin to collapse.

With alveolar collapse, ventilation is decreased and hypoxia develops. The resulting pulmonary injury and inflammatory reaction lead to edema and swelling of the interstitial space, thus impeding gas exchange between the capillaries and the functional alveoli. The inflammation also stimulates production of hyaline membranes composed of white fibrin accumulation in the alveoli. These deposits further reduce gas exchange in the lung and decrease lung compliance, resulting in increased work of breathing.

Decreased alveolar ventilation results in decreased ventilation-perfusion ratio and pulmonary arteriolar vasoconstriction. The pulmonary vasoconstriction can result in increased right cardiac volume and pressure, causing blood to be shunted from the right atrium through a patent foramen ovale to the left atrium. Increased pulmonary resistance also results in deoxygenated blood passing through the ductus arteriosus, totally bypassing the lungs, and causing a right-to-left shunt. The shunt further increases hypoxia.

Because of immature lungs and an already increased metabolic rate, the neonate must expend more energy to ventilate collapsed alveoli. This further increases oxygen demand and contributes to cyanosis. The neonate attempts to compensate with rapid shallow breathing, causing an initial respiratory alkalosis as carbon dioxide is expelled. The increased effort at lung expansion causes respirations to slow and respiratory acidosis to occur, leading to respiratory failure.

SIGNS AND SYMPTOMS
Signs and symptoms of RDS may include:

CLINICAL ALERT
Suspect RDS of the newborn in a patient with a history that includes preterm birth (before 28 weeks' gestation), cesarean delivery, maternal history of diabetes, or antepartum hemorrhage.

- rapid, shallow respirations from hypoxia
- intercostal, subcostal, or sternal retractions from hypoxia and increased work of breathing
- nasal flaring from hypoxia
- audible expiratory grunting (The grunting is a natural compensatory mechanism that produces positive end-expiratory pressure [PEEP] to prevent further alveolar collapse.)
- hypotension from cardiac failure
- peripheral edema from cardiac failure
- oliguria from vasoconstriction of the kidneys.

In severe cases, signs and symptoms may include:
- apnea from respiratory failure
- bradycardia from cardiac failure
- cyanosis from hypoxemia, right-to-left shunting through the foramen ovale, or right-to-left shunting through the atelectatic lung areas
- pallor from decreased circulation
- frothy sputum from pulmonary edema and atelectasis
- low body temperature, resulting from an immature nervous system and inadequate subcutaneous fat
- diminished air entry and crackles on auscultation because of atelectasis.

COMPLICATIONS
Possible complications of RDS of the newborn include:
- respiratory failure
- cardiac failure
- bronchopulmonary dysplasia.

DIAGNOSIS
These tests help diagnose RDS of the newborn:
- Chest X-rays may be normal for the first 6 to 12 hours in 50% of patients, although later films show a fine reticulonodular pattern and dark streaks, indicating air-filled, dilated bronchioles.
- Arterial blood gas analysis reveals a diminished partial pressure of arterial oxygen level; a normal, decreased, or increased partial pressure of arterial carbon dioxide level; and a reduced pH, indicating a combination of respiratory and metabolic acidosis.
- Lecithin-sphingomyelin ratio helps to assess prenatal lung development and infants at risk for this syndrome; this test is usually ordered if a cesarean delivery will be performed before 36 weeks' gestation.

TREATMENT
Correcting RDS of the newborn typically involves:
- warm, humidified, oxygen-enriched gases administered by oxygen hood or, if such treatment fails, by mechanical ventilation to promote adequate oxygenation and reverse hypoxia
- administration of surfactant by an endotracheal tube to prevent atelectasis
- mechanical ventilation with PEEP or continuous positive airway pressure administered by nasal prongs (This forces the alveoli to remain open on expiration and promotes increased surface area for exchange of oxygen and carbon dioxide.)
- high-frequency oscillation ventilation if the neonate can't maintain adequate gas exchange (This provides satisfactory minute volume [the total air breathed in 1 minute] with lower airway pressures.)
- radiant warmer or an Isolette to help maintain thermoregulation and reduce metabolic demands
- I.V. fluids to promote adequate hydration and maintain circulation with capillary refill of less than 2 seconds (Fluid and electrolyte balance is also maintained.)
- sodium bicarbonate to control acidosis
- tube feedings or total parenteral nutrition
- prophylactic antibiotics for underlying infections
- diuretics to reduce pulmonary edema

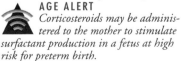

AGE ALERT
Corticosteroids may be administered to the mother to stimulate surfactant production in a fetus at high risk for preterm birth.

■ delayed delivery of a neonate (if premature labor) to possibly prevent RDS.

Sudden infant death syndrome

Sudden infant death syndrome (SIDS) is the leading cause of death among apparently healthy infants, ages 1 month to 1 year. Also called *crib death,* it occurs at a rate of 2 in every 1,000 live births; about 7,000 infants die of SIDS in the United States each year. The peak incidence occurs between ages 2 and 4 months.

CULTURAL DIVERSITY
The incidence of SIDS is slightly higher in preterm neonates, Inuit infants, disadvantaged Black infants, infants of mothers younger than age 20, and infants of multiple births. The incidence is also 10 times higher in SIDS siblings and in infants of mothers who are drug addicts.

CAUSES
Common causes of SIDS include:
■ hypoxemia, possibly from apnea or an immature respiratory system
■ rebreathing of carbon dioxide, as occurs when an infant is placed face down on the mattress.

PATHOPHYSIOLOGY
It has been suggested that the infant with SIDS may have damage to the respiratory control center in the brain from chronic hypoxemia. The infant may also have periods of sleep apnea and eventually die during an episode.

Normally, increased carbon dioxide levels stimulate the respiratory center to initiate breathing until very high levels actually depress the ventilatory effort. In infants who experience SIDS or near-miss episodes of SIDS, the child may not respond to increasing carbon dioxide levels, showing only depressed ventilation. In these infants, an episode of apnea may occur and carbon dioxide levels increase; however, the child isn't stimulated to breathe. Apnea continues until very high levels of carbon dioxide completely suppress the ventilatory effort and the child ceases to breathe.

SIGNS AND SYMPTOMS
Signs and symptoms of SIDS may include:
■ history indicating that the infant was found not breathing
■ mottling of the skin from cyanosis
■ apnea and absence of a pulse from severe hypoxemia and hypoxia.

COMPLICATIONS
Possible complications of SIDS include:
■ death
■ brain damage from a near-miss episode.

DIAGNOSIS
An autopsy is performed to rule out other causes of death.

TREATMENT
Treatment of SIDS typically involves:
■ resuscitation to restore circulation and oxygenation (usually futile)
■ emotional support to the family
■ prevention of SIDS in high-risk infants or those who have had near-miss episodes.

AGE ALERT
Infants at risk for SIDS should be monitored at home on an apnea monitor until the age of vulnerability has passed. Also, parents should be educated in prompt emergency treatment of detected apnea.

Nervous system

The nervous system coordinates and organizes the functions of all body systems. This intricate network of interlocking receptors and transmitters is a dynamic system that controls and regulates every mental and physical function. It has three main divisions:

■ *central nervous system (CNS)*—the brain and spinal cord (see *Reviewing the central nervous system*)

■ *peripheral nervous system*—the motor and sensory nerves, which carry messages between the CNS and remote parts of the body (see *Reviewing the peripheral nervous system,* pages 253 and 254)

■ *autonomic nervous system*—actually part of the peripheral nervous system, regulates involuntary functions of the internal organs.

The fundamental unit that participates in all nervous system activity is the *neuron*. A neuron is a highly specialized cell that receives and transmits electro-chemical nerve impulses through delicate, threadlike fibers that extend from the central cell body. Axons carry impulses away from the cell body; dendrites carry impulses to it. Most neurons have several dendrites but only one axon.

■ Sensory (or afferent) neurons transmit impulses from receptors to the spinal cord or the brain.

■ Motor (or efferent) neurons transmit impulses from the CNS to regulate the activity of muscles or glands.

■ Interneurons, also known as *connecting* or *association* neurons, carry signals through complex pathways between sensory and motor neurons. Interneurons account for 99% of all the neurons in the nervous system.

From birth to death, the nervous system efficiently organizes and controls the smallest action, thought, or feeling; monitors communication and the instinct for survival; and allows introspection, wonder, abstract thought, and self-awareness. Together, the CNS and peripheral nervous system (the part of the nervous system that is outside the CNS) keep a person alert, awake, oriented, and able to move about freely without discomfort and with all body systems working to maintain homeostasis.

Thus, any disorder affecting the nervous system can cause signs and symptoms in any and all body systems. Patients with nervous system disorders commonly have signs and symptoms that are elusive, subtle, and sometimes latent.

PATHOPHYSIOLOGIC CHANGES

Typically, disorders of the nervous system involve some alteration in arousal, cognition, movement, muscle tone, homeostatic mechanisms, or pain. Most disorders cause more than one alteration, and the close intercommunication between the CNS and peripheral nervous system means that one alteration may lead to another.

Reviewing the central nervous system

The central nervous system includes the brain and spinal cord. The brain consists of the cerebrum, cerebellum, brain stem, and primitive structures that lie below the cerebrum: the diencephalon, limbic system, and reticular activating system (RAS). The spinal cord is the primary pathway for messages between peripheral areas of the body and the brain. It also mediates reflexes.

CEREBRUM
The left and right cerebral hemispheres are joined by the corpus callosum, a mass of nerve fibers that allows communication between corresponding centers in the right and left hemispheres. Each hemisphere is divided into four lobes, based on anatomic landmarks and functional differences. The lobes are named for the cranial bones that lie over them (frontal, temporal, parietal, and occipital):
◆ *frontal lobe* — influences personality, judgment, abstract reasoning, social behavior, language expression, and movement (in the motor portion)
◆ *temporal lobe* — controls hearing, language comprehension, and storage and recall of memories (although memories are stored throughout the brain)
◆ *parietal lobe* — interprets and integrates sensations, including pain, temperature, and touch; also interprets size, shape, distance, and texture (The parietal lobe of the nondominant hemisphere, usually the right, is especially important for awareness of body shape.)
◆ *occipital lobe* — functions primarily in interpreting visual stimuli.
    The cerebral cortex, the thin surface layer of the cerebrum, is composed of gray matter (unmyelinated cell bodies). The surface of the cerebrum has convolutions (gyri) and creases or fissures (sulci).

CEREBELLUM
The cerebellum, which also has two hemispheres, maintains muscle tone, coordinates muscle movement, and controls balance.

BRAIN STEM
Composed of the pons, midbrain, and medulla oblongata, the brain stem relays messages between upper and lower levels of the nervous system. The cranial nerves originate from the pons, midbrain, and medulla oblongata:
◆ *pons* — connects the cerebellum with the cerebrum and the midbrain to the medulla oblongata, and contains one of the respiratory centers
◆ *midbrain* — mediates the auditory and visual reflexes
◆ *medulla oblongata* — regulates respiratory, vasomotor, and cardiac function.

PRIMITIVE STRUCTURES
The diencephalon contains the thalamus and hypothalamus, which lie beneath the cerebral hemispheres. The thalamus relays all sensory stimuli (except olfactory) as they ascend to the cerebral cortex. Thalamic functions include primitive awareness of pain, screening of incoming stimuli, and focusing of attention. The hypothalamus controls or affects body temperature, appetite, water balance, pituitary secretions, emotions, and autonomic functions, including sleep and wake cycles.
    The limbic system lies deep within the temporal lobe. It initiates primitive drives (hunger, aggression, and sexual and emotional arousal) and screens all sensory messages traveling to the cerebral cortex.
    The RAS, a diffuse network of hyperexcitable neurons fanning out from the brain stem through the cerebral cortex, screens all incoming sensory information and channels it to appropriate areas of the brain for interpretation. RAS activity also stimulates wakefulness.

(continued)

Reviewing the central nervous system *(continued)*

SPINAL CORD

The spinal cord joins the brain stem at the level of the foramen magnum and terminates near the second lumbar vertebra.

A cross section of the spinal cord reveals a central H-shaped mass of gray matter divided into dorsal (posterior) and ventral (anterior) horns. Gray matter in the dorsal horns relays sensory (afferent) impulses; in the ventral horns, motor (efferent) impulses. White matter (myelinated axons of sensory and motor nerves) surrounds these horns and forms the ascending and descending tracts.

Arousal

Arousal refers to the level of consciousness or state of awareness. A person who is aware of himself and the environment and can respond to the environment in specific ways is said to be fully conscious. Full consciousness requires that the reticular activating system (RAS), higher systems in the cerebral cortex, and thalamic connections be intact and functioning properly. Several mechanisms can alter arousal:

■ direct destruction of the RAS and its pathways
■ destruction of the entire brain stem, either directly by invasion or indirectly by impairment of its blood supply
■ compression of the RAS by a disease process, either from direct pressure or compression as structures expand or herniate.

Those mechanisms may result from structural, metabolic, or psychogenic disturbances:

■ Structural changes include infections, vascular problems, neoplasms, trauma, and developmental and degenerative conditions. They usually are identified by their location relative to the tentorial plate, the double fold of dura that supports the temporal and occipital lobes and separates the cerebral hemispheres from the brain stem and cerebellum. Those above the tentorial plate are called *supratentorial,* and those below are called *infratentorial.*
■ Metabolic changes that affect the nervous system include hypoxia, electrolyte disturbances, hypoglycemia, drugs, and toxins (endogenous and exogenous). Es-

sentially any systemic disease can affect the nervous system.

■ Psychogenic changes are commonly associated with mental and psychiatric illnesses. Ongoing research has linked neuroanatomy and neurophysiology of the CNS and supporting structures, including neurotransmitters, with certain psychiatric illnesses. For example, dysfunction of the limbic system has been linked to schizophrenia, depression, and anxiety disorders.

Decreased arousal may be a result of diffuse or localized dysfunction in supratentorial areas:

■ Diffuse dysfunction reflects damage to the cerebral cortex or underlying subcortical white matter. Disease is the most common cause of diffuse dysfunction; other causes include neoplasms, closed head trauma with subsequent bleeding, and pus accumulation.
■ Localized dysfunction reflects mechanical forces on the thalamus or hypothalamus. Masses (such as bleeding, infarction, emboli, and tumors) may directly impinge on the deep diencephalic structures or herniation may compress them.

STAGES OF ALTERED AROUSAL

An alteration in arousal usually begins with some interruption or disruption in the *diencephalon.* When this occurs, the patient shows evidence of dullness, confusion, lethargy, and stupor. Continued decreases in arousal result from midbrain dysfunction and are evidenced by a deepening of the stupor. Eventually, if the medulla and pons are affected, coma results.

Reviewing the peripheral nervous system

The peripheral nervous system consists of the cranial nerves (CNs), the spinal nerves, and the autonomic nervous system (ANS).

CRANIAL NERVES

The 12 pairs of CNs transmit motor or sensory messages, or both, primarily between the brain or brain stem and the head and neck. All CNs, except for the olfactory and optic nerves, originate from the midbrain, pons, or medulla oblongata. The CNs are sensory, motor, or both, as follows:

◆ olfactory (CN I) — Sensory: smell
◆ optic (CN II) — Sensory: vision
◆ oculomotor (CN III) — Motor: extraocular eye movement (superior, medial, and inferior lateral), pupillary constriction, and upper eyelid elevation
◆ trochlear (CN IV) — Motor: extraocular eye movement (inferior medial)
◆ trigeminal (CN V) — Sensory: transmitting stimuli from face and head, corneal reflex; motor: chewing, biting, and lateral jaw movements
◆ abducens (CN VI) — Motor: extraocular eye movement (lateral)
◆ facial (CN VII) — Sensory: taste receptors (anterior two-thirds of tongue); motor: Facial muscle movement, including muscles of expression (those in the forehead and around the eyes and mouth)
◆ acoustic (CN VIII) — Sensory: hearing, sense of balance
◆ glossopharyngeal (CN IX) — Sensory: sensations of throat; taste receptors (posterior one-third of tongue); motor: swallowing movements
◆ vagus (CN X) — Sensory: sensations of throat, larynx, and thoracic and abdominal viscera (heart, lungs, bronchi, and GI tract); motor: movement of palate, swallowing, gag reflex; activity of the thoracic and abdominal viscera, such as heart rate and peristalsis
◆ spinal accessory (CN XI) — Motor: shoulder movement, head rotation
◆ hypoglossal (CN XII) — Motor: tongue movement.

SPINAL NERVES

The 31 pairs of spinal nerves are named according to the vertebra immediately below their exit point from the spinal cord. Each spinal nerve consists of afferent (sensory) and efferent (motor) neurons, which carry messages to and from particular body regions, called dermatomes.

AUTONOMIC NERVOUS SYSTEM

The ANS innervates all internal organs. Sometimes known as the visceral efferent nerves, autonomic nerves carry messages to the viscera from the brain stem and neuroendocrine system. The ANS has two major divisions: the sympathetic (thoracolumbar) nervous system and the parasympathetic (craniosacral) nervous system.

Sympathetic nervous system

Sympathetic nerves exit the spinal cord between the levels of the 1st thoracic and 2nd lumbar vertebrae; hence the name thoracolumbar. These preganglionic neurons enter small relay stations (ganglia) near the cord. The ganglia form a chain that disseminates the impulse to postganglionic neurons, which reach many organs and glands, and can produce widespread, generalized responses.

The physiologic effects of sympathetic activity include:

◆ vasoconstriction
◆ elevated blood pressure
◆ enhanced blood flow to skeletal muscles
◆ increased heart rate and contractility
◆ heightened respiratory rate
◆ smooth muscle relaxation of the bronchioles, GI tract, and urinary tract
◆ sphincter contraction
◆ pupillary dilation and ciliary muscle relaxation
◆ increased sweat gland secretion
◆ reduced pancreatic secretion.

(continued)

Reviewing the peripheral nervous system *(continued)*

Parasympathetic nervous system
The fibers of the parasympathetic, or craniosacral, nervous system leave the central nervous system (CNS) by way of the CNs from the midbrain and medulla and with the spinal nerves between the 2nd and 4th sacral vertebrae (S2 to S4).

After leaving the CNS, the long preganglionic fiber of each parasympathetic nerve travels to a ganglion near a particular organ or gland, and the short postganglionic fiber enters the organ or gland. Parasympathetic nerves have a specific response involving only one organ or gland.

The physiologic effects of parasympathetic system activity include:

◆ reduced heart rate, contractility, and conduction velocity
◆ bronchial smooth muscle constriction
◆ increased GI tract tone and peristalsis with sphincter relaxation
◆ urinary system sphincter relaxation and increased bladder tone
◆ vasodilation of external genitalia, causing erection
◆ pupillary constriction
◆ increased pancreatic, salivary, and lacrimal secretions.

The parasympathetic system has little effect on mental or metabolic activity.

A patient may move back and forth between stages or levels of arousal, depending on the cause of the altered arousal state, the start of treatment, and response to treatment. Typically, if the underlying problem isn't or can't be corrected, then the patient will progress through the various stages of decreased consciousness (called *rostral-caudal progression*).

Six levels of altered arousal or consciousness have been identified. (See *Stages of altered arousal.*)

Typically, five areas of neurologic function are evaluated to help identify the cause of altered arousal:

■ level of consciousness (includes awareness and cognitive functioning, which indicate cerebral status)
■ pattern of breathing (helps localize the cause to the cerebral hemisphere or brain stem)
■ pupillary changes (reflects the level of brain stem function; the brain stem areas that control arousal are anatomically next to the areas that control the pupils)
■ eye movement and reflex responses (help identify the level of brain stem dysfunction and its mechanism, such as destruction or compression)
■ motor responses (help identify the level, side, and severity of brain dysfunction).

Cognition

Cognition is the ability to be aware and to perceive, reason, judge, remember, and use intuition. It reflects higher functioning of the cerebral cortex, including the frontal, parietal, and temporal lobes and portions of the brain stem. Typically, an alteration in cognition results from direct destruction by ischemia and hypoxia or from indirect destruction by compression or the effects of toxins and chemicals.

Altered cognition may appear as agnosia, aphasia, or dysphasia:
■ Agnosia is a defect in the ability to recognize the form or nature of objects. Usually, agnosia involves only one sense — hearing, vision, or touch.
■ Aphasia is loss of the ability to comprehend or produce language.
■ Dysphasia is impairment to the ability to comprehend or use symbols in either verbal or written language, or to produce language.

Dysphasia typically arises from the left cerebral hemisphere, usually the frontotemporal region, but different types of dysphasia occur, depending on the specific area of the brain involved. For example, a dysfunction in the posteroinferior frontal lobe (Broca's area) causes a motor dysphasia in which the patient can't move the

Stages of altered arousal

This table highlights the six stages of altered arousal and their characteristics.

STAGE	CHARACTERISTICS
Confusion	◆ Loss of ability to think rapidly and clearly ◆ Impaired judgment and decision making
Disorientation	◆ Beginning loss of consciousness ◆ Disorientation to time progresses to include disorientation to place ◆ Impaired memory ◆ Lack of recognition of self (last to go)
Lethargy	◆ Limited spontaneous movement or speech ◆ Easy to arouse by normal speech or touch ◆ Possible disorientation to time, place, or person
Obtundation	◆ Mild to moderate reduction in arousal ◆ Limited responsiveness to environment ◆ Ability to fall asleep easily without verbal or tactile stimulation from others ◆ Ability to answer questions with minimum response
Stupor	◆ State of deep sleep or unresponsiveness ◆ Arousable (motor or verbal response only to vigorous and repeated stimulation) ◆ Withdrawal or grabbing response to stimulation
Coma	◆ Lack of motor or verbal response to external environment or any stimuli ◆ No response to noxious stimuli such as deep pain ◆ Inability to be aroused by any stimulus

muscles, necessary to say words and has difficulty writing and repeating words. Dysfunction in the pathways connecting the primary auditory area to the auditory association areas in the middle third of the left superior temporal gyrus causes a form of dysphasia called "word deafness": the patient has fluent speech, but his comprehension of the spoken word and ability to repeat speech are impaired. Rather than hearing words, the patient hears meaningless noise, even though reading comprehension and writing ability are intact.

DEMENTIA

Dementia is the loss of more than one intellectual or cognitive function, which interferes with the ability to function in daily life. The patient may experience a problem with orientation, general knowledge and information, vigilance (attentiveness, alertness, and watchfulness), recent memory, remote memory, concept formulation, abstraction (the ability to generalize about nonconcrete thoughts and ideas), reasoning, or language use.

The underlying mechanism is a defect in the neuron circuitry of the brain. The extent of dysfunction reflects the total quantity of neurons lost and the area where this loss occurred. Processes that have been associated with dementia include:

- degeneration
- cerebrovascular disorders
- compression
- effects of toxins
- metabolic conditions

CLOSER LOOK
Reviewing motor impulse transmission

Motor impulses that originate in the motor cortex of the frontal lobe travel through upper motor neurons of the pyramidal or extrapyramidal tract to the lower motor neurons of the peripheral nervous system.

In the pyramidal tract, most impulses from the motor cortex travel through the internal capsule to the medulla, where they cross (decussate) to the opposite side and continue down the spinal cord as the lateral corticospinal tract, ending in the anterior horn of the gray matter at a specific spinal cord level. Some fibers don't cross in the medulla but continue down the anterior corticospinal tract and cross near the level of termination in the anterior horn. The fibers of the pyramidal tract are considered upper motor neurons. In the anterior horn of the spinal cord, upper motor neurons relay impulses to the lower motor neurons, which carry them via the spinal and peripheral nerves to the muscles, producing a motor response.

Motor impulses that regulate involuntary muscle tone and muscle control travel along the extrapyramidal tract from the premotor area of the frontal lobe to the pons of the brain stem, where they cross to the opposite side. The impulses then travel down the spinal cord to the anterior horn, where they're relayed to lower motor neurons for ultimate delivery to the muscles.

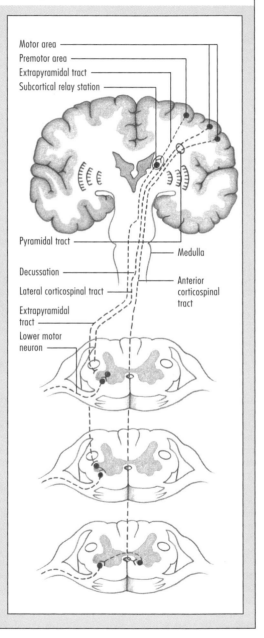

Motor area
Premotor area
Extrapyramidal tract
Subcortical relay station

Pyramidal tract

Medulla

Decussation

Lateral corticospinal tract

Anterior corticospinal tract

Extrapyramidal tract

Lower motor neuron

- biochemical imbalances
- demyelinization
- infection.

Three major types of dementia have been identified: amnestic, intentional, and cognitive. Each type affects a specific area of the brain, resulting in characteristic impairments:

- Amnestic dementia typically results from defective neuronal circuitry in the temporal lobe. Characteristically, the patient exhibits difficulty in naming things, loss of recent memory, and loss of language comprehension.
- Intentional dementia results from a defect in the frontal lobe. The patient is easily distracted and, although able to follow simple commands, can't carry out such sequential executive functions as planning, initiating, and regulating behavior or achieving specific goals. The patient may exhibit personality changes and a flat affect (lack of signs expressing emotion). He may appear accident prone, and he may lose motor function — indicated by a wide shuffling gait, small steps, rigid muscles, abnormal reflexes, incontinence of bowel and bladder and, possibly, total immobility.
- Cognitive dementia reflects dysfunctional neuronal circuitry in the cerebral cortex. Typically, the patient loses remote memory, language comprehension, and mathematical skills, and has difficulty with visual-spatial relationships.

Movement

Movement involves a complex array of activities controlled by the cerebral cortex, the pyramidal system, the extrapyramidal system, and the motor units (the axon of the lower motor neuron from the anterior horn cell of the spinal cord and the muscles innervated by it). A problem in any one of these areas can affect movement. (See *Reviewing motor impulse transmission.*)

For movement to occur, the muscles must change their state from one of contraction to relaxation or vice versa. A change in muscle innervation anywhere along the motor pathway will affect movement. Certain neurotransmitters, such as dopamine, play a role in altered movement.

Alterations in movement typically include excessive movement (hyperkinesia) or decreased movement (hypokinesia). Hyperkinesia is a broad category that includes many different types of abnormal movements. Each type of hyperkinesia is associated with a specific underlying pathophysiologic mechanism affecting the brain or motor pathway. (See *Types of hyperkinesia,* pages 258 and 259.)

Hypokinesia usually involves loss of voluntary control, even though peripheral nerve and muscle functions are intact. The types of hypokinesia include paresis, akinesia, bradykinesia, and loss of associated movement.

PARESIS

Paresis is a partial loss of motor function (paralysis) and muscle power, which the patient will commonly describe as weakness. Paresis can result from the dysfunction of the:

- upper motor neurons in the cerebral cortex, subcortical white matter, the internal capsule, brain stem, or spinal cord
- lower motor neurons in the brain stem motor nuclei and anterior horn of the spinal cord, or problems with their axons as they travel to the skeletal muscle
- motor units affecting the muscle fibers or the neuromuscular junction.

Upper motor neurons

Upper motor neuron dysfunction reflects an interruption in the pyramidal tract and consequent decreased activation of the lower motor neurons innervating one or more areas of the body. Upper motor neuron dysfunction usually affects more than one muscle group and generally affects distal muscle groups more severely than proximal groups. Onset of spastic muscle tone over several days to weeks commonly accompanies upper motor neuron paresis, unless the dysfunction is acute. In acute dysfunction, flaccid tone and loss of deep tendon reflexes indicates spinal shock, caused by a severe, acute lesion below the foramen magnum. Incoordination resulting from upper motor neuron paresis causes slow, coarse movement with abnormal rhythm.

Types of hyperkinesia

This table summarizes some of the most common types of hyperkinesias, their characteristics, and the underlying mechanisms involved in their development.

TYPE	CHARACTERISTICS
Akathisia	◆ Ranges from mildly compulsive movement (usually the legs) to severely frenzied motion ◆ Partly voluntary, with ability to suppress for short periods ◆ Relief obtained by performing motion
Asterixis	◆ Irregular flapping-hand movement ◆ More prominent when arms outstretched
Athetosis	◆ Slow, sinuous, irregular movements in the distal extremities ◆ Characteristic hand posture ◆ Slow, fluctuating grimaces
Ballism	◆ Severe, wild, flinging, stereotypical limb movements ◆ Present when awake or asleep ◆ Usually on one side of the body
Chorea	◆ Random, irregular, involuntary, rapid contractions of muscle groups ◆ Nonrepetitive ◆ Diminishes with rest, disappears during sleep ◆ Increases during emotional stress or attempts at voluntary movement
Hyperactivity	◆ Prolonged, generalized, increased activity ◆ Mainly involuntary but possibly subject to voluntary control ◆ Continual changes in body posture or excessive performance of a simple activity at inappropriate times
Intentional cerebellar tremor	◆ Tremor secondary to movement ◆ Most severe when nearing end of the movement
Myoclonus	◆ Shocklike contractions ◆ Throwing limb movements ◆ Random occurrence ◆ Triggered by startle ◆ Present even during sleep
Parkinsonian tremor	◆ Regular, rhythmic, slow flexion and extension contraction ◆ Primarily affects metacarpophalangeal and wrist joints ◆ Disappears with voluntary movement
Wandering	◆ Moving about without attention to environment

MECHANISMS

Possible association with impaired dopaminergic transmission

Believed to result from buildup of toxins not broken down by the liver (such as ammonia)

Believed to result from injury to the putamen of the basal ganglion

Injury to subthalamus nucleus, causing inhibition of the nucleus

Excess concentration or heightened sensitivity to dopamine in the basal ganglia

Possibly from injury to frontal lobe and reticular activating system (RAS)

Errors in the feedback from the periphery and goal-directed movement caused by disease of dentate nucleus and superior cerebellar peduncle

Irritability of nervous system and spontaneous discharge of neurons in the cerebral cortex, cerebellum, RAS, and spinal cord

Loss of inhibitory effects of dopamine in basal ganglia

Possibly from bilateral injury to globus pallidus or putamen

Lower motor neurons

Lower motor neurons are of two basic types: large (alpha) and small (gamma). Dysfunction of the large motor neurons of the anterior horn of the spinal cord, the motor nuclei of the brain stem, and their axons, causes impairment of voluntary and involuntary movement. The extent of paresis is directly correlated to the number of large lower motor neurons affected. If only a small portion of the large motor neurons are involved, paresis occurs; if all motor units are affected, the result is paralysis.

The small motor neurons play two necessary roles in movement: maintaining muscle tone and protecting the muscle from injury. Usually when the large motor neurons are affected, dysfunction of the small motor neurons causes reduced or absent muscle tone, flaccid paresis, and paralysis.

Motor units

The muscles innervated by motor neurons in the anterior horn of the spinal cord may also be affected. Paresis results from a decrease in the number or force of activated muscle fibers in the motor unit. The action potential of each motor unit decreases so that additional motor units are needed more quickly to produce the power necessary to move the muscle. Dysfunction of the neuromuscular junction causes paresis in a similar way, but the functional capability of the motor units to function is lost, not the actual number of units.

AKINESIA

Akinesia is a partial or complete loss of voluntary and associated movements as well as a disturbance in the time needed to perform a movement. Commonly caused by dysfunction of the extrapyramidal tract, akinesia is associated with dopamine deficiency at the synapse or a defect in the postsynaptic receptors for dopamine.

BRADYKINESIA

Bradykinesia refers to slow voluntary movements that are labored, deliberate, and hard to initiate. The patient has difficulty performing movements consecutively and at the same time. Like akinesia, bradykinesia involves a disturbance in the time needed to perform a movement.

LOSS OF ASSOCIATED MOVEMENT
Movement involves not only the innervation of specific muscles to accomplish an action, but also the work of other innervated muscles that enhance the action. Loss of associated neurons involves alterations in movement that accompany the usual habitual voluntary movements for skill, grace, and balance. For example, when a person expresses emotion, the muscles of the face and the posture change. Loss of neurons associated with emotional expression would result in a flat, blank expression and a stiff posture. Loss of neurons needed for locomotion would result in a decrease in arm and shoulder movement, hip swinging, and rotation of the cervical spine.

Muscle tone

Like movement, muscle tone involves complex activities controlled by the cerebral cortex, pyramidal system, extrapyramidal system, and motor units. Normal muscle tone is the slight resistance that occurs in response to passive movement. When one muscle contracts, reciprocal muscles relax to permit movement with only minimal resistance. For example, when the elbow is flexed, the biceps muscle contracts and feels firm and the triceps muscle is somewhat relaxed and soft; with continued flexion, the biceps relax and the triceps contract. Thus, when a joint is moved through range of motion, the resistance is normally smooth, even, and constant.

The two major types of altered muscle tone are hypotonia (decreased muscle tone) and hypertonia (increased muscle tone).

HYPOTONIA
Hypotonia (also referred to as *muscle flaccidity*) typically reflects cerebellar damage, but rarely it may result from pure pyramidal tract damage.

Hypotonia is thought to involve a decrease in muscle spindle activity as a result of a decrease in neuron excitability. Flaccidity generally occurs with loss of nerve impulses from the motor unit responsible for maintaining muscle tone.

It may be localized to a limb or muscle group, or it may be generalized, affecting the entire body. Flaccid muscles can be moved rapidly with little or no resistance; eventually they become limp and atrophy.

HYPERTONIA
Hypertonia is increased resistance to passive movement. There are four types of hypertonia:
- Spasticity is hyperexcitability of stretch reflexes caused by damage to the lateral corticospinal tract and the motor, premotor, and supplementary motor areas. (See *How spasticity develops*.)
- Paratonia (gegenhalten) is variance in resistance to passive movement in direct proportion to the force applied; the cause is frontal lobe injury.
- Dystonia is sustained, involuntary twisting movements resulting from slow muscle contraction; the cause is lack of appropriate inhibition of reciprocal muscles.
- Rigidity, or constant, involuntary muscle contraction, is resistance in both flexion and extension; the causes are damage to basal ganglion ("cog-wheel" or "lead-pipe" rigidity) or loss of cerebral cortex inhibition or cerebellar control (gamma and alpha rigidity).

Hypertonia usually leads to atrophy of unused muscles, but in some cases, if the motor reflex arc remains functional but isn't inhibited by the higher centers, the overstimulated muscles may hypertrophy.

Homeostatic mechanisms

For proper function, the brain must maintain and regulate pressure inside the skull — intracranial pressure (ICP) — as it also maintains the flow of oxygen and nutrients to its tissues. Both of these are accomplished by balancing changes in blood flow and cerebrospinal fluid (CSF) volume.

Constriction and dilation of the cerebral blood vessels help regulate ICP and delivery of nutrients to the brain. These vessels respond to changes in levels of carbon dioxide (CO_2), oxygen, and hydrogen ions (H^+). For example, if the CO_2 level in blood increases, the gas combines with

CLOSER LOOK
How spasticity develops

Motor activity is controlled by pyramidal and extrapyramidal tracts that originate in the motor cortex, basal ganglia, brain stem, and spinal cord. Nerve fibers from the various tracts converge and synapse at the anterior horn of the spinal cord. Together they maintain segmental muscle tone by modulating the stretch reflex arc. This arc, shown in a simplified version below, is basically a negative feedback loop in which muscle stretch (stimu- lation) causes reflexive contraction (inhibition), thus maintaining muscle length and tone.

Damage to certain tracts results in loss of inhibition and disruption of the stretch reflex arc. Uninhibited muscle stretch produces exaggerated, uncontrolled muscle activity, accentuating the reflex arc, and eventually resulting in spasticity.

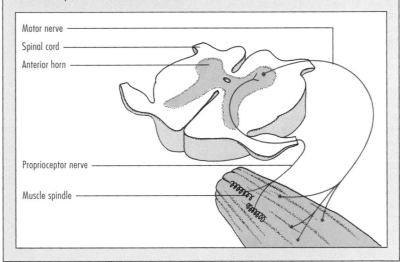

Motor nerve
Spinal cord
Anterior horn
Proprioceptor nerve
Muscle spindle

body fluids to form carbonic acid, which eventually releases H+. An increase in H+ level causes the cerebral vessels to dilate, increasing blood flow to the brain and cerebral perfusion and, subsequently, causing a drop in H+ level. A decrease in oxygen level also stimulates cerebral vasodilation, increasing blood flow and oxygen delivery to the brain.

Should these normal autoregulatory mechanisms fail, the abnormal blood chemistry stimulates the sympathetic nervous system to cause vasoconstriction of the large and medium-sized cerebral arteries. This helps prevent increases in blood pressure from reaching the smaller cerebral vessels.

CSF volume remains relatively constant, but if ICP rises, even as little as 5 mm Hg, the arachnoid villi open and excess CSF drains into the venous system.

The blood-brain barrier also helps maintain homeostasis in the brain. This barrier is composed of tight junctions between the endothelial cells of the cerebral vessels and neuroglial cells (nonneural cellular elements of the central and peripheral nervous systems) and is relatively impermeable to most substances. Some substances required for metabolism do pass through the blood-brain barrier, depending on their size, solubility, and electrical charge. This barrier also regulates water flow from the blood, thus helping maintain the volume within the skull.

INCREASED ICP

The pressure exerted by the brain tissue, CSF, and cerebral blood (intracranial components) against the skull is the ICP. The skull is a rigid structure; therefore, a change in the volume of the intracranial contents triggers a reciprocal change in one or more of the intracranial components to maintain a consistent pressure. Any condition that alters the normal balance of the intracranial components — including increased brain volume, increased blood volume, or increased CSF volume — can increase ICP.

At first the body uses its compensatory mechanisms (described earlier) to attempt to maintain homeostasis and lower ICP. If these mechanisms become overwhelmed and are no longer effective, ICP continues to rise. Cerebral perfusion pressure falls and cerebral blood flow decreases. Ischemia leads to cellular hypoxia, which initiates vasodilation of cerebral blood vessels to try to increase cerebral blood flow. Unfortunately, this only causes the ICP to rise more. As the pressure continues to rise, compression of brain tissue and cerebral vessels further impairs cerebral blood flow.

If ICP continues to rise, the brain begins to shift under the extreme pressure and may herniate to an area of lesser pressure. When the herniating brain tissue's blood supply is compromised, cerebral ischemia and hypoxia worsen. The herniation increases pressure in the area where the pressure was lower, thus impairing its blood supply. As ICP approaches systemic blood pressure, cerebral perfusion slows even more, ceasing when ICP equals systemic blood pressure. (See *What happens when ICP rises.*)

CEREBRAL EDEMA

Cerebral edema is an increase in the fluid content of brain tissue that leads to an increase in the intracellular or extracellular fluid volume. Cerebral edema may result from an initial injury to the brain tissue or

 CLOSER LOOK

What happens when ICP rises

Intracranial pressure (ICP) is the pressure exerted within the intact skull by the intracranial volume — about 10% blood, 10% cerebrospinal fluid (CSF), and 80% brain tissue. The rigid skull has little space for expansion of these substances.

The brain compensates for increases in ICP by regulating the volume of the three substances in the following ways:
◆ limiting blood flow to the head
◆ displacing CSF into the spinal canal
◆ increasing absorption or decreasing production of CSF — withdrawing water from brain tissue and excreting it through the kidneys.

When compensatory mechanisms become overworked, small changes in volume lead to large changes in pressure. The following flowchart outlines the pathophysiology of increased ICP.

it may develop in response to cerebral ischemia, hypoxia, and hypercapnia.

Cerebral edema is classified in four types — vasogenic, cytotoxic, ischemic, or

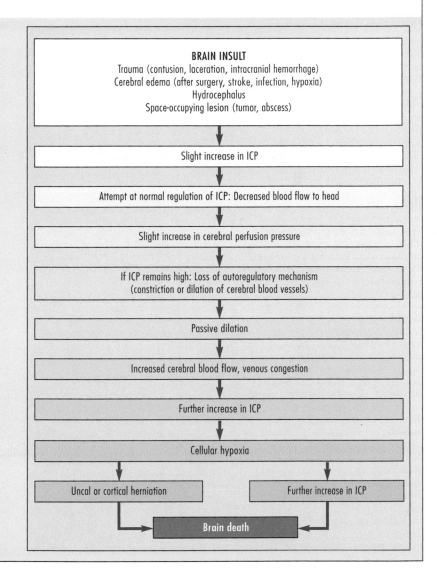

BRAIN INSULT
Trauma (contusion, laceration, intracranial hemorrhage)
Cerebral edema (after surgery, stroke, infection, hypoxia)
Hydrocephalus
Space-occupying lesion (tumor, abscess)

↓

Slight increase in ICP

↓

Attempt at normal regulation of ICP: Decreased blood flow to head

↓

Slight increase in cerebral perfusion pressure

↓

If ICP remains high: Loss of autoregulatory mechanism
(constriction or dilation of cerebral blood vessels)

↓

Passive dilation

↓

Increased cerebral blood flow, venous congestion

↓

Further increase in ICP

↓

Cellular hypoxia

↓   ↓

Uncal or cortical herniation   Further increase in ICP

↓   ↓

Brain death

interstitial — depending on the underlying mechanism responsible for the increased fluid content:

■ *Vasogenic* — Injury to the vasculature increases capillary permeability and disruption of the blood-brain barrier; leakage of plasma proteins into the extracellular spaces pulls water into the brain parenchyma.

■ *Cytotoxic (metabolic)* — Toxins cause failure of the active transport mechanisms. Loss of intracellular potassium and influx of sodium (and water) cause cells in the brain to swell.

■ *Ischemic* — Caused by cerebral infarction and initially confined to intracellular compartment; after several days, released lysosomes from necrosed cells disrupt blood-brain barrier.

■ *Interstitial* — Movement of CSF from brain's ventricles to extracellular spaces increases brain volume.

Regardless of the type of cerebral edema, blood vessels become distorted and brain tissue is displaced, ultimately leading to herniation.

Pain

Pain is the result of a complex series of steps from a site of injury to the brain, which interprets the stimuli as pain. Pain that originates outside the nervous system is termed *nociceptive* pain; pain in the nervous system is *neurogenic* or *neuropathic* pain.

NOCICEPTION

Nociception begins when noxious stimuli reach pain fibers. Sensory receptors called nociceptors — which are free nerve endings in the tissues — are stimulated by various agents, such as chemicals, temperature, or mechanical pressure. If a stimulus is sufficiently strong, impulses travel via the afferent nerve fibers along sensory pathways to the spinal cord, where they initiate autonomic and motor reflexes. The information also continues to travel to the brain, which perceives it as pain. Several theories have been developed in an attempt to explain pain. (See *Theories of pain.*)

Nociception consists of four steps: transduction, transmission, modulation, and perception.

Transduction

Transduction is the conversion of noxious stimuli into electrical impulses and subsequent depolarization of the nerve membrane. These electrical impulses are created by algesic substances that sensitize the nociceptors and are released at the site of injury or inflammation. Examples include hydrogen and potassium ions, serotonin, histamine, prostaglandins, bradykinin, and substance P.

Transmission

A-delta fibers and C fibers transmit pain sensations from the tissues to the central nervous system (CNS).

A-delta fibers are small-diameter, lightly myelinated fibers. Mechanical or thermal stimuli elicit a rapid or "fast" response. These fibers transmit localized, sharp, stinging, or pinpricking type pain sensations. A-delta fibers connect with secondary neuron groupings on the dorsal horn of the spinal cord.

C fibers are smaller and unmyelinated. They connect with second-order neurons in lamina I and II (the latter includes the substantia gelatinosa, an area in which pain is modulated). C fibers respond to chemical stimuli, rather than heat or pressure, triggering a slow pain response, usually within 1 second. This dull ache or burning sensation isn't localized and leads to two responses: an acute response transmitted immediately through fast pain pathways, which prompts the person to evade the stimulus, and lingering pain transmitted through slow pathways, which persists or worsens.

The A-delta and C fibers carry the pain signal from the peripheral tissues to the dorsal horn of the spinal cord. Excitatory and inhibitory interneurons and projection cells (neurons that connect pathways in the cerebral cortex of the CNS and peripheral nervous system) carry the signal to the brain by way of crossed and uncrossed pathways. An example of a crossed pathway is the spinothalamic tract, which enters the brain stem and ends in the thalamus. Sensory impulses travel from the medial and lateral lemniscus (tract) to the thalamus and brain stem. From the thalamus, other neurons carry the information to the sensory cortex, where pain is perceived and understood.

Another example of a crossed pathway is the ascending spinoreticulothalamic tract, which is responsible for the psycho-

Theories of pain

Over the years, numerous theories have attempted to explain the sensation of pain and describe how it occurs. This table highlights some of the major theories about pain.

THEORY	MAJOR ASSUMPTIONS	COMMENT
Specificity	◆ Four types of cutaneous sensation (touch, warmth, cold, pain) exist; each results from stimulation of specific skin receptor sites and neural pathways. Specific pain neurons transmit pain sensation along specific pain fibers. ◆ At synapses in the substantia gelatinosa, pain impulses cross to the opposite side of the cord and ascend the specific pain pathways of the spinothalamic tract to the thalamus and the pain receptor areas of the cerebral cortex.	◆ Focuses on the direct relationship between the pain stimulus and perception; doesn't account for adaptation to pain and the psychosocial factors modulating it.
Intensity	◆ Pain results from excessive stimulation of sensory receptors. Disorders or processes causing pain create an intense summation of non-noxious stimuli.	◆ Doesn't explain the existence of intense stimuli not perceived as pain.
Pattern	◆ Nonspecific receptors transmit specific patterns (characterized by the length of the pain sensation, the amount of involved tissue, and the summation of impulses) from the skin to the spinal cord, leading to pain perception.	◆ Includes some components of the intensity theory; pain possibly a response to intense stimulation of the sensory receptors regardless of receptor type or pathway.
Neuromatrix	◆ A pattern theory (sensations imprinted in the brain) — sensory inputs may trigger a pattern of sensation from the neuromatrix (a proposed network of neurons looping between the thalamus and the cortex, and the cortex and the limbic system). ◆ Sensation pattern is possible without the sensory trigger.	◆ Explains the existence of phantom pain.
Gate control	◆ Pain is transmitted from skin via the small-diameter A-delta and C fibers to the cells of the substantia gelatinosa in the dorsal horn, where interconnections between other sensory pathways exist. Stimulation of the large-diameter, fast, myelinated A-beta and A-alpha fibers "closes the gate," which restricts transmission of the impulse to the central nervous system (CNS) and diminishes pain perception. ◆ Large-fiber stimulation is possible through massage, scratching or rubbing the skin, or through electrical stimulation. Concurrent firing of pain	◆ Provides the basis for use of massage and electrical stimulation in pain management; is being used to develop additional theories and models.

(continued)

Theories of pain *(continued)*

THEORY	MAJOR ASSUMPTIONS	COMMENT
Gate control *(continued)*	and touch paths reduces transmission and perception of the pain impulses but not of touch impulses. ◆ An increase in small-fiber activity inhibits the substantia gelatinosa cells, "opening the gate" and increasing pain transmission and perception. ◆ The substantia gelatinosa acts as a gate-control system to inhibit the flow of nerve impulses from peripheral fibers to the CNS. ◆ Central T cells act as a CNS control to stimulate selective brain processes that influence the gate-control system. Inhibition of T cells closes the gate, and pain impulses aren't transmitted to the brain. ◆ T-cell activation of neural mechanisms in the brain is responsible for pain perception and response; transmitters partly regulate the release of substance P, the peptide that conveys pain information. Pain modulation is also partly controlled by the neurotransmitters enkephalin and serotonin. ◆ Persistent pain initiates a gradual decline in the fraction of impulses that pass through the various gates. ◆ Descending efferent impulses from the brain may be responsible for closing, partially opening, or completely opening the gate.	
Melzack-Casey Conceptual Model of Pain	◆ Three major psychological dimensions of pain exist: sensory-discriminative from thalamus and somatosensory cortex, motivational-affective from the reticular formation, and cognitive-evaluative. ◆ Interactions among the three produce descending inhibitory influences that alter pain input to the dorsal horn and ultimately modify the sensory pain experience and motivational-affective dimensions. ◆ Pain is localized and identified by its characteristics, evaluated by past experiences, and undergoes further cognitive processing. The complex sensory, motivational, and cognitive interactions determine motor activities and behaviors associated with the pain experience.	◆ Takes into account the powerful role of psychological functioning in determining the quality and intensity of pain.

logical components of pain and arousal. At this site, neurons synapse with interneurons before they cross to the opposite side of the cord and make their way to the medulla and, eventually, the reticular activating system, mesencephalon, and thalamus. Impulses then are transmitted to the cerebral cortex, limbic system, and basal ganglia.

After stimuli are delivered to the brain, responses from the brain must be relayed back to the original site. Several pathways carry the information in the dorsolateral white columns to the dorsal horn of the spinal cord. Some corticospinal tract neurons end in the dorsal horn and allow the brain to pay selective attention to certain stimuli while ignoring others. This allows transmission of the primary signal while suppressing the tendency for signals to spread to adjacent neurons.

Modulation

Modulation refers to modifications in pain transmission. Some neurons from the cerebral cortex and brain stem activate inhibitory processes, thus modifying the transmission. Specific substances — such as serotonin from the mesencephalon, norepinephrine from the pons, and endorphins from the brain and spinal cord — inhibit pain transmission by decreasing the release of nociceptive neurotransmitters. Spinal reflexes involving motor neurons may initiate a protective action such as withdrawal from a pinprick or may enhance the pain, such as when trauma causes a muscle spasm in the injured area.

Perception

Perception is the end result of pain transduction, transmission, and modulation. It encompasses the emotional, sensory, and subjective aspects of the pain experience. Pain perception is thought to occur in the cortical structures of the somatosensory cortex and limbic system. Alertness, arousal, and motivation are believed to result from the action of the reticular activating system and limbic system. Cardiovascular responses and typical fight or flight responses are thought to involve the medulla and hypothalamus.

The following three variables contribute to the wide variety of individual pain experiences:

■ *pain threshold* — level of intensity at which a stimulus is perceived as pain
■ *perceptual dominance* — existence of pain at another location that is given more attention
■ *pain tolerance* — duration or intensity of pain to be endured before a response is initiated.

NEUROGENIC PAIN
Neurogenic pain is associated with neural injury. Pain results from spontaneous discharges from the damaged nerves, spontaneous dorsal root activity, or degeneration of modulating mechanisms. Neurogenic pain doesn't activate nociceptors, and there's no typical pathway for transmission.

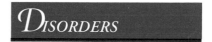

Disorders

Alzheimer's disease
Alzheimer's disease is a degenerative disorder of the cerebral cortex, especially the frontal lobe, which accounts for more than half of all cases of dementia.

AGE ALERT
Although primarily found in the elderly population, 1% to 10% of cases start in middle age.

Because this is a primary progressive dementia, the prognosis for a patient with this disease is poor.

CAUSES
The exact cause of Alzheimer's disease is unknown. Factors that have been linked to its development include the following types:

■ *neurochemical* — deficiencies in the neurotransmitters acetylcholine, somatostatin, substance P, and norepinephrine
■ *environmental* — repeated head trauma; exposure to aluminum or manganese
■ *genetic* — autosomal dominant form of Alzheimer's disease associated with early onset and death and the established risk factors of a family history of the disease or

the presence of Down syndrome in the patient.

PATHOPHYSIOLOGY
The brain tissue of patients with Alzheimer's disease exhibits three distinct and characteristic features:
- neurofibrillatory tangles (fibrous proteins)
- neuritic plaques (composed of degenerating axons and dendrites)
- granulovascular changes.

Additional structural changes include cortical atrophy, ventricular dilation, deposition of amyloid (a glycoprotein) around the cortical blood vessels, and reduced brain volume. Also found is a selective loss of cholinergic neurons in the pathways to the frontal lobes and hippocampus, areas that are important for memory and cognitive functions. Examination of the brain after death commonly reveals an atrophic brain, typically weighing less than 1,000 g (normal, 1,380 g).

SIGNS AND SYMPTOMS
The typical signs and symptoms reflect neurologic abnormalities associated with the pathophysiologic changes of the disease, such as:
- gradual loss of recent and remote memory, loss of sense of smell, and a "flattening" of mood and personality
- difficulty with learning new information
- deterioration in personal hygiene
- inability to concentrate
- increasing difficulty with abstraction and judgment
- impaired communication
- severe deterioration in memory, language, and motor function
- loss of coordination
- inability to write or speak
- personality changes
- wandering away
- nocturnal awakenings
- loss of eye contact, a fearful look
- signs of anxiety such as hand-wringing
- acute confusion, agitation, compulsiveness, or fearfulness when overwhelmed with anxiety
- disorientation and emotional lability (rapidly changing emotions)

- progressive deterioration of physical and intellectual ability.

COMPLICATIONS
The most common complications include:
- injury caused by violent behavior or wandering
- pneumonia and other infections
- malnutrition
- dehydration
- aspiration
- death.

DIAGNOSIS
Alzheimer's disease is diagnosed by exclusion; that is, by ruling out other disorders as the cause for the patient's signs and symptoms. The only true way to confirm Alzheimer's disease is by finding pathologic changes in the brain at autopsy, but the following diagnostic tests may be useful:
- Positron emission tomography shows changes in the metabolism of the cerebral cortex.
- Computed tomography scan shows evidence of early brain atrophy in excess of that which occurs in normal aging.
- Magnetic resonance imaging shows no lesion as the cause of the dementia.
- EEG shows evidence of slowed brain waves in the later stages of the disease.
- Cerebral blood flow studies show abnormalities in blood flow.

TREATMENT
No cure or definitive treatment exists for Alzheimer's disease. Therapy may include:
- N-methyl-D-aspartate (NMDA) receptor antagonists to improve memory and learning in those with moderate to severe Alzheimer's disease
- antipsychotics to treat hallucinations, delusions, aggression, hostility, and uncooperativeness
- anxiolytics for anxiety, restlessness, verbally disruptive behavior, and resistance
- antidepressants, if depression seems to worsen the dementia
- tacrine, an anticholinesterase agent, to help improve memory deficits
- antioxidants to delay disease effects
- behavioral interventions (simplifying environment, tasks, and routine) to prevent agitation.

Amyotrophic lateral sclerosis

Commonly called *Lou Gehrig disease,* after the New York Yankees' first baseman who died of this disorder, amyotrophic lateral sclerosis (ALS) is the most common of the motor neuron diseases causing muscular atrophy. Other motor neuron diseases include progressive muscular atrophy and progressive bulbar palsy. Onset is usually between ages 40 and 70. A chronic, progressively debilitating disease, ALS may be fatal in less than 1 year or continue for 10 years or more, depending on the muscles affected. More than 30,000 people in the United States have ALS; about 5,000 new cases are diagnosed each year; and the disease affects three times as many men as women.

CAUSES

The exact cause of ALS is unknown, but about 5% to 10% of cases have a genetic component — an autosomal dominant trait that affects men and women equally.

Several mechanisms have been postulated, including:
- slow-acting virus
- nutritional deficiency related to a disturbance in enzyme metabolism
- metabolic interference in nucleic acid production by the nerve fibers
- autoimmune disorders that affect immune complexes in the renal glomerulus and basement membrane.

Factors that may bring on acute deterioration include any severe stress, such as myocardial infarction, trauma, viral infections, and physical exhaustion.

PATHOPHYSIOLOGY

ALS progressively destroys the upper and lower motor neurons. It doesn't affect cranial nerves III, IV, and VI and, therefore, some facial movements such as blinking persist. Intellectual and sensory functions aren't affected.

Some believe that glutamate — the primary excitatory neurotransmitter of the central nervous system — builds to toxic levels at the nerve synapses. The affected motor units are no longer innervated and progressive degeneration of axons causes loss of myelin. Some nearby motor nerves may sprout axons in an attempt to maintain function but, ultimately, nonfunctional scar tissue replaces normal neuronal tissue.

SIGNS AND SYMPTOMS

Typical signs and symptoms of ALS include:
- fasciculations (involuntary contractions, or twitchings, of bundles of muscle fibers) accompanied by spasticity, atrophy, and weakness, caused by degeneration of the upper and lower motor neurons, and loss of functioning motor units, especially in the muscles of the forearms and the hands
- impaired speech, difficulty chewing and swallowing, choking, and excessive drooling from degeneration of cranial nerves V, IX, X, and XII
- difficulty breathing, especially if the brain stem is affected
- muscle atrophy caused by loss of innervation.

Mental deterioration doesn't usually occur, but patients may become depressed as a reaction to the disease. Progressive bulbar palsy may cause crying spells or inappropriate laughter.

COMPLICATIONS

The most common complications include:
- respiratory infections
- respiratory failure
- aspiration.

DIAGNOSIS

Although no diagnostic tests are specific to ALS, the following may aid in the diagnosis:
- Electromyography shows abnormalities of electrical activity in involved muscles.
- Muscle biopsy shows atrophic fibers interspersed between normal fibers.
- Nerve conduction studies show normal results.
- Computed tomography scan and EEG show normal results and thus rule out multiple sclerosis, spinal cord neoplasm, polyarteritis, syringomyelia, myasthenia gravis, progressive muscular dystrophy, and progressive stroke.

TREATMENT

ALS has no cure. Treatment is supportive and may include:

- diazepam, dantrolene, or baclofen to decrease spasticity
- quinidine to relieve painful muscle cramps
- thyrotropin-releasing hormone (I.V. or intrathecally) to temporarily improve motor function (successful only in some patients)
- riluzole to modulate glutamate activity and to slow disease progression
- respiratory, speech, and physical therapy to maintain function as much as possible
- psychological support to help cope with this progressive, fatal illness.

Arteriovenous malformations

Arteriovenous malformations (AVMs) are tangled masses of thin-walled, dilated blood vessels between arteries and veins that don't connect by capillaries. AVMs are common in the brain, primarily in the posterior portion of the cerebral hemispheres. Abnormal channels between the arterial and venous system mix oxygenated and unoxygenated blood and, thereby, prevent adequate perfusion of brain tissue.

AVMs range in size from a few millimeters to large malformations extending from the cerebral cortex to the ventricles. Commonly more than one AVM is present. Males and females are affected equally, and some evidence exists that AVMs occur in families. Most AVMs are present at birth, but symptoms typically don't occur until the person is age 10 to 20.

CAUSES

Causes of AVMs may be:
- congenital, caused by a hereditary defect
- acquired from penetrating injuries such as trauma.

PATHOPHYSIOLOGY

AVMs lack the typical structural characteristics of the blood vessels. The vessels of an AVM are very thin; one or more arteries feed into the AVM, causing it to appear dilated and torturous. The typically high-pressured arterial flow moves into the venous system through the connecting channels to increase venous pressure, engorging and dilating the venous structures. An

aneurysm may develop. If the AVM is large enough, the shunting can deprive the surrounding tissue of adequate blood flow. Additionally, the thin-walled vessels may ooze small amounts of blood or actually rupture, causing hemorrhage into the brain or subarachnoid space.

SIGNS AND SYMPTOMS

Typically the patient experiences few, if any, signs and symptoms unless the AVM is large, leaks, or ruptures. Possible signs and symptoms include:
- chronic mild headache and confusion from AVM dilation, vessel engorgement, and increased pressure
- seizures caused by compression of the surrounding tissues by the engorged vessels
- systolic bruit over the carotid artery, mastoid process, or orbit, indicating turbulent blood flow
- focal neurologic deficits (depending on the location of the AVM) resulting from compression and diminished perfusion
- symptoms of intracranial (intracerebral, subarachnoid, or subdural) hemorrhage, including sudden severe headache, seizures, confusion, lethargy, and meningeal irritation from bleeding into the brain tissue or subarachnoid space
- hydrocephalus from AVM extension into the ventricular lining.

COMPLICATIONS

Complications depend on the severity (location and size) of the AVM. They include:
- aneurysm development and resulting rupture
- hemorrhage (intracerebral, subarachnoid, or subdural, depending on the location of the AVM)
- hydrocephalus.

DIAGNOSIS

A definitive diagnosis depends on these diagnostic tests:
- Cerebral arteriogram confirms the presence of AVMs and evaluates blood flow.
- Doppler ultrasonography of cerebrovascular system indicates abnormal, turbulent blood flow.

TREATMENT

Treatment can be supportive, corrective, or both, including:

- support measures, including aneurysm precautions to prevent possible rupture
- surgery—block dissection, laser, or ligation—to repair the communicating channels and remove the feeding vessels
- embolization or radiation therapy if surgery isn't possible, to close the communicating channels and feeder vessels and thus reduce the blood flow to the AVM.

Bell's palsy

Bell's palsy is a disease of cranial nerve VII (facial) that produces unilateral or bilateral facial weakness or paralysis. The onset of symptoms is rapid. Although it affects all age-groups, Bell's palsy occurs most commonly in people younger than age 60. In 80% to 90% of patients, it subsides spontaneously, with complete recovery in 1 to 8 weeks, but recovery may be delayed in elderly people. If recovery is partial, contractures may develop on the paralyzed side of the face. Bell's palsy may recur on the same or opposite side of the face.

CAUSES

Bell's palsy may result from:

- infection
- hemorrhage
- tumor
- meningitis
- local trauma.

PATHOPHYSIOLOGY

Bell's palsy reflects an inflammatory reaction around the seventh cranial nerve, usually at the internal auditory meatus where the nerve leaves bony tissue. This inflammatory reaction produces a conduction block that inhibits appropriate neural stimulation to the muscle by the motor fibers of the facial nerve, resulting in the characteristic unilateral or bilateral facial weakness. (See *Neurologic dysfunction in Bell's palsy,* page 272.)

SIGNS AND SYMPTOMS

The signs and symptoms exhibited by the patient typically reflect interference in motor function associated with the seventh cranial nerve. Bell's palsy usually produces unilateral facial weakness, occasionally with aching pain around the angle of the jaw or behind the ear. On the weak side, the mouth droops (causing the patient to drool saliva from the corner of his mouth), and taste perception is distorted over the affected anterior portion of the tongue. The forehead appears smooth, and the patient's ability to close his eye on the weak side is markedly impaired. When he tries to close this eye, it rolls upward (Bell's phenomenon) and shows excessive tearing. Although Bell's phenomenon also occurs in people who are otherwise healthy, it isn't apparent because the eyelids close completely and cover this eye motion. In Bell's palsy, incomplete eye closure makes this upward motion obvious. Other symptoms may include loss of taste and ringing in the ear.

COMPLICATIONS

Complications may include:

- corneal abrasion
- infection (masked by steroid use)
- poor functional recovery.

DIAGNOSIS

Diagnosis is based on clinical presentation: distorted facial appearance and inability to raise the eyebrow, close the eyelid, smile, show the teeth, or puff out the cheek on the affected side. After 10 days, electromyography helps predict the level of expected recovery by distinguishing temporary conduction defects from a pathologic interruption of nerve fibers.

TREATMENT

Treatment consists of prednisone, an oral corticosteroid that reduces facial nerve edema and improves nerve conduction and blood flow. After the 14th day of prednisone therapy, electrotherapy may help prevent atrophy of facial muscles. Persistent paralysis may require surgical treatment.

Cerebral palsy

The most common cause of physical disability in children, cerebral palsy (CP) is a group of neuromuscular disorders caused by prenatal, perinatal, or postnatal damage to the upper motor neurons. Although

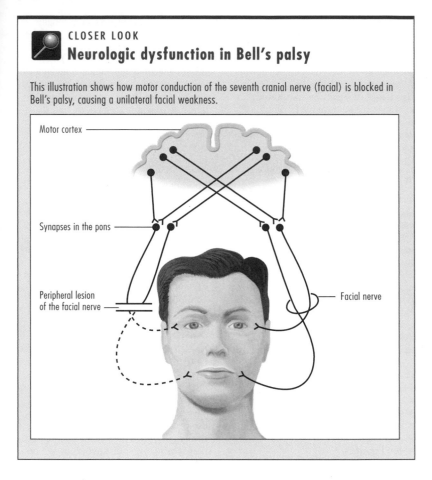

CLOSER LOOK

Neurologic dysfunction in Bell's palsy

This illustration shows how motor conduction of the seventh cranial nerve (facial) is blocked in Bell's palsy, causing a unilateral facial weakness.

Motor cortex

Synapses in the pons

Peripheral lesion of the facial nerve

Facial nerve

nonprogressive, these disorders may become more obvious as an affected infant grows.

The three major types of cerebral palsy — spastic, athetoid, and ataxic — may occur alone or in combination. Motor impairment may be minimal (sometimes apparent only during physical activities such as running) or severely disabling. Common associated defects are seizures, speech disorders, and mental retardation.

CP occurs in about 7,000 live births every year. Incidence is highest in premature neonates (anoxia plays the greatest role in contributing to cerebral palsy) and in those who are small for gestational age. Almost half the children with CP are

mentally retarded, about one-fourth have seizure disorders, and more than three-fourths have impaired speech. Additionally, children with CP commonly have dental abnormalities, vision and hearing defects, and reading disabilities.

CP is more common in whites than in other ethnic groups. The prognosis varies. Treatment may make a near-normal life possible for children with mild impairment. Those with severe impairment require special services and schooling.

CAUSES
The exact cause of CP is unknown, but conditions resulting in cerebral anoxia, hemorrhage, or other central nervous system

damage are probably responsible. Potential causes vary with time of damage.

Prenatal causes include:
- maternal infection (especially rubella)
- exposure to radiation
- anoxia
- toxemia
- maternal diabetes
- abnormal placental attachment
- malnutrition
- isoimmunization.

Perinatal and birth factors may include:
- forceps delivery
- breech presentation
- placenta previa
- abruptio placentae
- depressed maternal vital signs from general or spinal anesthesia
- prolapsed cord with delay in blood delivery to the head
- premature birth
- prolonged or unusually rapid labor
- multiple births (especially infants born last)
- infection or trauma during infancy.

Postnatal causes include:
- kernicterus resulting from erythroblastosis fetalis
- brain infection or tumor
- head trauma
- prolonged anoxia
- cerebral circulatory anomalies causing blood vessel rupture
- systemic disease resulting in cerebral thrombosis or embolus.

PATHOPHYSIOLOGY

In the early stages of brain development, a lesion or abnormality causes structural and functional defects that in turn cause impaired motor function or cognition. Even though the defects are present at birth, problems may not be apparent until months later, when the axons have become myelinated and the basal ganglia are mature.

SIGNS AND SYMPTOMS

Shortly after birth, the neonate with CP may exhibit some typical signs and symptoms reflecting impaired motor function, including:
- excessive lethargy or irritability
- high-pitched cry

- poor head control
- weak sucking reflex.

Additional physical findings reflecting structural and functional brain defects suggestive of CP include:
- delayed motor development (inability to meet major developmental milestones)
- abnormal head circumference, typically smaller than normal for age (because the head grows as the brain grows)
- abnormal postures, such as straightening legs when on his back, toes down; holding his head higher than normal when prone, caused by arching of his back
- abnormal reflexes (neonatal reflexes lasting longer than expected, extreme reflexes, or clonus)
- abnormal muscle tone and performance (scooting on his back to crawl, toe-first walking).

Each type of CP typically produces a distinctive set of clinical features, although some children display a mixed form of the disease. (See *Assessing signs of CP,* page 274.)

COMPLICATIONS

Complications depend on the type of CP and the severity of the involvement. Possible complications include:
- contractures
- skin breakdown and ulcer formation
- muscle atrophy
- malnutrition
- seizure disorders
- speech, hearing, and vision problems
- language and perceptual deficits
- mental retardation
- dental problems
- respiratory difficulties, including aspiration from poor gag and swallowing reflexes.

DIAGNOSIS

No diagnostic tests are specific to CP, but neurologic screening will exclude other possible conditions, such as infection, spina bifida, or muscular dystrophy. Diagnostic tests that may be performed include:
- developmental screening reveals delay in achieving milestones
- vision and hearing screening demonstrates degree of impairment

Assessing signs of CP

Each type of cerebral palsy (CP) shows specific signs. This table highlights the major signs and symptoms associated with each type of CP. The characteristics reflect impaired upper motor neuron function and disruption of the normal stretch reflex.

TYPE OF CP	SIGNS AND SYMPTOMS
Spastic CP (from impairment of the pyramidal tract [most common type])	◆ Hyperactive deep tendon reflexes ◆ Increased stretch reflexes ◆ Rapid alternating muscle contraction and relaxation ◆ Muscle weakness ◆ Underdevelopment of affected limbs ◆ Muscle contraction in response to manipulation ◆ Tendency toward contractures ◆ Typical walking on toes with a scissors gait, crossing one foot in front of the other

Athetoid CP (from impairment of the extrapyramidal tract)	◆ Involuntary movements (usually affecting arms more severely than legs), including:
	  – grimacing
	  – wormlike writhing
	  – dystonia
	  – sharp jerks
	◆ Difficulty with speech because of involuntary facial movements
	◆ Increasing severity of movements during stress; decreased with relaxation and disappearing entirely during sleep

Ataxic CP (from impairment of the extrapyramidal tract)	◆ Disturbed balance ◆ Incoordination (especially of the arms) ◆ Hypoactive reflexes ◆ Nystagmus ◆ Muscle weakness ◆ Tremor ◆ Lack of leg movement during infancy ◆ Wide gait as the child begins to walk ◆ Sudden or fine movements impossible (because of ataxia)
Mixed CP	◆ Spasticity and athetoid movements ◆ Ataxic and athetoid movements (resulting in severe impairment)

■ EEG identifies the source of seizure activity.

CLINICAL ALERT
Suspect CP whenever an infant shows an alteration in neurologic function during clinical observation. This may include difficulty in sucking or moving voluntarily. Infants particularly at risk are those with a low birth weight, low Apgar score at 5 minutes, seizures, and metabolic disturbances. All infants should have a screening test for CP as a regular part of their 6-month checkup.

TREATMENT
CP can't be cured, but proper treatment can help affected children reach their full potential within the limits set by this dis-

order. Such treatment requires a comprehensive and cooperative effort that involves physicians, nurses, teachers, psychologists, the child's family, and occupational, physical, and speech therapists. Home care is usually possible. Treatment typically includes:

- braces, casts, or splints and special appliances, such as adapted eating utensils and a low toilet seat with arms, to help the child perform activities of daily living independently
- an artificial urinary sphincter for the incontinent child who can use the hand controls
- range-of-motion exercises to minimize contractures
- an anticonvulsant agent to control seizures
- muscle relaxants (sometimes) to reduce spasticity
- surgery to decrease spasticity or correct contractures
- muscle transfer or tendon-lengthening surgery to improve function of joints
- rehabilitation, including occupational, physical, and speech therapy to maintain or improve functional abilities, along with referrals to supportive community organizations.

Guillain-Barré syndrome

Also known as *infectious polyneuritis, Landry-Guillain-Barré syndrome,* or *acute idiopathic polyneuritis,* Guillain-Barré syndrome is an acute, rapidly progressive, and potentially fatal form of polyneuritis that causes muscle weakness and mild distal sensory loss.

This syndrome can occur at any age but is most common between ages 30 and 50. It affects both sexes equally. Recovery is spontaneous and complete in about 95% of patients, although mild motor or reflex deficits may persist in the feet and legs. The prognosis is best when symptoms clear within 20 days after onset.

This syndrome occurs in three phases:
- Acute phase begins with the onset of the first definitive symptom and ends 1 to 3 weeks later. Further deterioration doesn't occur after the acute phase.
- Plateau phase lasts several days to 2 weeks.

- Recovery phase is believed to coincide with remyelinization and regrowth of axonal processes. It extends over 4 to 6 months but may last up to 3 years if the disease is severe.

CAUSES
The precise cause of Guillain-Barré syndrome is unknown, but it may be a cell-mediated immune response to a virus.

About 50% of patients with Guillain-Barré syndrome have a recent history of minor fever-causing illness, usually an upper respiratory tract infection or, less commonly, gastroenteritis. When infection precedes the onset of Guillain-Barré syndrome, signs of infection subside before neurologic features appear.

Other possible precipitating factors include:
- surgery
- rabies or swine influenza vaccination
- Hodgkin's disease or other malignant disease
- systemic lupus erythematosus.

PATHOPHYSIOLOGY
The major pathologic characteristic is segmental demyelination of the peripheral nerves. This prevents normal transmission of electrical impulses along the sensorimotor nerve roots. Because this syndrome causes inflammation and degenerative changes in both the posterior (sensory) and the anterior (motor) nerve roots, signs of sensory and motor losses occur at the same time. (See *Understanding sensorimotor nerve degeneration,* page 276.) Additionally, autonomic nerve transmission may be impaired.

SIGNS AND SYMPTOMS
Symptoms are progressive and include:
- symmetrical muscle weakness (major neurologic sign) appearing in the legs first (ascending type) and then extending to the arms and facial nerves in 24 to 72 hours as a result of impaired anterior nerve root transmission
- muscle weakness developing in the arms first (descending type) or in the arms and legs at the same time, from impaired anterior nerve root transmission

> ### 🔍 CLOSER LOOK
> # Understanding sensorimotor nerve degeneration
>
> Guillain-Barré syndrome attacks the peripheral nerves so that they can't transmit messages to the brain correctly. Here's what goes wrong.
>
> The myelin sheath degenerates for unknown reasons. This sheath covers the nerve axons and conducts electrical impulses along the nerve pathways. Degeneration brings inflammation, swelling, and patchy demyelination. As this disorder destroys myelin, the nodes of Ranvier (at the junction of the myelin sheaths) widen. This delays and impairs impulse transmission along the dorsal and anterior nerve roots.
>
> Because the dorsal nerve roots handle sensory function, the patient may experience tingling and numbness. Similarly, because the anterior nerve roots are responsible for motor function, impairment causes varying weakness, immobility, and paralysis.

- muscle weakness absent or affecting only the cranial nerves (in mild forms)
- paresthesia, sometimes preceding muscle weakness but vanishing quickly, from impairment of the dorsal nerve root transmission
- diplegia, possibly with ophthalmoplegia (eye paralysis), from impaired motor nerve root transmission and involvement of cranial nerves III, IV, and VI
- dysphagia or dysarthria and, less common, weakness of the muscles supplied by cranial nerve XI (spinal accessory nerve)
- hypotonia and areflexia from interruption of the reflex arc.

COMPLICATIONS
Common complications include:
- thrombophlebitis
- pressure ulcers
- muscle wasting
- sepsis
- joint contractures
- aspiration
- respiratory tract infections
- mechanical respiratory failure
- sinus tachycardia or bradycardia
- hypertension and postural hypotension
- loss of bladder and bowel sphincter control.

DIAGNOSIS
The following tests may aid in the diagnosis:
- Cerebrospinal fluid (CSF) analysis by lumbar puncture reveals elevated protein levels, peaking in 4 to 6 weeks, probably as a result of widespread inflammation of the nerve roots; the CSF white blood cell count remains normal, but in severe disease, CSF pressure may rise above normal.
- Complete blood count shows leukocytosis with immature forms early in the illness, and then quickly returns to normal.
- Electromyography possibly shows repeated firing of the same motor unit, instead of widespread sectional stimulation.
- Nerve conduction velocities show slowing soon after paralysis develops.
- Serum immunoglobulin levels reveal elevated levels from inflammatory response.

TREATMENT
Treatment is primarily supportive; it may include:
- Endotracheal intubation or tracheotomy may be performed if respiratory muscle involvement causes difficulty in clearing secretions.
- Trial dose (7 days) of prednisone is given to reduce inflammatory response if the disease is relentlessly progressive; if prednisone produces no noticeable improvement, the drug is discontinued.
- Plasmapheresis is useful during the initial phase but of no benefit if begun 2 weeks after onset.
- Continuous electrocardiogram monitoring alerts for possible arrhythmias from autonomic dysfunction; propranolol treats tachycardia and hypertension, or atropine

is given for bradycardia; volume replacement is provided for severe hypotension.

Headache

The most common patient complaint, headache usually occurs as a symptom of an underlying disorder. Ninety percent of all headaches are vascular or muscle-contractile, or a combination; 10% are caused by underlying intracranial, systemic, or psychological disorders. Migraine headaches, probably the most intensely studied, are throbbing vascular headaches that usually begin to appear in childhood or adolescence and recur throughout adulthood. Affecting up to 10% of people in the United States, they're more common in females and have a strong familial incidence.

CAUSES

Most chronic headaches result from tension (muscle contraction), which may be caused by:

- emotional stress or fatigue
- menstruation
- environmental stimuli (noise, crowds, or bright lights).

Other possible causes include:

- glaucoma
- inflammation of the eyes or mucosa of the nasal or paranasal sinuses
- diseases of the scalp, teeth, extracranial arteries, or external or middle ear
- vasodilators (nitrates, alcohol, and histamine)
- systemic disease
- hypertension
- increased intracranial pressure (ICP)
- head trauma or tumor
- intracranial bleeding, abscess, or aneurysm.

PATHOPHYSIOLOGY

Headaches are believed to be associated with constriction and dilation of intracranial and extracranial arteries. During a migraine attack, certain biochemical abnormalities, including local leakage of a vasodilator polypeptide called neurokinin through the dilated arteries and a decrease in the plasma level of serotonin are thought to occur.

Headache pain may emanate from the pain-sensitive structures of the skin, scalp, muscles, arteries, and veins; cranial nerves V, VII, IX, and X or cervical nerves 1, 2, and 3. Intracranial mechanisms of headaches include traction or displacement of arteries, venous sinuses, or venous tributaries and inflammation or direct pressure on the cranial nerves with afferent pain fibers.

Four headache phases

The evolution of a headache has four distinct phases:

(Cerebral and temporal arteries are innervated extracranially; parenchymal arteries are noninnervated.)

- *Vasoconstriction (aura)* — Stress-related neurogenic local vasoconstriction of innervated cerebral arteries reduces cerebral blood flow (localized ischemia). Systematically, the prostaglandin thromboxane causes increased platelet aggregation and release of serotonin, a potent vasoconstrictor, and, possibly, other vasoactive substances.

- *Parenchymal artery dilation* — Noninnervated parenchymal vessels dilate in response to local acidosis and anoxia (ischemia). Neurogenic or biologic factors may cause preformed arteriovenous shunts to open. Increased blood flow, increased internal pressure, and enhanced pulsations short-circuit the normal nutritive capillaries and cause pain.

- *Vasodilation (headache)* — Compensatory mechanisms cause marked vasodilation of the innervated arteries resulting in headache. Systemic platelet aggregation decreases, and falling serotonin levels result in vasodilation. A painful, sterile perivascular inflammation develops.

- *Perivascular inflammation (post-headache)* — Painful perivascular inflammation persists after the headache goes away.

SIGNS AND SYMPTOMS

Initially, *migraine headaches* usually produce unilateral, pulsating pain, which later becomes more generalized. They're commonly preceded by a glittering scotoma (isolated area of the visual field, with absent or depressed vision), hemianopsia

Features of migraine headaches

TYPE	SIGNS AND SYMPTOMS
COMMON MIGRAINE (MOST PREVALENT)	
Usually occurs on weekends and holidays	◆ Prodromal symptoms, including fatigue, nausea, vomiting, and fluid imbalance, that precede headache by about 1 day ◆ Sensitivity to light and noise (most prominent feature) ◆ Headache pain (unilateral or bilateral, aching or throbbing)
CLASSIC MIGRAINE	
Usually occurs in people with compulsive personalities and within families	◆ Prodromal symptoms, including vision disturbances, such as zigzag lines and bright lights (most common), sensory disturbances (tingling of face, lips, and hands), or motor disturbances (staggering gait) ◆ Recurrent, periodic headaches
HEMIPLEGIC AND OPHTHALMOPLEGIC MIGRAINE (RARE)	
Usually occurs in young adults	◆ Severe, unilateral pain ◆ Extraocular muscle palsies (involving third cranial nerve [CN III]) and ptosis ◆ With repeated headaches, possible permanent CN III injury ◆ In hemiplegic migraine, neurologic deficits (hemiparesis, hemiplegia) that may persist after headache subsides
BASILAR ARTERY MIGRAINE	
Occurs in young women before their menstrual periods	◆ Prodromal symptoms, including partial vision loss followed by vertigo, ataxia, dysarthria, tinnitus and, sometimes, tingling of fingers and toes; these may last from several minutes to almost an hour ◆ Headache pain, severe occipital throbbing, vomiting

(blindness in one-half the field of vision in one or both eyes), unilateral paresthesia, or speech disorders. The person may experience irritability, anorexia, nausea, vomiting, and extreme sensitivity to light. (See *Features of migraine headaches.*)

Both *muscle contraction and traction-inflammatory vascular headaches* produce a dull, persistent ache, tender spots on the head and neck, and a feeling of tightness around the head, with a characteristic "hat-band" distribution. The pain is typically severe and unrelenting. If caused by intracranial bleeding, headache may result in neurologic deficits, such as paresthesia and muscle weakness; opioids may fail to relieve pain in these cases. If caused by a

tumor, pain is most severe when the patient awakens.

COMPLICATIONS

Complications may include:
- results of misdiagnosis
- status migraines
- drug dependency
- disruption of lifestyle.

DIAGNOSIS

Diagnosis requires:
- review of the history of recurrent headache
- physical examination of the head and neck. Such examination includes percussion, auscultation for bruits, inspection for

signs of infection, and palpation for defects, crepitus, or tender spots (especially after trauma).

Definitive diagnosis also requires a complete neurologic examination, assessment for other systemic diseases, and a psychosocial evaluation when such factors are suspected.

Diagnostic tests include:

- cervical spine and sinus X-rays
- EEG
- computed tomography scan — performed before lumbar puncture to rule out increased ICP — or magnetic resonance imaging.

A lumbar puncture isn't done if there's evidence of increased ICP or if a brain tumor is suspected because rapidly reducing pressure, by removing spinal fluid, can cause brain herniation.

TREATMENT
Depending on the type of headache, analgesics — ranging from aspirin to codeine or meperidine — may provide symptomatic relief. Other measures include identification and elimination of causative factors and, possibly, psychotherapy for headaches caused by emotional stress. Chronic tension headaches may also require muscle relaxants.

For migraine headaches, ergotamine alone or with caffeine may be an effective treatment. It's important to remember that these medications can't be taken by pregnant women because they stimulate uterine contractions. These drugs and others, such as metoclopramide or naproxen, work best when taken early in the course of an attack. If nausea and vomiting make oral administration impossible, drugs may be given as rectal suppositories.

Drugs in the class of sumatriptan are considered by many clinicians to be the drug of choice for acute migraine attacks or cluster headaches. Drugs that can help prevent migraine headaches include propranolol, atenolol, clonidine, and amitriptyline.

Head trauma

Head trauma describes any traumatic insult to the brain that results in physical, intellectual, emotional, social, or vocational changes. Young children age 6 months to 2 years, persons age 15 to 24, and elderly people are at highest risk for head trauma. The risk for men is double the risk for women.

Head trauma is generally categorized as *closed* or *open* trauma. Closed trauma, or blunt trauma as it's sometimes called, is more common. It typically occurs when the head strikes a hard surface or a rapidly moving object strikes the head. The dura is intact, and no brain tissue is exposed to the external environment. In open trauma, as the name suggests, an opening in the scalp, skull, meninges, or brain tissue, including the dura, exposes the cranial contents to the environment, and the risk of infection is high.

Mortality from head trauma has declined with advances in preventive measures, such as seat belts, airbags, and quicker response and transport times, and improved treatment, including the development of regional trauma centers. Advances in technology have increased the effectiveness of rehabilitative services, even for patients with severe head injuries.

CAUSES
Causes of head trauma may include:

- transportation or automobile accident (number one cause)
- falls
- sports-related injuries
- crime and assaults.

PATHOPHYSIOLOGY
The brain is shielded by the cranial vault (hair, skin, bone, meninges, and cerebrospinal fluid (CSF), which intercepts the force of a physical blow. Below a certain level of force (the absorption capacity), the cranial vault prevents energy (force) from affecting the brain. The degree of traumatic head injury usually is proportional to the amount of force reaching the cranial tissues. Furthermore, unless ruled out, neck injuries should be presumed present in patients with traumatic head injury.

Closed trauma is typically a sudden acceleration-deceleration or coup and contrecoup injury. In coup and contrecoup, the head hits a relatively stationary object, injuring cranial tissues near the point of impact (coup); then the remaining force pushes the brain against the opposite side of the skull, causing a second impact and injury (contrecoup). Contusions and lacerations may also occur during contrecoup as the brain's soft tissues slide over the rough bone of the cranial cavity. In addition, the cerebrum may endure rotational shear, damaging the upper midbrain and areas of the frontal, temporal, and occipital lobes.

Open trauma may penetrate the scalp, skull, meninges, or brain. Open head injuries are usually associated with skull fractures, and bone fragments commonly cause hematomas and meningeal tears with consequent loss of CSF.

SIGNS AND SYMPTOMS
Types of head trauma include concussion, contusion, epidural hematoma, subdural hematoma, intracerebral hematoma, and skull fractures. Each is associated with specific signs and symptoms. (See *Types of head trauma,* pages 282 to 285.)

COMPLICATIONS
Complications may include:
- increased intracranial pressure
- infection (in open trauma)
- respiratory depression and failure
- brain herniation.

DIAGNOSIS
Each type of head trauma is associated with specific diagnostic findings. (See *Types of head trauma,* pages 282 to 285.)

TREATMENT
Surgical treatment includes:
- evacuation of the hematoma or a craniotomy to elevate or remove fragments that have been driven into the brain, and to extract foreign bodies and necrotic tissue, thereby reducing the risk of infection and further brain damage from fractures.

Supportive treatment includes:
- close observation to detect changes in neurologic status suggesting further damage or expanding hematoma
- cleaning and debridement of any wounds associated with skull fractures

- diuretics, such as mannitol, to reduce cerebral edema
- analgesics, such as acetaminophen and codeine (for severe headache), to relieve headache
- anticonvulsants such as phenytoin to prevent and treat seizures
- respiratory support, including mechanical ventilation and endotracheal intubation, as indicated, for respiratory failure from brain stem involvement
- prophylactic antibiotics to prevent the onset of meningitis from CSF leakage associated with skull fractures.

Herniated intervertebral disk
Also called a *ruptured* or *slipped disk* or a *herniated nucleus pulposus,* a herniated disk occurs when all or part of the nucleus pulposus — the soft, gelatinous, central portion of an intervertebral disk — is forced through the disk's weakened or torn outer ring (anulus fibrosus).

Herniated disks usually occur in adults (mostly men) under age 45. About 90% of herniated disks occur in the lumbar and lumbosacral regions, 8% occur in the cervical area, and 1% to 2% occur in the thoracic area. Patients with a congenitally small lumbar spinal canal or with osteophyte formation along the vertebrae may be more susceptible to nerve root compression and more likely to have neurologic symptoms.

CAUSES
The two major causes of herniated intervertebral disk are:
- severe trauma or strain
- intervertebral joint degeneration.

 AGE ALERT
In older patients whose disks have begun to degenerate, minor trauma may cause herniation.

PATHOPHYSIOLOGY
An intervertebral disk has two parts: the soft center called the nucleus pulposus and the tough, fibrous surrounding ring called the anulus fibrosus. The nucleus pulposus acts as a shock absorber, distributing the mechanical stress applied to the spine when the body moves. Physical stress, usu-

ally a twisting motion, can tear or rupture the anulus fibrosus so that the nucleus pulposus herniates into the spinal canal. The vertebrae move closer together and the ruptured disk material exerts pressure on the nerve roots, causing pain and, possibly, sensory and motor loss. A herniated disk also can occur with intervertebral joint degeneration. If the disk has begun to degenerate, minor trauma may cause herniation.

Herniation occurs in three steps:
- *protrusion* — nucleus pulposus presses against the anulus fibrosus
- *extrusion* — nucleus pulposus bulges forcibly though the anulus fibrosus, pushing against the nerve root
- *sequestration* — anulus gives way as the disk's core bursts and presses against the nerve root.

SIGNS AND SYMPTOMS
Signs and symptoms include:
- severe lower back pain to the buttocks, legs, and feet, usually unilaterally, from compression of nerve roots supplying these areas
- sudden pain after trauma, subsiding in a few days, and then recurring at shorter intervals and with progressive intensity because of nerve root compression
- sciatic pain after trauma, beginning as a dull pain in the buttocks; Valsalva's maneuver, coughing, sneezing, and bending intensify the pain, which is typically accompanied by muscle spasms from pressure and irritation of the sciatic nerve root
- sensory and motor loss in the area innervated by the compressed spinal nerve root and, in later stages, weakness and atrophy of leg muscles.

COMPLICATIONS
Complications are dependent on the severity and the specific site of herniation. Common complications include:
- neurologic deficits
- bowel and bladder problems.

DIAGNOSIS
- Straight-leg raising test is positive only if the patient has posterior leg (sciatic) pain, not back pain

- Lasègue's test reveals resistance and pain as well as loss of ankle or knee-jerk reflex, indicating spinal root compression.
- Spinal X-rays rule out other abnormalities but may not diagnose a herniated disk because a marked disk prolapse may not be apparent on a regular X-ray.
- Myelogram, computed tomography scan, and magnetic resonance imaging show spinal canal compression by herniated disk material.

TREATMENT
Treatment may include:
- heat applications to decrease muscle spasm and aid in pain relief
- exercise program to strengthen associated muscles and prevent further deterioration
- corticosteroids such as dexamethasone for an initial, short course or anti-inflammatories, such as aspirin and nonsteroidal anti-inflammatory drugs, to reduce inflammation and edema at the site of injury; muscle relaxants, such as diazepam, methocarbamol, and cyclobenzaprine, to minimize muscle spasm from nerve root irritation; epidural injections at the level of the protrusion to relieve pain
- surgery, including laminectomy to remove the extruded disk, spinal fusion to overcome segmental instability, or both to stabilize the spine.

Huntington's disease
Also called *Huntington's chorea, hereditary chorea, chronic progressive chorea,* and *adult chorea,* Huntington's disease is a hereditary disorder in which degeneration of the cerebral cortex and basal ganglia causes chronic progressive chorea (involuntary and irregular movements) and cognitive deterioration, ending in dementia.

Huntington's disease usually strikes people between ages 25 and 55 (the average age is 35), but 2% of cases occur in children, and 5% occur as late as age 60. It affects men and women equally. Death usually results 10 to 15 years after onset from suicide, heart failure, or pneumonia.

(Text continues on page 284.)

Types of head trauma

This table summarizes the signs and symptoms and diagnostic test findings for the different types of head trauma.

TYPE	DESCRIPTION
Concussion (closed head injury)	◆ A blow to the head hard enough to make the brain hit the skull, but not hard enough to cause a cerebral contusion, causes temporary neural dysfunction. ◆ Recovery is usually complete in 24 to 48 hours. ◆ Repeated injuries exact a cumulative toll on the brain.
Contusion (bruising of brain tissue; more serious than concussion)	◆ Most common in people ages 20 to 40. ◆ Typically results from arterial bleeding. ◆ Blood commonly accumulates between skull and dura. Injury to middle meningeal artery in parietotemporal area is the most common and is usually accompanied by linear skull fractures in temporal region over middle meningeal artery. ◆ Less commonly arises from dural venous sinuses.
Epidural hematoma	◆ Acceleration-deceleration or coup-contrecoup injuries disrupt normal nerve functions in bruised area. ◆ Injury is directly beneath the site of impact when the brain rebounds against the skull from the force of a blow (a beating with a blunt instrument, for example), when the force of the blow drives the brain against the opposite side of the skull, or when the head is hurled forward and stopped abruptly (as in an automobile crash when a driver's head strikes the windshield). ◆ Brain continues moving and slaps against the skull (acceleration), then rebounds (deceleration). Brain may strike bony prominences inside the skull (especially the sphenoidal ridges), causing intracranial hemorrhage or hematoma that may result in tentorial herniation.

SIGNS AND SYMPTOMS	DIAGNOSTIC TEST FINDINGS
◆ Short-term loss of consciousness caused by disruption of reticular activating system (RAS), possibly because of abrupt pressure changes in the areas responsible for consciousness, changes in polarity of the neurons, ischemia, or structural distortion of neurons ◆ Vomiting from localized injury and compression ◆ Anterograde and retrograde amnesia (patient can't recall events immediately after the injury or events that led up to the traumatic incident) correlating with severity of injury; all related to disruption of RAS ◆ Irritability or lethargy from localized injury and compression ◆ Behavior out of character because of focal injury ◆ Dizziness, nausea, or severe headache caused by focal injury and compression	◆ Computed tomography (CT) scan reveals no sign of fracture, bleeding, or other nervous system lesion.
◆ Severe scalp wounds from direct injury ◆ Labored respiration and loss of consciousness caused by increased pressure from bruising ◆ Drowsiness, confusion, disorientation, agitation, or violence from increased intracranial pressure (ICP) associated with trauma ◆ Hemiparesis related to interrupted blood flow to the site of injury ◆ Decorticate or decerebrate posturing from cortical damage or hemispheric dysfunction ◆ Unequal pupillary response from brain stem involvement	◆ CT scan shows changes in tissue density, possible displacement of the surrounding structures, and evidence of ischemic tissue, hematomas, and fractures. ◆ EEG recordings directly over area of contusion reveal progressive abnormalities by appearance of high-amplitude theta and delta waves.
◆ Brief period of unconsciousness after injury reflecting the concussive effects of head trauma, followed by a lucid interval varying from 10 to 15 minutes to hours or, rarely, days ◆ Severe headache ◆ Progressive loss of consciousness and deterioration in neurologic signs resulting from expanding lesion and extrusion of medial portion of temporal lobe through tentorial opening ◆ Compression of brain stem by temporal lobe, causing characteristics of intracranial hypertension ◆ Deterioration in level of consciousness resulting from compression of brain stem reticular formation as temporal lobe herniates on its upper portion ◆ Respirations, initially deep and labored, becoming shallow and irregular as brain stem is impacted ◆ Contralateral motor deficits reflecting compression of corticospinal tracts that pass through the brain stem ◆ Ipsilateral (same-side) pupillary dilation caused by compression of third cranial nerve (CN III) ◆ Seizures possible from high ICP ◆ Continued bleeding leading to progressive neurologic degeneration, evidenced by bilateral pupillary dilation, bilateral decerebrate response, increased systemic blood pressure, decreased pulse, and profound coma with irregular respiratory patterns	◆ CT scan or magnetic resonance imaging (MRI) identifies abnormal masses or structural shifts within the cranium.

(continued)

Types of head trauma *(continued)*

TYPE	DESCRIPTION
Subdural hematoma	◆ Meningeal hemorrhages, resulting from accumulation of blood in subdural space (between dura mater and arachnoid) are most common. ◆ May be acute, subacute, and chronic; unilateral or bilateral. ◆ Usually associated with torn connecting veins in cerebral cortex; rarely from arteries. ◆ Acute hematomas are a surgical emergency.
Intracerebral hematoma	◆ Subacute hematomas have better prognosis because venous bleeding tends to be slower. ◆ Traumatic or spontaneous disruption of cerebral vessels in brain parenchyma cause neurologic deficits, depending on site and amount of bleeding. ◆ Shear forces from brain movement frequently cause vessel laceration and hemorrhage into the parenchyma. ◆ Frontal and temporal lobes are common sites. Trauma is associated with few intracerebral hematomas; most caused by hypertension.
Skull fractures	◆ Four types: linear, comminuted, depressed, and basilar. ◆ Fractures of anterior and middle fossae are associated with severe head trauma and are more common than those of posterior fossa. ◆ Blow to the head causes one or more of the types. May not be problematic unless brain is exposed or bone fragments are driven into neural tissue.

CAUSES

The actual cause of this disorder is unknown, but it's transmitted as an autosomal dominant trait, which either sex can transmit and inherit. Each child of an affected parent has a 50% chance of inheriting it; the child who doesn't inherit it can't transmit it. Huntington's disease is prevalent in areas where affected families have lived for several generations because of hereditary transmission and delayed expression. Genetic testing is now available to families with a known history of the disease.

PATHOPHYSIOLOGY

Huntington's disease involves a disturbance in neurotransmitter substances, primarily gamma-aminobutyric acid (GABA) and dopamine. In the basal ganglia, frontal cortex, and cerebellum, GABA neurons are destroyed and replaced by

SIGNS AND SYMPTOMS	DIAGNOSTIC TEST FINDINGS
◆ Similar to epidural hematoma but significantly slower in onset because bleeding is typically of venous origin	◆ CT scan, X-rays, and arteriography reveal mass and altered blood flow in the area, confirming hematoma. ◆ CT scan or MRI reveals evidence of masses and tissue shifting. ◆ CSF is yellow and has relatively low protein (chronic subdural hematoma).
◆ Immediate unresponsiveness or a lucid period before person lapses into a coma from increasing ICP and mass effect of hemorrhage ◆ Possible motor deficits and decorticate or decerebrate responses from compression of corticospinal tracts and brain stem	◆ CT scan or cerebral arteriography identifies bleeding site. CSF is pressure elevated; fluid may appear bloody or xanthochromic (yellow or straw-colored) from hemoglobin breakdown.
◆ May produce no symptoms, depends on underlying brain trauma ◆ Discontinuity and displacement of bone structure with severe fracture ◆ Motor sensory and CN dysfunction with associated facial fractures ◆ With anterior fossa basilar skull fractures: possible periorbital ecchymosis ("raccoon eyes"), anosmia (loss of smell caused by CN I involvement), and pupil abnormalities (CN II and III involvement) ◆ With middle fossa basilar skull fractures: Cerebrospinal fluid (CSF) rhinorrhea (leakage through nose), CSF otorrhea (leakage from the ear), hemotympanum (blood accumulation at the tympanic membrane), ecchymosis over the mastoid bone (Battle's sign), and facial paralysis (CN VII injury) ◆ With posterior fossa basilar skull fracture: signs of medullary dysfunction, such as cardiovascular and respiratory failure	◆ CT scan and MRI reveal intracranial hemorrhage from ruptured blood vessels and swelling. ◆ Skull X-ray may reveal fracture. ◆ Lumbar puncture is contraindicated by expanding lesions.

glial cells. The consequent deficiency of GABA (an inhibitory neurotransmitter) results in a relative excess of dopamine and abnormal neurotransmission along the affected pathways.

SIGNS AND SYMPTOMS
The onset of this disease is insidious. The patient eventually becomes totally dependent—emotionally and physically—through loss of musculoskeletal control.

Neurologic characteristics include:
■ progressively severe choreic movements, which are caused by the relative excess of dopamine. Such movements are rapid, typically violent, and purposeless.
■ choreic movements are initially unilateral and more prominent in the face and arms than in the legs. They progress from mild fidgeting to grimacing, tongue smacking, dysarthria (indistinct speech), emotion-related athetoid (slow, twisting,

snakelike) movements (especially of the hands) from injury to the basal ganglion, and torticollis from shortening of neck muscles.
- bradykinesia (slow movement), commonly accompanied by rigidity.
- impairment of voluntary and involuntary movement caused by the combination of chorea, bradykinesia, and muscle dysfunction.
- dysphagia caused by impaired reflexes occurs in most patients in the advanced stages.
- dysarthria may be complicated by perseveration (persistent repetition of a reply), oral apraxia (difficulty coordinating movement of the mouth), and aprosody (inability to accurately reproduce or interpret the tone of language).

Cognitive signs and symptoms may include:
- dementia, an early indication of the disease, from dysfunction of the subcortex without significant impairment of immediate memory
- problems with recent memory because of retrieval problems rather than encoding problems
- deficits of executive function (planning, organizing, regulating, and programming) from frontal lobe involvement
- impaired impulse control.

The patient may also exhibit psychiatric symptoms, commonly before movement problems occur. Psychiatric symptoms may include:
- depression and possible mania (earliest symptom) related to altered levels of dopamine and GABA
- personality changes including irritability, lability, impulsiveness, and aggressive behavior.

COMPLICATIONS

Common complications of Huntington's disease include:
- choking
- aspiration
- pneumonia
- heart failure
- infections.

DIAGNOSIS

- Genetic testing reveals autosomal dominant trait.
- Positron emission tomography confirms disorder.
- Computed tomography scan and magnetic resonance imaging show brain atrophy in caudate nuclei and putamen and ventricular enlargement.

TREATMENT

No known cure exists for Huntington's disease. Treatment is symptom-based, supportive, and protective. It may include:
- haloperidol or diazepam to modify choreic movements and control behavioral characteristics and depression
- psychotherapy to decrease anxiety and stress and manage psychiatric symptoms
- institutionalization to manage progressive mental deterioration and self-care deficits.

Hydrocephalus

An excessive accumulation of cerebrospinal fluid (CSF) within the ventricular spaces of the brain, hydrocephalus occurs most commonly in neonates. It can also occur in adults as a result of injury or disease. In infants, hydrocephalus enlarges the head and, in both infants and adults, the resulting compression can damage brain tissue.

With early detection and surgical intervention, the prognosis improves but remains guarded. Even after surgery, complications may persist, such as developmental delay, impaired motor function, and vision loss. Without surgery, the prognosis is poor. Death may result from increased intracranial pressure (ICP) in people of all ages; infants may die of infection and malnutrition.

CAUSES

Hydrocephalus may result from:
- obstruction in CSF flow (noncommunicating hydrocephalus)
- faulty absorption of CSF (communicating hydrocephalus).

Risk factors associated with the development of hydrocephalus in infants may include:
- intrauterine infection

■ intracranial hemorrhage from birth trauma or prematurity.

In older children and adults, risk factors may include:
■ meningitis
■ mastoiditis
■ chronic otitis media
■ brain tumors or intracranial hemorrhage.

PATHOPHYSIOLOGY

In noncommunicating hydrocephalus, the obstruction occurs most frequently between the third and fourth ventricles, at the aqueduct of Sylvius, but it can also occur at the outlets of the fourth ventricle (foramina of Luschka and Magendie) or, rarely, at the foramen of Monro. This obstruction may result from faulty fetal development, infection (syphilis, granulomatous diseases, meningitis), a tumor, a cerebral aneurysm, or a blood clot (after intracranial hemorrhage).

In communicating hydrocephalus, faulty absorption of CSF may result from surgery to repair a myelomeningocele, adhesions between meninges at the base of the brain, or meningeal hemorrhage. Rarely, a tumor in the choroid plexus causes overproduction of CSF and consequent hydrocephalus.

In either type, both CSF pressure and volume increase. Obstruction in the ventricles causes dilation, stretching, and disruption of the lining. Underlying white matter atrophies. Compression of brain tissue and cerebral blood vessels leads to ischemia and, eventually, cell death.

SIGNS AND SYMPTOMS

In infants, the signs and symptoms typically include:
■ enlargement of the head clearly disproportionate to the infant's growth (most characteristic sign) from the increased CSF volume
■ distended scalp veins from increased CSF pressure
■ thin, shiny, fragile-looking scalp skin from the increase in CSF pressure
■ underdeveloped neck muscles from increased weight of the head

■ depressed orbital roof with downward displacement of the eyes and prominent sclerae from increased pressure
■ high-pitched shrill cry, irritability, and abnormal muscle tone in the legs from neurologic compression
■ projectile vomiting from increased ICP
■ skull widening to accommodate increased pressure.

In adults and older children, indicators of hydrocephalus include:
■ decreased level of consciousness from increasing ICP
■ ataxia from increased pressure leading to compression of the motor areas
■ incontinence caused by increased pressure affecting neurologic control over bowel and bladder function
■ impaired intellect.

COMPLICATIONS

Complications may include:
■ mental retardation
■ impaired motor function
■ vision loss
■ brain herniation
■ infection
■ malnutrition
■ shunt infection (after surgery)
■ septicemia (after shunt insertion)
■ paralytic ileus, adhesions, peritonitis, and intestinal perforation (after shunt insertion)
■ death from increased ICP.

DIAGNOSIS

■ Skull X-rays show thinning of the skull with separation of the sutures and widening of the fontanels.
■ Angiography shows vessel abnormalities caused by stretching.
■ Computed tomography scan and magnetic resonance imaging reveal variations in tissue density and fluid in the ventricular system.
■ Lumbar puncture reveals increased fluid pressure from communicating hydrocephalus.
■ Ventriculography shows ventricular dilation with excess fluid.

▲ AGE ALERT
In infants, abnormally large head size for the patient's age strongly suggests hydrocephalus. Measurement of the

CLOSER LOOK
Most common sites of cerebral aneurysm

Cerebral aneurysms usually arise at the arterial bifurcation in the Circle of Willis and its branches. This illustration shows the most common sites around this circle.

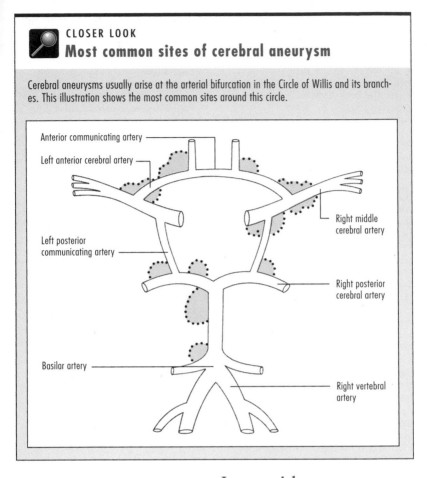

- Anterior communicating artery
- Left anterior cerebral artery
- Left posterior communicating artery
- Basilar artery
- Right middle cerebral artery
- Right posterior cerebral artery
- Right vertebral artery

head circumference is the most important diagnostic technique.

TREATMENT
The only treatment for hydrocephalus is surgical correction, by insertion of:
- ventriculoperitoneal shunt, which carries excess fluid from the lateral ventricle into the peritoneal cavity
- ventriculoatrial shunt (less common), which drains fluid from the brain's lateral ventricle into the right atrium of the heart, where the fluid makes its way into the venous circulation.

Supportive care is also warranted.

Intracranial aneurysm

An intracranial, or cerebral, aneurysm is a weakness in the wall of a cerebral artery that causes localized dilation. Its most common form is the berry aneurysm, a saclike outpouching in a cerebral artery. Cerebral aneurysms usually arise at an arterial junction in the Circle of Willis, the circular anastomosis forming the major cerebral arteries at the base of the brain. (See *Most common sites of cerebral aneurysm.*) Cerebral aneurysms commonly rupture and cause subarachnoid hemorrhage.

The incidence is slightly higher in women than in men, especially those in their late 40s or early to mid-50s, but a cerebral aneurysm may occur at any age in either sex. The prognosis is guarded. About one-half of all patients who suffer a subarachnoid hemorrhage die immediately. Of those who survive untreated, 40% die from the effects of hemorrhage and another 20% die later from recurring hemorrhage. New treatments are improving the prognosis.

CAUSES
Causes may include:
- congenital defect
- degenerative process
- combination of congenital defect and degenerative process
- trauma.

PATHOPHYSIOLOGY
Blood flow exerts pressure against a congenitally weak arterial wall, stretching it like an overblown balloon and making it likely to rupture. Such a rupture is followed by a subarachnoid hemorrhage, in which blood spills into the space normally occupied by cerebrospinal fluid. Sometimes, blood also spills into brain tissue, where a clot can cause potentially fatal increased intracranial pressure (ICP) and brain tissue damage.

SIGNS AND SYMPTOMS
Occasionally, the patient may exhibit premonitory symptoms resulting from oozing of blood into the subarachnoid space. These symptoms include:
- headache, intermittent nausea
- nuchal rigidity
- stiff back and legs.

Usually the rupture occurs abruptly and without warning, causing:
- sudden severe headache caused by increased pressure from bleeding into a closed space
- nausea and projectile vomiting related to increased pressure
- altered level of consciousness, including deep coma, depending on the severity and location of bleeding, from increased pressure caused by increased cerebral blood volume
- meningeal irritation, resulting in nuchal rigidity, back and leg pain, fever, restlessness, irritability, occasional seizures, pho-

---

Determining severity of an intracranial aneurysm rupture

The severity of symptoms varies from patient to patient, depending on the site and amount of bleeding. Five grades characterize a ruptured cerebral aneurysm:
◆ *Grade I: minimal bleeding* — The patient is alert with no neurologic deficit; he may have a slight headache and nuchal rigidity.
◆ *Grade II: mild bleeding* — The patient is alert, with a mild to severe headache and nuchal rigidity; he may have third-nerve palsy.
◆ *Grade III: moderate bleeding* — The patient is confused or drowsy, with nuchal rigidity and, possibly, a mild focal deficit.
◆ *Grade IV: severe bleeding* — The patient is stuporous, with nuchal rigidity and, possibly, mild to severe hemiparesis.
◆ *Grade V: moribund (commonly fatal)* — If the rupture is nonfatal, the patient is in a deep coma or decerebrate.

---

tophobia, and blurred vision, caused by bleeding into the meninges
- hemiparesis, hemisensory defects, dysphagia, and visual defects from bleeding into the brain tissues
- diplopia, ptosis, dilated pupil, and inability to rotate the eye caused by compression on the oculomotor nerve if the aneurysm is near the internal carotid artery.

Typically, the severity of a ruptured intracranial aneurysm is graded according to the patient's signs and symptoms. (See *Determining severity of an intracranial aneurysm rupture*.)

COMPLICATIONS
The major complications associated with cerebral aneurysm include:
- death from increased ICP and brain herniation
- rebleeding
- vasospasm.

DIAGNOSIS
- Cerebral angiography reveals altered cerebral blood flow, vessel lumen dilation, and differences in arterial filling.
- Computed tomography scan reveals subarachnoid or ventricular bleeding with blood in subarachnoid space and displaced midline structures.
- Magnetic resonance imaging shows a cerebral blood flow void.
- Skull X-rays may reveal calcified wall of the aneurysm and areas of bone erosion.

TREATMENT
Treatment to reduce the risk of rupture if it hasn't occurred may include:
- bed rest in a quiet, darkened room with minimal stimulation
- avoidance of coffee, other stimulants, and aspirin to reduce the risk of blood pressure elevation
- codeine or another analgesic as needed to maintain rest and minimize risk of pressure changes
- hydralazine or another antihypertensive agent, if the patient is hypertensive
- phenobarbital or another sedative to prevent agitation leading to hypertension.
Other treatment may include:
- surgical repair by clipping, ligation, or wrapping (before or after rupture)
- calcium channel blockers to decrease spasm and subsequent rebleeding
- corticosteroids to manage headache in subarachnoid hemorrhage
- phenytoin or another anticonvulsant to prevent or treat seizures caused by pressure and tissue irritation from bleeding
- aminocaproic acid, an inhibitor of fibrinolysis, to minimize the risk of rebleeding by delaying blood clot lysis (drug's effectiveness is under dispute).

Meningitis
In meningitis, the brain and the spinal cord meninges become inflamed, usually as a result of bacterial infection. Such inflammation may involve all three meningeal membranes — the dura mater, arachnoid, and pia mater.

If the disease is recognized early and the infecting organism responds to treatment, the prognosis is good and complications are rare. The prognosis is poorer for in-fants and elderly patients. Mortality in untreated meningitis is 70% to 100%.

CAUSES
Meningitis is almost always a complication of bacteremia, especially from:
- pneumonia
- empyema
- osteomyelitis
- endocarditis.
Other infections associated with the development of meningitis include:
- sinusitis
- otitis media
- encephalitis
- myelitis
- brain abscess, usually caused by *Neisseria meningitidis, Haemophilus influenzae, Streptococcus pneumoniae,* and *Escherichia coli.*
Meningitis may follow trauma or invasive procedures, including:
- skull fracture
- penetrating head wound
- lumbar puncture
- ventricular shunting.
Aseptic meningitis may result from a virus or other organism. Sometimes no causative organism can be found.

PATHOPHYSIOLOGY
Meningitis commonly begins as an inflammation of the pia-arachnoid, which may progress to congestion of adjacent tissues and destroy some nerve cells.

The microorganism typically enters the central nervous system by one of four routes:
- the blood (most common)
- a direct opening between the cerebrospinal fluid (CSF) and the environment as a result of trauma
- along the cranial and peripheral nerves
- through the mouth or nose.

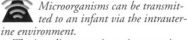

AGE ALERT
Microorganisms can be transmitted to an infant via the intrauterine environment.

The invading organism triggers an inflammatory response in the meninges. In an attempt to ward off the invasion, neutrophils gather in the area and produce an exudate in the subarachnoid space, causing the CSF to thicken. The thickened

CSF flows less readily around the brain and spinal cord, and it can block the arachnoid villi, obstructing flow of CSF and causing hydrocephalus.

The exudate also:
- worsens the inflammatory response, increasing the pressure in the brain
- can extend to the cranial and peripheral nerves, triggering additional inflammation
- irritates the meninges, disrupting their cell membranes and causing edema.

The consequences are elevated intracranial pressure (ICP), engorged blood vessels, disrupted cerebral blood supply, possible thrombosis or rupture and, if ICP isn't reduced, cerebral infarction. Encephalitis may also ensue as a secondary infection of the brain tissue.

In aseptic meningitis, lymphocytes infiltrate the pia-arachnoid layers, but usually not as severely as in bacterial meningitis, and no exudate is formed. Thus, this type of meningitis is self-limiting.

SIGNS AND SYMPTOMS

Signs of meningitis typically include:
- fever, chills, and malaise resulting from infection and inflammation
- headache, vomiting and, rarely, papilledema (inflammation and edema of the optic nerve) from increased ICP.

Signs of meningeal irritation include:
- nuchal rigidity
- positive Brudzinski's and Kernig's signs
- exaggerated and symmetrical deep tendon reflexes
- opisthotonos (a spasm in which the back and extremities arch backward so that the body rests on the head and heels).

Other features of meningitis may include:
- sinus arrhythmias from irritation of the nerves of the autonomic nervous system
- irritability from increasing ICP
- photophobia, diplopia, and other vision problems from cranial nerve irritation
- delirium, deep stupor, and coma from increased ICP and cerebral edema.

CLINICAL ALERT
Be especially alert for a temperature increase up to 102° F (38.8° C), deteriorating LOC, onset of seizures, and altered respirations, all of which may signal an impending crisis.

AGE ALERT
An infant may show signs of infection, but most infants are simply fretful and refuse to eat. In an infant, vomiting can lead to dehydration, which prevents formation of a bulging fontanelle, an important sign of increased ICP.

As the illness progresses, twitching, seizures (in 30% of infants), or coma may develop. Most older children have the same symptoms as adults. In subacute meningitis, onset may be insidious.

COMPLICATIONS

Complications may include:
- increased ICP
- hydrocephalus
- cerebral infarction
- cranial nerve deficits including optic neuritis and deafness
- encephalitis
- paresis or paralysis
- endocarditis
- brain abscess
- syndrome of inappropriate antidiuretic hormone
- seizures
- coma.

In children, additional complications may include:
- mental retardation
- epilepsy
- unilateral or bilateral sensory hearing loss
- subdural effusions.

DIAGNOSIS

- Lumbar puncture shows elevated CSF pressure (from obstructed CSF outflow at the arachnoid villi), cloudy or milky-white CSF, high protein level, positive Gram stain and culture (unless a virus is responsible), and decreased glucose level.
- Positive Brudzinski's and Kernig's signs indicate meningeal irritation.
- Cultures of blood, urine, and nose and throat secretions reveal the offending organism.
- Chest X-ray may reveal pneumonitis or lung abscess, tubercular lesions, or granulomas caused by a fungal infection
- Sinus and skull X-rays may identify cranial osteomyelitis or paranasal sinusitis as the underlying infectious process, or skull

fracture as the mechanism for entrance of microorganism.

■ White blood cell count reveals leukocytosis.

■ Computed tomography scan may reveal hydrocephalus or rule out cerebral hematoma, hemorrhage, or tumor as the underlying cause.

TREATMENT

Treatment may include:

■ appropriate I.V. antibiotics for at least 2 weeks, followed by oral antibiotics selected by culture and sensitivity testing (usual treatment)

■ digoxin, to control arrhythmias

■ mannitol to decrease cerebral edema

■ anticonvulsant (usually given I.V.) or a sedative to reduce restlessness and prevent or control seizure activity

■ aspirin or acetaminophen to relieve headache and fever.

Supportive measures include:

■ bed rest to prevent increases in ICP

■ fever reduction to prevent hyperthermia and increased metabolic demands that may increase ICP

■ fluid therapy (given cautiously if cerebral edema and increased ICP are present) to prevent dehydration

■ appropriate therapy for any coexisting conditions, such as endocarditis or pneumonia

■ possible prophylactic antibiotics after ventricular shunting procedures, skull fracture, or penetrating head wounds, to prevent infection (use is controversial).

CLINICAL ALERT
Use droplet precautions (in addition to standard precautions) for meningitis caused by H. influenzae *and* N. meningitidis, *until 24 hours after the start of effective therapy.*

Multiple sclerosis

Multiple sclerosis (MS) causes demyelination of the white matter of the brain and spinal cord and damage to nerve fibers and their targets. Characterized by exacerbations and remissions, MS is a major cause of chronic disability in young adults. It usually becomes symptomatic between ages 20 and 40 (the average age of onset is

27). A family history of MS and living in a cold, damp climate increase the risk.

CULTURAL DIVERSITY
MS affects three women for every two men and five whites for every nonwhite. Incidence is generally higher among urban populations and upper socioeconomic groups.

The prognosis varies. MS may progress rapidly, disabling the patient by early adulthood or causing death within months of onset, but 70% of patients lead active, productive lives with prolonged remissions.

Several types of MS have been identified. Terms to describe MS types include:

■ *relapsing-remitting* — clear relapses (or acute attacks or exacerbations) with full recovery or partial recovery and lasting disability (The disease doesn't worsen between the attacks.)

■ *primary progressive* — steady progression from the onset with minor recovery or plateaus (This form is uncommon and may involve different brain and spinal cord damage than other forms.)

■ *secondary progressive* — begins as a pattern of clear-cut relapses and recovery (This form becomes steadily progressive and worsens between acute attacks.)

■ *progressive relapsing* — steadily progressive from the onset, but also has acute attacks. (This form is rare.)

CAUSES

The exact cause of MS is unknown, but current theories suggest that a slow-acting or latent viral infection triggers an autoimmune response. Other theories suggest that environmental and genetic factors may also be linked to MS.

Certain conditions appear to precede onset or exacerbation, including:

■ emotional stress

■ fatigue (physical or emotional)

■ pregnancy

■ acute respiratory infections.

PATHOPHYSIOLOGY

In MS, sporadic patches of axon demyelination and nerve fiber loss occur throughout the central nervous system (CNS), inducing widely disseminated and varied

CLOSER LOOK
How myelin breaks down

Myelin speeds electrical impulses to the brain for interpretation. This lipoprotein complex formed of glial cells or oligodendrocytes protects the neuron's axon much like the insulation on an electrical wire. Its high electrical resistance and low capacitance allow the myelin to conduct nerve impulses from one node of Ranvier to the next.

Myelin is susceptible to injury — for example, by hypoxemia, toxic chemicals, vascular insufficiencies, or autoimmune responses. The sheath becomes inflamed, and the membrane layers break down into smaller components that become well-circumscribed plaques (filled with microglial elements, macroglia, and lymphocytes). This process is called *demyelination.*

The damaged myelin sheath can't conduct normally. The partial loss or dispersion of the action potential causes neurologic dysfunction.

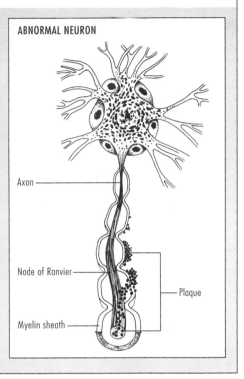

ABNORMAL NEURON

Axon

Node of Ranvier

Plaque

Myelin sheath

---

neurologic dysfunction. (See *How myelin breaks down.*)

New evidence of nerve fiber loss may provide an explanation for the invisible neurologic deficits experienced by many patients with MS. The axons determine the presence or absence of function; loss of myelin doesn't correlate with loss of function.

SIGNS AND SYMPTOMS
Signs and symptoms depend on the extent and site of myelin destruction, the extent of remyelination, and the adequacy of subsequent restored synaptic transmission. Flares may be transient, or they may last for hours or weeks, possibly waxing and waning with no predictable pattern, varying from day to day, and being bizarre and difficult for the patient to describe. Clinical effects may be so mild that the patient is unaware of them or so intense that they're debilitating.

Typical first signs and symptoms related to conduction deficits and impaired impulse transmission along the nerve fiber include:
- vision problems
- sensory impairment, such as burning, pins and needles, and electrical sensations
- fatigue.

Other characteristic changes include:
- *ocular disturbances* — optic neuritis, diplopia, ophthalmoplegia, blurred vision, and nystagmus from impaired cranial nerve dysfunction and conduction deficits to the optic nerve

■ *muscle dysfunction*—weakness, paralysis ranging from monoplegia to quadriplegia, spasticity, hyperreflexia, intention tremor, and gait ataxia from impaired motor reflex
■ *urinary disturbances*—incontinence, frequency, urgency, and frequent infections from impaired transmission involving sphincter innervation
■ *bowel disturbances*—involuntary evacuation or constipation from altered impulse transmission to internal sphincter
■ *fatigue*—commonly the most debilitating symptom
■ *speech problems*—poorly articulated or scanning speech and dysphagia from impaired transmission to the cranial nerves and sensory cortex.

COMPLICATIONS
Complications may include:
■ injuries from falls
■ urinary tract infection
■ constipation
■ joint contractures
■ pressure ulcers
■ rectal distention
■ pneumonia
■ depression.

DIAGNOSIS
Because early symptoms may be mild, years may elapse between onset and diagnosis. Diagnosis of this disorder requires evidence of two or more neurologic attacks. Periodic testing and close observation are necessary, perhaps for years, depending on the course of the disease. Spinal cord compression, foramen magnum tumor (which may mimic the exacerbations and remissions of MS), multiple small strokes, syphilis or another infection, thyroid disease, and chronic fatigue syndrome must be ruled out.

The following tests may be useful:
■ Magnetic resonance imaging reveals multifocal white matter lesions.
■ EEG reveals abnormalities in brain waves in one-third of patients.
■ Lumbar puncture shows normal total cerebrospinal fluid (CSF) protein but elevated immunoglobulin (Ig) G (gamma globulin); IgG reflects hyperactivity of the immune system caused by chronic demyelination. Elevated CSF IgG is significant only when serum IgG is normal. CSF white blood cell count may be elevated.
■ CSF electrophoresis detects bands of IgG in most patients, even when the percentage of IgG in CSF is normal. Presence of kappa light chains provide additional support to the diagnosis.
■ Evoked potential studies (visual, brain stem, auditory, and somatosensory) reveal slowed conduction of nerve impulses in most patients.

TREATMENT
The aim of treatment is threefold: Treat the acute exacerbation, treat the disease process, and treat the related signs and symptoms.
■ I.V. methylprednisolone followed by oral therapy reduces edema of the myelin sheath (speeds recovery from acute attacks). Other drugs, such as azathioprine or methotrexate and cyclophosphamide may be used.
■ Immune system therapy consisting of interferon and glatiramer (a combination of 4 amino acids) reduces frequency and severity of relapses, and may possibly slow CNS damage.
■ Stretching and range-of-motion exercises, coupled with correct positioning, may relieve the spasticity resulting from opposing muscle groups relaxing and contracting at the same time; helpful in relaxing muscles and maintaining function.
■ Baclofen and tizanidine may be used to treat spasticity. For severe spasticity, botulinum toxin injections, intrathecal injections, nerve blocks, and surgery may be necessary.
■ Frequent rest periods, aerobic exercise, and cooling techniques (air conditioning, breezes, water sprays) may minimize fatigue. Fatigue is characterized by an overwhelming feeling of exhaustion that can occur at any time of the day without warning. The cause is unknown. Changes in environmental conditions, such as heat and humidity, can aggravate fatigue.
■ Amantadine, pemoline, and methylphenidate have proven beneficial, as have antidepressants to manage fatigue.
■ Bladder problems (failure to store urine, failure to empty the bladder or, more commonly, both) are managed by such

strategies as drinking cranberry juice or insertion of an indwelling catheter and suprapubic tubes. Intermittent self-catheterization and postvoid catheterization programs are helpful, as are anticholinergic medications in some patients.

■ Bowel problems (constipation and involuntary evacuation) are managed by such measures as increasing fiber intake and using bulking agents, and bowel-training strategies, such as daily suppositories and rectal stimulation.

■ Low-dose tricyclic antidepressants, phenytoin, or carbamazepine may manage sensory symptoms, such as pain, numbness, burning, and tingling sensations.

■ Adaptive devices and physical therapy help with motor dysfunction, such as problems with balance, strength, and muscle coordination.

■ Beta-adrenergic blockers, sedatives, or diuretics may be used to alleviate tremors.

■ Speech therapy may manage dysarthria.

■ Antihistamines, vision therapy, or exercises may minimize vertigo.

■ Vision therapy or adaptive lenses may manage visual problems.

Myasthenia gravis

Myasthenia gravis causes sporadic but progressive weakness and abnormal fatigability of striated (skeletal) muscles; symptoms get worse with exercise and repeated movement and are relieved by anticholinesterase drugs. Usually, this disorder affects muscles innervated by the cranial nerves (face, lips, tongue, neck, and throat), but it can affect any muscle group.

Myasthenia gravis follows an unpredictable course of periodic exacerbations and remissions. There's no known cure. Drug treatment has improved the prognosis and allows patients to lead relatively normal lives, except during exacerbations. When the disease involves the respiratory system, it may be life threatening.

Myasthenia gravis affects 1 in 25,000 people at any age, but incidence peaks between ages 20 and 40. It's three times more common in women than in men in this age group, but after age 40 the incidence among women and men is similar.

About 20% of neonates born to mothers with myasthenia gravis have transient (or occasionally persistent) myasthenia. This disease may coexist with immune and thyroid disorders; 15% of patients with myasthenia gravis have thymomas. Remissions occur in about 25% of patients.

CAUSES
The exact cause of myasthenia gravis is unknown, but it's believed to be the result of:

■ autoimmune response
■ ineffective acetylcholine release
■ inadequate muscle fiber response to acetylcholine.

PATHOPHYSIOLOGY
Myasthenia gravis causes a failure in transmission of nerve impulses at the neuromuscular junction. The site of action is the postsynaptic membrane. Theoretically, antireceptor antibodies block, weaken, or reduce the number of acetylcholine receptors available at each neuromuscular junction and thereby impair muscle depolarization necessary for movement. (See *Impaired transmission in myasthenia gravis,* page 296.)

SIGNS AND SYMPTOMS
Myasthenia gravis may occur gradually or suddenly. Signs and symptoms include:

■ weak eye closure, ptosis, and diplopia from impaired neuromuscular transmission to the cranial nerves supplying the eye muscles (may be only symptom present)

■ skeletal muscle weakness and fatigue, increasing through the day but decreasing with rest (initially, easy fatigability of certain muscles may be only symptom; fatigability may later become severe enough to cause paralysis)

■ progressive muscle weakness and accompanying loss of function depending on muscle group affected; becoming more intense during menses and after emotional stress, prolonged exposure to sunlight or cold, or infections

■ blank and expressionless facial appearance and nasal vocal tones caused by impaired transmission of cranial nerves innervating the facial muscles

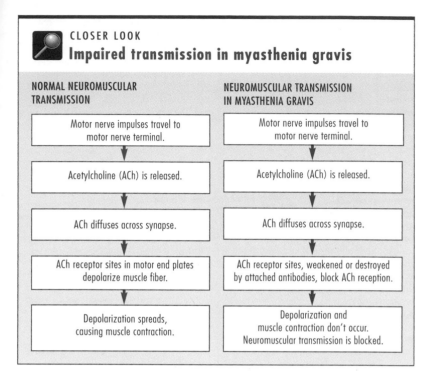

CLOSER LOOK
Impaired transmission in myasthenia gravis

NORMAL NEUROMUSCULAR TRANSMISSION

Motor nerve impulses travel to motor nerve terminal.

↓

Acetylcholine (ACh) is released.

↓

ACh diffuses across synapse.

↓

ACh receptor sites in motor end plates depolarize muscle fiber.

↓

Depolarization spreads, causing muscle contraction.

NEUROMUSCULAR TRANSMISSION IN MYASTHENIA GRAVIS

Motor nerve impulses travel to motor nerve terminal.

↓

Acetylcholine (ACh) is released.

↓

ACh diffuses across synapse.

↓

ACh receptor sites, weakened or destroyed by attached antibodies, block ACh reception.

↓

Depolarization and muscle contraction don't occur. Neuromuscular transmission is blocked.

- frequent nasal regurgitation of fluids and difficulty chewing and swallowing from cranial nerve involvement
- drooping eyelids from weakness of facial and extraocular muscles
- weakened neck muscles with head tilting back to see (neck muscles may become too weak to support the head without bobbing)
- weakened respiratory muscles, decreased tidal volume and vital capacity from impaired transmission to the diaphragm making breathing difficult and predisposing the patient to pneumonia and other respiratory tract infections
- respiratory muscle weakness (myasthenic crisis) possibly severe enough to require an emergency airway and mechanical ventilation.

COMPLICATIONS
Complications may include:
- respiratory distress
- pneumonia
- aspiration
- myasthenic crisis.

DIAGNOSIS
- Tensilon test confirms diagnosis of myasthenia gravis, revealing temporarily improved muscle function in 30 to 60 seconds after I.V. injection of edrophonium or neostigmine and lasting up to 30 minutes.
- Electromyography with repeated neural stimulation shows progressive decrease in muscle fiber contraction.
- Serum antiacetylcholine antibody titer may be elevated.
- Chest X-ray reveals thymoma (in about 15% of patients).

TREATMENT
Treatment may include:
- anticholinesterase drugs, such as neostigmine and pyridostigmine, to counteract fatigue and muscle weakness and allow about 80% of normal muscle function (drugs are less effective as disease worsens)
- immunosuppressant therapy with corticosteroids, azathioprine, cyclosporine, and cyclophosphamide used in a progressive fashion (when the previous drug response

is poor, the next one is used) to decrease the immune response toward acetylcholine receptors at the neuromuscular junction
- immunoglobulin G during acute relapses or plasmapheresis in severe exacerbations to suppress the immune system
- thymectomy to remove thymomas and possibly induce remission in some cases of adult-onset myasthenia
- tracheotomy, positive-pressure ventilation, and vigorous suctioning to remove secretions for treatment of acute exacerbations that cause severe respiratory distress
- discontinuation of anticholinesterase drugs in myasthenic crisis, until respiratory function improves — myasthenic crisis requires immediate hospitalization and vigorous respiratory support.

Parkinson's disease

Named for James Parkinson, the English physician who wrote the first accurate description of the disease in 1817, Parkinson's disease (also known as *shaking palsy*) characteristically produces progressive muscle rigidity, akinesia, and involuntary tremor. Deterioration is a progressive process. Death may result from complications, such as aspiration pneumonia or some other infection.

Parkinson's disease is one of the most common disabling diseases in the United States. It strikes 1 in every 100 people over age 60 and affects men more typically than women. Roughly, 60,000 new cases are diagnosed annually in the United States alone, and incidence is predicted to increase as the population ages.

CAUSES

The cause of Parkinson's disease is unknown, but study of the extrapyramidal brain nuclei (corpus striatum, globus pallidus, substantia nigra) has established the following:
- Dopamine deficiency prevents affected brain cells from performing their normal inhibitory function in the central nervous system.
- Some cases are caused by exposure to toxins, such as manganese dust or carbon monoxide.

PATHOPHYSIOLOGY

Parkinson's disease is a degenerative process involving the dopaminergic neurons in the substantia nigra (the area of the basal ganglia that produces and stores the neurotransmitter dopamine). This area plays an important role in the extrapyramidal system, which controls posture and coordination of voluntary motor movements.

Normally, stimulation of the basal ganglia results in refined motor movement because acetylcholine (excitatory) and dopamine (inhibitory) release are balanced. Degeneration of the dopaminergic neurons and loss of available dopamine leads to an excess of excitatory acetylcholine at the synapse and consequent rigidity, tremors, and bradykinesia.

Other nondopaminergic neurons may be affected, possibly contributing to depression and the other nonmotor symptoms of this disease. The basal ganglia are interconnected to the hypothalamus, potentially affecting autonomic and endocrine function as well.

Current research on the pathogenesis of Parkinson's disease focuses on damage to the substantia nigra from oxidative stress. Oxidative stress is believed to diminish brain iron content; impair mitochondrial function; inhibit antioxidant and protective systems; reduce glutathione secretion; and damage lipids, proteins, and deoxyribonucleic acid. Brain cells are less capable of repairing oxidative damage than are other tissues.

SIGNS AND SYMPTOMS

Signs and symptoms may include:
- muscle rigidity, akinesia, and an insidious tremor beginning in the fingers (unilateral "pill-roll" tremor) that increases during stress or anxiety and decreases with purposeful movement and sleep; caused by loss of inhibitory dopamine activity at the synapse
- muscle rigidity with resistance to passive muscle stretching, which may be uniform ("lead-pipe" rigidity) or jerky ("cogwheel" rigidity) caused by dopamine depletion
- akinesia causing difficulty walking (gait that lacks normal parallel motion and may

be retropulsive or propulsive) from impaired dopamine action
■ high-pitched, monotone voice caused by dopamine depletion
■ drooling caused by impaired regulation of motor function
■ masklike facial expression because of facial motor dysfunction caused by dopamine depletion
■ loss of posture control (the patient walks with body bent forward) from loss of motor control caused by dopamine depletion
■ dysarthria, dysphagia, or both
■ oculogyric crises (eyes are fixed upward, with involuntary tonic movements) or blepharospasm (eyelids are completely closed)
■ excessive sweating from impaired autonomic dysfunction
■ decreased motility of GI and genitourinary smooth muscle from impaired autonomic transmission
■ orthostatic hypotension from impaired vascular smooth muscle response
■ oily skin caused by inappropriate androgen production controlled by the hypothalamus pituitary axis.

COMPLICATIONS
Complications may include:
■ injury from falls
■ aspiration
■ urinary tract infections
■ pressure ulcers.

DIAGNOSIS
Diagnostic tests are usually of little value in identifying Parkinson's disease. Diagnosis is based on the patient's age and history and on the characteristic signs and symptoms. Urinalysis may support the diagnosis by revealing decreased dopamine levels.

A conclusive diagnosis is possible only after ruling out other causes of tremor, involutional depression, cerebral arteriosclerosis, and, in patients under age 30, intracranial tumors, Wilson's disease, or phenothiazine or other drug toxicity.

TREATMENT
The aim of treatment is to relieve symptoms and keep the patient functional as long as possible. Treatment includes:
■ levodopa, a dopamine replacement most effective during early stages and given in increasing doses until symptoms are relieved or side effects appear. (Because adverse effects can be serious, levodopa is usually given in combination with carbidopa to halt peripheral dopamine synthesis.) Dopamine agonists may be used early in the disease or in combination with levodopa to enhance response or decrease adverse effects. (Such agents include pramipexole, ropinirole, pergolide, and bromocriptine.)
■ alternative drug therapy, including anticholinergics such as trihexyphenidyl; antihistamines such as diphenhydramine; and amantadine, an antiviral agent, or selegiline, an enzyme-inhibiting agent, when levodopa is ineffective, to conserve dopamine and enhance the therapeutic effect of levodopa.
■ stereotactic neurosurgery (to prevent involuntary movement), which is most effective in young, otherwise healthy persons with unilateral tremor or muscle rigidity, when drug therapy fails, to destroy the ventrolateral nucleus of the thalamus (used only to relieve symptoms, not cure the disease); deep brain stimulation, an alternative for patients in whom conventional treatment fails, in which neurostimulator and electrodes are implanted that stimulate the globus pallidus subthalamic nucleus to decrease tremors and allow normal function; or fetal cell transplantation (controversial), in which fetal brain tissue is injected into the patient's brain, in the hope that injected cells will grow, allowing the brain to process dopamine, thereby halting or reducing the disease progression.
■ physical therapy, as adjunct to drugs and neurosurgery maintain normal muscle tone and function; including active and passive range-of-motion exercises, routine daily activities, walking, and baths and massage to help relax muscles.

Reye's syndrome
Reye's syndrome is an acute childhood illness that causes fatty infiltration of the liver, with concurrent hyperammonemia, encephalopathy, and increased intracranial pressure (ICP). In addition, fatty infiltration of the kidneys, brain, and myocardium may occur. Reye's syndrome affects

children from infancy to adolescence and occurs equally in boys and girls.

Prognosis depends on the severity of central nervous system (CNS) depression. Until recently, mortality was as high as 90%. Today, ICP monitoring and, consequently, early treatment of increased ICP, along with other treatment measures, have reduced mortality to about 20%. Death is usually a result of cerebral edema or respiratory arrest. Comatose patients who survive may have residual brain damage.

Incidence commonly rises during influenza outbreaks and may be linked to aspirin use. For this reason, use of aspirin for children under age 15 isn't recommended.

CAUSES

Reye's syndrome typically begins in 1 to 3 days of an acute viral infection, such as an upper respiratory tract infection, type B influenza, or varicella (chickenpox).

PATHOPHYSIOLOGY

In Reye's syndrome, damaged hepatic mitochondria disrupt the urea cycle, which normally changes ammonia to urea for its excretion from the body. This disruption results in hyperammonemia, hypoglycemia (in 15% of cases), and an increase in short-chain fatty acids, leading to encephalopathy. Simultaneously, fatty infiltration occurs in renal tubular cells, neuronal tissue, and muscle tissue, including the heart.

SIGNS AND SYMPTOMS

The severity of a child's signs and symptoms varies with the degree of encephalopathy and cerebral edema. In any case, Reye's syndrome develops in five stages. After the initial viral infection, a brief recovery period follows when the child doesn't seem seriously ill. A few days later, he develops intractable vomiting; lethargy; rapidly changing mental status (mild to severe agitation, confusion, irritability, and delirium); rising blood pressure, respiratory rate, and pulse rate; and hyperactive reflexes.

Reye's syndrome commonly progresses to coma. As coma deepens, seizures develop, followed by decreased tendon reflexes and, usually, respiratory failure.

COMPLICATIONS

Increased ICP, a serious complication, is now considered the result of an increased cerebral blood volume causing intracranial hypertension. The increased ICP may develop as a result of acidosis, increased cerebral metabolic rate, and an impaired autoregulatory mechanism. Other complications may include respiratory failure and death.

DIAGNOSIS

A history of a recent viral disorder with typical features strongly suggests Reye's syndrome. An increased serum ammonia level, abnormal results in clotting studies, and hepatic dysfunction confirm it. Testing serum salicylate levels rules out aspirin use. Absence of jaundice, despite increased liver aminotransferase levels, rules out acute hepatic failure and hepatic encephalopathy.

Abnormal test results may include:

■ *liver function studies* — aspartate aminotransferase and alanine aminotransferase levels are elevated to twice normal levels; bilirubin level is usually normal

■ *liver biopsy* — fatty droplets are uniformly distributed throughout cells

■ *cerebrospinal fluid (CSF) analysis* — white blood cell count is less than 10/µl; with coma, increased CSF pressure.

■ *coagulation studies* — prolonged prothrombin time and partial thromboplastin time

■ *blood values* — elevated serum ammonia levels; normal or low (in 15% of cases) serum glucose levels; increased serum fatty acid and lactate levels.

TREATMENT

For treatment guidelines, see *Stages of treatment for Reye's syndrome,* pages 300 and 301.

Seizure disorder

Seizure disorder, or epilepsy, is a condition of the brain characterized by susceptibility to recurrent seizures (paroxysmal events associated with abnormal electrical discharges of neurons in the brain). Primary seizure disorder or epilepsy is idiopathic without apparent structural changes in the brain. Secondary epilepsy, characterized by structural changes or metabolic alterations

Stages of treatment for Reye's syndrome

SIGNS AND SYMPTOMS	BASELINE TREATMENT	BASELINE INTERVENTION
STAGE I		
Vomiting, lethargy, hepatic dysfunction	◆ To decrease intracranial pressure (ICP) and brain edema, give I.V. fluids at ⅔ maintenance level. Also give an osmotic diuretic or furosemide. ◆ To treat hypoprothrombinemia, give vitamin K; if vitamin K is unsuccessful, give fresh frozen plasma. ◆ Monitor serum ammonia and blood glucose levels and plasma osmolality every 4 to 8 hours to check progress.	◆ Monitor vital signs and check level of consciousness for increasing lethargy. Take vital signs more often as the patient's condition deteriorates. ◆ Monitor fluid intake and output to prevent fluid overload. Maintain urine output at 1 ml/kg per hour; plasma osmolality, 290 mOsm; and blood glucose, 150 mg/ml. (Goal: Keep glucose level high, osmolality normal to high, and ammonia level low.) Also, restrict protein.
STAGE II		
Hyperventilation, delirium, hepatic dysfunction, hyperactive reflexes	◆ Continue baseline treatment from stage I.	◆ Maintain seizure precautions. ◆ Immediately report any signs of coma that require invasive, supportive therapy, such as intubation. ◆ Keep head of bed at 30-degree angle.
STAGE III		
Coma, hyperventilation, decorticate rigidity, hepatic dysfunction	◆ Continue baseline treatment from stage I. ◆ Monitor ICP with a subarachnoid screw or other invasive device; treat seizures. ◆ Provide endotracheal intubation and mechanical ventilation to control partial pressure of arterial carbon dioxide ($Paco_2$) levels. A paralyzing agent, such as atracurium or pancuronium I.V., may help maintain ventilation. ◆ Give mannitol I.V. or glycerol by nasogastric tube.	◆ Monitor ICP (should be < 20 mm Hg before suctioning) or give a barbiturate I.V., as ordered; hyperventilate the patient as necessary. ◆ When ventilating the patient, maintain $Paco_2$ between 25 and 30 mm Hg and partial pressure of arterial oxygen between 80 and 100 mm Hg. ◆ Closely monitor cardiovascular status with a pulmonary artery catheter or central venous pressure line. ◆ Give good skin and mouth care and range-of-motion exercises.

Stages of treatment for Reye's syndrome (continued)

SIGNS AND SYMPTOMS	BASELINE TREATMENT	BASELINE INTERVENTION
STAGE IV		
Deepening coma; decerebrate rigidity; large, fixed pupils; minimal hepatic function	◆ Continue baseline treatment from stage I and supportive care. ◆ If all previous measures fail, some pediatric centers use barbiturate coma, decompressive craniotomy, hypothermia, or exchange transfusion.	◆ Check patient for loss of reflexes and signs of flaccidity. ◆ Give the family the extra support they need, considering their child's poor prognosis.
STAGE V		
Seizures, loss of deep tendon reflexes, flaccidity, respiratory arrest, ammonia level above 300 mg/dl	◆ Continue baseline treatment from stage I and supportive care.	◆ Help the family to face the patient's impending death.

of the neuronal membranes, causes increased automaticity.

About 2.5 million people in the United States have epilepsy. The incidence is highest in childhood and among elderly people. The prognosis is good if a person adheres strictly to prescribed treatment.

CAUSES

About one-half of all seizure disorder cases are idiopathic; possible causes of other cases include:

- birth trauma (inadequate oxygen supply to the brain, blood incompatibility between mother and fetus, neonatal hemorrhage, or maternal hemorrhage during delivery)
- perinatal infection
- anoxia
- infectious diseases (meningitis, encephalitis, or brain abscess)
- ingestion of toxins (mercury or lead) or exposure to carbon monoxide
- brain tumors
- inherited disorders or degenerative disease, such as phenylketonuria or tuberous sclerosis

- head injury or trauma
- metabolic disorders, such as hypoglycemia and hypoparathyroidism
- stroke (hemorrhage, thrombosis, or embolism).

PATHOPHYSIOLOGY

Some neurons in the brain may depolarize easily or be hyperexcitable; this epileptogenic focus fires more readily than normal when stimulated. In these neurons, the membrane potential at rest is less negative or inhibitory connections are missing, possibly as a result of decreased gamma-aminobutyric acid activity or localized shifts in electrolytes.

On stimulation, the epileptogenic focus fires and spreads electrical current to surrounding cells. These cells fire in turn and the impulse cascades to one side of the brain (a partial seizure), both sides of the brain (a generalized seizure), or cortical, subcortical, and brain stem areas.

The brain's metabolic demand for oxygen increases dramatically during a seizure. If this demand isn't met, hypoxia and brain damage ensue. Firing of inhibitory

Types of seizures

The various types of seizures — partial, generalized, status epilepticus, and unclassified — have distinct signs and symptoms.

PARTIAL SEIZURES

Arising from a localized area of the brain, partial seizures cause focal symptoms. These seizures are classified by their effect on consciousness and whether they spread throughout the motor pathway, causing a generalized seizure.

◆ A *simple partial seizure* begins locally and generally doesn't cause an alteration in consciousness. It may cause sensory symptoms (lights flashing, smells, auditory hallucinations), autonomic symptoms (sweating, flushing, pupil dilation), and psychic symptoms (dream states, anger, fear). The seizure lasts for a few seconds and occurs without preceding or provoking events. This type can be motor or sensory.

◆ A *complex partial seizure* alters consciousness. Amnesia for events that occur during and immediately after the seizure is a differentiating characteristic. During the seizure, the patient may follow simple commands. This seizure generally lasts for 1 to 3 minutes.

GENERALIZED SEIZURES

As the term suggests, generalized seizures cause a generalized electrical abnormality within the brain. They can be convulsive or nonconvulsive and include several types:

◆ *Absence seizures* occur most commonly in children, although they may affect adults. They usually begin with a brief change in level of consciousness, indicated by blinking or rolling of the eyes, a blank stare, and slight mouth movements. The patient retains his posture and continues preseizure activity without difficulty. Typically, each seizure lasts from 1 to 10 seconds. If not properly treated, seizures can recur as often as 100 times per day. An absence seizure is a nonconvulsive seizure, but it may progress to a generalized tonic-clonic seizure.

◆ *Myoclonic seizures* (bilateral massive epileptic myoclonus) are brief, involuntary muscular jerks of the body or extremities, which may be rhythmic. Consciousness isn't usually affected.

◆ *Generalized tonic-clonic seizures* typically begin with a loud cry, precipitated by air rushing from the lungs through the vocal cords. The patient then loses consciousness and falls to the ground. The body stiffens (tonic phase) and then alternates between episodes of muscle spasm and relaxation (clonic phase). Tongue biting, incontinence, labored breathing, apnea, and subsequent cyanosis may occur. The seizure stops in 2 to 5 minutes, when abnormal electrical conduction ceases. When the patient regains consciousness, he's confused and may have difficulty talking. If he can talk, he may complain of drowsiness, fatigue, headache, muscle soreness, and arm or leg weakness. He may fall into a deep sleep after the seizure.

◆ *Atonic seizures* are characterized by a general loss of postural tone and a temporary loss of consciousness. They occur in young children and are sometimes called "drop attacks" because they cause the child to fall.

STATUS EPILEPTICUS

Status epilepticus is a continuous seizure state that can occur in all seizure types. The most life-threatening example is generalized tonic-clonic status epilepticus, a continuous generalized tonic-clonic seizure. Status epilepticus is accompanied by respiratory distress leading to hypoxia or anoxia. It can result from abrupt withdrawal of anticonvulsant medications, hypoxic encephalopathy, acute head trauma, metabolic encephalopathy, or septicemia secondary to encephalitis or meningitis.

UNCLASSIFIED SEIZURES

This category is reserved for seizures that don't fit the characteristics of partial or generalized seizures or status epilepticus. Included as unclassified are events that lack the data to make a more definitive diagnosis.

neurons causes the excitatory neurons to slow their firing and eventually stop. If this inhibitory action doesn't occur, the result is status epilepticus: one seizure occurring right after another and another; without treatment the anoxia is fatal.

SIGNS AND SYMPTOMS
The hallmark of epilepsy is recurring seizures, which can be classified as partial, generalized, status epilepticus, or unclassified (some patients may be affected by more than one type). (See *Types of seizures*.)

COMPLICATIONS
Complications may include:
- hypoxia or anoxia from airway occlusion
- traumatic injury
- brain damage
- depression and anxiety.

DIAGNOSIS
Clinically, the diagnosis of epilepsy is based on the occurrence of one or more seizures and proof or the assumption that the condition that caused them is still present. Diagnostic tests that help support the findings include:
- Computed tomography scan or magnetic resonance imaging reveal abnormalities.
- EEG reveals paroxysmal abnormalities to confirm the diagnosis and provide evidence of the continuing tendency to have seizures. In tonic-clonic seizures, high, fast voltage spikes are present in all leads; in absence seizures, rounded spike wave complexes are diagnostic. A negative EEG doesn't rule out epilepsy because the abnormalities occur intermittently.
- Skull X-ray may show evidence of fractures or shifting of the pineal gland, bony erosion, or separated sutures.
- Serum chemistry blood studies may reveal hypoglycemia, electrolyte imbalances, elevated liver enzymes, and elevated alcohol levels, providing clues to underlying conditions that increase the risk of seizure activity.

TREATMENT
Treatment may include:

- drug therapy specific to the type of seizure, including phenytoin, carbamazepine, phenobarbital, gabapentin, and primidone for generalized tonic-clonic seizures and complex partial seizures — I.V. fosphenytoin is an alternative to phenytoin and is just as effective, with a long half-life and minimal central nervous system depression (stable for 120 days at room temperature and compatible with many frequently used I.V. solutions; can be administered rapidly without the adverse cardiovascular effects that occur with phenytoin)
- valproic acid, clonazepam, and ethosuximide for absence seizures
- gabapentin and felbamate as other anticonvulsants
- surgical removal of a demonstrated focal lesion, if drug therapy is ineffective
- surgery to remove the underlying cause, such as a tumor, abscess, or vascular problem
- vagus nerve stimulator implant to possibly help reduce the incidence of focal seizure
- I.V. diazepam, lorazepam, phenytoin, or phenobarbital for status epilepticus
- administration of dextrose (when seizures are caused by hypoglycemia) or thiamine (in chronic alcoholism or withdrawal).

Spinal cord trauma
Spinal injuries include fractures, contusions, and compressions of the vertebral column, usually as the result of trauma to the head or neck. The real danger lies in spinal cord damage — cutting, pulling, twisting, or compressing. Damage may involve the entire cord or be restricted to one half, and it can occur at any level. Fractures of the fifth, sixth, or seventh cervical, twelfth thoracic, and first lumbar vertebrae are most common.

CAUSES
The most serious spinal cord traumas typically result from:
- automobile accidents
- falls
- sports injuries
- diving into shallow water
- gunshot or stab wounds.

Types of spinal cord injury

Injury to the spinal cord can be classified as complete or incomplete. An incomplete spinal injury may be a central cord syndrome, an anterior cord syndrome, or Brown-Sequard syndrome, depending on the area of the cord affected. This table highlights the characteristic signs and symptoms of each.

TYPE	DESCRIPTION	SIGNS AND SYMPTOMS
Complete transection	◆ All tracts of the spinal cord completely disrupted ◆ All functions involving the spinal cord below the level of transection lost ◆ Complete and permanent loss	◆ Loss of motor function: quadriplegia in cervical cord transection; paraplegia in thoracic cord transection ◆ Muscle flaccidity ◆ Loss of all reflexes and sensory function below level of injury ◆ Bladder and bowel atony ◆ Paralytic ileus ◆ Loss of vasomotor tone in lower body parts with low and unstable blood pressure ◆ Loss of perspiration below level of injury ◆ Dry, pale skin ◆ Respiratory impairment
Incomplete transection: Central cord syndrome	◆ Center portion of cord affected ◆ Typically from hyperextension injury	◆ Motor deficits greater in upper than in lower extremities ◆ Variable degree of bladder dysfunction
Incomplete transection: Anterior cord syndrome	◆ Occlusion of anterior spinal artery ◆ Occlusion from pressure of bone fragments	◆ Loss of motor function below level of injury ◆ Loss of pain and temperature sensations below level of injury ◆ Intact touch, pressure, position, and vibration senses
Incomplete transection: Brown-Sequard syndrome	◆ Hemisection of cord affected ◆ Most common in stab and gunshot wounds ◆ Damage to cord on only one side	◆ Ipsilateral paralysis or paresis below level of injury ◆ Ipsilateral loss of touch, pressure, vibration, and position senses below level of injury ◆ Contralateral loss of pain and temperature sensations below level of injury

Less serious injuries commonly occur from:
- lifting heavy objects
- minor falls.

PATHOPHYSIOLOGY

Like head trauma, spinal cord trauma results from acceleration, deceleration, or other deforming forces usually applied from a distance. Mechanisms involved with spinal cord trauma include:
- hyperextension from acceleration-deceleration forces and sudden reduction in the anteroposterior diameter of the spinal cord
- hyperflexion from sudden and excessive force, propelling the neck forward or causing an exaggerated movement to one side

- vertical compression from force being applied from the top of the cranium along the vertical axis through the vertebra
- rotational forces from twisting, which adds shearing forces.

Injury causes microscopic hemorrhages in the gray matter and pia-arachnoid. The hemorrhages gradually increase in size until all of the gray matter is filled with blood, which causes necrosis. From the gray matter, the blood enters the white matter, where it impedes the circulation within the spinal cord. Ensuing edema causes compression and decreases the blood supply. Thus, the spinal cord loses perfusion and becomes ischemic. The edema and hemorrhage are greatest at and about two segments above and below the injury. The edema temporarily adds to the patient's dysfunction by increasing pressure and compressing the nerves. Edema near the third to fifth cervical vertebrae may interfere with phrenic nerve impulse transmission to the diaphragm and inhibit respiratory function.

In the white matter, circulation usually returns to normal in about 24 hours, but in the gray matter, an inflammatory reaction prevents restoration of circulation. Phagocytes appear at the site within 36 to 48 hours after the injury. Macrophages engulf degenerating axons, and collagen replaces the normal tissue. Scarring and meningeal thickening leaves the nerves in the area blocked or tangled.

SIGNS AND SYMPTOMS

- Muscle spasm and back pain that worsens with movement. In cervical fractures, pain may cause point tenderness; in thoracic and lumbar fractures, it may radiate to other body areas such as the legs.
- Mild paresthesia to quadriplegia and shock, if the injury damages the spinal cord. In milder injury, such symptoms may be delayed several days or weeks. Specific signs and symptoms depend on injury type and degree. (See *Types of spinal cord injury.*)

COMPLICATIONS

Complications include:
- autonomic dysreflexia

- spinal shock
- neurogenic shock. (See *Complications of spinal cord injury,* page 306.)

DIAGNOSIS

- Spinal X-rays, the most important diagnostic measure, detect spinal fracture.
- Thorough neurologic evaluation locates the level of injury and detects cord damage.
- Lumbar puncture may show increased cerebrospinal fluid pressure from a lesion or trauma in cases of spinal compression.
- Computed tomography scan or magnetic resonance imaging reveals spinal cord edema and compression and may reveal a spinal mass.

TREATMENT

Treatment may include:
- immediate immobilization to stabilize the spine and prevent cord damage (primary treatment); use of sandbags on both sides of the patient's head, a hard cervical collar, or skeletal traction with skull tongs or a halo device for cervical spine injuries
- high doses of methylprednisolone to reduce inflammation with evidence of cord injury
- bed rest on firm support (such as a bed board), analgesics, and muscle relaxants for treatment of stable lumbar and thoracic fractures for several days until the fracture stabilizes
- plaster cast or a turning frame to treat unstable thoracic or lumbar fracture
- laminectomy and spinal fusion for severe lumbar fractures
- neurosurgery to relieve the pressure when the damage results in compression of the spinal column — if the cause of compression is a metastatic lesion, chemotherapy and radiation may relieve it
- treatment of surface wounds accompanying the spinal injury; tetanus prophylaxis unless the patient has had recent immunization
- exercises to strengthen the back muscles and a back brace or corset to provide support while walking
- rehabilitation to maintain or improve functional level.

Complications of spinal cord injury

Of the following three sets of complications, only autonomic dysreflexia requires emergency attention.

AUTONOMIC DYSREFLEXIA

Also known as *autonomic hyperreflexia*, autonomic dysreflexia is a serious medical condition that occurs after resolution of spinal shock. Emergency recognition and management is essential.

Autonomic dysreflexia should be suspected in the patient with:
◆ spinal cord trauma at or above level T6
◆ bradycardia
◆ hypertension and a severe pounding headache
◆ cold or goose-fleshed skin below the lesion.

Autonomic dysreflexia is an exaggerated autonomic response to noxious stimuli, most commonly a distended bladder or skin lesion. Treatment focuses on eliminating the stimulus; rapid identification and removal may avoid the need for pharmacologic control of the headache and hypertension.

SPINAL SHOCK

Spinal shock is the loss of autonomic, reflex, motor, and sensory activity below the level of the cord lesion. It occurs because of damage to the spinal cord.

Signs of spinal shock include:
◆ flaccid paralysis
◆ loss of deep tendon and perianal reflexes
◆ loss of motor and sensory function.

Until spinal shock has resolved (usually 1 to 6 weeks after injury), the extent of actual cord damage can't be assessed. The earliest indicator of resolution is the return of reflex activity.

NEUROGENIC SHOCK

Neurogenic shock is an abnormal vasomotor response that occurs because of disruption of sympathetic impulses from the brain stem to the thoracolumbar area and is seen most commonly in patients with cervical cord injury. This temporary loss of autonomic function below the level of injury causes cardiovascular changes.

Signs of neurogenic shock include:
◆ orthostatic hypotension
◆ bradycardia
◆ loss of the ability to sweat below the level of the lesion.

Treatment is symptomatic. Symptoms resolve when spinal cord edema resolves.

Stroke

A stroke, also known as a *cerebrovascular accident* or *brain attack,* is a sudden impairment of cerebral circulation in one or more blood vessels. A stroke interrupts or lessens the oxygen supply and commonly causes serious damage or necrosis in the brain tissues. The sooner the circulation returns to normal after a stroke, the better the chances are for a complete recovery. About one-half of the patients who survive a stroke remain permanently disabled and experience a recurrence within weeks, months, or years. It's the leading cause of admission to long-term care.

Stroke is the third most common cause of death in the United States and the most common cause of neurologic disability. It strikes more than 500,000 people per year and is fatal in about one-half of these people.

 AGE ALERT
Although strokes may occur in younger persons, most patients experiencing strokes are over age 65. In fact, the risk of stroke doubles with each passing decade after age 55.

CULTURAL DIVERSITY
The incidence of stroke is higher in Blacks than in Whites. In fact, Blacks have a 60% higher risk of stroke than Whites or Hispanics of the same age. This higher risk is believed to be the result of an increased prevalence of hypertension in Blacks. In addition, strokes in Blacks usually result from disease in the small cerebral vessels, whereas strokes in Whites are typically the result of disease in the

Types of stroke

Strokes are typically classified as ischemic or hemorrhagic depending on the underlying cause. This table describes the major types of stroke.

TYPE OF STROKE	DESCRIPTION
Ischemic: Thrombotic	◆ Most common cause of stroke ◆ Frequently the result of atherosclerosis; also associated with hypertension, smoking, diabetes ◆ Thrombus in extracranial or intracranial vessel blocks blood flow to the cerebral cortex ◆ Carotid artery most commonly affected extracranial vessel ◆ Common intracranial sites include bifurcation of the carotid arteries, distal intracranial portion of vertebral arteries, and proximal basilar arteries ◆ May occur during sleep or shortly after awakening, during surgery, or after a myocardial infarction
Ischemic: Embolic	◆ Second most common type of stroke ◆ Embolus from heart or extracranial arteries floats into cerebral bloodstream and lodges in middle cerebral artery or one of its branches ◆ Embolus commonly originates during atrial fibrillation ◆ Typically occurs during activity ◆ Develops rapidly
Ischemic: Lacunar	◆ Subtype of thrombotic stroke ◆ Hypertension creates cavities deep in white matter of the brain, affecting the internal capsule, basal ganglia, thalamus, and pons ◆ Lipid coating lining the small penetrating arteries thickens and weakens wall, causing microaneurysms and dissections
Hemorrhagic	◆ Third most common type of stroke ◆ Typically caused by hypertension or rupture of aneurysm ◆ Diminished blood supply to area supplied by ruptured artery and compression by accumulated blood

large carotid arteries. Mortality for Blacks from stroke is twice the rate for Whites.

CAUSES

Stroke typically results from one of three causes:

■ thrombosis of the cerebral arteries supplying the brain or of the intracranial vessels, occluding blood flow (see *Types of stroke*)

■ embolism from thrombus outside the brain, such as in the heart, aorta, or common carotid artery

■ hemorrhage from an intracranial artery or vein, such as from hypertension, ruptured aneurysm, arteriovenous malformations, trauma, hemorrhagic disorder, or septic embolism.

Risk factors that have been identified as predisposing a patient to stroke include:

■ hypertension

■ family history of stroke

■ history of transient ischemic attacks (TIAs) (see *Understanding TIAs,* page 308)

■ cardiac disease, including arrhythmias, coronary artery disease, acute myocardial

Understanding TIAs

A transient ischemic attack (TIA) is an episode of neurologic deficit resulting from cerebral ischemia. The attack may last from seconds to an hour and commonly recurs. It's usually considered a warning sign for stroke. In 14% of patients who experience a TIA, another TIA or a full stroke will occur within 1 year.

In a TIA, microemboli released from a thrombus may temporarily interrupt blood flow, especially in the small distal branches of the brain's arterial tree. Small spasms in those arterioles may impair blood flow and also precede a TIA.

The most distinctive features of TIAs are transient focal deficits with complete return of function. The deficits usually involve some degree of motor or sensory dysfunction. They may range to loss of consciousness and loss of motor or sensory function, but only for a brief time. Commonly the patient experiences weakness in the lower part of the face and arms, hands, fingers, and legs on the side opposite the affected region. Other characteristics may include transient dysphagia, numbness or tingling of the face and lips, double vision, slurred speech, and dizziness.

bral blood flow remains impaired for more than a few minutes, oxygen deprivation leads to infarction of brain tissue. The brain cells cease to function because they can neither store glucose or glycogen for use nor engage in anaerobic metabolism.

A thrombotic or embolic stroke causes ischemia. Some of the neurons served by the occluded vessel die from lack of oxygen and nutrients. This results in cerebral infarction, in which tissue injury triggers an inflammatory response that in turn increases intracranial pressure (ICP). Injury to the surrounding cells disrupts metabolism and leads to changes in ionic transport, localized acidosis, and free radical formation. Calcium, sodium, and water accumulate in the injured cells, and excitatory neurotransmitters are released. Consequent continued cellular injury and swelling set up a vicious cycle of further damage.

When hemorrhage is the cause, impaired cerebral perfusion causes infarction, and the blood itself acts as a space-occupying mass, exerting pressure on the brain tissues. The brain's regulatory mechanisms attempt to maintain equilibrium by increasing blood pressure to maintain cerebral perfusion pressure. The increased ICP forces cerebrospinal fluid (CSF) out, thus restoring the balance. If the hemorrhage is small, this may be enough to keep the patient alive with only minimal neurologic deficits. If the bleeding is heavy, ICP increases rapidly and perfusion stops. Even if the pressure returns to normal, many brain cells die.

Initially, the ruptured cerebral blood vessels may constrict to limit the blood loss. This vasospasm further compromises blood flow, leading to more ischemia and cellular damage. If a clot forms in the vessel, decreased blood flow also promotes ischemia. If the blood enters the subarachnoid space, meningeal irritation occurs. The blood cells that pass through the vessel wall into the surrounding tissue also may break down and block the arachnoid villi, causing hydrocephalus.

infarction, dilated cardiomyopathy, and valvular disease
- diabetes
- familial hyperlipidemia
- cigarette smoking
- increased alcohol intake
- obesity, sedentary lifestyle
- use of hormonal contraceptives.

PATHOPHYSIOLOGY
Regardless of the cause, the underlying event is deprivation of oxygen and nutrients. Normally, if the arteries become blocked, autoregulatory mechanisms help maintain cerebral circulation until collateral circulation develops to deliver blood to the affected area. If the compensatory mechanisms become overworked or cere-

SIGNS AND SYMPTOMS
The features of stroke vary according to the affected artery and the region of the

brain it supplies, the severity of the damage, and the extent of collateral circulation developed. A stroke in one hemisphere causes signs and symptoms on the opposite side of the body; a stroke that damages cranial nerves affects structures on the same side as the infarction.

General symptoms of a stroke reflect the underlying neurologic dysfunction and include:

- unilateral limb weakness
- speech difficulties
- unilateral numbness
- headache
- vision disturbances (diplopia, hemianopsia, ptosis)
- dizziness
- anxiety
- altered level of consciousness (LOC).

Symptoms are usually classified by the artery affected. Signs and symptoms of middle cerebral artery involvement include:

- aphasia
- dysphasia
- visual field deficits
- hemiparesis of affected side (more severe in the face and arm than in the leg).

Symptoms of carotid artery involvement include:

- weakness
- paralysis
- numbness
- sensory changes
- vision disturbances on the affected side
- altered LOC
- bruits
- headache
- aphasia
- ptosis.

Symptoms of vertebrobasilar artery involvement include:

- weakness on the affected side
- numbness around lips and mouth
- visual field deficits
- diplopia
- poor coordination
- dysphagia
- slurred speech
- dizziness
- nystagmus
- amnesia
- ataxia.

Signs and symptoms of anterior cerebral artery involvement include:

- confusion
- weakness
- numbness, especially in the legs on the affected side
- incontinence
- loss of coordination
- impaired motor and sensory functions
- personality changes.

Signs and symptoms of posterior cerebral artery involvement include:

- visual field deficits (homonymous hemianopsia)
- sensory impairment
- dyslexia
- perseveration (abnormally persistent replies to questions)
- coma
- cortical blindness
- absence of paralysis (usually).

COMPLICATIONS

Complications vary with the severity and type of stroke, but may include:

- unstable blood pressure (from loss of vasomotor control)
- cerebral edema
- fluid imbalances
- sensory impairment
- infections such as pneumonia
- altered LOC
- aspiration
- contractures
- pulmonary embolism
- death.

DIAGNOSIS

- Computed tomography (CT) scan identifies an ischemic stroke within the first 72 hours of onset of symptoms and identifies evidence of a hemorrhagic stroke (lesions larger than 1 cm) immediately.
- Magnetic resonance imaging helps identify areas of ischemia or infarction and cerebral swelling.
- Cerebral angiography reveals disruption or displacement of the cerebral circulation by occlusion, such as stenosis or acute thrombus, or hemorrhage.
- Digital subtraction angiography shows evidence of occlusion of cerebral vessels, lesions, or vascular abnormalities.

DISRUPTING DISEASE
Treating ischemic stroke

In an ischemic stroke, a thrombus occludes a cerebral vessel or one of its branches and blocks blood flow to the brain. This flowchart shows how these drugs disrupt an ischemic stroke, thus minimizing the effects of cerebral ischemia and infarction. Keep in mind that thrombolytic agents should be used within 3 hours after onset of the patient's symptoms.

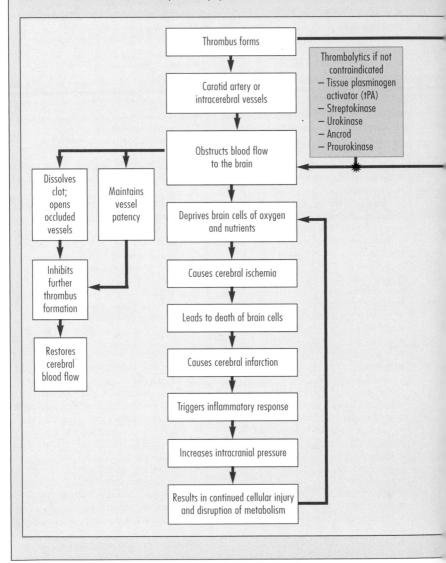

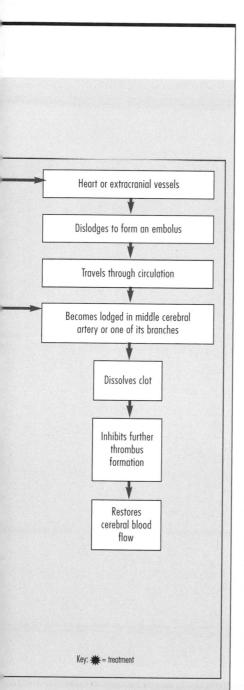

Heart or extracranial vessels

↓

Dislodges to form an embolus

↓

Travels through circulation

↓

Becomes lodged in middle cerebral artery or one of its branches

↓

Dissolves clot

↓

Inhibits further thrombus formation

↓

Restores cerebral blood flow

Key: ✳ = treatment

■ Carotid duplex scan identifies the degree of stenosis.

■ Brain scan shows ischemic areas but may not be conclusive for up to 2 weeks after a stroke.

■ Single photon emission CT and positron emission tomography scans identify areas of altered metabolism surrounding lesions not yet detectible by other diagnostic tests.

■ Transesophageal echocardiogram reveals cardiac disorders, such as atrial thrombi, atrial septal defect, or patent foramen ovale, as causes of thrombotic stroke.

■ Lumbar puncture (performed if there are no signs of increased ICP) reveals bloody CSF when stroke is hemorrhagic.

■ Ophthalmoscopy may identify signs of hypertension and atherosclerotic changes in retinal arteries.

■ EEG helps identify damaged areas of the brain.

TREATMENT

Treatment is supportive to minimize and prevent further cerebral damage. Measures include:

■ ICP management with monitoring, hyperventilation (to decrease the partial pressure of arterial carbon dioxide to lower ICP), osmotic diuretics (mannitol, to reduce cerebral edema), and corticosteroids (dexamethasone, to reduce inflammation and cerebral edema)

■ stool softeners to prevent straining, which increases ICP

■ anticonvulsants to treat or prevent seizures

■ surgery for large cerebellar infarction to remove infarcted tissue and decompress remaining live tissue

■ aneurysm repair to prevent further hemorrhage

■ percutaneous transluminal angioplasty or stent insertion to open occluded vessels.

■ rehabilitation therapy to address any residual deficits

Treatment for ischemic stroke includes:

■ thrombolytic therapy (tPA, alteplase) within the first 3 hours after the onset of symptoms to dissolve the clot, remove occlusion, and restore blood flow, thus minimizing cerebral damage (see *Treating ischemic stroke*)

■ anticoagulant therapy (heparin, warfarin) to maintain vessel patency and prevent further clot formation in cases of high-grade carotid stenosis or in newly diagnosed cardiovascular disease.

Treatment for hemorrhagic stroke includes:

■ analgesics, such as acetaminophen, to relieve headache associated with hemorrhagic stroke.

Treatment for TIAs includes:

■ antiplatelet agents (aspirin, ticlopidine, dipyridamole-aspirin combination to reduce the risk of platelet aggregation and subsequent clot formation

■ carotid endarterectomy to open partially (greater than 70%) occluded carotid arteries.

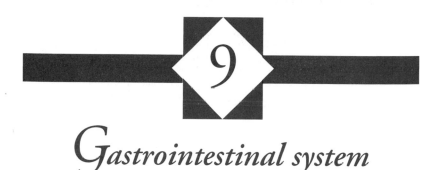

Gastrointestinal system

The GI system supplies essential nutrients to fuel all the physiologic and pathophysiologic activities of the body. Its functioning profoundly affects the quality of life through its impact on overall health. The GI system has two major components: the alimentary canal, or GI tract, and the accessory organs. A malfunction anywhere in the system can produce far-reaching metabolic effects, eventually threatening life.

The alimentary canal is a hollow muscular tube that begins in the mouth, ends at the anus, and includes the pharynx, esophagus, stomach, and small and large intestines. Peristalsis propels food and fluids along the tract; sphincters prevent reflux. Accessory organs and glands include the salivary glands, liver, biliary duct system (gallbladder and bile ducts), and pancreas.

Together, the GI tract and accessory organs serve two major functions: digestion (breaking down food and fluids into simple chemicals that can be absorbed into the bloodstream and carried throughout the body) and elimination of waste products from the body through defecation.

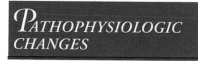

PATHOPHYSIOLOGIC CHANGES

Disorders of the GI system typically appear as vague, nonspecific complaints or problems that reflect disruption in one or more of the system's functions. For example, movement through the GI tract can be slowed, accelerated, or blocked, and secretion, absorption, or motility can be altered. As a result, one patient may experience several GI problems at once, most commonly anorexia, constipation, diarrhea, dysphagia (difficulty swallowing), jaundice, nausea, and vomiting.

Anorexia

Anorexia is a loss of appetite or a lack of desire for food. Nausea, abdominal pain, and diarrhea may go along with it. Anorexia can result from dysfunction or disease in the GI system or other systems, such as cancer, heart disease, or renal disease.

Normally, a physiologic stimulus is responsible for the sensation of hunger. Falling blood glucose levels stimulate the hunger center in the hypothalamus; rising lipid and amino acid levels help satisfy hunger. Hunger is also stimulated by contraction of an empty stomach and suppressed when the GI tract becomes distended, possibly as a result of stimulation of the vagus nerve. Sight, touch, and smell play subtle roles in controlling the appetite center.

In anorexia, the physiologic stimuli are present, but the person has no appetite or desire to eat. Slow gastric emptying or gastric stasis can cause anorexia. High levels of neurotransmitters such as serotonin (which may contribute to appetite satisfaction) and excess cortisol levels (which may suppress hypothalamic control of hunger) also have been linked to anorexia.

Constipation

Constipation is a condition in which bowel movements are incomplete or infrequent, as defined by a decrease in the number of stools per week. It's defined individually because normal bowel habits range from two to three stools per day to one per week. Causes of constipation include dehydration, a low-fiber diet, a sedentary lifestyle, lack of regular exercise, and frequent repression of the urge to defecate.

When a person is dehydrated or delays defecation, more fluid is absorbed from the intestine, the stool becomes harder, and constipation occurs. High-fiber diets cause water to be drawn into the stool by osmosis, keeping the stool soft and encouraging its movement through the intestine. High-fiber diets also cause intestinal dilation, which stimulates peristalsis.

 AGE ALERT
Elderly people usually have decreased intestinal motility and a slowing and dulling of neural impulses in the GI tract. Many older persons restrict fluid intake to prevent waking at night to use the bathroom or because of a fear of incontinence. This places them at risk for dehydration and constipation.

A sedentary lifestyle, lack of exercise, limitations in physical activity, or inability to be physically active can cause constipation because exercise stimulates the GI tract and promotes defecation. Antacids, opiates, and other drugs that inhibit bowel motility also lead to constipation.

Stress stimulates the sympathetic nervous system, and GI motility slows. Absence or degeneration in the neural pathways of the large intestine also contribute to constipation. Other conditions, such as spinal cord trauma, multiple sclerosis, intestinal neoplasms, and hypothyroidism, can also cause constipation.

Diarrhea

Diarrhea is an increase in the fluidity or volume of feces and the frequency of defecation. Factors that affect stool vol-

ume and consistency include water content of the colon and the presence of unabsorbed food, unabsorbable material, and intestinal secretions. Large-volume diarrhea is usually the result of an excessive amount of water, secretions, or both in the intestines. Small-volume diarrhea is usually caused by excessive intestinal motility. Diarrhea may also be caused by a parasympathetic stimulation of the intestine started by psychological factors, such as fear or stress.

The three major mechanisms of diarrhea include:

■ *osmotic diarrhea*—The presence of a nonabsorbable substance such as synthetic sugar or increased numbers of osmotic particles in the intestine increases osmotic pressure and draws excess water into the intestine, thereby increasing the weight and volume of the stool.
■ *secretory diarrhea*—A pathogen or tumor irritates the muscle and mucosal layers of the intestine. The result is an increase in motility and secretions (water, electrolytes, and mucus) causing diarrhea.
■ *motility diarrhea*—Inflammation, neuropathy, or obstruction causes a reflex increase in intestinal motility that may expel the irritant or clear the obstruction.

Dysphagia

Dysphagia—difficulty swallowing—can be caused by a mechanical obstruction of the esophagus or by impaired esophageal motility caused by another disorder. Mechanical obstruction is characterized as intrinsic or extrinsic.

Intrinsic obstructions originate in the esophagus itself. Causes of intrinsic obstructions include tumors, strictures, and diverticular herniations. Extrinsic obstructions originate outside of the esophagus and narrow the lumen by exerting pressure on the esophageal wall. Most extrinsic obstructions result from a tumor.

Distention and spasm at the site of the obstruction during swallowing may cause pain. Upper esophageal obstruction causes pain 2 to 4 seconds after swallowing; lower esophageal obstructions, 10 to 15 seconds after swallowing. If a tumor is present, dysphagia begins with difficulty swallowing solids and eventually progress-

How swallowing occurs

Before peristalsis can begin, the neural pattern to initiate swallowing, illustrated here, must occur:

◆ Food reaching the back of the mouth stimulates swallowing receptors that surround the pharyngeal opening.

◆ The receptors transmit impulses to the brain by way of the sensory portions of the

trigeminal (V) and glossopharyngeal (IX) nerves.

◆ The brain's swallowing center relays motor impulses to the esophagus by way of the trigeminal (V), glossopharyngeal (IX), vagus (X), and hypoglossal (XII) nerves.

◆ Swallowing occurs.

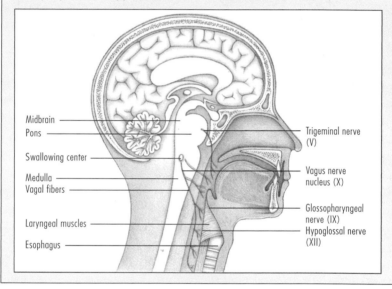

Midbrain
Pons
Swallowing center
Medulla
Vagal fibers
Laryngeal muscles
Esophagus

Trigeminal nerve (V)
Vagus nerve nucleus (X)
Glossopharyngeal nerve (IX)
Hypoglossal nerve (XII)

es to difficulty swallowing semisolids and liquids. Impaired motor function makes both liquids and solids more difficult to swallow.

Neural or muscular disorders can also interfere with voluntary swallowing or peristalsis. This is known as functional dysphagia. Causes of functional dysphagia include dermatomyositis, stroke, Parkinson's disease, or achalasia. (See *How swallowing occurs*.) Malfunction of the upper esophageal striated muscles interferes with the voluntary phase of swallowing.

In achalasia, the esophageal ganglionic cells are thought to have degenerated, and the cardiac sphincter (muscle fibers

around the opening of the esophagus into the stomach) can't relax. The lower end of the esophagus loses neuromuscular coordination and muscle tone, and food accumulates, causing hypertrophy and dilation. Eventually, accumulated food raises the hydrostatic pressure and forces the sphincter open, and small amounts of food slowly move into the stomach.

Jaundice

Jaundice—yellow pigmentation of the skin and sclera (white outer coating of the eyeball)—is caused by an excess accumulation of bilirubin in the blood. Bilirubin, a product of red blood cell (RBC) break-

CLOSER LOOK
Jaundice: Impaired bilirubin metabolism

Jaundice occurs in three forms: prehepatic, hepatic, and posthepatic. In all three, bilirubin levels in the blood increase.

PREHEPATIC JAUNDICE
Certain conditions and disorders, such as transfusion reactions and sickle cell anemia, cause massive hemolysis.
◆ Red blood cells rupture faster than the liver can conjugate bilirubin.
◆ Large amounts of unconjugated bilirubin pass into the blood.
◆ Intestinal enzymes convert bilirubin to water-soluble urobilinogen for excretion in urine and stools. (Unconjugated bilirubin is insoluble in water, so it can't be directly secreted in urine.)

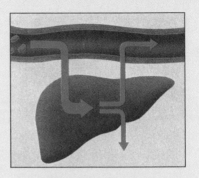

HEPATIC JAUNDICE
The liver becomes unable to conjugate or excrete bilirubin, leading to increased blood levels of conjugated and unconjugated bilirubin. This occurs in such disorders as hepatitis, cirrhosis, and metastatic cancer, and during prolonged use of drugs metabolized by the liver.

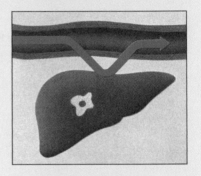

POSTHEPATIC JAUNDICE
In biliary and pancreatic disorders, bilirubin forms at its normal rate.
◆ Inflammation, scar tissue, tumor, or gallstones block the flow of bile into the intestines.
◆ Water-soluble conjugated bilirubin accumulates in the blood.
◆ The bilirubin is excreted in urine.

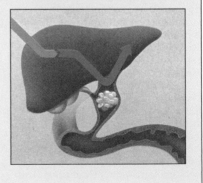

down, accumulates when production exceeds metabolism and excretion. This imbalance can result from excessive release of bilirubin precursors into the bloodstream or from impairment of its hepatic uptake, metabolism, or excretion. (See *Jaundice: Impaired bilirubin metabolism.*)

Jaundice occurs when bilirubin levels exceed 2 to 2.5 mg/dl, about twice the upper limit of the normal range. Lower levels of bilirubin may cause detectable jaundice in persons with fair skin, and jaundice may be difficult to detect in patients with dark skin.

CULTURAL DIVERSITY
Jaundice in dark-skinned persons may appear as yellow staining in the sclera, hard palate, and palmar or plantar surfaces.

The three main types of jaundice are hemolytic, hepatocellular, and obstructive:
■ *hemolytic jaundice*—When RBC lysis exceeds the liver's capacity to conjugate bilirubin (binding bilirubin to a polar group makes it water soluble and able to be excreted by the kidneys), hemolytic jaundice occurs. Causes include transfusion reactions, sickle cell anemia, thalassemia, and autoimmune disease.
■ *hepatocellular jaundice*—Hepatocyte dysfunction limits uptake and conjugation of bilirubin. Liver dysfunction can occur in hepatitis, cancer, cirrhosis, or congenital disorders; it can also be caused by some drugs.
■ *obstructive jaundice*—When the flow of bile out of the liver through the hepatic duct or through the bile duct is blocked, the liver can conjugate bilirubin, but the bilirubin can't reach the small intestine. Blockage of the hepatic duct by calculi ("stones") or a tumor is considered an intrahepatic cause of obstructive jaundice. A blocked bile duct is an extrahepatic cause that may be attributed to gallstones or a tumor.

Nausea

Nausea is feeling the urge to vomit. It may occur independently of vomiting, or it may precede or accompany it. Specific neural pathways haven't been identified, but increased salivation, diminished functional activities of the stomach, and altered small-intestine motility have been linked to nausea. Nausea may also be stimulated by high brain centers.

Vomiting

Vomiting is the forceful oral expulsion of gastric contents through the esophagus. The gastric musculature provides the ejection force. The gastric fundus and gastroesophageal sphincter relax, and forceful contractions of the diaphragm and abdominal wall muscles increase intraabdominal pressure. This, combined with the annular contraction of the gastric pylorus, forces gastric contents into the esophagus. Increased intrathoracic pressure then moves the gastric content from the esophagus to the mouth.

Vomiting is controlled by two centers in the medulla: the vomiting center and the chemoreceptor trigger zone (CTZ). The vomiting center initiates the actual act of vomiting. It's stimulated by the GI tract, from higher brain stem and cortical centers and from the CTZ. The CTZ can't induce vomiting by itself. Various stimuli or drugs activate the zone, such as apomorphine, levodopa, digitalis, bacterial toxins, radiation, and metabolic abnormalities. The activated zone sends impulses to the medullary vomiting center, and the following sequence begins:
■ The abdominal muscles and diaphragm contract.
■ Reverse peristalsis begins, causing intestinal material to flow back into the stomach, distending it.
■ The stomach pushes the diaphragm into the thoracic cavity, raising the intrathoracic pressure.
■ The pressure forces the upper esophageal sphincter open, the glottis closes, and the soft palate blocks the nasopharynx.
■ The pressure also forces the material up through the sphincter and out through the mouth.

Nausea and vomiting are characteristics of other disorders, such as acute abdominal emergencies, infections of the intestinal tract, central nervous system disorders, myocardial infarction, heart failure, metabolic and endocrinologic disorders, or as the adverse effect of many drugs. Nausea and vomiting can also be present in pregnancy. Vomiting can also be psychogenic, resulting from emotional or psychological disturbance.

Disorders

Appendicitis

The most common disease requiring emergency surgery, appendicitis is inflammation and obstruction of the vermiform appendix (a blind pouch attached to the cecum). Appendicitis may occur at any age and usually affects both sexes equally, but between puberty and age 25 it's more prevalent in men. Since the advent of antibiotics, the frequency of and death rate from complications resulting from appendicitis have declined; if untreated, this disease is invariably fatal.

CAUSES
Causes can include:
- mucosal ulceration
- fecal mass
- stricture in the GI tract
- barium ingestion
- viral infection.

PATHOPHYSIOLOGY
Mucosal ulceration of the appendix triggers inflammation, which temporarily obstructs the appendix. The obstruction blocks mucus outflow. Pressure in the now-distended appendix increases, and the appendix contracts. Bacteria multiply, and inflammation and pressure continue to increase, restricting blood flow to the pouch and causing severe abdominal pain.

SIGNS AND SYMPTOMS
Signs and symptoms may include:
- abdominal pain, caused by inflammation of the appendix and bowel obstruction and distention, begins in the epigastric region, and then shifts to the right lower quadrant

- anorexia after the onset of pain — because of pain, distention, and obstruction
- nausea or vomiting caused by the inflammation
- low-grade fever from systemic manifestation of inflammation and leukocytosis
- tenderness from inflammation.

COMPLICATIONS
Complications may include:
- wound infection
- intra-abdominal abscess
- fecal fistula
- intestinal obstruction
- incisional hernia
- peritonitis
- death.

DIAGNOSIS
- White blood cell count is moderately high with an increased number of immature cells.
- X-ray with radiographic contrast agent reveals failure of the appendix to fill with contrast.

TREATMENT
Treatment may include:
- maintenance of nothing-by-mouth status until surgery
- Fowler's position to aid in pain relief
- GI intubation for decompression
- appendectomy
- antibiotics to treat infection if peritonitis occurs
- parental replacement of fluid and electrolytes to reverse possible dehydration resulting from surgery or nausea and vomiting.

Cholecystitis

Cholecystitis — acute or chronic inflammation causing painful distention of the gallbladder — is usually linked to a gallstone impacted in the cystic duct.

Cholecystitis accounts for 10% to 25% of all patients requiring gallbladder surgery. The acute form is most common among middle-aged women; the chronic form, among elderly people. The prognosis is good with treatment.

CAUSES

Causes may include:

- gallstones (the most common cause)
- poor or absent blood flow to the gallbladder
- abnormal metabolism of cholesterol and bile salts.

PATHOPHYSIOLOGY

In acute cholecystitis, inflammation of the gallbladder wall usually develops after a gallstone lodges in the cystic duct. (See *Understanding gallstone formation,* pages 320 and 321.)

When bile flow is blocked, the gallbladder becomes inflamed and distended. Bacterial growth, usually *Escherichia coli,* may contribute to the inflammation. Edema of the gallbladder (and sometimes the cystic duct) obstructs bile flow, which chemically irritates the gallbladder. Cells in the gallbladder wall may become oxygen starved and die as the distended organ presses on vessels and impairs blood flow. The dead cells slough off, and an exudate covers ulcerated areas, causing the gallbladder to adhere to surrounding structures.

SIGNS AND SYMPTOMS

Signs and symptoms may include:

- acute abdominal pain in the right upper quadrant that may radiate to the back, between the shoulders, or to the front of the chest from inflammation and irritation of nerve fibers
- colic caused by the passage of gallstones along the bile duct
- nausea and vomiting triggered by the inflammatory response
- chills related to inflammation and fever
- low-grade fever caused by inflammation
- jaundice from obstruction of the common bile duct by calculi.

COMPLICATIONS

Complications include:

- perforation and abscess formation
- fistula formation
- gangrene
- empyema
- cholangitis
- hepatitis
- pancreatitis

- gallstone ileus
- carcinoma.

DIAGNOSIS

- X-ray reveals gallstones if they contain enough calcium to be radiopaque; also helps disclose porcelain gallbladder (hard, brittle gallbladder because of calcium deposited in wall), limy bile, and gallstone ileus.
- Ultrasonography detects gallstones as small as 2 mm and distinguishes between obstructive and nonobstructive jaundice.
- Technetium-labeled scan reveals cystic duct obstruction and acute or chronic cholecystitis if ultrasound doesn't provide a picture of the gallbladder.
- Percutaneous transhepatic cholangiography supports the diagnosis of obstructive jaundice and reveals calculi in the ducts.
- Levels of serum alkaline phosphate, lactate dehydrogenase, aspartate aminotransferase, and total bilirubin are high; serum amylase level slightly elevated; and icteric index elevated.
- White blood cell counts are slightly elevated during cholecystitis attack.

TREATMENT

Treatment may include:

- cholecystectomy to surgically remove the inflamed gallbladder
- choledochostomy to surgically create an opening into the common bile duct for drainage
- percutaneous transhepatic cholecystostomy
- endoscopic retrograde cholangiopancreatography for removal of gallstones
- lithotripsy to break up gallstones and relieve obstruction
- oral chenodeoxycholic acid or ursodeoxycholic acid to dissolve calculi
- low-fat diet to prevent attacks
- vitamin K to relieve itching, jaundice, and bleeding tendencies caused by vitamin K deficiencies
- antibiotics for use during acute attack for treatment of infection
- nasogastric tube insertion during acute attack for abdominal decompression.

CLOSER LOOK
Understanding gallstone formation

Abnormal metabolism of cholesterol and bile salts plays an important role in gallstone formation. The liver makes bile continuously. The gallbladder concentrates and stores it until the duodenum signals it needs it to help digest fat. Changes in the composition of bile may allow gallstones to form. Changes in the absorptive ability of the gallbladder lining may also contribute to gallstone formation.

TOO MUCH CHOLESTEROL
Certain conditions, such as obesity, increasing age, and estrogen imbalance, cause the liver to secrete bile that's abnormally high in cholesterol or lacking in the proper concentration of bile salts.

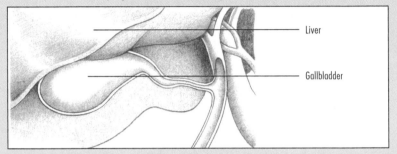

Liver

Gallbladder

INSIDE THE GALLBLADDER
When the gallbladder concentrates this bile, inflammation may occur. Excessive reabsorption of water and bile salts makes the bile less soluble. Cholesterol, calcium, and bilirubin precipitate into gallstones.

 Fat entering the duodenum causes the intestinal mucosa to secrete the hormone cholecystokinin, which stimulates the gallbladder to contract and empty. If a stone lodges in the cystic duct, the gallbladder contracts but can't empty.

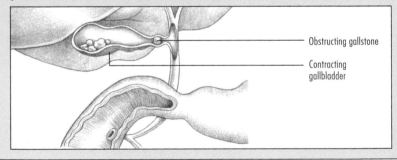

Obstructing gallstone

Contracting gallbladder

Cirrhosis
Cirrhosis is a chronic disease characterized by diffuse destruction and fibrotic regeneration of hepatic cells. As necrotic tissue yields to fibrosis, this disease damages liver tissue and normal vasculature, impairs blood and lymph flow, and ultimately causes hepatic insufficiency. It's twice as common in men as in women, and is especially prevalent among malnourished persons over age 50 with chronic alcoholism. Mortality is high; many patients die within 5 years of onset.

JAUNDICE, IRRITATION, INFLAMMATION

If a stone lodges in the common bile duct, the bile can't flow into the duodenum. Bilirubin is absorbed into the blood and causes jaundice.

Biliary narrowing and swelling of the tissue around the stone can also cause irritation and inflammation of the common bile duct.

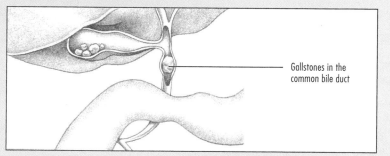

Gallstones in the common bile duct

UP THE BILIARY TREE

Inflammation can progress up the biliary tree into any of the bile ducts. This causes scar tissue, fluid accumulation, cirrhosis, portal hypertension, and bleeding.

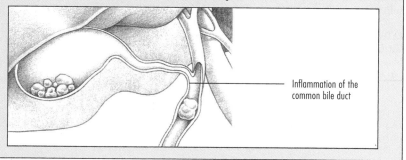

Inflammation of the common bile duct

CAUSES

Cirrhosis may be a result of a wide range of diseases. The following types of cirrhosis reflect its diverse etiology.

Hepatocellular disease

This group includes the following disorders:

■ *Postnecrotic cirrhosis* accounts for 10% to 30% of patients and stems from various types of hepatitis (such as types A, B, C, and D viral hepatitis) or toxic exposures.

■ *Laënnec's cirrhosis,* also called portal, nutritional, or alcoholic cirrhosis, is the most common type and is primarily caused by hepatitis C and alcoholism. Liver damage results from malnutrition (especially dietary protein) and chronic alcohol intake. Fibrous tissue forms in portal areas and around central veins.

■ Autoimmune disease, such as sarcoidosis or chronic inflammatory bowel disease, may cause cirrhosis.

Cholestatic diseases

Cholestatic diseases include diseases of the biliary tree (biliary cirrhosis resulting from bile duct diseases that suppress bile flow) and sclerosing cholangitis.

Metabolic diseases

Metabolic diseases include such disorders as Wilson's disease, alpha$_1$-antitrypsin, and hemochromatosis (pigment cirrhosis).

Other types of cirrhosis

Other types of cirrhosis include Budd-Chiari syndrome (epigastric pain, liver enlargement, and ascites [accumulation of fluid in the abdomen] from hepatic vein obstruction), cardiac cirrhosis, and cryptogenic cirrhosis (cirrhosis of unknown origin). Cardiac cirrhosis is rare; the liver damage results from right-sided heart failure.

PATHOPHYSIOLOGY

Cirrhosis begins with hepatic scarring or fibrosis. The scar begins as an increase in extracellular matrix components — fibril-forming collagens, proteoglycans, fibronectin, and hyaluronic acid. The site of collagen deposition varies with the cause. Hepatocyte function is eventually impaired as the matrix changes. Fat-storing cells are believed to be the source of the new matrix components. Contraction of these cells may also contribute to disruption of the lobular architecture and obstruction of the flow of blood or bile. Cellular changes producing bands of scar tissue also disrupt the lobular structure.

SIGNS AND SYMPTOMS

Signs and symptoms of the early stages include:

■ anorexia because of distaste for certain foods

■ nausea and vomiting caused by inflammatory response and systemic effects of liver inflammation

■ diarrhea from malabsorption

■ dull abdominal ache caused by liver inflammation.

Signs and symptoms of the late stages include:

■ *respiratory* — pleural effusion, limited thoracic expansion because of abdominal ascites; interferes with efficient gas exchange, which causes hypoxia

■ *central nervous system* — progressive signs or symptoms of hepatic encephalopathy, including lethargy, mental changes, slurred speech, asterixis, peripheral neuritis, paranoia, hallucinations, extreme obtundation, and coma — caused by the loss of ammonia-to-urea conversion and consequent delivery of toxic ammonia to the brain

■ *hematologic* — bleeding tendencies (nosebleeds, easy bruising, bleeding gums), splenomegaly, anemia resulting from thrombocytopenia (caused by splenomegaly and decreased vitamin K absorption), and portal hypertension

■ *endocrine* — testicular atrophy, menstrual irregularities, gynecomastia, and loss of chest and axillary hair from decreased hormone metabolism

■ *skin* — abnormal pigmentation, spider angiomas, palmar erythema, and jaundice related to impaired hepatic function; severe pruritus from jaundice caused by bilirubinemia; extreme dryness and poor tissue turgor related to malnutrition

■ *hepatic* — jaundice from decreased bilirubin metabolism; hepatomegaly caused by liver scarring and portal hypertension; ascites and edema of the legs from portal hypertension and decreased plasma proteins; hepatic encephalopathy from ammonia toxicity; and hepatorenal syndrome from advanced liver disease and subsequent renal failure

■ *miscellaneous* — musty breath from ammonia buildup; enlarged superficial abdominal veins caused by portal hyperten-

CLOSER LOOK
What happens in portal hypertension

Portal hypertension (elevated pressure in the portal vein) occurs when blood flow meets increased resistance. This common result of cirrhosis may also stem from mechanical obstruction and occlusion of the hepatic veins (Budd-Chiari syndrome).

As the pressure in the portal vein rises, blood backs up into the spleen and flows through collateral channels to the venous system, bypassing the liver. Thus, portal hypertension causes:

◆ splenomegaly with thrombocytopenia

◆ dilated collateral veins (esophageal varices, hemorrhoids, or prominent abdominal veins)
◆ ascites.

In many patients, the first sign of portal hypertension is bleeding esophageal varices (dilated tortuous veins in the submucosa of the lower esophagus). Esophageal varices commonly cause massive hematemesis, requiring emergency care to control hemorrhage and prevent hypovolemic shock.

Superior vena cava
Right atrium
Azygos vein
Esophagus
Esophageal varices
Inferior vena cava
Hepatic vein
Enlarged spleen
Short gastric vein
Left gastric vein
Relative increase in hepatic artery flow
Portal vein pressure rises to 20 mm Hg or more
Splenic vein

sion; pain in the right upper abdominal quadrant that worsens when patient sits up or leans forward, caused by inflammation and irritation of area nerve fibers; palpable liver or spleen caused by organomegaly; temperature of 101° to 103° F (38.3° to 39.4° C) from inflammatory response; hemorrhage because of esophageal varices resulting from portal hypertension. (See *What happens in portal hypertension.*)

COMPLICATIONS
Complications can include:
■ respiratory compromise
■ ascites
■ portal hypertension
■ jaundice
■ coagulopathy
■ hepatic encephalopathy
■ bleeding esophageal varices; acute GI bleeding
■ liver failure
■ renal failure.

DIAGNOSIS

The following tests help to diagnose cirrhosis:

- Liver biopsy reveals tissue destruction and fibrosis.
- Abdominal X-ray shows enlarged liver, cysts, or gas within the biliary tract or liver, liver calcification, and massive ascites.
- Computed tomography and liver scans show liver size, abnormal masses, and hepatic blood flow and obstruction.
- Esophagogastroduodenoscopy reveals bleeding esophageal varices, stomach irritation or ulceration, or duodenal bleeding and irritation.
- Blood studies reveal elevated levels of liver enzymes, total serum bilirubin, and indirect bilirubin; decreased levels of total serum albumin and protein; prolonged prothrombin time; decreased hemoglobin, hematocrit, and electrolyte levels; and deficiency of vitamins A, C, and K.
- Urine studies show increased bilirubin and urobilirubinogen level.
- Fecal studies show decreased fecal urobilirubinogen level.

TREATMENT

Treatment may include:

- vitamins and nutritional supplements to help heal damaged liver cells and improve nutritional status
- antacids to reduce gastric distress and decrease the potential for GI bleeding
- potassium-sparing diuretics to reduce fluid accumulation
- vasopressin to treat esophageal varices
- esophagogastric intubation with multilumen tubes (tubes with several chambers) to control bleeding from esophageal varices or other hemorrhage sites, using balloons to exert pressure on the bleeding site.
- gastric lavage until the contents are clear; with antacids and histamine antagonists if the bleeding is caused by a gastric ulcer
- esophageal balloon tamponade to compress bleeding vessels and stop blood loss from esophageal varices
- paracentesis to relieve abdominal pressure and remove ascitic fluid
- surgical shunt placement to divert ascitic fluid into venous circulation, leading to weight loss, decreased abdominal girth, increased sodium excretion from the kidneys, and improved urine output
- sclerosing agents injected into oozing vessels to cause clotting and sclerosis
- insertion of portosystemic shunts to control bleeding from esophageal varices and decrease portal hypertension (diverts a portion of the portal vein blood flow away from the liver; seldom performed).

Crohn's disease

Crohn's disease, also known as *regional enteritis* or *granulomatous colitis,* is inflammation of any part of the GI tract (usually the proximal portion of the colon and less commonly the terminal ileum), extending through all layers of the intestinal wall. It may also involve regional lymph nodes and the mesentery. Crohn's disease is most prevalent in adults age 20 to 40.

CAUSES

The exact cause is unknown but conditions that may contribute include:

- lymphatic obstruction
- allergies
- immune disorders
- infection
- genetic predisposition.

PATHOPHYSIOLOGY

Whatever the cause of Crohn's disease, inflammation spreads slowly and progressively. Enlarged lymph nodes block lymph flow in the submucosa. Lymphatic obstruction leads to edema, mucosal ulceration and fissures, abscesses, and sometimes granulomas. Mucosal ulcerations are called "skipping lesions" because they aren't continuous, as in ulcerative colitis.

Oval, elevated patches of closely packed lymph follicles — called *Peyer's patches* — develop in the lining of the small intestine. Subsequent fibrosis thickens the bowel wall and causes stenosis, or narrowing of the lumen. (See *Bowel changes in Crohn's disease.*)

The serous membrane becomes inflamed (serositis), inflamed bowel loops adhere to other diseased or normal loops, and diseased bowel segments become interspersed with healthy ones. Finally, dis-

CLOSER LOOK
Bowel changes in Crohn's disease

As Crohn's disease progresses, fibrosis thickens the bowel wall and narrows the lumen. Narrowing — or stenosis — can occur in any part of the intestine and cause varying degrees of intestinal obstruction. At first, the mucosa may appear normal, but as the disease progresses it takes on a "cobblestone" appearance, as shown.

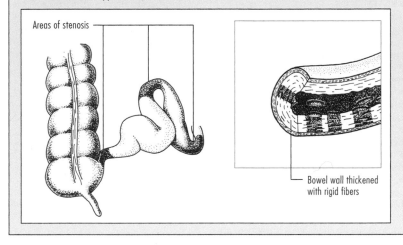

Areas of stenosis

Bowel wall thickened with rigid fibers

eased parts of the bowel become thicker, narrower, and shorter.

SIGNS AND SYMPTOMS
Signs and symptoms include:
- steady, colicky pain in the right lower quadrant caused by acute inflammation and nerve fiber irritation
- cramping caused by acute inflammation
- tenderness caused by acute inflammation
- palpable mass in the right lower quadrant because of bowel thickening
- weight loss caused by diarrhea and malabsorption
- diarrhea from bile salt malabsorption, loss of healthy intestinal surface area, and bacterial growth
- steatorrhea caused by fat malabsorption
- bloody stools from the bleeding caused by bowel inflammation and ulceration.

COMPLICATIONS
Complications may include:

- anal fistula
- perineal abscess
- fistulas to the bladder or vagina or to the skin in an old scar area
- intestinal obstruction
- nutrient deficiencies from poor digestion and malabsorption of bile salts and vitamin B_{12}
- fluid imbalances.

DIAGNOSIS
The following tests help to diagnose Crohn's disease:
- Fecal occult test reveals minute amounts of blood in stools.
- Small-bowel X-ray shows irregular mucosa, ulceration, and stiffening.
- Barium enema reveals the string sign (segments of stricture separated by normal bowel) and possibly fissures and narrowing of the bowel.
- Sigmoidoscopy and colonoscopy reveal patchy areas of inflammation (helps to rule out ulcerative colitis), with cobble-

stone-like mucosal surface. When colon is involved, ulcers may be seen.
- Biopsy reveals granulomas in up to one-half of all specimens.
- Blood tests reveal increased white blood cell count and erythrocyte sedimentation rate, and decreased potassium, calcium, magnesium, and hemoglobin levels.

TREATMENT
Treatment measures for Crohn's disease include:
- corticosteroids to reduce inflammation and, thus, diarrhea, pain, and bleeding
- immunosuppressants to suppress the response to antigens
- sulfasalazine to reduce inflammation
- metronidazole to treat perianal complications
- antidiarrheal agents (not used for patients with significant bowel obstruction)
- opioid analgesics to control pain and diarrhea
- stress reduction and reduced physical activity to rest the bowel and allow it to heal
- vitamin supplements to replace and compensate for the bowel's inability to absorb vitamins
- dietary changes (elimination of fruits, vegetables, high fiber foods, dairy products, spicy and fatty foods, foods that irritate the mucosa, carbonated or caffeinated beverages, and other foods or liquids that stimulate excessive intestinal activity); goal is to decrease bowel activity while still providing adequate nutrition
- surgery, if necessary, to repair bowel perforation and correct massive hemorrhage, fistulas or acute intestinal obstruction; colectomy with ileostomy in patients with extensive disease of the large intestine and rectum.

Diverticular disease
In diverticular disease, bulging pouches (diverticula) in the GI wall push the mucosal lining through the surrounding muscle. Although the most common site for diverticula is in the sigmoid colon, they may develop anywhere, from the proximal end of the pharynx to the anus. Other typical sites include the duodenum, near the pancreatic border or the ampulla of Vater, and the jejunum.

CULTURAL DIVERSITY
Diverticular disease is common in Western countries, suggesting that a low-fiber diet reduces stool bulk and leads to diminished colonic motility. The consequent increased intraluminal pressure causes herniation of the mucosa.

Diverticular disease of the stomach is rare and is usually a precursor of peptic or neoplastic disease. Diverticular disease of the ileum (Meckel's diverticulum) is the most common congenital anomaly of the GI tract.

Diverticular disease has two forms:
- diverticulosis, in which diverticula are present but don't cause symptoms
- diverticulitis, in which diverticula are inflamed and may cause potentially fatal obstruction, infection, or hemorrhage.

AGE ALERT
Diverticular disease is most prevalent in men over age 40 and people who eat a low-fiber diet. More than one-half of all people over age 50 have colonic diverticula.

CAUSES
Causes may include:
- diminished colonic motility and increased intraluminal pressure
- low-fiber diet
- defects in colon wall strength.

PATHOPHYSIOLOGY
Diverticula probably result from high intraluminal pressure on an area of weakness in the GI wall, where blood vessels enter. Diet may be a contributing factor because insufficient fiber reduces fecal residue, narrows the bowel lumen, and leads to high intra-abdominal pressure during defecation.

In diverticulitis, retained undigested food and bacteria accumulate in the diverticular sac. This hard mass cuts off the blood supply to the thin walls of the sac, making them more susceptible to attack by colonic bacteria. Inflammation follows and may lead to perforation, abscess, peritonitis, obstruction, or hemorrhage. Occasionally, the inflamed colon segment may adhere to the bladder or other organs and cause a fistula.

SIGNS AND SYMPTOMS

Typically, a person with diverticulosis has no symptoms and may never have them unless diverticulitis develops.

Mild diverticulitis

In mild diverticulitis, signs and symptoms include:
- moderate left lower abdominal pain caused by inflammation of diverticula
- low-grade fever caused by trapping of bacteria-rich stool in the diverticula
- leukocytosis from infection caused by trapping of bacteria-rich stool in the diverticula.

Severe diverticulitis

In severe diverticulitis, signs and symptoms include:
- abdominal rigidity from rupture of the diverticula, abscesses, and peritonitis
- left lower quadrant pain caused by rupture of the diverticula and the resulting inflammation and infection
- high fever, chills, hypotension from sepsis, and shock caused by the release of fecal material from the rupture site
- microscopic or massive hemorrhage from rupture of diverticulum near a vessel.

Chronic diverticulitis

In chronic diverticulitis, signs and symptoms include:
- constipation, ribbon-like stools, intermittent diarrhea, and abdominal distention resulting from intestinal obstruction (possible when fibrosis and adhesions narrow the bowel's lumen)
- abdominal rigidity and pain, diminishing or absent bowel sounds, nausea, and vomiting caused by intestinal obstruction.

COMPLICATIONS

Complications include:
- perforation
- peritonitis
- bowel obstruction
- abscess
- fistulas.

DIAGNOSIS

The following tests help with diagnosis:
- Upper GI series confirms or rules out diverticulosis of the esophagus and upper bowel
- Barium enema reveals filling of diverticula, which confirms diagnosis.
- Biopsy reveals evidence of benign disease, ruling out cancer.
- Blood studies show an elevated erythrocyte sedimentation rate in diverticulitis.

TREATMENT

Treatment may include:
- liquid or bland diet, stool softeners, and occasional doses of mineral oil for symptomatic diverticulosis to relieve symptoms, minimize irritation, and lessen the risk of progression to diverticulitis
- high-residue diet for treatment of diverticulosis after pain has subsided to help decrease intra-abdominal pressure during defecation
- exercise to increase the rate of stool passage
- antibiotics to treat infection of the diverticula
- analgesics, such as meperidine or morphine, to control pain and to relax smooth muscle
- antispasmodic agents to control muscle spasms
- colon resection with removal of involved segment to correct cases refractory to medical treatment
- temporary colostomy if necessary to drain abscesses and rest the colon in diverticulitis accompanied by perforation, peritonitis, obstruction, or fistula
- blood transfusions if necessary to treat blood loss from hemorrhage, and fluid replacement as needed.

Gastroesophageal reflux disease

Popularly known as *heartburn,* gastroesophageal reflux disease (GERD) refers to backflow of gastric or duodenal contents or both into the esophagus and past the lower esophageal sphincter (LES), without associated belching or vomiting. The reflux of gastric contents causes acute epigastric pain, usually after a meal. The pain may radiate to the chest or arms. It com-

CLOSER LOOK
How gastroesophageal reflux disease occurs

Hormonal fluctuations, mechanical stress, and the effects of certain foods and drugs can decrease lower esophageal sphincter (LES) pressure. When LES pressure falls and intra-abdominal or intragastric pressure rises, the normally contracted LES relaxes inappropriately and allows reflux of gastric acid or bile secretions into the lower esophagus. There, the reflux irritates and inflames the esophageal mucosa, causing pyrosis.

Persistent inflammation can cause LES pressure to decrease even more and may trigger a recurrent cycle of reflux and pyrosis.

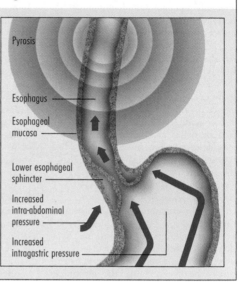

Pyrosis

Esophagus

Esophageal mucosa

Lower esophageal sphincter

Increased intra-abdominal pressure

Increased intragastric pressure

monly occurs in pregnant or obese persons. Lying down after a meal also contributes to reflux.

CAUSES
Causes of GERD include:
- weakened esophageal sphincter
- increased abdominal pressure, such as with obesity or pregnancy
- hiatal hernia
- medications, such as morphine, diazepam, calcium channel blockers, meperidine, and anticholinergic agents
- alcohol, cigarettes, or food that lowers LES pressure
- nasogastric intubation for more than 4 days.

PATHOPHYSIOLOGY
Normally, the LES maintains enough pressure around the lower end of the esophagus to close it and prevent reflux. Typically, the sphincter relaxes after each swallow to allow food into the stomach. In GERD, the sphincter doesn't remain closed (usually because of deficient LES

pressure or pressure within the stomach that exceeds LES pressure) and the pressure in the stomach pushes the stomach contents into the esophagus. The high acidity of the stomach contents causes irritation and pyrosis (burning pain, "heartburn") when it enters the esophagus. (See *How gastroesophageal reflux disease occurs.*)

SIGNS AND SYMPTOMS
Signs and symptoms include:
- burning pain in the epigastric area, possibly radiating to the arms and chest, from the reflux of gastric contents into the esophagus causing irritation and esophageal spasm
- pain, usually after a meal or when lying down, from increased abdominal pressure causing reflux
- feeling of fluid accumulation in the throat (without a sour or bitter taste) from hypersecretion of saliva.

COMPLICATIONS
Complications include:
- reflux esophagitis

- esophageal stricture
- esophageal ulceration
- chronic pulmonary disease caused by aspiration of gastric contents in the throat.

DIAGNOSIS

Diagnostic tests are aimed at determining the underlying cause of GERD:

- Esophageal acidity test evaluates the competence of the LES and provides objective measure of reflux.
- Acid perfusion test confirms esophagitis and distinguishes it from cardiac disorders.
- Esophagoscopy allows visual examination of the lining of the esophagus to reveal the extent of the disease and confirm pathologic changes in mucosa.
- Barium swallow identifies hiatal hernia as the cause.
- Upper GI series detects hiatal hernia or motility problems.
- Esophageal manometry evaluates resting pressure of LES and determines sphincter competence.

TREATMENT

Treatment may include:

- diet therapy with frequent, small meals and avoidance of eating before going to bed, to reduce abdominal pressure and reduce the incidence of reflux
- positioning—sitting up during and after meals and sleeping with head of bed elevated—to reduce abdominal pressure and prevent reflux
- increased fluid intake to wash gastric contents out of the esophagus
- antacids to neutralize acidic content of the stomach and minimize irritation
- histamine-2 receptor antagonists to inhibit gastric acid secretion
- proton pump inhibitors to reduce gastric acidity
- cholinergic agents to increase LES pressure
- smoking cessation to improve LES pressure (nicotine lowers LES pressure)
- surgery if hiatal hernia is the cause or patient has refractory symptoms.

Hemorrhoids

Hemorrhoids are varicosities in the superior or inferior hemorrhoidal venous plexus. Dilation and enlargement of the superior plexus of the superior hemorrhoidal veins above the dentate line cause internal hemorrhoids. Enlargement of the plexus of the inferior hemorrhoidal veins below the dentate line causes external hemorrhoids, which may protrude from the rectum. Hemorrhoids occur in both sexes. Prevalence is usually highest between ages 20 and 50.

CAUSES

Causes may include:

- prolonged sitting
- straining at defecation
- constipation, low-fiber diet
- pregnancy
- obesity.

PATHOPHYSIOLOGY

Hemorrhoids result from activities that increase intravenous pressure, causing distention and engorgement. Predisposing factors include prolonged sitting, straining at defecation, constipation, low-fiber diet, pregnancy, and obesity. Other factors include hepatic disease, such as cirrhosis, amebic abscesses, or hepatitis; alcoholism; and anorectal infections.

Hemorrhoids are classified as first, second, third, or fourth degree, depending on their severity. First-degree hemorrhoids are confined to the anal canal. Second-degree hemorrhoids prolapse during straining but reduce spontaneously. Third-degree hemorrhoids are prolapsed hemorrhoids that require manual reduction after each bowel movement. Fourth-degree hemorrhoids are irreducible. Signs and symptoms vary accordingly.

SIGNS AND SYMPTOMS

Signs and symptoms include:

- painless, intermittent bleeding during defecation from irritation and injury to the hemorrhoid mucosa
- bright red blood on stool or toilet tissue from injury to hemorrhoid mucosa
- anal itching from poor anal hygiene and pressure
- vague feeling of anal discomfort when bleeding occurs
- prolapse of rectal mucosa from straining
- pain from thrombosis of external hemorrhoids.

COMPLICATIONS

Complications include:

- constipation
- local infection
- thrombosis of hemorrhoids
- secondary anemia from severe or recurrent bleeding.

DIAGNOSIS

- Physical examination confirms external hemorrhoids.
- Anoscopy and flexible sigmoidoscopy visualizes internal hemorrhoids.

TREATMENT

Treatment depends on the type and severity of the hemorrhoids:

- high-fiber diet, increased fluid intake, and bulking agents to relieve constipation
- avoidance of prolonged sitting on the toilet, to prevent venous congestion
- local anesthetic agents to decrease local swelling and pain
- hydrocortisone cream and suppositories to reduce edematous, prolapsed hemorrhoids, and itching
- warm sitz baths to relieve pain
- injection sclerotherapy or rubber band ligation to reduce prolapsed hemorrhoids
- hemorrhoidectomy by cauterization or excision.

Hepatitis, nonviral

Nonviral hepatitis is an inflammation of the liver that usually results from exposure to certain chemicals or drugs. Most patients recover from this illness, although a few develop fulminating hepatitis or cirrhosis.

CAUSES

Causes include:

- hepatotoxic chemicals
- hepatotoxic drugs.

PATHOPHYSIOLOGY

Various hepatotoxins—such as carbon tetrachloride, acetaminophen, trichloroethylene, poisonous mushrooms, and vinyl chloride—can cause hepatitis. After exposure to these agents, hepatic cellular necrosis, scarring, Kupffer cell hyperplasia, and infiltration by mononuclear phagocytes do occur with varying severity. Alco-

hol, anoxia, and preexisting liver disease worsen the effects of some toxins.

Drug-induced (idiosyncratic) hepatitis may begin with a hypersensitivity reaction unique to the individual, unlike toxic hepatitis, which appears to affect all exposed people indiscriminately. Possible causes of drug-induced hepatitis include niacin, halothane, sulfonamides, isoniazid, acetaminophen, methyldopa, and phenothiazines (cholestasis-induced hepatitis). Symptoms of hepatic dysfunction can appear at any time during or after exposure to these drugs, but drug-induced hepatitis usually occurs after 2 weeks of drug exposure.

SIGNS AND SYMPTOMS

Signs and symptoms include:

- anorexia, nausea, and vomiting from systemic effects of liver inflammation
- jaundice from decreased bilirubin metabolism, leading to hyperbilirubinemia
- dark urine from elevated urobilinogen
- hepatomegaly caused by inflammation
- possible abdominal pain from liver inflammation
- clay-colored stool from decreased bile in the GI tract from liver necrosis
- pruritus from jaundice and hyperbilirubinemia.

COMPLICATIONS

Complications include:

- cirrhosis
- hepatic failure.

DIAGNOSIS

- Liver enzymes, such as serum aspartate aminotransferase and alanine aminotransferase levels, are elevated.
- Total and direct bilirubin levels are elevated.
- Alkaline phosphatase levels are elevated.
- White blood cell count and eosinophil count are elevated.
- Liver biopsy identifies underlying pathology, especially infiltration with white blood cells and eosinophils.

TREATMENT

Treatment includes:

■ lavage, catharsis, or hyperventilation, depending on the route of exposure, to remove the causative agent
■ acetylcysteine as an antidote for acetaminophen poisoning
■ corticosteroid to relieve symptoms of drug-induced nonviral hepatitis.

Hepatitis, viral

Viral hepatitis is a common infection of the liver, resulting in hepatic cell destruction, necrosis, and autolysis. In most patients, hepatic cells eventually regenerate with little or no residual damage, but old age and serious underlying disorders make complications more likely. The prognosis is poor if edema and hepatic encephalopathy develop.

Five major forms of hepatitis are currently recognized:
■ Type A (infectious or short-incubation hepatitis) is most common among male homosexuals and in people with human immunodeficiency virus (HIV) infection. It's commonly spread via the fecal-oral route by the ingestion of fecal contaminants.
■ Type B (serum or long-incubation hepatitis) also is most common among HIV-positive persons. Routine screening of donor blood for the hepatitis B surface antigen has reduced the incidence of post-transfusion cases, but transmission by needles shared by drug abusers remains a major problem.
■ Type C accounts for about 20% of all viral hepatitis cases and for most post-transfusion cases.
■ Type D (delta hepatitis) is responsible for about 50% of all cases of fulminant (sudden or severe) hepatitis, which has a high mortality. Developing in 1% of patients with viral hepatitis, fulminant hepatitis causes unremitting liver failure with encephalopathy. It progresses to coma and commonly leads to death within 2 weeks. In the United States, type D occurs only in people who are frequently exposed to blood and blood products, such as I.V. drug users and hemophilia patients. Type D hepatitis is found only in patients with an acute or chronic episode of hepatitis B and requires the presence of hepatitis B surface antigen. The type D virus depends on the double-shelled type B virus to replicate. (For this reason, type D infection can't outlast a type B infection.)
■ Type E (formerly grouped with types C and D under the name non-A, non-B hepatitis) occurs primarily among patients who have recently returned from an endemic area (such as India, Africa, Asia, or Central America). It's more common in young adults and more severe in pregnant woman. (See *Viral hepatitis from A to E*, pages 332 and 333.)
■ Other types continue to be identified with growing patient populations and sophisticated laboratory identification techniques.

CAUSES
The five major forms of viral hepatitis result from infection with the causative viruses: A, B, C, D, and E.

PATHOPHYSIOLOGY
Hepatic damage is usually similar in all types of viral hepatitis. Varying degrees of cell injury and necrosis occur.

On entering the body, the virus causes hepatocyte injury and hepatocyte death, either by directly killing the cells or by activating inflammatory and immune reactions. The inflammatory and immune reactions will, in turn, injure or destroy hepatocytes by lysing the infected or neighboring cells. Later, direct antibody attack against the viral antigens causes further destruction of the infected cells. Edema and swelling in the interstitium (interspaces) lead to collapse of capillaries and decreased blood flow, tissue hypoxia, and scarring and fibrosis.

SIGNS AND SYMPTOMS
Signs and symptoms reflect the stage of the disease.

Prodromal stage
Signs and symptoms of the prodromal stage include:
■ easy fatigue and generalized malaise caused by systemic effects of liver inflammation
■ anorexia and mild weight loss caused by systemic effects of liver inflammation on the GI system

Viral hepatitis from A to E

This table compares the features of each (characterized) type of viral hepatitis. Other types are emerging.

FEATURE	HEPATITIS A	HEPATITIS B
Incubation	15 to 45 days	30 to 180 days
Onset	Acute	Insidious
Age-group most affected	Children, young adults	Any age
Transmission	Fecal-oral, sexual (especially oral-anal contact), nonpercutaneous (sexual, maternal-neonatal), percutaneous (rare)	Blood-borne; parenteral route, sexual, maternal-neonatal; virus is shed in all body fluids
Severity	Mild	Usually severe
Prognosis	Generally good	Worsens with age and debility
Progression to chronicity	None	Occasional

■ arthralgia and myalgia caused by systemic effects of liver inflammation
■ nausea and vomiting from GI effects of liver inflammation
■ changes in the senses of taste and smell related to liver inflammation
■ fever from inflammatory process
■ right upper quadrant tenderness from liver inflammation and irritation of area nerve fibers
■ dark-colored urine from urobilinogen
■ clay-colored stools from decreased bile in the GI tract.

Clinical stage
Signs and symptoms of the clinical stage include:
■ worsening of all symptoms of prodromal stage

■ itching from increased bilirubin in the blood
■ abdominal pain or tenderness from continued liver inflammation
■ jaundice from elevated bilirubin in the blood.

Recovery stage
The patient's symptoms subside and appetite returns.

COMPLICATIONS
Complications may include:
■ chronic persistent hepatitis, which may prolong recovery up to 8 months
■ chronic active hepatitis
■ cirrhosis
■ hepatic failure and death
■ primary hepatocellular carcinoma.

HEPATITIS C	HEPATITIS D	HEPATITIS E
15 to 160 days	14 to 64 days	14 to 60 days
Insidious	Acute and chronic	Acute
More common in adults	Any age	Ages 20 to 40
Blood-borne; parenteral route	Parenteral route; most persons infected with hepatitis D are also infected with hepatitis B	Primarily fecal-oral
Moderate	Can be severe and lead to fulminant hepatitis	Highly virulent with common progression to fulminant hepatitis and hepatic failure, especially in a pregnant patient
Moderate	Fair, worsens in chronic cases; can lead to chronic hepatitis D and chronic liver disease	Good unless patient is pregnant
10% to 50% of cases	Occasional	None

DIAGNOSIS

■ Hepatitis profile study identifies antibodies specific to the causative virus, establishing the type of hepatitis.
■ Serum aspartate aminotransferase and alanine aminotransferase levels are increased in the prodromal stage.
■ Serum alkaline phosphatase level is slightly increased
■ Serum bilirubin level may remain high into late disease, especially in severe cases.
■ Prothrombin time is prolonged (greater than 3 seconds longer than normal indicates severe liver damage)
■ White blood cell counts reveal transient neutropenia and lymphopenia followed by lymphocytosis.
■ Liver biopsy confirms suspicion of chronic hepatitis.

TREATMENT

Treatment may include:
■ rest to minimize energy demands
■ avoiding alcohol or other drugs, to prevent further hepatic damage
■ diet therapy with small, high-calorie meals to combat anorexia
■ parenteral nutrition if the patient can't eat because of persistent vomiting
■ vaccination of the patient against hepatitis A and B to provide immunity to these viruses before transmission occurs.

Hirschsprung's disease

Hirschsprung's disease, also called *congenital megacolon* and *congenital aganglionic megacolon,* is a congenital disorder of the large intestine, characterized by the absence or marked reduction of parasympathetic ganglion cells in the colorectal wall.

Hirschsprung's disease appears in 1 in 2,000 to 1 in 5,000 live births. It's up to seven times more common in males than in females (although the aganglionic segment is usually shorter in males) and is most prevalent in whites. Total aganglionosis affects both sexes equally. Females with Hirschsprung's disease are at higher risk for having affected children. This disease usually coexists with other congenital anomalies, particularly trisomy 21 and anomalies of the urinary tract such as megaloureter.

Without prompt treatment, a neonate with colonic obstruction may die within 24 hours from enterocolitis that leads to severe diarrhea and hypovolemic shock. With prompt treatment, the prognosis is good.

CAUSES
Hirschsprung's disease is caused by familial congenital defect.

PATHOPHYSIOLOGY
In Hirschsprung's disease, parasympathetic ganglion cells in the colorectal wall are absent or markedly reduced in number. The aganglionic bowel segment contracts without the reciprocal relaxation needed to propel feces forward. Impaired intestinal motility causes severe, intractable constipation. Colonic obstruction can follow, causing bowel dilation and then occlusion of surrounding blood vessels and lymphatics. The resulting mucosal edema, ischemia, and infarction draw large amounts of fluid into the bowel, causing copious amounts of liquid stool. Continued infarction and destruction of the mucosa can lead to infection and sepsis.

SIGNS AND SYMPTOMS
In the neonate, signs and symptoms include:
■ failure to pass meconium within 24 to 48 hours of birth because of inability to propel intestinal contents forward
■ bile-stained or fecal vomiting as a result of bowel obstruction
■ abdominal distention from retention of intestinal contents and bowel obstruction
■ irritability because of abdominal distention

■ feeding difficulties and failure to thrive related to retention of intestinal contents and abdominal distention
■ dehydration related to feeding difficulties and inability to ingest adequate fluids
■ overflow diarrhea because of increased water secretion into bowel with bowel obstruction.

In children, signs and symptoms include:
■ intractable constipation caused by decreased GI motility
■ abdominal distention from retention of stool
■ easily palpated fecal masses from retention of stool
■ wasted extremities (in severe cases) from impaired intestinal motility and its effects on nutrition and intake
■ loss of subcutaneous tissue (in severe cases) caused by malnutrition
■ large protuberant abdomen caused by retention of stool and the resulting changes in fluid and electrolyte homeostasis.

In adults (occurs rarely and is more prevalent in men), signs and symptoms include:
■ abdominal distention from decreased bowel motility and constipation
■ chronic intermittent constipation caused by impaired intestinal motility.

COMPLICATIONS
Complications may include:
■ bowel perforation
■ electrolyte imbalances
■ nutritional deficiencies
■ enterocolitis
■ hypovolemic shock
■ sepsis.

DIAGNOSIS
The following measures aid in diagnosis:
■ Rectal biopsy confirms diagnosis by showing the absence of ganglion cells.
■ Barium enema, used in older infants, reveals a narrowed segment of distal colon with a saw-toothed appearance and a funnel-shaped segment above it. This confirms the diagnosis and assesses the extent of intestinal involvement.

- Rectal manometry detects failure of the internal anal sphincter to relax and contract.
- Upright plain abdominal X-rays show marked colonic distention.

TREATMENT
Treatment may include:
- corrective surgery to pull the normal ganglionic segment through to the anus (usually delayed until the infant is at least 10 months old)
- daily colonic lavage to empty the bowel of the infant until the time of surgery
- temporary colostomy or ileostomy to compress the colon in instances of total bowel obstruction.

Hyperbilirubinemia
Hyperbilirubinemia, also called *neonatal jaundice,* is the result of hemolytic processes in the neonate and is marked by elevated serum bilirubin levels and mild jaundice. It can be physiologic (with jaundice the only symptom) or pathologic (resulting from an underlying disease).

Physiologic jaundice usually develops 24 to 48 hours after birth and disappears by day 7 in full-term neonates and by day 9 or 10 in premature neonates. Serum unconjugated bilirubin levels don't exceed 12 mg/dl. Pathologic jaundice may appear anytime after the first day of life and may persist beyond 7 days. Serum bilirubin levels are greater than 12 mg/dl in a full-term neonate, greater than 15 mg/dl in a premature neonate, or increase more than 5 mg/dl in 24 hours in any neonate. Physiologic jaundice is self-limiting; the course of pathologic jaundice varies, depending on the underlying cause.

CAUSES
Causes of hyperbilirubinemia may include:
- mother-neonate blood type incompatibility
- intrauterine infection (rubella, cytomegalic inclusion disease, toxoplasmosis, syphilis, and, occasionally, bacteria such as *Escherichia coli, Staphylococcus, Pseudomonas, Klebsiella, Proteus,* and *Streptococcus)*
- infection (gram-negative bacteria)
- polycythemia
- enclosed hemorrhages (bruises, subdural hematoma)
- respiratory distress syndrome (hyaline membrane disease)
- Heinz-body anemia from drugs and toxins (vitamin K_3, sodium nitrate)
- transient neonatal hypoxia
- abnormal red blood cell (RBC) morphology
- deficiencies of RBC enzymes (glucose-6-phosphate dehydrogenase, hexokinase)
- breast-feeding
- maternal diabetes
- Crigler-Najjar syndrome
- Gilbert syndrome
- herpes simplex
- pyloric stenosis
- hypothyroidism
- neonatal giant cell hepatitis
- bile duct atresia
- galactosemia
- choledochal cyst.

PATHOPHYSIOLOGY
As erythrocytes break down at the end of their neonatal life cycle, hemoglobin separates into globin (protein) and heme (iron) fragments. Heme fragments form unconjugated (indirect) bilirubin, which binds to albumin for transport to liver cells to conjugate with glucuronide, forming direct bilirubin. Because unconjugated bilirubin is fat-soluble and can't be excreted in the urine or bile, it may escape to extravascular (outside the vessel) tissue, especially fatty tissue and the brain, causing hyperbilirubinemia.

Certain drugs (such as aspirin, tranquilizers, and sulfonamides) and conditions (such as hypothermia, anoxia, hypoglycemia, and hypoalbuminemia) can disrupt conjugation and take over albumin-binding sites.

Decreased hepatic function also reduces bilirubin conjugation. Biliary obstruction or hepatitis can cause hyperbilirubinemia by blocking normal bile flow.

Increased erythrocyte production or breakdown in hemolytic disorders or in Rh or ABO incompatibility can cause hyperbilirubinemia. Lysis releases bilirubin and stimulates cell agglutination. As a result, the liver's capacity to conjugate bilirubin becomes overloaded.

Finally, maternal enzymes in breast milk may inhibit the infant's glucuronyl-transferase conjugating activity.

SIGNS AND SYMPTOMS

Signs and symptoms include jaundice caused by the escape of unconjugated bilirubin to extravascular tissue (primary sign of hyperbilirubinemia).

COMPLICATIONS

Complications include:
- kernicterus
- cerebral palsy, epilepsy, or mental retardation
- perceptual-motor disabilities and learning disorders.

DIAGNOSIS

- Jaundice and elevated serum bilirubin levels confirm the diagnosis.
- A detailed patient history (including prenatal history), family history (paternal Rh factor, inherited red cell defects), present neonate status (prematurity, infection), and blood testing of infant and mother (blood group incompatibilities, hemoglobin levels, direct Coombs' test, hematocrit) help identify the underlying cause.

TREATMENT

Treatment may include:
- phototherapy (treatment of choice for physiologic jaundice and pathologic jaundice caused by erythroblastosis fetalis, after the initial exchange transfusion) with fluorescent lights to decompose bilirubin in the skin by oxidation (usually discontinued after bilirubin levels fall below 10 mg/dl and continue to decrease for 24 hours)
- exchange transfusion to replace the neonate's blood with fresh blood (less then 48 hours old), removing some of the unconjugated bilirubin in serum; indicated for conditions such as hydrops fetalis, polycythemia, erythroblastosis fetalis; marked reticulocytosis, drug toxicity, and jaundice that develops in the first 6 hours after birth

- albumin administration to provide additional albumin for binding unconjugated bilirubin
- phenobarbital administration (rare) to the mother before delivery and to the neonate several days after delivery to stimulate the hepatic glucuronide-conjugating system.

Inguinal hernia

A hernia occurs when part of an internal organ protrudes through an abnormal opening in the wall of the cavity that surrounds it. Most hernias occur in the abdominal cavity. Although many kinds of abdominal hernias are possible, inguinal hernias (also called *ruptures*) are most common. (See *Common sites of hernia*.) Inguinal hernias may be direct or indirect. Indirect are more common; they may develop at any age, are three times more common in males, and are especially prevalent in infants.

CAUSES

Causes include:
- *indirect*—weakness in fascial margin of internal inguinal ring
- *direct*—weakness in fascial floor of inguinal canal
- *either*—weak abdominal muscles (caused by congenital malformation, trauma, or aging) or increased intra-abdominal pressure (caused by heavy lifting, pregnancy, obesity, or straining).

PATHOPHYSIOLOGY

In an inguinal hernia, the large or small intestine, omentum, or bladder protrudes into the inguinal canal. In an indirect hernia, abdominal viscera leave the abdomen through the inguinal ring and follow the spermatic cord (in males) or round ligament (in females); they emerge at the external ring and extend down into the inguinal canal, often into the scrotum or labia.

In a direct inguinal hernia, instead of entering the canal through the internal ring, the hernia passes through the posterior inguinal wall, protrudes directly through the transverse fascia of the canal (in an area known as Hesselbach's triangle), and comes out at the external ring.

Common sites of hernia

The four common sites of hernia are umbilical, incisional, inguinal, and femoral. Below are descriptions of each type with an illustration demonstrating where each type is located.

UMBILICAL
Umbilical hernia results from abnormal muscular structures around the umbilical cord. This hernia is quite common in neonates, but also occurs in women who are obese or who have had several pregnancies. Because most umbilical hernias in neonates close spontaneously, surgery is warranted only if the hernia persists for longer than 5 years. Taping or binding the affected area or supporting it with a truss may relieve symptoms until the hernia closes. A severe congenital umbilical hernia allows the abdominal viscera to protrude outside the body. This condition requires immediate repair.

INCISIONAL
Incisional hernia (ventral) develops at the site of previous surgery, usually along vertical incisions. This hernia may result from a weakness in the abdominal wall, perhaps as a result of an infection or impaired wound healing. Inadequate nutrition, extreme abdominal distention, or obesity also predispose a person to incisional hernia. Palpation of an incisional hernia may reveal several defects in the surgical scar. Effective repair requires pulling the layers of the abdominal wall together without creating tension. If this isn't possible, surgical reconstruction uses Teflon, Marlex mesh, or tantalum mesh to close the opening.

INGUINAL
Inguinal hernia can be direct or indirect. A direct inguinal hernia results from a weakness in the fascial floor of the inguinal canal. An indirect inguinal hernia causes the abdominal viscera to protrude through the inguinal ring and follow the spermatic cord (in males) or round ligament (in females).

FEMORAL
Femoral hernia occurs where the femoral artery passes into the femoral canal. Typically, a fatty deposit within the femoral canal enlarges and eventually creates a hole big enough to accommodate part of the peritoneum and bladder. A femoral hernia appears as a swelling or bulge at the pulse point of the large femoral artery. It's usually a soft, pliable, reducible, nontender mass but commonly becomes incarcerated or strangulated.

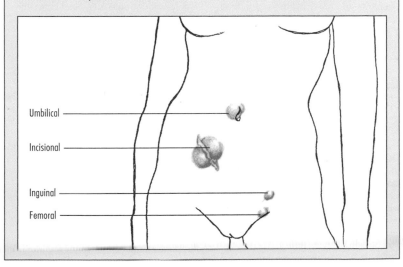

Umbilical

Incisional

Inguinal

Femoral

In a neonate, an inguinal hernia commonly coexists with an unde-scended testicle or hydrocele. In males, dur-ing the seventh month of gestation, the tes-ticle normally descends into the scrotum, preceded by the peritoneal sac. If the sac closes improperly, it leaves an opening through which the intestine can protrude.

Hernias can be reduced (if the hernia can be manipulated back into place with relative ease), incarcerated (if the hernia can't be reduced because adhesions have formed, obstructing the intestinal flow), or strangulated (part of the herniated intes-tine becomes twisted or edematous, seri-ously interfering with normal blood flow and peristalsis and, possibly, leading to in-testinal obstruction and necrosis).

SIGNS AND SYMPTOMS
Signs and symptoms of hernia include:
- A lump that appears over the herniated area when the patient stands or strains; it disappears when the patient is supine.
- Tension on the herniated contents may cause a sharp, steady pain in the groin, which fades when the hernia is reduced.
- Strangulation produces severe pain and may lead to partial or complete bowel ob-struction and even intestinal necrosis.
- Partial bowel obstruction may cause anorexia, vomiting, pain and tenderness in the groin, an irreducible mass, and dimin-ished bowel sounds.
- Complete obstruction may cause shock, high fever, absent bowel sounds, and bloody stools.

COMPLICATIONS
Complications may include:
- strangulation
- intestinal obstruction
- infection (after surgery).

DIAGNOSIS
In a patient with a large hernia, physical examination reveals an obvious swelling or lump in the inguinal area. In the patient with a small hernia, the affected area may simply appear full. Palpation of the in-guinal area while the patient is performing Valsalva's maneuver confirms the diagno-sis. To detect a hernia in a male patient, ask the patient to stand with his ipsilateral leg (on the same side as the hernia) slightly flexed and his weight resting on the other leg. Insert your index finger into the lower part of the scrotum and invaginate the scrotal skin so the finger advances through the external inguinal ring to the internal ring (about ½″ to 2″ [1 to 5 cm] through the inguinal canal). Tell the patient to cough. If the examiner feels pressure against the fingertip, an indirect hernia ex-ists; if pressure is felt against the side of the finger, a direct hernia exists.

A history of sharp or "catching" pain when lifting or straining may help confirm the diagnosis. Suspected bowel obstruc-tion requires X-rays and a white blood cell count (may be elevated).

TREATMENT
If the hernia is reducible, the pain may be temporarily relieved by pushing the hernia back into place. A truss may keep the ab-dominal contents from protruding into the hernial sac, although it won't cure the hernia. This device is especially beneficial for an elderly or debilitated patient for whom surgery might be hazardous.

For neonates, adults, and otherwise healthy elderly patients, herniorrhaphy is the treatment of choice. Herniorrhaphy replaces the contents of the hernial sac into the abdominal cavity and closes the opening. In many cases, this procedure is performed under local anesthesia in a short-procedure unit or as a single-day ad-mission. Another effective surgical proce-dure for repairing a hernia is hernioplasty, which reinforces the weakened area with steel mesh, fascia, or wire.

A strangulated or necrotic hernia neces-sitates bowel resection. Rarely, an extensive resection may require temporary colosto-my. In either case, bowel resection length-ens postoperative recovery and requires antibiotics, parenteral fluids, and elec-trolyte replacement.

Intestinal obstruction
Intestinal obstruction is the partial or complete blockage of the lumen in the small or large bowel. Small-bowel obstruc-

Paralytic ileus

Paralytic ileus is a physiologic form of intestinal obstruction that develops in the small bowel most commonly after abdominal surgery. It causes decreased or absent intestinal motility that usually corrects itself spontaneously after about 3 days. Clinical effects of paralytic ileus include severe abdominal distention, extreme distress and, possibly, vomiting. The patient may be severely constipated or may pass flatus and small liquid stools.

CAUSES

This condition can develop as a response to trauma, toxemia, or peritonitis or as a result of electrolyte deficiencies (especially hypokalemia) and the use of certain drugs, such as ganglionic blocking agents and anticholinergics. It can also result from vascular causes, such as thrombosis and embolism. Excessive air swallowing may contribute to it, but paralytic ileus brought on by this factor alone seldom lasts more than 24 hours.

TREATMENT

Paralytic ileus lasting longer than 48 hours requires intubation for decompression and nasogastric suctioning. Because of the absence of peristaltic activity, a long, weighted intestinal tube — called a *Miller-Abbott tube* — may be necessary for the patient with extraordinary abdominal distension. Such procedures must be used with extreme caution because any additional trauma to the bowel can aggravate paralytic ileus. When paralytic ileus results from surgical manipulation of the bowel, treatment may also include cholinergic agents, such as neostigmine or bethanechol.

When caring for a patient with paralytic ileus, the caregiver should warn the patient who's receiving cholinergic agents to expect certain paradoxical adverse effects, such as intestinal cramps and diarrhea. Remember that neostigmine produces cardiovascular adverse effects, usually bradycardia and hypotension. Check frequently for returning bowel sounds.

---

tion is far more common (90% of patients) and usually more serious. Complete obstruction in any part of the bowel, if untreated, can cause death within hours because of shock and vascular collapse. Intestinal obstruction is most likely to occur after abdominal surgery or in persons with congenital bowel deformities.

CAUSES

Adhesions and strangulated hernias usually cause small-bowel obstruction; large-bowel obstruction is typically caused by carcinomas. Mechanical intestinal obstruction results from foreign bodies (fruit pits, gallstones, or worms) or compression of the bowel wall from stenosis, intussusception, volvulus of the sigmoid or cecum, tumors, or atresia. Nonmechanical obstruction results from physiologic disturbances, such as paralytic ileus, electrolyte imbalances, toxicity (uremia or generalized infection), neurogenic abnormalities (spinal cord lesions), and thrombosis or embolism of mesenteric vessels. (See *Paralytic ileus.*)

PATHOPHYSIOLOGY

Intestinal obstruction develops in three forms:

- *simple*—Blockage prevents intestinal contents from passing, with no other complications.
- *strangulated*—Blood supply to part or all of the obstructed section is cut off, in addition to blockage of the lumen.
- *close-looped*—Both ends of a bowel section are occluded, isolating it from the rest of the intestine.

The physiologic effects are similar in all three forms of obstruction: When intestinal obstruction occurs, fluid, air, and gas collect near the site. Peristalsis increases temporarily as the bowel tries to force its contents through the obstruction, injuring intestinal mucosa and causing distention at and above the site of the obstruction.

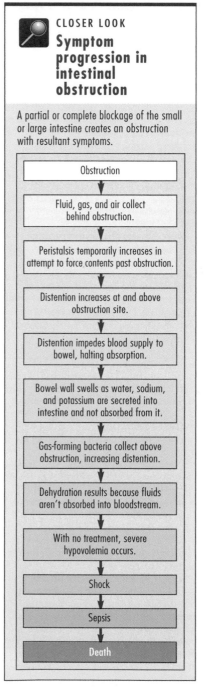

CLOSER LOOK

Symptom progression in intestinal obstruction

A partial or complete blockage of the small or large intestine creates an obstruction with resultant symptoms.

Obstruction

↓

Fluid, gas, and air collect behind obstruction.

↓

Peristalsis temporarily increases in attempt to force contents past obstruction.

↓

Distention increases at and above obstruction site.

↓

Distention impedes blood supply to bowel, halting absorption.

↓

Bowel wall swells as water, sodium, and potassium are secreted into intestine and not absorbed from it.

↓

Gas-forming bacteria collect above obstruction, increasing distention.

↓

Dehydration results because fluids aren't absorbed into bloodstream.

↓

With no treatment, severe hypovolemia occurs.

↓

Shock

↓

Sepsis

↓

Death

Distention blocks the flow of venous blood and halts normal absorptive processes; as a result, the bowel begins to secrete water, sodium, and potassium into the fluid pooled in the lumen.

Obstruction in the small intestine results in metabolic alkalosis from dehydration and loss of gastric hydrochloric acid; lower bowel obstruction causes slower dehydration and loss of intestinal alkaline fluids, resulting in metabolic acidosis. Ultimately, intestinal obstruction may lead to ischemia, necrosis, and death. (See *Symptom progression in intestinal obstruction.*)

CLINICAL ALERT
Watch for air-fluid lock syndrome in older adults who remain recumbent for extended periods. In this syndrome, fluid collects in the dependent bowel loops. Then, peristalsis is too weak to push fluid "uphill." The resulting obstruction primarily occurs in the large bowel.

SIGNS AND SYMPTOMS

Colicky pain, nausea, vomiting, constipation, and abdominal distention characterize small-bowel obstruction. It may also cause drowsiness, intense thirst, malaise, and aching and may dry up oral mucous membranes and the tongue.

Auscultation reveals bowel sounds, borborygmi (rumbling noise caused by gas being propelled through the intestine), and rushes caused by increased peristaltic activity; occasionally, these are loud enough to be heard without a stethoscope. Palpation elicits abdominal tenderness, with moderate distention; rebound tenderness occurs when obstruction has caused strangulation with ischemia. In late stages, signs of hypovolemic shock result from progressive dehydration and plasma loss.

In complete small-bowel obstruction, vigorous peristaltic waves propel bowel contents toward the mouth instead of the rectum. Spasms may occur every 3 to 5 minutes and last about 1 minute each, with persistent epigastric or periumbilical pain. Passage of small amounts of mucus and blood may occur. The higher the obstruction, the earlier and more severe the vomiting. Vomitus at first contains gastric juice, then bile, and, finally, contents of the ileum.

Symptoms of large-bowel obstruction develop more slowly because the colon can absorb fluid from its contents and distend well beyond its normal size. Constipation may be the only symptom for days. Colicky abdominal pain may then appear suddenly, producing spasms that last less than 1 minute each and recur every few minutes. Continuous hypogastric pain and nausea may develop, but vomiting is usually absent at first. Large-bowel obstruction can cause dramatic abdominal distention; loops of the large bowel may become visible on the abdomen. Eventually, complete large-bowel obstruction may cause fecal vomiting, continuous pain, or localized peritonitis.

Patients with partial obstruction may display any of the above signs and symptoms in a milder form, but leakage of liquid stool around the obstruction is common in partial obstruction.

COMPLICATIONS
Complications may include:
- perforation
- peritonitis
- septicemia
- secondary infection
- metabolic alkalosis or acidosis
- hypovolemic or septic shock
- if untreated, death.

DIAGNOSIS
Progressive, colicky, abdominal pain and distention, with or without nausea and vomiting, suggest bowel obstruction. X-rays confirm the diagnosis. Abdominal films show the presence and location of intestinal gas or fluid. In small-bowel obstruction, a typical "stepladder" pattern emerges, with alternating fluid and gas levels apparent in 3 to 4 hours. In large-bowel obstruction, barium enema reveals a distended, air-filled colon or a closed loop of sigmoid with extreme distention (in sigmoid volvulus).

Laboratory results that support this diagnosis include:
- decreased serum sodium, chloride, and potassium levels (because of vomiting)

- slightly elevated white blood cell count (in necrosis, peritonitis, or strangulation)
- increased serum amylase level (possibly from irritation of the pancreas by bowel loop).

TREATMENT
Preoperative therapy consists of correction of fluid and electrolyte imbalances, decompression of the bowel to relieve vomiting and distention, and treatment of shock and peritonitis. Strangulated obstruction usually necessitates blood replacement as well as I.V. fluid administration. Passage of a nasogastric (NG) tube, followed by use of the longer and weighted Miller-Abbott or Cantor tube, usually accomplishes decompression, especially in small-bowel obstruction.

Close monitoring of the patient's condition determines the duration of treatment; if the patient's condition doesn't improve or if his condition deteriorates, surgery is necessary. In large-bowel obstruction, surgical resection with anastomosis, colostomy, or ileostomy commonly follows decompression with an NG tube.

Total parenteral nutrition may be appropriate if the patient suffers a protein deficit from chronic obstruction, postoperative or paralytic ileus, or infection. Drug therapy includes analgesics, sedatives, and antibiotics for peritonitis caused by bowel strangulation or infarction.

Irritable bowel syndrome

Also referred to as *spastic colon* or *spastic colitis,* irritable bowel syndrome (IBS) is marked by chronic symptoms of abdominal pain, alternating constipation and diarrhea, excess flatus, a sense of incomplete bowel movement, and abdominal distention. IBS is a common, stress-related disorder, but 20% of persons with IBS never seek medical attention. IBS is a benign condition that has no anatomical abnormality or inflammatory component. It occurs in women twice as often as in men.

CAUSES
Causes include:
- psychological stress (most common cause)

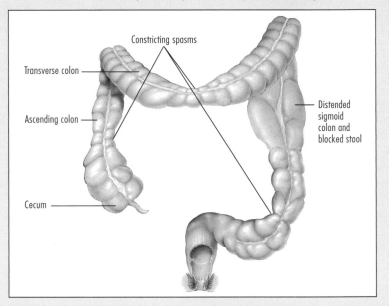

CLOSER LOOK
What happens in irritable bowel syndrome

Typically, the patient with irritable bowel syndrome (IBS) has a normal-appearing GI tract, but careful examination of the colon may reveal functional irritability — an abnormality in colonic smooth-muscle function marked by excessive peristalsis and spasms, even during remission.

Constricting spasms

Transverse colon

Ascending colon

Distended sigmoid colon and blocked stool

Cecum

INTESTINAL FUNCTION

To understand what happens in IBS, consider how smooth muscle controls bowel function. Normally, segmental muscle contractions mix intestinal contents while peristalsis propels the contents through the GI tract. Motor activity is most propulsive in the proximal (nearer the stomach) and the distal (sigmoid colon) portions of the intestines. Activity in the rest of the intestines is slower, permitting nutrient and water absorption.

In IBS, the autonomic nervous system, which innervates the large intestine, doesn't cause the alternating contractions and relaxations that propel stools smoothly toward the rectum.

The result is constipation or diarrhea or both.

Constipation

Some patients have spasmodic intestinal contractions that set up a partial obstruction by trapping gas and stools. This causes distention, bloating, gas pain, and constipation.

Diarrhea

Other patients have dramatically increased intestinal motility. Eating or cholinergic stimulation triggers a rush of the small intestine's contents into the large intestine, dumping watery stools and irritating the mucosa. The result is diarrhea.

Mixed symptoms

If further spasms trap liquid stools, the intestinal mucosa absorbs water from the stools, leaving them dry, hard, and difficult to pass. The result: a pattern of alternating diarrhea and constipation.

- ingestion of irritants (coffee, raw fruit, or vegetables)
- lactose intolerance
- abuse of laxatives
- hormonal changes (menstruation).

PATHOPHYSIOLOGY
IBS appears to reflect motor disturbances of the entire colon in response to stimuli. Some muscles of the small bowel are particularly sensitive to motor abnormalities and distention; others are particularly sensitive to certain foods and drugs. The patient may be hypersensitive to the hormones gastrin and cholecystokinin. The pain of IBS seems to be caused by abnormally strong contractions of the intestinal smooth muscle as it reacts to distention, irritants, or stress. (See *What happens in irritable bowel syndrome.*)

SIGNS AND SYMPTOMS
Signs and symptoms include:
- crampy lower abdominal pain from muscle contraction; usually occurs during the day and is relieved by defecation or passage of flatus
- pain that intensifies 1 to 2 hours after a meal from irritation of nerve fibers by the causative stimulus
- constipation alternating with diarrhea, with one dominant; caused by motor disturbances from the causative stimulus
- mucus passed through the rectum from altered secretion in intestinal lumen caused by motor abnormalities
- abdominal distention and bloating from flatus and constipation.

COMPLICATIONS
Complications include:
- fluid and electrolyte imbalances resulting from persistent diarrhea.

DIAGNOSIS
- Careful examination reveals contributing psychological factors such as a recent stressful life change.
- Stool samples for ova, parasites, bacteria, and blood rule out infection.
- Lactose intolerance test rules out lactose intolerance.
- Barium enema may reveal colon spasm and tubular appearance of descending colon without evidence of cancers or diverticulosis.
- Sigmoidoscopy or colonoscopy may reveal spastic contractions without evidence of colon cancer or inflammatory bowel disease.
- Rectal biopsy rules out malignancy.

TREATMENT
Treatment may include:
- stress-relief measures, including counseling or mild anxiolytics
- investigation, identification, and avoidance of food irritants
- application of heat to abdomen
- bulking agents to reduce episodes of diarrhea and minimize effect of nonpropulsive colonic contractions
- antispasmodics (propantheline or diphenoxylate with atropine sulfate) for pain
- loperamide to reduce urgency and fecal soiling in persistent diarrhea
- bowel training (if the cause of IBS is chronic laxative abuse) to regain muscle control.

Liver failure
Liver failure can be the end result of any liver disease. The liver performs more than 100 separate functions in the body. When the liver fails, a complex syndrome involving the impairment of many different organs and body functions begins. (See *Functions of the liver,* page 344.) Hepatic encephalopathy and hepatorenal syndrome are two conditions that occur in liver failure. The only cure for liver failure is a liver transplant.

CAUSES
Causes include:
- viral hepatitis
- nonviral hepatitis
- cirrhosis
- liver cancer.

PATHOPHYSIOLOGY
Conditions of liver failure include hepatic encephalopathy and hepatorenal syndrome.
Hepatic encephalopathy—a set of central nervous system disorders—results when the liver can no longer detoxify the

Functions of the liver

The liver is one of the most essential organs of the body. To understand how liver disease affects the body, it's best to understand its main functions:

◆ detoxifies poisonous chemicals, including alcohol, beer, wine, and drugs (prescribed and over-the-counter drugs as well as illegal substances)
◆ makes bile to help digest food
◆ stores energy by stockpiling sugar (carbohydrates, glucose, and fat) until needed
◆ stores iron reserves as well as vitamins and minerals
◆ manufactures new proteins
◆ produces important plasma proteins necessary for blood coagulation, including prothrombin and fibrinogen
◆ serves as a site for hematopoiesis during fetal development.

blood. Liver dysfunction and collateral vessels that shunt blood around the liver to the systemic circulation let toxins absorbed from the GI tract circulate freely to the brain. Ammonia, a by-product of protein metabolism, is one of the main toxins causing hepatic encephalopathy. The normal liver changes ammonia to urea, which the kidneys excrete. When the liver fails and can no longer change ammonia to urea, blood ammonia levels rise and the ammonia is delivered to the brain. Short-chain fatty acids, serotonin, tryptophan, and false neurotransmitters may also accumulate in the blood and contribute to hepatic encephalopathy.

Hepatorenal syndrome is kidney failure concurrent with liver disease; the kidneys appear to be normal but suddenly stop functioning. The syndrome causes an increase in blood volume, accumulation of hydrogen ions, and electrolyte disturbances. It's most common in patients with alcoholic cirrhosis or fulminating hepatitis. The cause may be the accumulation of vasoactive substances that cause inappropriate constriction of renal arterioles, leading to decreased glomerular filtration and

oliguria (diminished amount of urine in relation to fluid intake). The vasoconstriction may also be a compensatory response to portal hypertension and the pooling of blood in the splenic circulation.

SIGNS AND SYMPTOMS
Signs and symptoms include:
■ jaundice from the failure of the liver to conjugate bilirubin
■ abdominal pain or tenderness from liver inflammation
■ nausea and anorexia from systemic effects of inflammation
■ fatigue and weight loss from failure of hepatic metabolism
■ pruritus because of the accumulation of bilirubin in the skin
■ oliguria caused by constriction of the arterioles in the kidneys
■ splenomegaly because of portal hypertension
■ ascites caused by portal hypertension and decreased plasma proteins
■ peripheral edema from the accumulation of retained fluid caused by decreased plasma protein production and loss of albumin with ascites
■ varices of the esophagus, rectum, and abdominal wall caused by portal hypertension
■ bleeding tendencies because of thrombocytopenia (from blood accumulation in the spleen) and prolonged prothrombin time (caused by the impaired production of coagulation factors)
■ petechiae resulting from thrombocytopenia
■ amenorrhea caused by altered steroid hormone production and metabolism
■ gynecomastia in males from estrogen buildup caused by failure of hepatic biotransformation functions.

COMPLICATIONS
Complications include:
■ variceal bleeding
■ GI hemorrhage
■ coma
■ death.

DIAGNOSIS
■ Liver function tests reveal elevated levels of aspartate aminotransferase, alanine

aminotransferase, alkaline phosphatase, and bilirubin.

- Blood studies reveal anemia, impaired production of red blood cell, elevated bleeding and clotting times, low blood glucose levels, and increased serum ammonia levels.
- Urine osmolarity is increased.

TREATMENT

Treatment may include:
- liver transplantation
- low-protein, high-carbohydrate diet to correct nutritional deficiencies and prevent overtaxing the liver
- lactulose to reduce ammonia blood levels and help alleviate some symptoms of hepatic encephalopathy.

For ascites, treatment includes:
- salt restriction and potassium-sparing diuretics to increase water excretion
- potassium supplements to reverse the effects of high aldosterone level
- paracentesis to remove ascitic fluid and relieve abdominal discomfort
- shunt placement to help remove ascitic fluid and relieve abdominal discomfort.

For portal hypertension, treatment includes:
- shunt placement between the portal vein and another systemic vein to divert blood flow and relieve pressure.

For variceal bleeding, treatment includes:
- vasoconstrictor drugs to decrease blood flow
- balloon tamponade to control bleeding by exerting pressure on the varices using a balloon catheter
- surgery to tie off bleeding collateral veins sprouting from the portal vein
- vitamin K to control bleeding by decreasing prothrombin time.

Malabsorption

Malabsorption is failure of the intestinal mucosa to absorb single or multiple nutrients efficiently. Absorption of amino acids, fat, sugar, or vitamins may be impaired. The result is inadequate movement of nutrients from the small intestine to the bloodstream or lymphatic system. Signs and symptoms depend primarily on the substance being malabsorbed.

CAUSES

A wide variety of disorders result in malabsorption. (See *Causes of malabsorption,* page 346.)

Causes may include:
- prior gastric surgery
- pancreatic disorders
- hepatobiliary disease
- disease of the small intestine such as celiac disease
- hereditary disorder
- drug toxicity.

PATHOPHYSIOLOGY

The small intestine's inability to absorb nutrients efficiently may result from a variety of disease processes. The mechanism of malabsorption depends on the cause. Some common causes of malabsorption syndrome include celiac disease, lactase deficiency, gastrectomy, Zollinger-Ellison syndrome, and bacterial overgrowth in the duodenal stump.

In celiac sprue, dietary gluten — a product of wheat, barley, rye, and oats — is toxic to the patient, causing injury to the mucosal villi. The mucosa appear flat and have lost absorptive surface. Symptoms usually disappear when gluten is removed from the diet.

Lactase deficiency is a disaccharide deficiency syndrome. Lactase is an intestinal enzyme that splits nonabsorbable lactose (a disaccharide) into the absorbable monosaccharides glucose and galactose. Production may be deficient, or another intestinal disease may inhibit the enzyme.

After gastrectomy, poor mixing of chyme with gastric secretions may cause malabsorption.

In Zollinger-Ellison syndrome, increased acidity in the duodenum inhibits release of cholecystokinin, which stimulates pancreatic enzyme secretion. Pancreatic enzyme deficiency leads to decreased breakdown of nutrients and malabsorption.

Bacterial overgrowth in the duodenal stump (loop created in the Billroth II procedure) causes malabsorption of vitamin B_{12}.

SIGNS AND SYMPTOMS

Signs and symptoms include:

Causes of malabsorption

Many disorders — from systemic to organ-specific diseases — may give rise to malabsorption.

DISEASES OF THE SMALL INTESTINE
Primary small bowel disease
- Bacterial overgrowth caused by stasis in afferent loop after Billroth II gastrectomy
- Massive bowel resection
- Nontropical sprue (celiac disease)
- Regional enteritis
- Tropical sprue

Ischemic small bowel disease
- Chronic heart failure
- Mesenteric atherosclerosis

Small bowel infections and infestations
- Acute enteritis
- Giardiasis

Systemic disease involving small bowel
- Amyloidosis
- Lymphoma
- Sarcoidosis
- Scleroderma
- Whipple's disease

DRUG-INDUCED MALABSORPTION
- Calcium carbonate
- Neomycin

HEPATOBILIARY DISEASE
- Biliary fistula
- Biliary tract obstruction
- Cirrhosis and hepatitis

HEREDITARY DISORDER
- Primary lactase deficiency

PANCREATIC DISORDERS
- Chronic pancreatitis
- Cystic fibrosis
- Pancreatic cancer
- Pancreatic resection
- Zollinger-Ellison syndrome

PREVIOUS GASTRIC SURGERY
- Billroth II gastrectomy
- Pyloroplasty
- Total gastrectomy
- Vagotomy

- weight loss and generalized malnutrition from impaired absorption of carbohydrate, fat, and protein
- diarrhea from decreased absorption of fluids, electrolytes, bile acids, and fatty acids in the colon
- steatorrhea from decreased absorption of fat in the colon leading to excess fat in the stool
- flatulence and abdominal distention caused by fermentation of undigested lactose
- nocturia from delayed absorption of water
- weakness and fatigue from anemia and electrolyte depletion from diarrhea
- edema caused by impaired absorption of amino acids, resulting in protein depletion and hypoproteinemia
- amenorrhea caused by protein depletion leading to hypopituitarism
- anemia because of the impaired absorption of iron, folic acid, and vitamin B_{12}
- glossitis, cheilosis from a deficiency of iron, folic acid, vitamin B_{12}, and other vitamins
- peripheral neuropathy caused by a deficiency of vitamin B_{12} and thiamine
- bruising, bleeding tendency caused by vitamin K malabsorption and hypoprothrombinemia
- bone pain, skeletal deformities, fractures because of calcium malabsorption that leads to hypocalcemia; protein depletion leading to osteoporosis; and vitamin D malabsorption causing impaired calcium absorption
- tetany, paresthesias resulting from calcium malabsorption, leading to hypocalcemia; and magnesium malabsorption, leading to hypomagnesemia and hypokalemia.

COMPLICATIONS

Complications include:
- fractures
- anemias
- bleeding disorders
- tetany
- malnutrition.

DIAGNOSIS

Useful tests and their results include:
- Stool specimen for fat reveals excretion of greater than 6 g of fat per day.
- D-xylose absorption test shows less than 20% of 25 g of D-xylose in the urine after 5 hours (reflects disorders of proximal bowel).
- Schilling test reveals deficiency of vitamin B_{12} absorption.
- Culture of duodenal and jejunal contents confirms bacterial overgrowth in the proximal bowel.
- GI barium studies show characteristic features of the small intestine.
- Small intestine biopsy reveals the atrophy of mucosal villi.

TREATMENT

Treatment includes:
- identification of cause and appropriate correction
- gluten-free diet to stop progression of celiac disease and malabsorption
- lactose-free diet to treat lactase deficiency
- dietary supplementation to replace nutrient deficiencies
- vitamin B_{12} injections to treat vitamin B_{12} deficiency.

Pancreatitis

Pancreatitis, inflammation of the pancreas, may be acute or chronic. In men, this disease is commonly linked to alcoholism, trauma, or peptic ulcer; in women, to biliary tract disease. The prognosis is good for pancreatitis linked to biliary tract disease but poor when linked to alcoholism. Mortality is as high as 60% when pancreatitis is linked to necrosis and hemorrhage.

CAUSES

Causes include:
- biliary tract disease
- alcoholism
- abnormal organ structure
- metabolic or endocrine disorders, such as high cholesterol levels or overactive thyroid
- pancreatic cysts or tumors
- penetrating peptic ulcers
- blunt trauma or surgical trauma
- drugs, such as glucocorticoids, sulfonamides, thiazides, hormonal contraceptives, and nonsteroidal anti-inflammatory drugs
- kidney failure or transplantation
- endoscopic examination of the bile ducts and pancreas.

PATHOPHYSIOLOGY

Acute pancreatitis occurs in two forms: edematous (interstitial) and necrotizing (hemorrhagic). Edematous pancreatitis causes fluid accumulation and swelling. Necrotizing pancreatitis causes cell death and tissue damage. The inflammation that occurs with both types is caused by premature activation of enzymes, which causes tissue damage. Enzymes back up and spill out into the pancreatic tissue resulting in autodigestion of the pancreas.

Normally, the acini in the pancreas secrete enzymes in an inactive form. Two theories explain why enzymes become prematurely activated.

In one view, a toxic agent such as alcohol alters the way the pancreas secretes enzymes. Alcohol probably increases pancreatic secretion, alters the metabolism of the acinar cells, and encourages duct obstruction by causing pancreatic secretory proteins to precipitate.

Another theory is that a reflux of duodenal contents containing activated enzymes enters the pancreatic duct, activating other enzymes and setting up a cycle of more pancreatic damage.

In chronic pancreatitis, persistent inflammation produces irreversible changes in the structure and function of the pancreas. It sometimes follows an episode of acute pancreatitis. Protein precipitates block the pancreatic duct and eventually harden or calcify. Structural changes lead to fibrosis and atrophy of the glands. Growths called pseudocysts contain pancreatic enzymes and tissue debris.

An abscess results if pseudocysts become infected.

CLINICAL ALERT
Pancreatitis that damages the islets of Langerhans may lead to diabetes mellitus. Sudden severe pancreatitis may cause massive hemorrhage and total destruction of the pancreas, resulting in diabetic acidosis, shock, or coma.

SIGNS AND SYMPTOMS

Signs and symptoms include:
- midepigastric abdominal pain, which can radiate to the back, caused by the escape of inflammatory exudate and enzymes into the back of the peritoneum; edema and distention of the pancreatic capsule; and obstruction of the biliary tract
- persistent vomiting (in a severe attack) from hypermotility or paralytic ileus caused by pancreatitis or peritonitis
- abdominal distention (in a severe attack) from bowel hypermotility and the accumulation of fluids in the abdominal cavity
- diminished bowel activity (in severe attack) suggesting altered motility caused by peritonitis
- crackles at lung bases (in a severe attack) caused by heart failure
- left pleural effusion (in a severe attack) from circulating pancreatic enzymes
- mottled skin from hemorrhagic necrosis of the pancreas
- tachycardia caused by dehydration and possible hypovolemia
- low-grade fever resulting from the inflammatory response
- cold, sweaty extremities caused by cardiovascular collapse
- restlessness related to pain from acute pancreatitis
- extreme malaise (in chronic pancreatitis) related to malabsorption or diabetes.

COMPLICATIONS

Complications include:
- massive hemorrhage and shock
- pseudocysts
- biliary and duodenal obstruction
- portal and splenic vein thrombosis
- diabetes mellitus
- respiratory failure.

DIAGNOSIS

The following tests and results may aid or confirm diagnosis:
- Elevated serum amylase and lipase levels (confirm diagnosis).
- Blood and urine glucose tests reveal transient glucose in urine and hyperglycemia. In chronic pancreatitis, serum glucose levels may be transiently elevated.
- White blood cell count is elevated.
- Serum bilirubin levels are elevated in both acute and chronic pancreatitis.
- Blood calcium levels may be decreased.
- Stool analysis shows elevated lipid and trypsin levels in chronic pancreatitis.
- Abdominal and chest X-rays detect pleural effusions and differentiate pancreatitis from diseases that cause similar symptoms; may detect pancreatic calculi.
- Computed tomography scan and ultrasonography show enlarged pancreas with cysts and pseudocysts.
- Endoscopic retrograde cholangiopancreatography identifies ductal system abnormalities, such as calcification or strictures; helps differentiate pancreatitis from other disorders such as pancreatic cancer.

TREATMENT

Treatment may include:
- I.V. replacement of fluids, protein, and electrolytes to treat shock
- fluid volume replacement to help correct metabolic acidosis
- blood transfusions to replace blood loss from hemorrhage
- withholding of food and fluids to rest the pancreas and reduce pancreatic enzyme secretion
- nasogastric tube suctioning to decrease stomach distention and suppress pancreatic secretions
- antiemetics to reduce nausea and vomiting
- meperidine to relieve abdominal pain
- antacids to neutralize gastric secretions
- histamine antagonists to decrease hydrochloric acid production
- antibiotics to fight bacterial infections
- anticholinergics to reduce vagal stimulation, decrease GI motility, and inhibit pancreatic enzyme secretion
- insulin to correct hyperglycemia

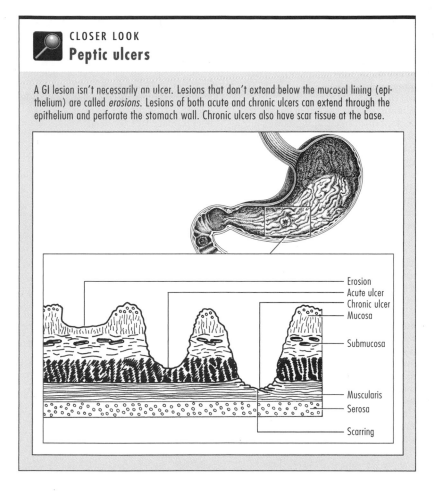

CLOSER LOOK
Peptic ulcers

A GI lesion isn't necessarily an ulcer. Lesions that don't extend below the mucosal lining (epithelium) are called *erosions*. Lesions of both acute and chronic ulcers can extend through the epithelium and perforate the stomach wall. Chronic ulcers also have scar tissue at the base.

Erosion
Acute ulcer
Chronic ulcer
Mucosa

Submucosa

Muscularis
Serosa

Scarring

- surgical drainage to treat a pancreatic abscess or pseudocyst or to reestablish drainage of the pancreas
- laparotomy (if biliary tract obstruction causes acute pancreatitis) to remove obstruction.

Peptic ulcers

Peptic ulcers, circumscribed lesions in the mucosal membrane extending below the epithelium, can develop in the lower esophagus, stomach, pylorus, duodenum, or jejunum. Although erosions are often referred to as ulcers, erosions are breaks in the mucosal membranes that don't extend below the epithelium. Ulcers may be acute

or chronic in nature. A chronic ulcer is identified by scar tissue at its base. (See *Peptic ulcers.*)

About 80% of all peptic ulcers are duodenal ulcers, which affect the proximal part of the small intestine and occur most commonly in men ages 20 to 50. Duodenal ulcers usually follow a chronic course with remissions and exacerbations; 5% to 10% of patients develop complications that necessitate surgery.

Gastric ulcers are most common in middle-aged and elderly men, especially in chronic users of nonsteroidal anti-inflammatory drugs (NSAIDs), alcohol, or tobacco.

CAUSES
Causes include:
- *Helicobacter pylori* infection
- use of NSAIDs
- pathologic hypersecretory disorders.

PATHOPHYSIOLOGY
Although the stomach contains acidic secretions that can digest substances, intrinsic defenses protect the gastric mucosal membrane from injury. A thick, tenacious layer of gastric mucus protects the stomach from autodigestion, mechanical trauma, and chemical trauma. Prostaglandins provide another line of defense. Gastric ulcers may be a result of destruction of the mucosal barrier.

The duodenum is protected from ulceration by the function of Brunner's glands. These glands produce a viscid, mucoid, alkaline secretion that neutralizes the acid chyme. Duodenal ulcers appear to result from excessive acid protection.

H. pylori releases a toxin that destroys the gastric and duodenal mucosa, reducing the epithelium's resistance to acid digestion and causing gastritis and ulcer disease.

Salicylates and other NSAIDs inhibit the secretion of prostaglandins (substances that block ulceration). Certain illnesses, such as pancreatitis, hepatic disease, Crohn's disease, preexisting gastritis, and Zollinger-Ellison syndrome also contribute to ulceration.

Besides peptic ulcer's main causes, several predisposing factors are acknowledged. They include blood type (gastric ulcers and type A; duodenal ulcers and type O) and other genetic factors. Exposure to irritants, such as alcohol, coffee, and tobacco, may contribute by accelerating gastric acid emptying and promoting mucosal breakdown. Emotional stress also contributes to ulcer formation because of increased stimulation of acid and pepsin secretion and decreased mucosal defense. Physical trauma and normal aging are additional predisposing conditions.

SIGNS AND SYMPTOMS
Symptoms vary by the type of ulcer. A gastric ulcer produces the following signs and symptoms:

- pain that worsens with eating because of stretching of the mucosa by food
- nausea and anorexia caused by mucosal stretching.

A duodenal ulcer produces the following signs and symptoms:
- epigastric pain that's gnawing, dull, aching, or hunger-like because of excessive acid production
- pain relieved by food or antacids (but usually recurring 2 to 4 hours later) because of food acting as a buffer for acid.

COMPLICATIONS
Complications include:
- hemorrhage
- shock
- gastric perforation
- gastric outlet obstruction.

DIAGNOSIS
The following tests are useful for diagnosis:
- Barium swallow or upper GI and small bowel series may reveal the presence of the ulcer. This is the first test performed on a patient when symptoms aren't severe.
- Esophagogastroduodenoscopy confirms the presence of an ulcer and permits cytologic studies and biopsy to rule out *H. pylori* or cancer.
- X-rays of the upper GI tract reveal mucosal abnormalities.
- Stool analysis may reveal occult blood.
- Serologic testing may disclose signs of infection, such as elevated white blood cell count.
- Gastric secretory studies show hyperchlorhydria.
- Urea breath test results reflect activity of *H. pylori*.

TREATMENT
Treatment may include:
- antimicrobial agents (tetracycline, bismuth subsalicylate, and metronidazole) to eradicate *H. pylori* infection (see *Treating peptic ulcers,* pages 352 and 353)
- misoprostol (a prostaglandin analog) to inhibit gastric acid secretion and increase carbonate and mucus production, to protect the stomach lining

POLYPS, INTESTINAL ◆ **351**

- antacids to neutralize acid gastric contents by elevating the gastric pH, thus protecting the mucosa and relieving pain
- avoiding caffeine and alcohol, to reduce stimulation of gastric acid secretion
- anticholinergic drugs to inhibit the effect of the vagal nerve on acid-secreting cells
- histamine-2 blockers to reduce acid secretion
- sucralfate, a mucosal protectant to form an acid-impermeable membrane that adheres to the mucous membrane and also accelerates mucus production
- proton gastric acid pump inhibitor (omeprazole) to decrease gastric acid secretion
- dietary therapy with small, frequent meals and avoidance of eating before bedtime to reduce gastric acid secretion
- insertion of a nasogastric tube (in those with GI bleeding) for gastric decompression and rest and, also, to permit iced saline lavage that may contain norepinephrine
- gastroscopy to allow visualization of a bleeding site; coagulation by laser or cautery to control bleeding
- surgery to repair perforation; to treat if conservative treatment is ineffective; or when malignancy is suspected.

Polyps, intestinal

A polyp is a small, tumorlike growth that projects from a mucous membrane surface. Polyps may develop in the colon or rectum, where they protrude into the GI tract. Polyps are classified according to tissue type. Common polyp types include:
- adenomatous polyps, such as tubular adenoma, tubulovillous adenoma, and villous adenoma
- nonadenomatous polyps, such as hyperplastic polyps, inflammatory polyps, and juvenile polyps.

Polyposis syndromes include familial adenomatous polyposis, hamartomatous polyposis syndromes, and acquired polyposis syndromes such as Cronkhite-Canada syndrome. Most polyps are benign, but villous and familial polyps show a marked inclination to become malignant. A striking feature of familial polyposis is its frequent link to rectosigmoid adenocarcinoma.

▲ **AGE ALERT**
Villous adenomas are most prevalent in men over age 55. Common polypoid adenomas are most prevalent in white women between age 45 and 60. The prevalence of adenomas in both sexes increases after age 70. Juvenile polyps occur most commonly in children under age 10 and are characterized by rectal bleeding.

CAUSES
The cause of polyps is unknown. Predisposing risk factors include:
- heredity
- increasing age (except for juvenile polyps)
- high-fat, low-fiber diet.

PATHOPHYSIOLOGY
Intestinal polyps are masses of tissue, resulting from unrestrained cell growth in the upper epithelium, that rise above the mucosal membrane and protrude into the GI tract.

Polyps may be described by their appearance: pedunculated (attached by a stalk to the intestinal wall) or sessile (attached to the intestinal wall with a broad base and no stalk).

Familial polyposis and the hamartomatous polyposis syndromes are rare, autosomal dominant inherited disorders. Cronkhite-Canada syndrome is also a rare disorder with unknown etiology.

SIGNS AND SYMPTOMS
Because intestinal polyps don't generally cause symptoms, they're usually discovered incidentally during a digital examination or rectosigmoidoscopy. Rectal bleeding is a common sign because of irritation of the GI tract; high rectal polyps leave a streak of blood on the stool, whereas low rectal polyps bleed freely.

Polyps vary in appearance. Hyperplastic polyps are usually less than 0.5 cm in diameter. Common polypoid adenomas are small, multiple lesions that are redder than normal mucosa. They're commonly slightly raised, pedunculated, and granular, with a red, lobular, or eroded surface.

DISRUPTING DISEASE
Treating peptic ulcers

Peptic ulcers can result from factors that increase gastric acid production or from factors that impair mucosal barrier protection. This illustration highlights the actions of the major treatments used for peptic ulcers and where they interfere with the pathophysiologic chain of events.

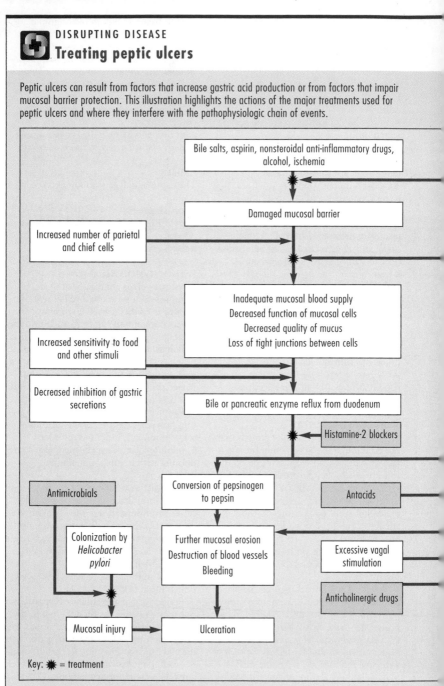

Key: ✳ = treatment

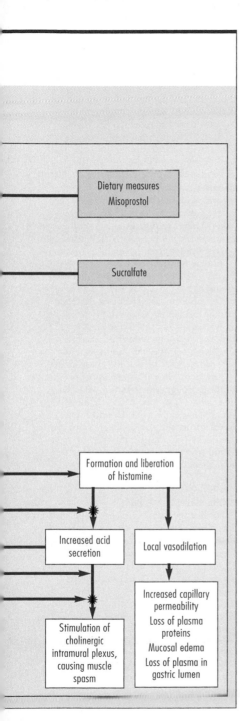

Dietary measures
Misoprostol

Sucralfate

Formation and liberation of histamine

Increased acid secretion

Local vasodilation

Increased capillary permeability

Loss of plasma proteins

Mucosal edema

Loss of plasma in gastric lumen

Stimulation of cholinergic intramural plexus, causing muscle spasm

Villous adenomas are usually sessile and usually less than 2 cm in diameter. They're soft, friable, and finely lobulated. They may grow large and cause painful defecation, but because adenomas are soft, they rarely cause bowel obstruction. Sometimes adenomas prolapse outside the anus, expelling parts of the adenoma with the feces. These polyps may cause diarrhea, bloody stools, and subsequent fluid and electrolyte depletion, with hypotension and oliguria.

In hereditary polyposis, rectal polyps resemble benign adenomas but occur as hundreds or thousands of 0.5-cm diameter lesions carpeting the entire mucosal surface. The signs include diarrhea, bloody stools, and anemia, resulting from mucosal irritation. In patients with familial polyposis, changes in bowel habits with abdominal pain usually signal rectosigmoid cancer.

Juvenile polyps appear as smooth, pedunculated cherry-red polyps and are generally large. Mucus-filled cysts cover their usually smooth surface.

Focal polypoid hyperplasia produces lesions that are less than 3 mm in diameter, granular, and sessile; they may be gray, translucent, or similar to the colon in color. They usually occur at the rectosigmoid junction.

COMPLICATIONS

Complications may include:
■ anemia resulting from slow-bleeding polyps
■ bowel obstruction resulting from large polyps
■ rectal bleeding
■ intussusception
■ colorectal cancer (villous adenomas and familial polyps).

DIAGNOSIS

Firm diagnosis of rectal polyps requires identification of the polyps by sigmoidoscopy or colonoscopy and rectal biopsy. Barium enema can help identify polyps that are located high in the colon. Supportive laboratory findings include occult blood in the stools, low hemoglobin level and hematocrit (with anemia) and, possibly, serum electrolyte imbalances in patients with villous adenomas.

TREATMENT

Treatment varies according to the type and size of the polyps and their location in the colon. Common polypoid adenomas less than 1 cm in size require polypectomy, commonly by fulguration (destruction by high-frequency electricity) during endoscopy. For common polypoid adenomas over 4 cm and all invasive villous adenomas, treatment usually consists of abdominoperineal resection or low anterior resection.

Focal polypoid hyperplasia can be obliterated by biopsy. Depending on GI involvement, hereditary polyps require total abdominoperineal resection with a permanent ileostomy, subtotal colectomy with ileoproctostomy, or ileoanal anastomosis. Juvenile polyps are prone to autoamputation, from spontaneous sloughing of the polyp; if this doesn't occur, snare removal during colonoscopy is the treatment of choice.

Tracheoesophageal fistula and esophageal atresia

Tracheoesophageal fistula is a developmental anomaly characterized by an abnormal connection between the trachea and the esophagus. It usually accompanies esophageal atresia, in which the esophagus is closed off at some point. Although these malformations have numerous anatomic variations, the most common, by far, is esophageal atresia with fistula to the distal segment. (See *Types of tracheoesophageal anomaly.*)

Two of the most serious surgical emergencies in neonates, these disorders need immediate diagnosis and correction. Esophageal atresia occurs in about 1 of every 4,000 live births; about one-third of these neonates are born prematurely.

CAUSES

These disorders are congenital anomalies that are commonly found in infants with other anomalies, such as:
- congenital heart disease
- imperforate anus
- genitourinary abnormalities

- intestinal atresia.

PATHOPHYSIOLOGY

Tracheoesophageal fistula and esophageal atresia result from failure of the embryonic esophagus and trachea to develop and separate correctly. Respiratory system development begins at about day 26 of gestation. Abnormal development of the septum (dividing wall) during this time can lead to tracheoesophageal fistula. The most common abnormality is type C, tracheoesophageal fistula with esophageal atresia, in which the upper section of the esophagus terminates in a blind pouch and the lower section ascends from the stomach and connects with the trachea by a short fistulous tract.

In type A atresia, both esophageal segments are blind pouches and neither is connected to the airway. In type E (or type H) tracheoesophageal fistula without atresia, the fistula may occur anywhere between the level of the cricoid cartilage of the trachea and the midesophagus but is usually higher in the trachea than in the esophagus. Such a fistula may be as small as a pinpoint. In type B, the upper portion of the esophagus opens into the trachea and the lower portion ends in a blind pouch. In type D, both the upper and lower portions of the esophagus open into the trachea via a fistula. Infants with type B and type D anomalies may experience life-threatening aspiration of saliva or food.

SIGNS AND SYMPTOMS

A neonate with type C tracheoesophageal fistula with esophageal atresia appears to swallow normally but soon after swallowing coughs, struggles, becomes cyanotic, and stops breathing as he aspirates fluids returning from the blind pouch of the esophagus through his nose and mouth. Stomach distention may cause respiratory distress; air and gastric contents (bile and gastric secretions) may reflux through the fistula into the trachea, resulting in chemical pneumonitis.

An infant with type A esophageal atresia appears normal at birth. The infant swallows normally, but as secretions fill the esophageal sac and overflow into the oro-

CLOSER LOOK
Types of tracheoesophageal anomaly

Congenital malformations of the esophagus occur in about 1 in 4,000 live births. The American Academy of Pediatrics classifies the anatomic variations of tracheoesophageal anomaly as follows:

◆ type A (7.7%) — esophageal atresia without fistula
◆ type B (0.8%) — esophageal atresia with tracheoesophageal fistula to the proximal segment
◆ type C (86.5%) — esophageal atresia with fistula to the distal segment
◆ type D (0.7%) — esophageal atresia with fistula to both segments
◆ type E (or H-Type) (4.2%) — tracheoesophageal fistula without atresia.

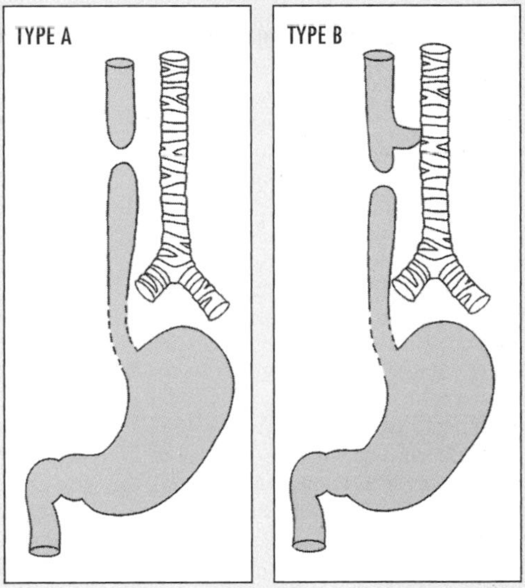

TYPE A

TYPE B

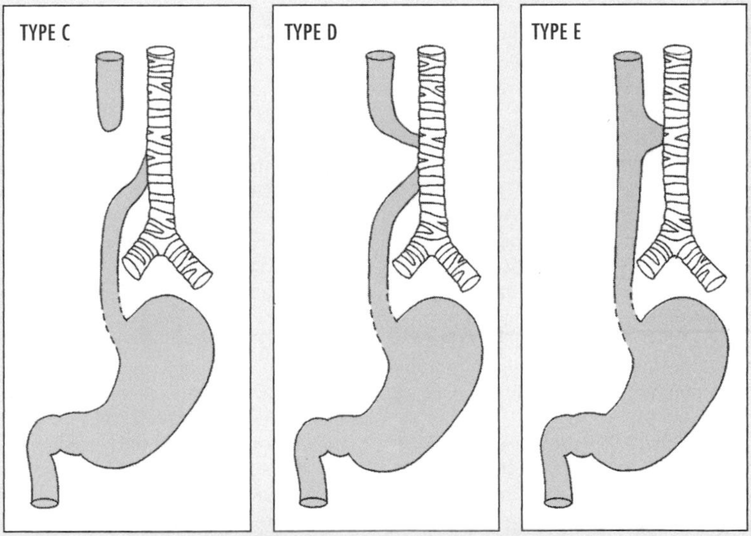

TYPE C

TYPE D

TYPE E

pharynx, he develops mucus in the oropharynx and drools excessively. When the infant is fed, regurgitation and respiratory distress follow aspiration. Suctioning the mucus and secretions temporarily relieves these symptoms. Excessive secretions and drooling in the newborn strongly suggest esophageal atresia.

Repeated episodes of pneumonitis, pulmonary infection, and abdominal distention may signal type E (or type H) tracheoesophageal fistula. When a child with this disorder drinks, he coughs, chokes, and becomes cyanotic. Excessive mucus builds up in the oropharynx. Crying forces air from the trachea into the esophagus, producing abdominal distention. Because such a child may appear normal at birth, this type of tracheoesophageal fistula may be overlooked, and diagnosis may be delayed as long as 1 year.

Both type B (proximal fistula) and type D (fistula to both segments) cause immediate aspiration of saliva into the airway, leading to bacterial pneumonitis.

COMPLICATIONS
Complications may include:
- aspiration of secretions into the lungs leading to respiratory distress, cessation of breathing, or pneumonia
- death, if untreated.

DIAGNOSIS
Respiratory distress and drooling in a neonate suggest tracheoesophageal fistula and esophageal atresia. The following procedures confirm it:
- A size 6 or size 8 French catheter passed through the nose meets an obstruction (esophageal atresia) about 4″ to 5″ (10 to 12.5 cm) from the nostrils. Aspirate of gastric contents is less acidic than normal.
- Chest X-ray with the catheter in place shows the position of the catheter and can also show a dilated, air-filled upper esophageal pouch, pneumonia in the right upper lobe, or bilateral pneumonitis. Both pneumonia and pneumonitis suggest aspiration.
- Abdominal X-ray shows gas in the bowel in a distal fistula (type C) but none in a proximal fistula (type B) or in atresia without fistula (type A).
- Cinefluorography allows visualization on a fluoroscopic screen. After a size 10 or 12 French catheter is passed through the patient's nostril into the esophagus, a small amount of contrast medium is instilled to

define the tip of the upper pouch and to differentiate between overflow aspiration from a blind end (atresia) and aspiration from passage of liquids through a tracheoesophageal fistula.

TREATMENT
Tracheoesophageal fistula and esophageal atresia require surgical correction and are usually surgical emergencies. The type and timing of the surgical procedure depend on the nature of the anomaly, the patient's general condition, and the presence of coexisting congenital defects.
- In premature neonates (nearly 33% of neonates with this anomaly are born prematurely), who are poor surgical risks, correction of combined *tracheoesophageal fistula and esophageal atresia* is done in two stages: first, gastrostomy (for gastric decompression, prevention of reflux, and feeding) and closure of the fistula; then, 1 to 2 months later, anastomosis of the esophagus. Before and after surgery, positioning varies with the physician's philosophy and the child's anatomy: The child may be placed supine, with his head low to facilitate drainage, or with his head elevated to prevent aspiration. The child should receive I.V. fluids, as necessary, and appropriate antibiotics for infection.

Postoperative complications after correction of tracheoesophageal fistula include recurrent fistulas, esophageal motility dysfunction, esophageal stricture, recurrent bronchitis, pneumothorax, and failure to thrive. After surgery to correct esophageal atresia, esophageal motility dysfunction or hiatal hernia may develop.
- Correction of *esophageal atresia* alone requires anastomosis of the proximal and distal esophageal segments in one or two stages. End-to-end anastomosis commonly produces postoperative stricture; end-to-side anastomosis is less likely to do so. If the esophageal ends are widely separated, treatment may include a colonic interposition (grafting a piece of the colon) or elongation of the proximal segment of the esophagus by bougienage. About 10 days after surgery, and again 1 and 3 months later, X-rays are required to evaluate the effectiveness of surgical repair. Postoperative

treatment includes placement of a suction catheter in the upper esophageal pouch to control secretions and prevent aspiration, keeping the infant in an upright position to avoid reflux of gastric juices into the trachea, I.V. fluids (nothing by mouth), gastrostomy to prevent reflux and allow feeding, and appropriate antibiotics for pneumonia.

Postoperative complications may include impaired esophageal motility (in one-third of patients), hiatal hernia, and reflux esophagitis.

Ulcerative colitis

Ulcerative colitis is an inflammatory, usually chronic, disease that affects the mucosa of the colon. It invariably begins in the rectum and sigmoid colon, and commonly extends upward into the entire colon, rarely affecting the small intestine. Ulcerative colitis produces edema (leading to mucosa that's easily crushed or pulverized) and ulcerations. Severity ranges from a mild, localized disorder to a fulminant disease that may cause a perforated colon, progressing to potentially fatal peritonitis and toxemia. The disease cycles between exacerbation and remission.

Ulcerative colitis occurs primarily in young adults, especially women.

CULTURAL DIVERSITY
Ulcerative colitis is more common among Ashkenazi Jews and in higher socioeconomic groups, and there seems to be a familial tendency.

The prevalence is unknown, but some studies suggest as many as 100 of 100,000 persons have the disease. Onset of symptoms seems to peak between ages 15 and 20 and between ages 55 and 60.

CAUSES
Specific causes of ulcerative colitis are unknown but may be caused by abnormal immune response in the GI tract, possibly associated with food or bacteria such as *Escherichia coli.*

PATHOPHYSIOLOGY
Ulcerative colitis usually begins as inflammation in the base of the mucosal layer of the large intestine. The colon's mucosal surface becomes dark, red, and velvety. Inflammation leads to erosions that coalesce and form ulcers. The mucosa becomes diffusely ulcerated, with hemorrhage, congestion, edema, and exudative inflammation. Ulcerations are continuous. Abscesses in the mucosa drain purulent exudate, become necrotic, and ulcerate. Sloughing causes bloody, mucus filled stools. As abscesses heal, scarring and thickening may appear in the bowel's inner muscle layer. As granulation tissue replaces the muscle layer, the colon narrows, shortens, and loses its characteristic pouches (haustral folds).

SIGNS AND SYMPTOMS
Signs and symptoms may include:
- recurrent bloody diarrhea (as many as 10 to 20 stools per day), typically containing pus and mucus (hallmark sign), from accumulated blood and mucus in the bowel resulting from mucosal sloughing, ulceration, congestion, and inflammation
- abdominal cramping and rectal urgency from increased pressure from accumulated blood and mucus
- weight loss caused by malabsorption
- weakness related to possible malabsorption and resulting anemia.

COMPLICATIONS
Complications may include:
- perforation
- toxic megacolon
- liver disease
- stricture formation
- colon cancer
- anemia.

DIAGNOSIS
- Sigmoidoscopy confirms rectal involvement: specifically, mucosal friability and flattening and thick, inflammatory exudate.
- Colonoscopy reveals extent of the disease, stricture areas, and pseudopolyps (procedure isn't performed when the patient has active signs and symptoms).
- Biopsy with colonoscopy confirms the diagnosis.
- Barium enema reveals the extent of the disease, detects complications, and identi-

fies cancer (not performed when the patient has active signs and symptoms).

■ Stool specimen analysis reveals blood, pus, and mucus but no disease-causing organisms.

■ Serology studies show decreased serum potassium, magnesium, and albumin levels; decreased white blood cell count; decreased hemoglobin level; and prolonged prothrombin time. Elevated erythrocyte sedimentation rate correlates with severity of the attack.

TREATMENT

Treatment includes:

■ corticotropin and adrenal corticosteroids to control inflammation

■ sulfasalazine for its anti-inflammatory and antimicrobial effects

■ antidiarrheal agents to relieve frequent, troublesome diarrhea in patients whose ulcerative colitis is otherwise under control

■ iron supplements to correct anemia

■ total parenteral nutrition and nothing by mouth for patients with severe disease, to rest the intestinal tract, decrease stool volume, and restore nitrogen balance

■ supplemental drinks to supplement nutrition in patients with moderate symptoms

■ I.V. hydration to replace fluid loss from diarrhea

■ surgery to correct massive dilation of the colon and to treat patients with symptoms that are unbearable or for which drugs and supportive measures aren't effective

■ proctocolectomy with ileostomy to divert stool and to allow rectal anastomosis to heal, removing all the potentially malignant epithelia of the rectum and colon.

10

*M*usculoskeletal system

The musculoskeletal system is a complex system of bones, joints, muscles, ligaments, tendons, and other tissues that gives the body form and shape. It also protects vital organs, makes movement possible, stores calcium and other minerals in the bony matrix for mobilization if deficiency occurs, and provides sites for hematopoiesis (blood cell production) in the marrow.

*B*ONES

The human skeleton contains 206 bones, which are composed of inorganic salts (primarily calcium and phosphate), embedded in a framework of collagen fibers.

Bone shape and structure
Bones are classified by shape as long, short, flat, or irregular. Long bones are found in the extremities and include the humerus, radius, and ulna of the arm; the femur, tibia, and fibula of the leg; and the phalanges, metacarpals, and metatarsals of the hands and feet. (See *Structure of long bones,* page 360.) Short bones include the tarsal and carpal bones of the feet and hands, respectively. Flat bones include the frontal and parietal bones of the cranium, ribs, sternum, scapulae, ilium, and pubis. Irregular bones include the bones of the spine (vertebrae, sacrum, coccyx) and certain bones of the skull (the temporal, sphenoid, ethmoid, and mandible).

Classified according to structure, bone is either cortical (compact) or cancellous (spongy or trabecular). Adult cortical bone consists of networks of interconnecting canals, or canaliculi. Each of these networks, or haversian systems, runs parallel to the bone's long axis and consists of a central haversian canal surrounded by layers (lamellae) of bone. Between adjacent lamellae are small openings called *lacunae,* which contain bone cells or osteocytes. The canaliculi, each containing one capillary or more, provide a route for tissue fluids transport; they connect all the lacunae.

Cancellous bone consists of thin plates (trabeculae) that form the interior meshwork of bone. These trabeculae are arranged in various directions to correspond with the lines of maximum stress or pressure. This gives the bone added structural strength. Chemically, inorganic salts (calcium and phosphate, with small amounts of sodium, potassium carbonate, and magnesium ions) make up 70% of the mature bone. The salts give bone its elasticity and ability to withstand compression.

Bone growth
Ongoing bone formation is affected by hormonal stimulation, dietary factors, and the amount of stress put on the bone. It's accomplished by the continual actions of bone-forming osteoblasts and bone-reabsorbing cells called osteoclasts.

Osteoblasts are present on the outer surface of and within bones. They respond to

Structure of long bones

Long bones are the weight-bearing bones of the body. Their structures provide maximal strength and minimal weight. Structure of a long bone in an adult is shown below.

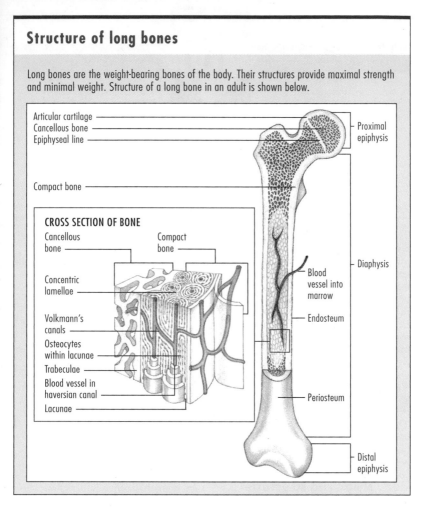

various stimuli to produce the bony matrix, or osteoid. As calcium salts precipitate on the organic matrix, the bone hardens. As the bone forms, a system of microscopic canals in the bone grows around the osteocytes.

Osteoclasts are phagocytic cells that digest old, weakened bone section by section. As they finish, osteoblasts simultaneously replace the cleared section with new, stronger bone. Vitamin D supports bone calcification by stimulating osteoblast activity and calcium absorption from the gut to make it available for bone building.

When serum calcium levels fall, the parathyroid gland releases parathyroid hormone, which then stimulates osteoclast activity and bone breakdown, freeing calcium into the blood. Parathyroid hormone also increases serum calcium by decreasing renal excretion of calcium and increasing renal excretion of phosphate ion.

Phosphates are essential to bone formation; bone contains about 85% of the body's phosphates. The intestine absorbs phosphates from dietary sources, but adequate levels of vitamin D are necessary for their absorption. Because calcium and phosphates interact reciprocally, renal excretion of phosphates increases or decreases in inverse proportion to serum calcium levels. Alkaline phosphatase (ALP) influences bone calcification and lipid and metabolite transport. Osteoblasts contain a large amount of ALP. A rise in serum ALP levels can identify skeletal diseases, mainly those that involve evident osteoblastic activity, such as bone metastases or Paget's disease. It can also identify biliary obstruction, hyperparathyroidism, and excessive intake of vitamin D.

In children and young adults, bone growth occurs in the epiphyseal plate, a layer of cartilage between the diaphysis and epiphysis of long bones. Osteoblasts deposit new bone in the area just beneath the epiphysis, making the bone longer, and osteoclasts model the new bone's shape by reabsorbing previously deposited bone. These remodeling activities promote longitudinal bone growth, which continues until the epiphyseal growth plates, located at both ends, close during adolescence. In adults, bone growth is complete, and the epiphyseal plate (cartilage) is replaced by bone, becoming the epiphyseal line.

Joints

The tendons, ligaments, cartilage, and other tissues that connect two bones constitute a joint. Depending on their structures, joints mainly permit motion or provide stability. Joints, like bones, are classified according to structure and function.

Classification of joints
The three structural types of joints are fibrous, cartilaginous, and synovial.
- Fibrous joints, or synarthroses, permit only the tiniest motion and thus provide stability when tight union is necessary, as in the sutures that join the cranial bones.
- Cartilaginous joints, or amphiarthroses, allow limited motion, as between vertebrae.
- Synovial joints, or diarthroses, are the most common and permit the greatest degree of movement. These joints include

Structure of a synovial joint

The metacarpophalangeal joint shown here permits angular motion between the finger and the hand. A synovial joint is characterized by a synovial pouch full of fluid that lubricates the two articulating bones.

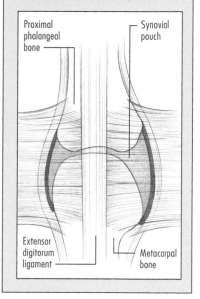

Proximal phalangeal bone

Synovial pouch

Extensor digitorum ligament

Metacarpal bone

the elbows and knees. (See *Structure of a synovial joint.*)

Synovial joints have distinct characteristics.
- The two articulating (joining) surfaces of the bones have a smooth hyaline covering (articular cartilage) that's resilient to pressure.
- Their opposing surfaces fit together well (are congruous) and glide smoothly on each other.
- A fibrous (articular) capsule holds them together.
- Beneath the capsule, lining the joint cavity, is the synovial membrane, which secretes a clear viscous fluid called synovial fluid. This fluid lubricates the two opposing bone surfaces during motion and nourishes the articular cartilage.

■ Surrounding a synovial joint are ligaments, muscles, and tendons, which strengthen and stabilize the joint but allow free movement.

Joint movement

The two types of synovial joint movement are angular and circular.

ANGULAR MOVEMENT

Joints of the knees, elbows, and phalanges (the bones of the fingers and toes) permit these angular movements:
■ flexion (closing of the joint angle)
■ extension (opening of the joint angle)
■ hyperextension (extension of the angle beyond the usual arc).

Other joints, including the shoulders and hips, permit these movements:
■ abduction (movement away from the body's midline)
■ adduction (movement toward the midline).

CIRCULAR MOVEMENTS

Circular movements include:
■ rotation (motion around a central axis), such as the ball-and-socket joints of the hips and shoulders
■ pronation (downward wrist or ankle motion)
■ supination (upward wrist motion).

Other kinds of movement are inversion (inward turning such as of the foot), eversion (outward turning such as of the foot), protraction (as in forward motion of the mandible), and retraction (returning protracted part into place).

MUSCLES

The most specialized feature of muscle tissue—*contractility*—makes the movement of bones and joints possible. Normal skeletal muscles contract in response to neural impulses. Appropriate contraction of muscle usually applies force to one or more tendons. The force pulls one bone toward, away from, or around a second bone, depending on the type of muscle contraction and the type of joint involved. Abnormal metabolism in the muscle may

result in inappropriate contractility. For example, when stored glycogen or lipids can't be used because of the lack of an enzyme necessary to convert energy for contraction, cramps, fatigue, and exercise intolerance may result.

Muscles permit and maintain body positions, such as sitting and standing. Muscles also pump blood through the body (cardiac contraction and vessel compression), move food through the intestines (peristalsis), and make breathing possible. Skeletal muscular activity produces heat; this feature is an important component in temperature regulation. Deep body temperature regulators are found in the abdominal viscera, spinal cord, and great veins. These receptors detect changes in the body core temperature and stimulate the hypothalamus to institute appropriate temperature-changing responses, such as shivering in response to cold. Muscle mass accounts for about 40% of an average man's weight.

Muscle classification

Muscles are classified according to structure, anatomic location, and function.
■ Skeletal muscles are attached to bone and have a striped (striated) appearance that reflects their cellular structures.
■ Visceral muscles move contents through internal organs and are smooth (nonstriated).
■ Cardiac muscles (smooth) constitute the heart wall.

When muscles are classified according to activity, they're called either *voluntary* or *involuntary*. (See chapter 8, Nervous system.) Voluntary muscles can be controlled at will and are under the influence of the somatic nervous system; these are the skeletal muscles. Involuntary muscles, controlled by the autonomic nervous system, include the cardiac and visceral muscles. Some organs contain voluntary and involuntary muscles.

Muscle contraction

Each skeletal muscle consists of many elongated muscle cells, called *muscle fibers,* through which run slender threads of protein, called *myofibrils.* Muscle fibers are held together in bundles by sheaths of fibrous tissues called *fascia.* Blood vessels and nerves pass into muscles through the fascia to reach the individual muscle fibers. Motor neurons synapse with the motor nerve fibers of voluntary muscles. These fibers reach the membranes of skeletal muscle cells at neuromuscular (myoneural) junctions. When an impulse reaches the myoneural junction, the junction releases the neurotransmitter, acetylcholine. Acetylcholine causes the release of calcium from the sarcoplasmic reticulum (a membranous network in the muscle fiber), which, in turn, triggers muscle contraction. Muscle contraction is isometric or isotonic. *Isometric* contraction results in an increase in tension without change in length. *Isotonic* contraction occurs when the muscle shortens as weight is lifted. The energy source for muscle contraction is adenosine triphosphate (ATP). ATP release is also triggered by the impulse at the myoneural junction. Relaxation of a muscle is believed to involve reversal of these mechanisms.

Muscle fatigue results when the sources of ATP in a muscle are depleted. If a muscle is deprived of oxygen, fatigue occurs rapidly. As the muscle fatigues, it switches to anaerobic metabolism of glycogen stores, in which the stored glycogen is split into glucose (glycolysis) without the use of oxygen. Lactic acid is a by-product of anaerobic glycolysis and may accumulate in the muscle and blood, causing intense or prolonged muscle contraction.

Tendons and Ligaments

Skeletal muscles are attached to bone directly or indirectly by fibrous cords known as *tendons.* The least movable end of the muscle attachment (usually proximal) is called the *point of origin;* the most movable end (usually distal) is called the *point of insertion.*

Ligaments are fibrous connections that control joint movement between two bones or cartilages. Their purpose is to support and strengthen joints.

Pathophysiologic Changes

Alterations of the normal functioning of bones and muscles are the cause or result of important interactions within the body. Most musculoskeletal disorders are caused by or profoundly affect other body systems.

Alterations in bone

Disease may alter density, growth, or bone strength.

DENSITY

In healthy young adults, the resorption and formation phases are tightly coupled for maintaining bone mass in a steady state. Bone loss occurs when the two phases become uncoupled, and resorption exceeds formation. The hormone estrogen not only regulates calcium uptake and release, it also regulates osteoblastic activity. Decreased estrogen levels may lead to a decrease in osteoblastic activity and loss of bone mass, called *osteoporosis.* In children, vitamin D deficiency prevents development of normal bone shape and structure and leads to rickets.

▲ **AGE ALERT**
Bone density and structural integrity (ability to withstand stress) decrease after age 30 in women and after age 45 in men. The relatively steady loss of bone matrix can be partially offset by exercise and appropriate dietary calcium intake.

CULTURAL DIVERSITY
Age, race, and sex affect bone mass, structural integrity, and bone loss. For example, Blacks commonly have denser bones than Whites, and men typically have denser bones than women.

GROWTH

The osteochondroses are a group of disorders characterized by avascular necrosis of the epiphyseal growth plates in growing children and adolescents. In these disorders, a lack of blood supply to the bone leads to septic necrosis, with softening and resorption of bone. Revascularization then initiates new bone formation in the bone, which leads to malformation.

BONE STRENGTH
Both cortical and trabecular bone contribute to skeletal strength. Any loss of the inorganic salts that make up the chemical structure of bone will weaken bone. Cancellous bone is more sensitive to metabolic influences, so conditions that produce rapid bone loss tend to affect cancellous bone more quickly than cortical bone.

Alterations of muscle
Pathologic effects on muscle include atrophy, fatigue, weakness, myotonia, and spasticity.

ATROPHY
Atrophy is a decrease in the size of a tissue or cell. In muscles, the myofibrils atrophy after prolonged inactivity from bed rest or trauma (casting), when local nerve damage makes movement impossible, or when illness removes needed nutrients from muscles. The effects of muscular deconditioning linked to lack of physical activity may be apparent in a matter of days. A person who's confined to bed loses muscle mass as well as muscle strength, from baseline levels at a rate of 3% per day. Conditioning and stretching exercises may help prevent atrophy. If reuse isn't restored within 1 year, regeneration of muscle fibers is unlikely.

AGE ALERT
Some degree of muscle atrophy is normal with aging.

FATIGUE
Pathologic muscle fatigue may be the result of impaired neural stimulation of muscle or energy metabolism or disruption of calcium flux. See chapter 4, Fluids and electrolytes, for a detailed discussion of these events.

WEAKNESS
Muscle weakness refers to a loss of strength (decrease in power) in one or more muscle groups. Muscle weakness can result from a malfunction in the cerebral hemispheres, brainstem, spinal cord, nerve

roots, peripheral nerves or myoneural junction.

AGE ALERT
Muscle mass and strength decrease in elderly people, usually as a result of muscle disuse. This decrease can be reversed with moderate, regular, weight-bearing exercise.

Periodic paralysis is a disorder that can be triggered by exercise or a process or chemical (such as medication) that increases serum potassium levels (hyperkalemia). This hyperkalemic periodic paralysis may be caused by a high-carbohydrate diet, emotional stress, prolonged bed rest, or hyperthyroidism. During an attack of periodic paralysis, the muscle membrane is unresponsive to neural stimuli, and the electrical charge needed to initiate the impulse (resting membrane potential) is reduced from −90 to −45 millivolts.

MYOTONIA AND SPASTICITY
Myotonia is delayed relaxation after a voluntary muscle contraction — such as grip, eye closure, or muscle percussion — along with prolonged depolarization of the muscle membrane. Depolarization is the reversal of the resting potential in stimulated cell membranes. It's the process by which the cell membrane "resets" its positive charge with respect to the negative charge outside the cell. Myotonia occurs in myotonic muscular dystrophy and some forms of periodic paralysis.

Stress-induced muscle tension, or spasticity, is presumably caused by increased activity in the reticular activating system and in the muscle fiber. The reticular activating system consists of multiple diffuse pathways in the brain that control wakefulness and response to stimuli. A pathologic contracture is permanent muscle shortening caused by muscle spasticity, seen in central nervous system injury or severe muscle weakness.

ᴅISORDERS

AGE ALERT
Patients with musculoskeletal disorders are commonly elderly, have

concurrent medical conditions, or have experienced trauma. Generally, they face prolonged immobilization. (See Managing a patient with musculoskeletal pain.*)*

Bone fracture

When a force exceeds a bone's compressive or tensile strength (the ability of the bone to hold together), a fracture will occur. (For an explanation of the terms used to identify fractures, see *Classifying fractures,* page 366.)

An estimated 25% of the population suffers traumatic musculoskeletal injury each year, and a significant number of these involve fractures.

The prognosis varies with the extent of disablement or deformity, amount of tissue and vascular damage, adequacy of reduction (correction of the fracture) and immobilization, and the patient's age, health, and nutritional status.

AGE ALERT
Children's bones usually heal rapidly and without deformity, but epiphyseal plate fractures in children are likely to cause deformity because they interfere with normal bone growth. In elderly people, underlying systemic illness, impaired circulation, or poor nutrition may cause slow or poor healing.

CAUSES

Risk factors for bone fractures include:
- falls
- automobile accidents
- sports
- use of drugs that impair judgment or mobility
- young age (immaturity of bone)
- bone tumors
- metabolic illnesses (such as hypoparathyroidism or hyperparathyroidism)
- medications that cause iatrogenic (caused by treatment) osteoporosis such as steroids.

AGE ALERT
The highest incidence of bone fractures occurs in young men between ages 15 and 24 (fractures of the tibia, clavicle, and lower humerus); these fractures are usually the result of trauma. In elderly people, fractures of the upper femur, upper humerus, forearm, wrist, vertebrae,

---

Managing a patient with musculoskeletal pain

Assess and treat a patient with a musculoskeletal disorder that causes chronic, nonmalignant pain in a stepped approach that includes:

◆ nonpharmacologic methods, such as heat, ice, elevation, and rest
◆ acetaminophen
◆ nonsteroidal anti-inflammatory drugs such as ibuprofen
◆ other nonopioid analgesics, such as tramadol or topical capsaicin
◆ tricyclic antidepressants, such as amitriptyline, to decrease the pain signal at the neurosynaptic junctions
◆ opioid analgesics alone or with a tricyclic antidepressant.

---

and pelvis are commonly linked to osteoporosis.

PATHOPHYSIOLOGY

When a bone is fractured, the periosteum and blood vessels in the cortex, marrow, and surrounding soft tissue are disrupted. A hematoma forms between the broken ends of the bone and beneath the periosteum, and granulation tissue eventually replaces the hematoma.

Damage to bone tissue triggers an intense inflammatory response in which cells from surrounding soft tissue and the marrow cavity invade the fracture area, and blood flow to the entire bone is increased. Osteoblasts in the periosteum, endosteum, and marrow produce osteoid (collagenous, young bone that hasn't yet calcified, also called *callus*), which hardens along the outer surface of the shaft and over the broken ends of the bone. Osteoclasts reabsorb material from previously formed bones and osteoblasts to rebuild bone. Osteoblasts then transform into osteocytes (mature bone cells).

SIGNS AND SYMPTOMS

Signs and symptoms of bone fracture may include:

Classifying fractures

One of the best-known systems for classifying fractures uses a combination of terms that describe general classification, fragment position, and fracture line — such as simple, nondisplaced, and oblique.

GENERAL CLASSIFICATION OF FRACTURES

◆ Simple (closed) — Bone fragments don't penetrate the skin.
◆ Compound (open) — Bone fragments penetrate the skin.
◆ Incomplete (partial) — Bone continuity isn't completely interrupted.
◆ Complete — Bone continuity is completely interrupted.

CLASSIFICATION BY FRAGMENT POSITION

◆ Comminuted — The bone breaks into small pieces.
◆ Impacted — One bone fragment is forced into another.
◆ Angulated — Fragments lie at an angle to each other.

◆ Displaced — Fracture fragments separate and are deformed.
◆ Nondisplaced — The two sections of bone maintain essentially normal alignment.
◆ Overriding — Fragments overlap, shortening the total bone length.
◆ Segmental — Fractures occur in two adjacent areas with an isolated central segment.
◆ Avulsed — Fragments are pulled from the normal position by muscle contractions or ligament resistance.

CLASSIFICATION BY FRACTURE LINE

◆ Linear — The fracture line runs parallel to the bone's axis.
◆ Longitudinal — The fracture line extends in a longitudinal (but not parallel) direction along the bone's axis.
◆ Oblique — The fracture line crosses the bone at about a 45-degree angle to the bone's axis.
◆ Spiral — The fracture line crosses the bone at an oblique angle, creating a spiral pattern.
◆ Transverse — The fracture line forms a right angle with the bone's axis.

■ deformity from unnatural alignment
■ swelling caused by vasodilation and infiltration by inflammatory leukocytes and mast cells
■ muscle spasm and tenderness related to the inflammatory response
■ impaired sensation distal to the fracture site caused by pinching or severing of neurovascular elements by the trauma or by bone fragments
■ limited range of motion because of misalignment, neurovascular compromise, swelling, and pain
■ crepitus, or "clicking" sounds on movement caused by shifting bone fragments.

COMPLICATIONS

Possible complications of bone fracture include:
■ permanent deformity and dysfunction if bones fail to heal (nonunion) or heal improperly (malunion)

■ aseptic (not caused by infection) necrosis of bone segments because of impaired circulation
■ hypovolemic shock as a result of blood vessel damage (especially with a fractured femur)
■ muscle contractures
■ compartment syndrome (see *Recognizing compartment syndrome*)
■ renal calculi resulting from the decalcification of bone caused by prolonged immobility
■ fat embolism caused by disruption of marrow and release of fat globules into the circulation after the trauma (may lead to respiratory or central nervous system distress).

DIAGNOSIS

Diagnosis of bone fracture includes:
■ history of traumatic injury and results of the physical examination, including

gentle palpation and a cautious attempt by the patient to move parts distal to the injury
■ X-rays of the suspected fracture and the joints above and below (confirm the diagnosis; after reduction, X-rays confirm bone alignment).

TREATMENT

For arm or leg fracture, emergency treatment consists of:
■ splinting the limb above and below the suspected fracture to immobilize it
■ applying a cold pack to reduce pain and edema
■ elevating the limb to reduce pain and edema.

 CLINICAL ALERT
The acronym RICE is useful to help remember treatment for a fracture in the first 24 hours:
R — *Rest*
I — *Ice*
C — *Compression*
E — *Elevation*

Treatment in severe bone fracture that causes blood loss includes:
■ direct pressure to control bleeding
■ fluid replacement as soon as possible to prevent or treat hypovolemic shock.

After a fracture is confirmed, treatment begins with reduction. *Closed reduction* involves:
■ manual manipulation
■ local anesthetic (such as lidocaine I.V.)
■ analgesic (such as morphine I.M.)
■ muscle relaxant (such as diazepam I.V.) or a sedative (such as midazolam I.V.) to facilitate the muscle stretching necessary to realign the bone.

When closed reduction isn't possible, *open reduction* by surgery involves:
■ immobilization of the fracture by means of rods, plates, or screws and application of a plaster cast
■ prophylactic tetanus
■ prophylactic antibiotics
■ surgery to repair soft tissue damage
■ thorough wound debridement
■ physical therapy after cast removal to restore limb mobility.

When a splint or cast fails to maintain the reduction, immobilization requires

Recognizing compartment syndrome

Compartment syndrome occurs when edema or bleeding increases pressure within a muscle compartment (a smaller section of a muscle), to the point of interfering with circulation. Crush injuries, burns, bites, and fractures requiring casts or dressings may cause this syndrome. Compartment syndrome most commonly occurs in the lower arm, hand, lower leg, or foot.

Symptoms include:
◆ increased pain
◆ decreased touch sensation
◆ increased weakness of the affected part
◆ increased swelling and pallor
◆ decreased pulses and capillary refill.

Treatment of compartment syndrome consists of:
◆ placing the limb at heart level
◆ removing constricting forces
◆ monitoring neurovascular status
◆ subfascial injection of hyaluronidase
◆ emergency fasciotomy.

skin or skeletal traction, using a series of weights and pulleys. This may involve:
■ elastic bandages and sheepskin coverings to attach traction devices to the patient's skin (skin traction)
■ pin or wire inserted through the bone distal to the fracture and attached to a weight to allow more prolonged traction (skeletal traction).

Carpal tunnel syndrome

Carpal tunnel syndrome, a form of repetitive stress injury, is the most common nerve entrapment syndrome. It poses a serious occupational health problem. Carpal tunnel syndrome typically occurs in women between ages 30 and 60; men employed as assembly line workers and packers and who repeatedly use poorly designed tools are just as likely to develop this disorder. Any strenuous use of the hands — sustained grasping, twisting, or flexing — aggravates this condition.

Carpal tunnel

The carpal tunnel is clearly visible in this palmar view and cross section of a right hand. Note the median nerve and flexor tendons of the fingers passing through the tunnel on their way from the forearm to the hand.

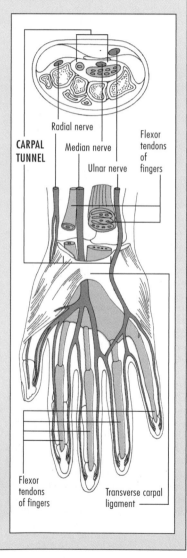

CARPAL TUNNEL

Radial nerve

Median nerve

Ulnar nerve

Flexor tendons of fingers

Flexor tendons of fingers

Transverse carpal ligament

CAUSES

Carpal tunnel syndrome is mainly idiopathic (of unknown cause), or it may result from one or more of the following:
- repetitive stress injury
- rheumatoid arthritis
- flexor tenosynovitis (commonly linked to rheumatic disease)
- nerve compression
- pregnancy
- multiple myeloma
- diabetes mellitus
- acromegaly
- hypothyroidism
- amyloidosis
- obesity
- benign tumor
- other conditions that increase fluid pressure in the wrist, including alterations in the endocrine or immune systems
- wrist dislocation or sprain, or Colles' fracture, followed by edema.

PATHOPHYSIOLOGY

The carpal bones and the transverse carpal ligament form the carpal tunnel. (See *Carpal tunnel.*) Inflammation or fibrosis of the tendon sheaths that pass through the carpal tunnel usually causes edema and compression of the median nerve. This compression neuropathy causes sensory and motor changes in the median distribution of the hands, initially impairing sensory transmission to the thumb, index finger, second finger, and inner part of the third finger.

SIGNS AND SYMPTOMS

The patient with carpal tunnel syndrome usually complains of weakness, pain, burning, numbness, or tingling in one or both hands. This paresthesia affects the thumb, forefinger, middle finger, and inner part of the fourth finger. The patient can't clench his hand into a fist; the nails may be atrophic, and the skin dry and shiny.

Because of vasodilatation and venous stasis, symptoms are typically worse at night and in the morning. The pain may spread to the forearm and, in severe cases, as far as the shoulder. The patient can usually relieve such pain by shaking or rubbing his hands vigorously or dangling his arms at his side.

COMPLICATIONS

Complications include:

■ continued use of the affected wrist may increase tendon inflammation, compression, and neural ischemia, causing a decrease in wrist function

■ untreated carpal tunnel syndrome can produce permanent nerve damage with loss of movement and sensation.

DIAGNOSIS

Physical examination reveals decreased sensation to light touch or pinpricks in the affected fingers. Thenar muscle atrophy (atrophy of the mound on the palm at the base of the thumb) occurs in about half of all cases of carpal tunnel syndrome but is usually a late sign.

The following tests provide rapid diagnosis of carpal tunnel syndrome:

■ Tinel's sign — tingling over the median nerve on light percussion

■ Phalen's maneuver — holding the forearms vertically and allowing both hands to drop into complete flexion at the wrists for 1 minute reproduces symptoms of carpal tunnel syndrome

■ compression test — blood pressure cuff inflated above systolic pressure on the forearm for 1 to 2 minutes provokes pain and paresthesia along the distribution of the median nerve.

Other tests include electromyography to detect a median nerve motor conduction delay of more than 5 msec and laboratory tests to identify underlying disease.

TREATMENT

Conservative treatment should be tried first, including resting the hands by splinting the wrist in neutral extension for 1 to 2 weeks. Nonsteroidal anti-inflammatory drugs usually provide symptomatic relief. Injection of the carpal tunnel with hydrocortisone and lidocaine may provide significant but temporary relief. If a definite link has been established between the patient's occupation and the development of repetitive stress injury, he may have to seek other work. Effective treatment may also

require correction of an underlying disorder. When conservative treatment fails, the only alternative is decompression of the nerve by resecting the entire transverse carpal tunnel ligament, by either conventional or endoscopic surgery. Neurolysis (freeing of the nerve fibers) may also be necessary.

Clubfoot

Clubfoot, also called *talipes deformity,* is the most common congenital disorder of the lower extremities. It's marked mainly by a deformed talus and shortened Achilles' tendon, which give the foot a characteristic clublike appearance. In talipes equinovarus, the foot points downward (equinus, or plantar flexion) and the heel turns inward from the midline of the leg (varus, or inversion), and the front of the foot curls medially (that is, toward the midline of the body — forefoot adduction).

Clubfoot affects about 1 in 1,000 births, is usually bilateral, and is twice as common in boys as in girls. Talipes equinovarus is by far the most common type. It may be linked with other birth anomalies, such as myelomeningocele, spina bifida, and arthrogryposis. Clubfoot is correctable with prompt treatment.

CAUSES

A combination of genetic and environmental factors in utero appears to cause clubfoot, including:

■ heredity (mechanism of transmission is undetermined; the sibling of a child born with clubfoot has 1 chance in 35 of being born with the same anomaly, and a child of a parent with clubfoot has 1 chance in 10)

■ interruption or halt in development during the 9th and 10th weeks of embryonic life when the feet are formed (children without a family history of clubfoot)

■ muscle abnormalities leading to variations in length and tendon insertions.

Paralysis, poliomyelitis, or cerebral palsy (older children), may also cause clubfoot; treatment includes management of the underlying disease.

PATHOPHYSIOLOGY

Abnormal development of the foot during fetal growth leads to abnormal muscles and joints and contracture of soft tissue. Clubfoot can also be a result of paralysis, poliomyelitis, or cerebral palsy. (The condition called *apparent clubfoot* results when a fetus maintains a position in utero that gives his feet a clubfoot appearance at birth; it can usually be corrected manually. Another form of apparent clubfoot is inversion of the feet, resulting from the denervation type of progressive muscular atrophy and progressive muscular dystrophy.)

SIGNS AND SYMPTOMS

Talipes equinovarus varies greatly in severity. Deformity may be so extreme that the toes touch the inside of the ankle, or it may be only vaguely noticeable.

Every case includes:
- deformed talus because of abnormal development
- shortened Achilles' tendon from contracture
- shortened and flattened calcaneus bone of the heel caused by abnormal development and contracture
- shortened, underdeveloped calf muscles and soft-tissue contractures at the site of the deformity (depending on degree of the varus deformity)
- foot tight in its deformed position, resisting manual efforts to push it back into normal position, because of shortening of muscles and contractures
- no pain, except in elderly, arthritic patients with secondary deformity.

COMPLICATIONS

Possible complications of talipes equinovarus include:
- chronic impairment from neglected clubfoot
- incomplete correction, when severe enough to require surgery.

DIAGNOSIS

Early diagnosis of clubfoot is usually no problem because the deformity is obvious, but in subtle deformity, true clubfoot must be distinguished from apparent clubfoot (such as metatarsus varus or "pigeon toe").

- X-rays shows superimposition of the talus and calcaneus and a ladderlike appearance of the metatarsals (true clubfoot).

TREATMENT

Treatment for clubfoot is done in three stages: correcting the deformity, maintaining the correction until the foot regains normal muscle balance, and observing the foot closely for several years to prevent the deformity from recurring.

Clubfoot deformities are usually corrected in sequential order: forefoot adduction first, then varus (or inversion), then equinus (or plantar flexion). Trying to correct all three deformities at once only results in a misshapen, "rocker-bottomed" foot.

Other essential parts of management include:
- stressing to parents the importance of prompt treatment and orthopedic supervision until growth is completed
- teaching parents cast care and how to recognize circulatory impairment, before a child in a clubfoot cast is discharged
- explaining to an older child and the parents that surgery can improve clubfoot with good function but can't totally correct it; the affected calf muscle will remain slightly underdeveloped
- emphasizing the need for long-term orthopedic care to maintain correction; correcting this condition permanently takes time and patience.

Developmental dysplasia of the hip

Developmental dysplasia of the hip (DDH), an abnormality of the hip joint present from birth, is the most common disorder affecting the hip joints in children younger than age 3. About 85% of affected infants are girls.

DDH can be unilateral or bilateral. This abnormality occurs in three forms of varying severity:
- Unstable dysplasia: the hip is positioned normally but can be dislocated by manipulation.
- Subluxation or incomplete dislocation: the femoral head rides on the edge of the acetabulum.

- Complete dislocation: the femoral head is totally outside the acetabulum.

CAUSES
Although the causes of DDH aren't clear, it's more likely to occur in the following circumstances:
- dislocation after breech delivery (malposition in utero, 10 times more common than after cephalic delivery)
- elevated maternal relaxin, the hormone secreted by the corpus luteum during pregnancy that causes relaxation of pubic symphysis and cervical dilation (may promote relaxation of the joint ligaments in the fetus, predisposing the neonate to DDH)
- large neonates and twins.

PATHOPHYSIOLOGY
The precise cause of DDH is unknown. Excessive or abnormal movement of the joint during a traumatic birth may cause dislocation. Displacement of bones within the joint may damage joint structures, including articulating surfaces, blood vessels, tendons, ligaments, and nerves. This may lead to ischemic necrosis because of the disruption of blood flow to the joint.

SIGNS AND SYMPTOMS
Signs and symptoms of DDH vary with age and include:
- no gross deformity or pain (in neonates)
- the hip riding above the acetabulum, causing the level of the knees to be uneven (complete dysplasia) caused by laxity of the hip joint
- limited abduction on the dislocated side (as the child grows older and begins to walk)
- swaying from side to side ("duck waddle") caused by uncorrected bilateral dysplasia)
- limp caused by uncorrected unilateral dysplasia.

COMPLICATIONS
If corrective treatment isn't begun until after age 2, DDH may cause:
- degenerative hip changes
- abnormal acetabular development

- lordosis (abnormally increased concave curvature of the lumbar and cervical spine)
- joint malformation
- sciatic nerve injury (paralysis)
- avascular necrosis of femoral head
- soft tissue damage
- permanent disability.

DIAGNOSIS
Diagnostic measures may include:
- X-rays to show the location of the femur head and a shallow acetabulum (also to monitor disease or treatment progress)
- sonography and magnetic resonance imaging to assess dislocation.

Observations during physical examination of the relaxed child that strongly suggest DDH include:
- restricted abduction of the affected hip
- the number of folds of skin over the thighs on each side when the child is placed on his back (a child in this position usually has an equal number of folds, but a child with subluxation or dislocation may have an extra fold on the affected side, which is also apparent when the child lies prone)
- buttock fold on the affected side higher with the child lying prone. (See *Ortolani's and Trendelenburg's signs of DDH*, page 372.)

TREATMENT
The earlier an infant receives treatment, the better the chances are for normal development. Treatment varies with the patient's age.

In infants younger than age 3 months, treatment includes:
- gentle manipulation to reduce the dislocation, followed by splint-brace or harness to hold the hips in a flexed and abducted position to maintain the reduction
- splint-brace or harness worn continuously for 2 to 3 months, then a night splint for another month to tighten and stabilize the joint capsule in correct alignment.

If treatment doesn't begin until after age 3 months, it may include:
- bilateral skin traction (in infants) or skeletal traction (in children who have

Ortolani's and Trendelenburg's signs of DDH

A positive Ortolani's or Trendelenburg's sign confirms developmental dysplasia of the hip (DDH).

ORTOLANI'S SIGN
◆ Place infant on his back, with hip flexed and in abduction. Adduct the hip while pressing the femur downward. This will dislocate the hip.
◆ Then abduct the hip while moving the femur upward. A click or a jerk (produced by the femoral head moving over the acetabular rim) indicates subluxation in a neonate younger than age 1 month and subluxation or complete dislocation in an infant older than age 1 month.

TRENDELENBURG'S SIGN
◆ When the child stands with his weight on the side of the dislocation and lifts his other knee, the pelvis drops on the normal side because abductor muscles in the affected hip are weak.
◆ When the child stands with his weight on the normal side and lifts his other knee, the pelvis remains horizontal.

started walking) to try to reduce the dislocation by gradually abducting the hips
■ Bryant's traction or divarication traction (both extremities placed in traction, even if only one is affected, to help maintain immobilization) for 2 to 3 weeks for children who are younger than age 3 and who weigh less than 35 lb (16 kg)
■ gentle closed reduction under general anesthesia to further abduct the hips, followed by a spica cast for the prescribed period (if traction fails)
■ between ages 6 and 12 months, immobilization in a spica cast for about 3 months, possibly as long as 9 months
■ in children older than age 18 months, open reduction and pelvic or femoral os-

teotomy to correct bony deformity, followed by immobilization in a spica cast for 6 to 8 weeks.

In children ages 2 to 5, treatment is difficult and includes:
■ skeletal traction and subcutaneous adductor tenotomy (surgical cutting of the tendon).

Treatment begun after age 5 rarely restores satisfactory hip function.

Gout

Gout, also called *gouty arthritis,* is a metabolic disease marked by urate deposits that cause painful arthritic joints. It's found mostly in the foot, especially the great toe, ankle, and midfoot, but may affect any joint. Gout follows an intermittent course, and patients may be completely free from symptoms for years between attacks. The prognosis is good with treatment.

CAUSES
Although the exact cause of primary gout remains unknown, it may be caused by:
■ genetic defect in purine metabolism, causing overproduction of uric acid (hyperuricemia), retention of uric acid, or both.

In secondary gout, which develops during the course of another disease (such as obesity, diabetes mellitus, hypertension, sickle cell anemia, and renal disease), the cause may be:
■ breakdown of nucleic acid causing hyperuricemia
■ result of drug therapy, especially after the use of hydrochlorothiazide or pyrazinamide, which decrease urate excretion (ionic form of uric acid).

⚠ **AGE ALERT**
Primary gout usually occurs in men after age 30 and in postmenopausal women; secondary gout occurs in elderly people.

PATHOPHYSIOLOGY
When uric acid becomes supersaturated in blood and other body fluids, it crystallizes and forms a precipitate of urate salts that accumulate in connective tissue throughout the body; these deposits are called *tophi.* The presence of the crystals triggers

an acute inflammatory response when neutrophils begin to ingest the crystals. Tissue damage begins when the neutrophils release their lysosomes (See chapter 12, Immune system). The lysosomes not only damage the tissues but also perpetuate the inflammation.

In gout that produces no symptoms, serum urate levels increase but don't crystallize or produce symptoms. As the disease progresses, it may cause hypertension or formation of urate kidney.

The first acute attack strikes suddenly and peaks quickly. Although it generally involves only one or a few joints, this first attack is extremely painful. Affected joints are tender and appear hot, inflamed, dusky red, or cyanotic. The metatarsophalangeal joint of the great toe usually becomes inflamed first (podagra), then the instep, ankle, heel, knee, or wrist joints. Sometimes a low-grade fever is present. Mild acute attacks often subside quickly but tend to recur at irregular intervals. Severe attacks may persist for days or weeks.

Intercritical periods are the symptom-free intervals between gout attacks. Most patients have a second attack in 6 months to 2 years; some second attacks, especially in untreated patients, may last longer and be more severe than first attacks. Such attacks are also polyarticular, invariably affecting joints in the feet and legs, and may be accompanied by fever. A migratory attack sequentially strikes various joints and the Achilles' tendon and is linked to subdeltoid or olecranon bursitis.

Eventually, chronic polyarticular gout sets in. This final, unremitting stage of the disease is marked by persistent painful polyarthritis, with large tophi in cartilage, synovial membranes, tendons, and soft tissue. Tophi form in fingers, hands, knees, feet, ulnar sides of the forearms, helices of the ears, Achilles' tendons, and, rarely, in internal organs, such as the kidneys and myocardium. The skin over the tophus may ulcerate and release a chalky, white exudate that's composed primarily of uric acid crystals.

SIGNS AND SYMPTOMS

Possible signs and symptoms of gout include:

- joint pain caused by uric acid deposits and inflammation
- redness and swelling in joints caused by uric acid deposits and irritation
- tophi in the great toe, ankle, and pinna of ear caused by urate deposits
- elevated skin temperature from inflammation.

COMPLICATIONS

Complications of gout may include:

- eventual erosions, deformity, and disability caused by chronic inflammation and tophi that cause secondary joint degeneration
- hypertension and albuminuria (in some patients)
- kidney involvement, with tubular damage from aggregates of urate crystals; progressively poorer excretion of uric acid and chronic renal dysfunction.

DIAGNOSIS

The following test results help diagnose gout:

- needlelike monosodium urate crystals in synovial fluid (shown by needle aspiration) or tissue sections of tophaceous deposits
- hyperuricemia (uric acid greater than 420 µmol/mmol of creatinine)
- elevated 24-hour urine uric acid (usually higher in secondary than in primary gout)
- X-rays initially normal; in chronic gout, damage of articular cartilage and subchondral bone. Outward displacement of the overhanging margin from the bone contour characterizes gout.

TREATMENT

The goals of treatment are to end the acute attack as quickly as possible, prevent recurring attacks, and prevent or reverse complications. Treatment for acute gout consists of:

- immobilization and protection of the inflamed, painful joints
- local application of heat or cold
- increased fluid intake (to 3 qt [3 L]/day, if not contraindicated by other conditions, to prevent renal calculi formation)
- treatment with colchicine (P.O. or I.V.) every hour for 8 hours to inhibit phagocy-

tosis of uric acid crystals by neutrophils, until the pain subsides or nausea, vomiting, cramping, or diarrhea develops (in acute inflammation)

■ nonsteroidal anti-inflammatory drugs (NSAIDs) for pain and inflammation.

AGE ALERT
Older patients are at risk for GI bleeding linked to the use of NSAIDs. Encourage the patient to take these drugs with meals, and monitor the patient's stool for occult blood.

Treatment for chronic gout aims to decrease serum uric acid levels, including:

■ maintenance dosage of allopurinol to suppress uric acid formation or control uric acid levels, preventing further attacks (use cautiously in patients with renal failure)

■ colchicine to prevent recurrent acute attacks until uric acid returns to its normal level (doesn't affect uric acid level)

■ uricosuric drugs (probenecid and sulfinpyrazone) to promote uric acid excretion and inhibit uric acid accumulation (of limited value in patients with renal impairment)

■ dietary restrictions, primarily avoiding alcohol and purine-rich foods (shellfish, liver, sardines, anchovies, and kidneys) that increase urate levels (adjunctive therapy).

Herniated disk

Herniated disk, also called *ruptured* or *slipped disk* and *herniated nucleus pulposus,* occurs when all or part of the nucleus pulposus—the soft, gelatinous, central portion of an intervertebral disk—is forced through the disk's weakened or torn outer ring (anulus fibrosus). Herniated disk usually occurs in adults (mostly men) younger than age 45. About 90% of herniated disks are lumbar or lumbosacral; 8%, cervical; and 1% to 2%, thoracic. A patient with a congenitally small lumbar spinal canal or with osteophyte formation along the vertebrae may be more susceptible to nerve root compression and more likely to have neurologic symptoms.

CAUSES

Causes may include:
■ severe trauma or strain

■ intervertebral joint degeneration.

AGE ALERT
In older people whose disks have begun to degenerate, even minor trauma can cause herniation.

PATHOPHYSIOLOGY

An intervertebral disk has two parts: the soft center called the *nucleus pulposus* and the tough, fibrous surrounding ring called the *anulus fibrosus.* The nucleus pulposus acts as a shock absorber, distributing the mechanical stress applied to the spine when the body moves.

Physical stress, usually a twisting motion, can tear or rupture the anulus fibrosus so that the nucleus pulposus herniates into the spinal canal. When this happens, the extruded disk may impinge on spinal nerve roots as they exit from the spinal canal or on the spinal cord itself, resulting in back pain and other signs of nerve root irritation. The vertebrae move closer together and in turn exert pressure on the nerve roots as they exit between the vertebrae. Pain and sensory and motor loss may follow. A herniated disk can also follow intervertebral joint degeneration; minor trauma may cause herniation.

Herniation occurs in three steps:

■ protrusion—nucleus pulposus presses against the anulus fibrosus

■ extrusion—nucleus pulposus bulges forcibly through the anulus fibrosus, pushing against the nerve root

■ sequestration—anulus fibrosus gives way as the disk's core bursts and presses against the nerve root. (See *How a herniated disk develops.*)

SIGNS AND SYMPTOMS

The main symptom of lumbar herniated disk is severe lower back pain that radiates to the buttocks, legs, and feet, usually unilaterally. When herniation follows trauma, the pain may begin suddenly, subside in a few days, and then recur at shorter intervals and with progressive intensity. Sciatic pain follows, beginning as a dull pain in the buttocks from pressure on the surrounding nerves. Valsalva's maneuver, coughing, sneezing, or bending intensifies the pain (resulting from increased pressure on the nerve from the activity), which is commonly accompanied by muscle spasms. Herniated disk may also cause sensory and motor loss in the area innervated by the compressed spinal nerve root and, in later stages, weakness and atrophy of leg muscles.

COMPLICATIONS
Complications may include:
■ neurologic deficits (most common)
■ bowel and bladder problems (with lumbar herniations).

DIAGNOSIS
Obtaining a detailed patient history is vital because the events that intensify disk pain are diagnostically significant.

The straight-leg-raising test and its variants are perhaps the best tests for herniated disk. For the straight-leg-raising test, the patient lies in a supine position while the examiner places one hand on the patient's ilium to stabilize the pelvis and the other hand under the ankle, then slowly raises the patient's leg. The test is positive only if the patient complains of posterior leg (sciatic) pain, not back pain. In testing for Lasègue's sign, the patient lies flat while the thigh and knee are flexed to a 90-degree angle. Resistance and pain as well as loss of ankle or knee-jerk reflex indicate spinal root compression.

X-rays of the spine are essential to rule out other abnormalities but may not diagnose herniated disk because marked disk prolapse can be present despite a normal X-ray result. A thorough check of the patient's peripheral vascular status—including posterior tibial and dorsalis pedis pulses and skin temperature of extremities—helps rule out ischemic disease, another cause of leg pain or numbness. After physical examination and X-rays, myelography, computed tomography and magnetic resonance imaging provide the most specific diagnostic information, showing spinal canal compression by herniated disk material. Magnetic resonance imaging is the method of choice to confirm the diagnosis and determine the exact level of herniation.

CLOSER LOOK
How a herniated disk develops

These illustrations show how herniation of an intervertebral disk develops.

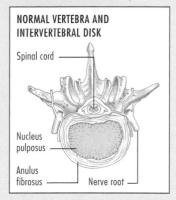

NORMAL VERTEBRA AND INTERVERTEBRAL DISK

Spinal cord

Nucleus pulposus

Anulus fibrosus

Nerve root

Physical stress, from severe trauma or strain, or intervertebral joint degeneration may cause herniation. Herniation occurs in three stages: protrusion, extrusion, and sequestration.

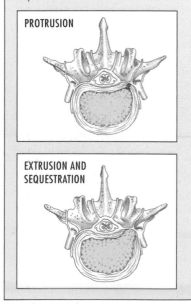

PROTRUSION

EXTRUSION AND SEQUESTRATION

TREATMENT

Unless neurologic impairment progresses rapidly, treatment is initially conservative and may consist of several weeks of bed rest (possibly with pelvic traction), administration of nonsteroidal anti-inflammatory drugs, heat applications, and an exercise program. Epidural corticosteroids, short-term oral corticosteroids, nerve root blocks, or physical therapy can be used to decrease pain. Muscle relaxants, such as diazepam, methocarbamol, or cyclobenzaprine may relieve muscle spasms.

If conservative treatment isn't effective, surgery may be necessary. The most common procedure, laminectomy, involves excision of a portion of the lamina (bone plates that make up a vertebral arch) and removal of the nucleus pulposus of the protruding disk. If laminectomy doesn't alleviate pain and disability, a spinal fusion may be necessary to overcome segmental instability. Laminectomy and spinal fusion are sometimes performed together to stabilize the spine. Microdiskectomy can also be used to remove fragments of nucleus pulposus.

Injection of chymopapain into the herniated disk produces a loss of water and proteoglycans from the disk, thereby reducing both the disk's size and the pressure on the nerve root. Chymopapain is most commonly used for herniations in the lumbar region.

Legg-Calvé-Perthes disease

Legg-Calvé-Perthes disease (also called *coxa plana*) is ischemic necrosis leading to eventual flattening of the head of the femur caused by vascular interruption. This condition occurs most commonly in boys ages 4 to 10 and tends to occur in families. It's typically unilateral but may be bilateral in 20% of patients.

Although this disease usually runs its course in 3 to 4 years, it may lead to premature osteoarthritis later in life because of misalignment of the acetabulum and flattening of the femoral head.

CAUSES

The exact vascular obstructive changes that start Legg-Calvé-Perthes disease are unknown. Current etiologic theories include:

- venous obstruction with secondary intraepiphyseal thrombosis
- trauma to retinacular vessels
- vascular irregularities (congenital or developmental)
- vascular occlusion caused by increased intracapsular pressure from acute transient synovitis
- increased blood viscosity resulting in stasis and decreased blood flow.

PATHOPHYSIOLOGY

The disease occurs in four stages. The first stage, synovitis, is characterized by synovial inflammation and increased joint fluid, and typically lasts 1 to 3 weeks. In the second (avascular) stage, vascular interruption causes necrosis of the ossification center of the femoral head (usually in several months to 1 year). In the third stage, revascularization, a new blood supply causes bone resorption and deposition of immature bone cells. New bone replaces necrotic bone and the femoral head gradually reforms. The final, or residual stage, involves healing and regeneration. Immature bone cells are replaced by normal bone cells, thereby fixing the joint's shape. There may be residual deformity, based on the degree of necrosis that occurred in stage two.

SIGNS AND SYMPTOMS

The first indication of Legg-Calvé-Perthes disease is usually a persistent thigh pain or limp that becomes progressively severe. This symptom appears when bone resorption and deformity begin. Other effects may include:

- mild pain in the hip, thigh, or knee—aggravated by activity and relieved by rest—caused by inflammation and increased joint fluid and avascular necrosis
- muscle spasm related to inflammation
- atrophy of muscles in the upper thigh, caused by necrosis
- slight shortening of the leg
- severely restricted abduction and internal rotation of the hip caused by pain and necrosis.

COMPLICATIONS

Complications result from misalignment of the acetabulum and the flattened femoral head and may include:

- permanent disability
- premature osteoarthritis.

DIAGNOSIS

A thorough physical examination and clinical history can suggest Legg-Calvé-Perthes disease. Hip X-rays taken every 3 to 4 months confirm the diagnosis, with findings that vary according to the stage of the disease. Anterior-posterior X-rays and magnetic resonance imaging allow visualization of articular surfaces and help with early diagnosis of necrosis.

Diagnostic evaluation must also differentiate between Legg-Calvé-Perthes disease (restriction of only the abduction and rotation of the hip) and infection or arthritis (restriction of all motion). Aspiration and culture of synovial fluid rule out joint sepsis.

TREATMENT

The aim of treatment is to protect the femoral head from further stress and damage by containing it within the acetabulum. After 1 to 2 weeks of bed rest, therapy may include reduced weight bearing by means of bed rest in bilateral split counterpoised traction, then application of hip abduction splint or cast, or weight bearing while a splint, cast, or brace holds the leg in abduction. Braces may remain in place for 6 to 18 months. Analgesics help relieve pain. Physical therapy with passive and active range-of-motion exercises after cast removal helps restore motion.

For a young child in the early stages of the disease, osteotomy and subtrochanteric internal rotation provide maximum confinement of the epiphysis within the acetabulum to allow return of the femoral head to normal shape and full range of motion. Proper placement of the epiphysis thus allows remolding with ambulation. Postoperatively, the patient requires a spica cast for about 2 months.

Muscular dystrophy

Muscular dystrophy is a group of congenital disorders characterized by progressive symmetric wasting of skeletal muscles without neural or sensory defects. Paradoxically, some wasted muscles tend to enlarge (pseudohypertrophy) because connective tissue and fat replace muscle tissue, giving a false impression of increased muscle strength. Genetic counseling regarding risk of transmitting disease for family members who are carriers is recommended.

The four main types of muscular dystrophy include:

- Duchenne's, or pseudohypertrophic; 50% of all cases
- Becker's, or benign pseudohypertrophic
- Landouzy-Dejerine, or facioscapulohumeral
- limb-girdle.

The prognosis varies with the form of disease. Duchenne muscular dystrophy strikes during early childhood and is usually fatal during the second decade of life. It mostly affects males, 13 to 33 per 100,000 people. Patients with Becker's muscular dystrophy can live into their 40s, and it mostly affects males, 1 to 3 per 100,000 people. Facioscapulohumeral and limb-girdle muscular dystrophies usually don't shorten life expectancy, and they affect both sexes equally.

CAUSES

Causes of muscular dystrophy include:

- various genetic mechanisms typically involving an enzymatic or metabolic defect
- X-linked recessive disorders caused by defects in the gene coding, mapped genetically to the Xp21 locus, for the muscle protein dystrophin, which is essential for maintaining muscle cell membrane; muscle cells deteriorate or die without it (Duchenne's and Becker's muscular dystrophies)
- autosomal dominant disorder (facioscapulohumeral muscular dystrophy)
- autosomal recessive disorder (limb-girdle muscular dystrophy).

PATHOPHYSIOLOGY

Abnormally permeable cell membranes allow leakage of a variety of muscle enzymes, particularly creatine kinase. This metabolic defect that causes the muscle cells to die is present from fetal life on-ward. The absence of progressive muscle wasting at birth suggests that other factors compensate for the effect of dystrophin deficiency. The specific trigger is un-known, but phagocytosis of the muscle cells by inflammatory cells causes scarring and loss of muscle function.

As the disease progresses, skeletal mus-cle becomes almost totally replaced by fat and connective tissue. The skeleton even-tually becomes deformed, causing progres-sive immobility. Cardiac and smooth mus-cle of the GI tract typically become fibrot-ic. No consistent structural abnormalities are seen in the brain.

SIGNS AND SYMPTOMS

Signs and symptoms of Duchenne's mus-cular dystrophy include:
- insidious onset between ages 3 and 5
- initial effect on legs, pelvis, and shoulders
- waddling gait, toe-walking, and lumbar lordosis caused by muscle weakness
- difficulty climbing stairs, frequent falls because of muscular weakness resulting from inflammation
- enlarged, firm calf muscles from muscle replacement by fat and connective tissue
- progressive immobility and skeletal de-formities (use of a wheelchair is usually necessary by age 12).

Signs and symptoms of Becker's (be-nign pseudohypertrophic) muscular dys-trophy are:
- similar to those of Duchenne's muscular dystrophy but with slower progression.

Signs of facioscapulohumeral (Landouzy-Dejerine) muscular dystrophy include:
- weakened face, shoulder, and upper arm muscles (initial sign) because of scar-ring and loss of muscle function
- pendulous lip and absent nasolabial fold because of muscular weakness
- inability to pucker mouth or whistle be-cause of muscular weakness
- abnormal facial movements and ab-sence of facial movements when laughing or crying, because of muscle weakness and scarring

- diffuse facial flattening leading to a masklike expression resulting from pro-gressive muscle scarring
- inability to raise arms above the head because of extreme muscle weakness.

Signs and symptoms of limb-girdle muscular dystrophy include:
- weakness in upper arms and pelvis first
- lumbar lordosis with abdominal protru-sion because of loss of muscular support
- "winging" of the scapulae
- waddling gait because of muscle weak-ness
- poor balance because of muscle weak-ness
- inability to raise the arms caused by progressive muscle weakness.

COMPLICATIONS

Possible complications include:
- weakened cardiac and respiratory mus-cles leading to tachycardia, electrocardio-graphic abnormalities, and pulmonary complications
- death commonly caused by sudden heart failure, respiratory failure, or infection.

DIAGNOSIS

Diagnosis depends on typical clinical find-ings, family history, and diagnostic test findings. If another family member has muscular dystrophy, its clinical character-istics can suggest the type of dystrophy thepatient has and how he may be affect-ed. The following tests may help in the diagnosis:
- electromyograph showing short, weak bursts of electrical activity in affected muscles
- muscle biopsy showing a combination of muscle cell degeneration and regenera-tion (in later stages, showing fat and con-nective tissue deposits)
- immunologic and molecular biological techniques (now available in specialized medical centers) to help with accurate prenatal and postnatal diagnosis of Duchenne's and Becker's muscular dys-trophies (replacing muscle biopsy and elevated serum creatine kinase levels in diagnosis).

TREATMENT

No treatment can stop the progressive muscle impairment. Supportive treatments include:
- having the patient cough and do deep-breathing exercises and diaphragmatic breathing
- teaching parents to recognize early signs of respiratory complications
- orthopedic appliances, exercise, physical therapy, and surgery to correct contractures (to help preserve mobility and independence)
- adequate fluid intake, increased dietary bulk, and stool softener for constipation caused by inactivity
- low-calorie, high-protein, high-fiber diet (physical inactivity put patient at risk for obesity)
- surgery to promote or maintain motility, such as tendon releases for contractures and spinal fusions for scoliosis.

Osteoarthritis

Osteoarthritis (commonly referred to as *degenerative joint disease*), the most common form of arthritis, is a chronic condition causing the deterioration of joint cartilage and the formation of reactive new bone at the margins and subchondral areas of the joints. It usually affects weight-bearing joints (knees, feet, hips, lumbar vertebrae). Osteoarthritis is widespread (affecting more than 60 million people in the United States) and is most common in women. Typically, its earliest symptoms appear in middle-age and progress from there.

Disability depends on the site and severity of involvement and can range from minor limitation of finger movement to severe disability in people with hip or knee involvement. The rate of progression varies, and joints may remain stable for years in an early stage of deterioration.

CAUSES

The primary defect in both idiopathic and secondary osteoarthritis is loss of articular cartilage caused by functional changes in chondrocytes (cells responsible for the formation of the proteoglycans, glycoproteins that act as cementing material in the cartilage, and collagen).

Idiopathic osteoarthritis, a normal part of aging, results from many factors, including:
- metabolic factors (endocrine disorders such as hyperparathyroidism) and genetic factors (decreased collagen synthesis)
- chemical factors (drugs that stimulate the collagen-digesting enzymes in the synovial membrane such as steroids)
- mechanical factors (repeated stress on the joint).

Secondary osteoarthritis usually follows an identifiable predisposing event that leads to degenerative changes, such as:
- trauma (most common cause)
- congenital deformity
- obesity.

PATHOPHYSIOLOGY

Osteoarthritis occurs in synovial joints. The joint cartilage deteriorates, and reactive new bone forms at the margins and subchondral areas of the joints. The degeneration results from damage to the chondrocytes. Cartilage softens with age, narrowing the joint space. Mechanical injury erodes articular cartilage, leaving the underlying bone unprotected. This causes sclerosis, or thickening and hardening of the bone underneath the cartilage.

Cartilage flakes irritate the synovial lining, which becomes fibrotic and limits joint movement. Synovial fluid may be forced into defects in the bone, causing cysts. New bone, called *osteophyte* (bone spur), forms at joint margins as the articular cartilage erodes, causing gross alteration of the bony contours and enlargement of the joint.

SIGNS AND SYMPTOMS

Symptoms, which increase with poor posture, obesity, and occupational stress, include:
- deep, aching joint pain caused by degradation of the cartilage, inflammation, and bone stress, particularly after exercise or weight bearing (the most common symptom, usually relieved by rest)
- stiffness in the morning and after exercise (relieved by rest) caused by degradation of the cartilage, inflammation, and bone stress

Specific care for arthritic joints

Specific care depends on the affected joint.
◆ Hand: Apply hot soaks and paraffin dips to relieve pain.
◆ Lumbar and sacral spine: Recommend a firm mattress or bed board to decrease morning pain.
◆ Cervical spine: If patient uses a cervical collar, check for constriction; watch for skin redness with prolonged use.
◆ Hip: Use moist heat pads to relieve pain, and give antispasmodics. Assist with range-of-motion (ROM) and strengthening exercises, always making sure the patient gets proper rest afterward. Check crutches, cane, braces, and walker for proper fit, and teach the patient to use them correctly. For example, the patient with unilateral joint involvement should use an orthopedic appliance (such as a cane or walker) on the unaffected side. Advise use of cushions for sitting and use of an elevated toilet seat.
◆ Knee: Assist with ROM exercises, exercises to maintain muscle tone, and progressive re-sistance exercises to increase muscle strength. Provide elastic supports or braces, if needed.

To minimize the long-term effects of osteoarthritis, teach the patient to:
◆ plan for adequate rest during the day, after exertion, and at night
◆ take medication exactly as prescribed and report adverse effects immediately
◆ avoid overexertion, take care to stand and walk correctly, minimize weight-bearing activities, and be especially careful when stooping or picking up objects
◆ always wear well-fitting supportive shoes and avoid letting the heels become too worn down
◆ use safety devices at home, such as guardrails in the bathroom
◆ perform ROM exercises as gently as possible
◆ maintain proper body weight to reduce strain on joints
◆ avoid percussive activities.

■ crepitus, or "grating" of the joint during motion because of cartilage damage
■ Heberden's nodes (bony enlargements of the distal interphalangeal joints) caused by repeated inflammation
■ altered gait because of contractures from overcompensation of the muscles supporting the joint
■ decreased range of motion because of pain and stiffness
■ joint enlargement caused by stress on the bone and disordered bone growth
■ localized headaches (may be a direct result of cervical spine arthritis).

COMPLICATIONS
Complications of osteoarthritis include:
■ irreversible joint changes and node formation (nodes eventually becoming red, swollen, and tender, causing numbness and loss of finger dexterity)
■ subluxation of the joint
■ decreased joint range of motion
■ joint contractures

■ pain (can be debilitating in later stages)
■ loss of independence in activities of daily living.

DIAGNOSIS
Findings that help diagnose osteoarthritis include:
■ absence of systemic symptoms (ruling out inflammatory joint disorder)
■ arthroscopy showing bone spurs, narrowing of joint space
■ increased erythrocyte sedimentation rate (in extensive synovitis).

X-rays of the affected joint help confirm the diagnosis but may appear normal in the early stages. X-ray may require many views and typically shows:
■ narrowing of joint space or margin
■ cystlike bony deposits in joint space and margins, sclerosis of the subchondral space
■ joint deformity caused by degeneration or articular damage
■ bony growths at weight-bearing areas
■ joint fusion.

TREATMENT

The goal of treatment is to relieve pain, maintain or improve mobility, and minimize disability. Treatment may include:

- weight loss to reduce stress on the joint
- a balance of rest and exercise
- medications, including aspirin, fenoprofen, ibuprofen, indomethacin, phenylbutazone, and other nonsteroidal anti-inflammatory drugs; propoxyphene, celecoxib, and glucosamine (see *Specific care for arthritic joints*)
- support or stabilization of joint with crutches, braces, cane, walker, cervical collar, or traction to reduce stress
- intra-articular injections of corticosteroids (every 4 to 6 months) to possibly delay node development in the hands (if used too frequently, corticosteroids may accelerate arthritic progression by depleting the normal ground substance of the cartilage).

Surgical treatment, reserved for patients with severe disability or uncontrollable pain, may include:

- arthroplasty (partial or total replacement of deteriorated part of joint with prosthetic appliance)
- arthrodesis (surgical fusion of bones, primarily in spine)
- osteoplasty (scraping and lavage of deteriorated bone from joint)
- osteotomy (cutting of bone) to relieve stress on the bone by cutting it or removing a wedge to realign the bone.

Osteogenesis imperfecta

Osteogenesis imperfecta (also called *brittle bone disease*) is a genetic disease in which bones are thin, poorly developed, and fracture easily.

The expression of the disease varies, depending on whether the defect is carried as a trait or is clinically obvious. (See chapter 5, Genetics.) If it's inherited as an autosomal dominant disorder, a heterozygote may eventually express the disease, which occurs in about 1 in 30,000 people. If inheritance is as an autosomal recessive disorder, the homozygous child will likely die before, during, or soon after birth from multiple fractures sustained in utero or during delivery.

CAUSES

Causes of osteogenesis imperfecta include:

- genetic disease, typically autosomal dominant (characterized by a defect in the synthesis of connective tissue)
- autosomal recessive carriage of gene defects that produce osteogenesis imperfecta in homozygotes (osteoporosis in some).

PATHOPHYSIOLOGY

Most forms of the disease appear to be caused by mutations in the genes that determine the structure of collagen. Possible mutations in other genes may cause variations in the assembly and maintenance of bone and other connective tissues. Collectively or alone, these mutated genes lead to pathologic fractures and impaired healing.

SIGNS AND SYMPTOMS

Signs and symptoms include (in the autosomal dominant disorder, some of these symptoms may not be apparent until the child's mobility increases):

- frequent fractures and poor healing from falls as toddler begins to walk
- short stature caused by multiple fractures from minor physical stress
- deformed cranial structure and limbs from multiple fractures
- thin skin and bluish sclera of the eyes; thin collagen fibers of the sclera allowing the choroid layer to be seen
- abnormal tooth and enamel development because of improper deposition of dentine
- middle ear deafness caused by bone deformity interfering with sound transmission.

COMPLICATIONS

Possible complications of osteogenesis imperfecta include:

- deafness caused by bone deformity and scarring of the middle and inner ear
- stillbirth or death within the first year of life (in autosomal-recessive disorder).

DIAGNOSIS

Diagnosis involves:

- fractures early in life, hearing loss, and blue sclera, showing that mutation in on

pressed in more than one kind of connective tissue
■ elevated serum alkaline phosphatase levels (during periods of rapid bone formation and cellular injury)
■ skin culture showing abnormally low quantity of fibroblasts
■ echocardiography, possibly showing mitral insufficiency or floppy mitral valves.

TREATMENT
Possible treatments are:
■ prevention of fractures with splints and supports
■ internal fixation of fractures to ensure stabilization and prevent deformities.

Osteomalacia and rickets

In vitamin D deficiency, bone can't calcify normally; the result is called *rickets* in infants and young children and *osteomalacia* in adults. This abnormal calcification may cause bone deformity.

Once a common childhood disease, rickets is now rare in the United States. It does appear occasionally in breast-fed infants who don't receive a vitamin D supplement or in infants fed a formula with a nonfortified milk base. Rickets also occurs in overcrowded, urban areas where smog limits sunlight penetration.

CULTURAL DIVERSITY
Incidence of rickets is highest in children with black or dark brown skin, who, because of their pigmentation, absorb less sunlight.

With treatment, the prognosis is good. In osteomalacia, bone deformities may disappear. They usually persist in children with rickets.

CAUSES
Causes of osteomalacia and rickets include:
■ inadequate dietary intake of vitamin D
■ malabsorption of vitamin D
■ inadequate exposure to sunlight (solar ultraviolet rays irradiate 7-dehydrocholesterol, a precursor of vitamin D, to form calciferol, important in the prevention and treatment of vitamin D deficiency)
■ inherited impairment of renal tubular reabsorption of phosphate (from vitamin D insensitivity) in vitamin D–resistant

rickets (refractory rickets, familial hypophosphatemia)
■ conditions that reduce the absorption of fat-soluble vitamin D (such as chronic pancreatitis, celiac disease, Crohn's disease, cystic fibrosis, gastric or small-bowel resections, fistulas, colitis, and biliary obstruction)
■ hepatic or renal disease (interfering with hydroxylated calciferol formation, needed to form a calcium-binding protein in intestinal absorption sites)
■ malfunctioning parathyroid gland (decreased secretion of parathyroid hormone), contributing to calcium deficiency and interfering with activation of vitamin D in the kidneys (see "Pathophysiology").

PATHOPHYSIOLOGY
Vitamin D regulates the absorption of calcium ions from the intestine. When vitamin D is lacking, falling serum calcium concentration stimulates synthesis and secretion of parathyroid hormone, causing release of calcium from bone, decreasing renal calcium excretion, and increasing renal phosphate excretion. When the concentration of phosphate in the bone decreases, osteoid may be produced, but mineralization can't proceed normally. Large quantities of osteoid accumulate, coating the trabeculae and linings of the haversian canals and areas beneath the periosteum.

When mineralization of bone matrix is delayed or inadequate, bone is disorganized in structure and lacks density. The result is gross deformity of both spongy and compact bone.

SIGNS AND SYMPTOMS
Osteomalacia may be asymptomatic until a fracture occurs. Chronic vitamin D deficiency induces numerous bone malformations caused by bone softening, such as:
■ bow legs
■ knock knees
■ rachitic rosary (beading of ends of ribs)
■ enlarged wrists and ankles
■ "pigeon breast" (protruding ribs and sternum)
■ delayed closing of fontanels
■ softening skull
■ bulging forehead

- kyphoscoliosis.
  Other possible signs and symptoms include:
- pain in the legs and lower back caused by vertebral collapse
- poorly developed muscles (pot belly)
- difficulty walking and climbing stairs caused by bone deformities.

COMPLICATIONS
Complications of osteomalacia and rickets may include:
- spontaneous multiple fractures
- tetany in infants
- bone deformities.

DIAGNOSIS
Physical examination, dietary history, and laboratory tests establish the diagnosis. Test results that suggest vitamin D deficiency include:
- serum calcium concentration less than 7.5 mg/dl
- serum inorganic phosphorus concentration less than 3 mg/dl
- serum citrate level less than 2.5 mg/dl, and alkaline phosphatase level less than 4 Bodansky units/dl
- X-rays showing characteristic bone deformities and abnormalities such as Looser's zones (radiolucent bands perpendicular to the surface of the bones indicating reduced bone ossification; confirms the diagnosis).

TREATMENT
Possible treatments include:
- massive oral doses of vitamin D or cod liver oil (for osteomalacia and rickets, except when caused by malabsorption)
- 25-hydroxycholecalciferol, 1,25-dihydroxycholecalciferol, or a synthetic analogue of active vitamin (for rickets refractory to vitamin D or rickets accompanied by hepatic or renal disease)
- foods high in vitamin D (fortified milk, fish liver oils, herring, liver, and egg yolks) and sufficient sun exposure
- supplemental aqueous preparations of vitamin D for chronic fat malabsorption, hydroxylated cholecalciferol for refractory rickets, and supplemental vitamin D for breast-fed infants (to prevent rickets)

- possible surgical intervention for intestinal disease.

Osteomyelitis

Osteomyelitis is a bone infection characterized by progressive inflammatory destruction after formation of new bone. It may be chronic or acute. It commonly results from a combination of local trauma—usually trivial but causing a hematoma—and an acute infection originating elsewhere in the body. Although osteomyelitis often remains localized, it can spread through the bone to the marrow, cortex, and periosteum. Acute osteomyelitis is usually a blood-borne disease and most commonly affects rapidly growing children. Chronic osteomyelitis, which is rare, is characterized by draining sinus tracts and widespread lesions.

AGE ALERT
Osteomyelitis occurs more commonly in children (especially boys) than in adults—usually as a complication of an acute localized infection. Typical sites in children are the lower end of the femur and the upper ends of the tibia, humerus, and radius. The most common sites in adults are the pelvis and vertebrae, generally after surgery or trauma.

The incidence of both chronic and acute osteomyelitis is declining, except in drug abusers.

With prompt treatment, the prognosis for acute osteomyelitis is very good; for chronic osteomyelitis, prognosis remains poor.

CAUSES
The most common pyogenic (pus-producing) organism in osteomyelitis is *Staphylococcus aureus.*
Others include:
- *Streptococcus pyogenes*
- pneumococcus
- *Pseudomonas aeruginosa*
- *Escherichia coli*
- *Proteus vulgaris*
- *Pasteurella multocida* (part of the normal mouth flora of cats and dogs).

PATHOPHYSIOLOGY
Typically, these organisms find a culture site in a hematoma from recent trauma or

DISRUPTING DISEASE
Avoiding osteomyelitis

Bones are essentially isolated from the body's natural defense system once an organism gets through the periosteum. Bones have only limited ability to replace necrotic tissue caused by infection, which may lead to chronic osteomyelitis.

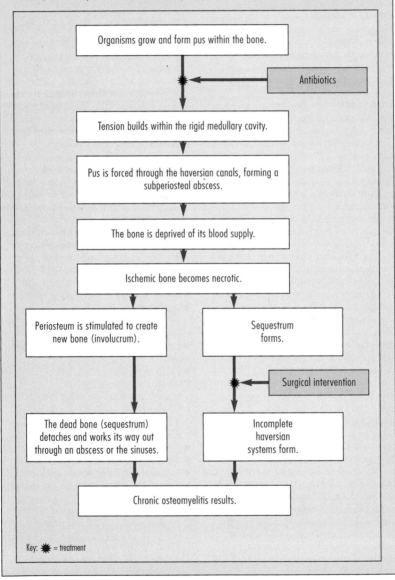

Organisms grow and form pus within the bone.

Antibiotics

Tension builds within the rigid medullary cavity.

Pus is forced through the haversian canals, forming a subperiosteal abscess.

The bone is deprived of its blood supply.

Ischemic bone becomes necrotic.

Periosteum is stimulated to create new bone (involucrum).

Sequestrum forms.

Surgical intervention

The dead bone (sequestrum) detaches and works its way out through an abscess or the sinuses.

Incomplete haversian systems form.

Chronic osteomyelitis results.

Key: ✹ = treatment

in a weakened area, such as the site of local infection (for example, furunculosis), and travel through the bloodstream to the metaphysis, the section of a long bone that's continuous with the epiphysis plates, where the blood flows into sinusoids. (See *Avoiding osteomyelitis.*)

SIGNS AND SYMPTOMS

Clinical features of chronic and acute osteomyelitis are generally the same and may include:
- rapid onset of acute osteomyelitis, with sudden pain in the affected bone and tenderness, heat, swelling, erythema, guarding of affected region of the limb, and restricted movement caused by inflammation and infection
- chronic infection persisting intermittently for years, flaring after minor trauma or persisting as drainage of pus from an old pocket in a sinus tract
- accompanying fever and tachycardia resulting from the infectious process
- dehydration (in young patients) resulting from effects of the infectious process
- irritability and poor feeding (in infants).

COMPLICATIONS

Possible complications of osteomyelitis include:
- amputation (of an arm or leg when resistant chronic osteomyelitis causes severe, unrelenting pain and decreases function)
- weakened bone cortex, predisposing the bone to pathologic fracture
- halted growth of an extremity (in children with severe disease).

DIAGNOSIS

Diagnosis must rule out septicemia, foreign bodies, poliomyelitis (rare), rheumatic fever, myositis (inflammation of voluntary muscle), and bone fracture. Patient's history, physical examination, and laboratory tests that help confirm osteomyelitis may include:
- history of a urinary tract, respiratory tract, ear, or skin infection; human or animal bite; or other penetrating trauma
- white blood cell count showing leukocytosis
- elevated erythrocyte sedimentation rate

- blood cultures showing causative organism
- magnetic resonance imaging to delineate bone marrow from soft tissue (facilitates diagnosis)
- X-rays (may not show bone involvement until the disease has been active for 2 to 3 weeks)
- bone scans to detect early infection.

TREATMENT

Treatment for acute osteomyelitis should begin before definitive diagnosis and includes:
- large doses of antibiotics I.V. (usually a penicillinase-resistant penicillin, such as nafcillin or oxacillin) after blood cultures are taken
- early surgical drainage to relieve pressure and abscess formation
- immobilization of the affected body part by cast, traction, or bed rest to prevent failure to heal or recurrence
- supportive measures, such as analgesics for pain and I.V. fluids to maintain hydration
- incision and drainage with a culture of the drainage (if an abscess or sinus tract forms).

Antibiotic therapy to control infection may include:
- systemic antibiotics
- intracavitary instillation of antibiotics through closed-system continuous irrigation with low intermittent suction
- limited irrigation with blood drainage system with suction (Hemovac)
- packed, wet, antibiotic-soaked dressings.

Chronic osteomyelitis care may include:
- surgery, usually required to remove dead bone and promote drainage (prognosis remains poor even after surgery)
- hyperbaric oxygen to stimulate normal immune mechanisms
- skin, bone, and muscle grafts to fill in dead space and increase blood supply.

Osteoporosis

Osteoporosis is a metabolic bone disorder in which the rate of bone resorption accelerates while the rate of bone formation slows, causing a loss of bone mass. Bones affected by this disease lose calcium and phosphate salts and become porous, brittle, and abnormally vulnerable to fractures. Osteoporosis may be primary or secondary, caused by an underlying disease, such as Cushing's syndrome or hyperthyroidism. It primarily affects the weight-bearing vertebrae. Only when the condition is advanced or severe, as in secondary disease, do similar changes occur in the skull, ribs, and long bones. Usually, the femoral heads and pelvic acetabula are selectively affected.

Primary osteoporosis is often called *postmenopausal osteoporosis* because it usually develops in postmenopausal women.

CAUSES
The cause of primary osteoporosis is unknown, but contributing factors include:
■ mild but prolonged negative calcium balance because of inadequate dietary intake of calcium (may be an important contributing factor)
■ declining gonadal and adrenal function
■ faulty protein metabolism caused by relative or progressive estrogen deficiency (estrogen stimulates osteoblastic activity and limits the osteoclastic-stimulating effects of parathyroid hormones)
■ sedentary lifestyle.

The many causes of secondary osteoporosis include:
■ prolonged therapy with steroids or heparin (heparin promotes bone resorption by inhibiting collagen synthesis or enhancing collagen breakdown)
■ total immobilization or disuse of a bone (as in hemiplegia)
■ alcoholism
■ malnutrition
■ malabsorption
■ scurvy
■ lactose intolerance
■ endocrine disorders such as hyperthyroidism, hyperparathyroidism, Cushing's syndrome, diabetes mellitus (plasma calcium and phosphate concentrations are maintained by the endocrine system)
■ osteogenesis imperfecta
■ Sudeck's atrophy (localized to hands and feet, with recurring attacks)
■ medications (aluminum-containing antacids, corticosteroids, anticonvulsants)
■ cigarette smoking.

PATHOPHYSIOLOGY
In normal bone, the rates of bone formation and resorption are constant; replacement follows resorption immediately, and the amount of bone replaced equals the amount of bone resorbed. Osteoporosis develops when the remodeling cycle is interrupted, and new bone formation falls behind resorption.

When bone is resorbed faster than it forms, the bone becomes less dense. Men have about 30% greater bone mass than women, which may explain why osteoporosis develops later in men.

SIGNS AND SYMPTOMS
The signs and symptoms seen with osteoporosis result from the loss of bone density. Osteoporosis is typically discovered suddenly, such as:
■ a postmenopausal woman bends to lift something, hears a snapping sound, then feels a sudden pain in her lower back
■ vertebral collapse causes back pain that radiates around the trunk (the most common presenting feature) and is aggravated by movement or jarring.

In another common pattern, osteoporosis can develop insidiously, showing:
■ increasing deformity, kyphosis, loss of height, decreased exercise tolerance, and a markedly aged appearance
■ spontaneous wedge (compression fracture of only the anterior part of a vertebrae, resulting in a wedge-shaped vertebra) fractures, pathologic fractures of the neck and femur, Colles' fractures of the distal radius after a minor fall, and hip fractures (common as bone is lost from the femoral neck).

COMPLICATIONS
Possible complications of osteoporosis include:
■ spontaneous fractures as the bones lose volume and become brittle and weak
■ shock, hemorrhage, or fat embolism (fatal complications of fractures).

DIAGNOSIS
Differential diagnosis must exclude other causes of bone loss, especially those affecting the spine, such as metastatic cancer or advanced multiple myeloma. History is

the key to identify the specific cause of osteoporosis. Diagnosis may include:

- dual- or single-photon absorptiometry to measure bone mass of the extremities, hips, and spine
- X-rays showing typical degeneration in the lower thoracic and lumbar vertebrae (vertebral bodies may appear flattened and may look denser than normal; bone mineral loss is evident in only later stages)
- computed tomography scan to assess spinal bone loss
- normal serum calcium, phosphorus, and alkaline phosphatase levels, possibly elevated parathyroid hormone
- bone biopsy showing thin, porous, but otherwise normal-looking bone.

TREATMENT
Treatment to control bone loss, prevent fractures, and control pain may include:

- physical therapy emphasizing gentle exercise and activity and regular, moderate weight-bearing exercise to slow bone loss and possibly reverse demineralization (the mechanical stress of exercise stimulates bone formation)
- supportive devices such as a back brace
- surgery, if indicated, for pathologic fractures
- hormone replacement therapy with estrogen and progesterone to slow bone loss and prevent occurrence of fractures
- analgesics and local heat to relieve pain.
  Other medications include:
- calcium and vitamin D supplements to support normal bone metabolism
- calcitonin to reduce bone resorption and slow the decline in bone mass
- bisphosphonates (such as etidronate to increase bone density and restore lost bone
- fluoride (such as alendronate) to stimulate bone formation; requires strict dosage precautions, and can cause gastric distress
- vitamin C, calcium, and protein to support skeletal metabolism (through a balanced diet rich in nutrients).
  Other measures include:
- early mobilization after surgery or trauma
- decreased alcohol and tobacco consumption
- careful observation for signs of malabsorption (fatty stools, chronic diarrhea)

- prompt, effective treatment of the underlying disorder (in secondary osteoporosis).

Paget's disease

Paget's disease, also called *osteitis deformans,* is a slowly progressive metabolic bone disease characterized by accelerated patterns of bone remodeling. An initial phase of excessive bone resorption (osteoclastic phase) is followed by a reactive phase of excessive abnormal bone formation (osteoblastic phase). Chronic accelerated remodeling eventually enlarges and softens the affected bones. The new bone structure, which is chaotic, fragile, and weak, causes painful deformities of both external contour and internal structure. Paget's disease usually localizes in one or several areas of the skeleton (most frequently the lumbosacral spine, skull, pelvis, femur, or tibia), but occasionally skeletal deformity is more widely distributed.

In the United States, Paget's disease affects about 2.5 million people older than age 40 (mostly men). It can be fatal, particularly when linked to heart failure (widespread disease creates a continuous need for high cardiac output), bone sarcoma, or giant-cell tumors.

CAUSES
Although the exact cause of Paget's disease is unknown, one theory is that early viral infection causes a dormant skeletal infection that erupts many years later as Paget's disease.

Other possible causes include:

- benign or malignant bone tumors
- vitamin D deficiency during the bone-developing years of childhood
- autoimmune disease
- estrogen deficiency.

PATHOPHYSIOLOGY
Repeated episodes of accelerated osteoclastic resorption of spongy bone occur. The trabeculae diminish, and vascular fibrous tissue replaces marrow. This is followed by short periods of rapid, abnormal bone formation. The collagen fibers in this new bone are disorganized, and glycoprotein levels in the matrix decrease. The partially

resorbed trabeculae thicken and enlarge because of excessive bone formation, and the bone becomes soft and weak.

SIGNS AND SYMPTOMS

Clinical effects of Paget's disease vary. Early stages may not produce symptoms. When signs and symptoms do appear, they may include:

■ usually severe and persistent pain intensifying with weight bearing, possibly with impaired movement caused by impingement of abnormal bone on the spinal cord or sensory nerve root (pain may also result from the constant inflammation accompanying cell breakdown)

■ characteristic cranial enlargement over frontal and occipital areas (hat size may increase) because of excessive bone formation, and possibly headaches, sensory abnormalities, and impaired motor function (with skull involvement) caused by abnormal bone impinging on brain.

Other deformities include:

■ kyphosis (spinal curvature caused by compression fractures of vertebrae)

■ "barrel" chest

■ asymmetric bowing of the tibia and femur (commonly reduces height)

■ waddling gait (from softening of pelvic bones)

■ warm and tender disease sites susceptible to pathologic fractures after minor trauma

■ slow and usually incomplete healing of pathologic fractures.

COMPLICATIONS

Possible complications of Paget's disease include:

■ blindness and hearing loss with tinnitus and vertigo caused by bony impingement on the cranial nerves

■ pathologic fractures

■ hypertension

■ renal calculi

■ hypercalcemia

■ gout

■ heart failure caused by high blood flow demands of remodeling bones

■ respiratory failure caused by deformed thoracic bones

■ malignant changes in involved bone (1% of the patients).

DIAGNOSIS

Diagnostic tests for Paget's disease may include:

■ X-rays, computed tomography scan, and magnetic resonance imaging — done before symptoms develop — showing increased bone expansion and density

■ radionuclide bone scan (more sensitive than X-rays) clearly showing early Paget's lesions (radioisotope concentrates in areas of active disease)

■ bone biopsy showing characteristic mosaic pattern.

Laboratory findings include:

■ anemia

■ elevated serum alkaline phosphatase level (an index of osteoblastic activity and bone formation)

■ elevated 24-hour urine level of hydroxyproline (amino acid excreted by kidneys and an index of osteoclastic hyperactivity)

■ normal or elevated serum calcium level.

TREATMENT

Primary treatment consists of drug therapy and includes one of the following regimens:

■ bisphosphonates (alendronate, etidronate) to inhibit osteoclast-mediated bone resorption

■ calcitonin, a hormone, and etidronate to retard bone resorption and reduce serum alkaline phosphate and urinary hydroxyproline secretion (calcitonin requires long-term maintenance therapy, but improvement is noticeable after the first few weeks of treatment; etidronate produces improvement after 1 to 3 months)

■ plicamycin (formerly mithramycin), a cytotoxic antibiotic, to decrease serum calcium, urinary hydroxyproline, and serum alkaline phosphatase levels; it produces remission of symptoms within 2 weeks and biochemical improvement in 1 to 2 months but may destroy platelets or compromise renal function.

Other treatment varies according to symptoms and includes:

■ surgery to reduce or prevent pathologic fractures, correct secondary deformities, and relieve neurologic impairment

■ joint replacement (difficult because bonding material [methyl methacrylate] doesn't set properly on pagetic bone)

- aspirin, indomethacin, or ibuprofen to control pain.

Rhabdomyolysis

Rhabdomyolysis, the breakdown of muscle tissue, may cause myoglobinuria, in which varying amounts of muscle protein (myoglobin) appear in the urine. Rhabdomyolysis usually follows major muscle trauma, especially a muscle crush injury. Long-distance running, certain severe infections, and exposure to electric shock can cause extensive muscle damage and excessive release of myoglobin. Prognosis is good if contributing causes are stopped or disease is checked before damage has progressed to an irreversible stage. Unchecked, it can cause renal failure.

CAUSES

Possible causes of rhabdomyolysis include:
- familial tendency
- strenuous exertion
- infection
- anesthetics (halothane) causing intraoperative rigidity
- heat stroke
- electrolyte disturbances
- cardiac arrhythmias
- excessive muscular activity associated with status epilepticus, electroconvulsive therapy, or high-voltage electrical shock.

PATHOPHYSIOLOGY

Muscle trauma that compresses tissue causes ischemia and necrosis. The ensuing local edema further increases compartment pressure and tamponade; pressure from severe swelling causes blood vessels to collapse, leading to tissue hypoxia, muscle infarction, neural damage in the area of the trauma, and release of myoglobin from the necrotic muscle fibers into the circulation.

SIGNS AND SYMPTOMS

Signs and symptoms of rhabdomyolysis include:
- tenderness, swelling, and muscle weakness caused by muscle trauma and pressure
- dark, reddish-brown urine from myoglobin.

COMPLICATIONS

Possible complications of rhabdomyolysis include:
- renal failure as myoglobin is trapped in renal capillaries or tubules
- amputation if muscle necrosis is substantial.

DIAGNOSIS

Diagnosis may include:
- urine myoglobin level greater than 0.5 mg/dl (evident with damage to only 200 g of muscle)
- elevated creatinine kinase level (0.5 to 0.95 mg/dl) caused by muscle damage
- elevated serum potassium, phosphate, creatinine, and creatine levels
- hypocalcemia in early stages, hypercalcemia in later stages
- computed tomography scan, magnetic resonance imaging, and bone scintigraphy to detect muscle necrosis
- intracompartmental venous pressure measurements using a wick catheter, needle, or slit catheter inserted into the muscle.

TREATMENT

Treatment of rhabdomyolysis may include:
- treating the underlying disorder
- preventing renal failure
- bed rest
- anti-inflammatories
- corticosteroids (in extreme cases)
- analgesics for pain
- immediate fasciotomy and debridement (if compartment venous pressure is greater than 25 mm Hg).

Scoliosis

Scoliosis is a lateral curvature of the thoracic, lumbar, or thoracolumbar spine. The curve may be convex to the right (more common in thoracic curves) or to the left (more common in lumbar curves). Rotation of the vertebral column around its axis may cause rib cage deformity. Scoliosis is commonly associated with kyphosis (humpback) and lordosis (swayback).

About 2% to 3% of adolescents have scoliosis. In general, the greater the magnitude of the curve and the younger the child at the time of diagnosis, the greater the risk for progression of the spinal abnormality. Favorable outcomes are usually achieved with optimal treatment.

Types of structural scoliosis are:
- congenital, such as wedge vertebrae, fused ribs or vertebrae, or hemivertebrae
- paralytic or musculoskeletal, developing several months after asymmetric paralysis of the trunk muscles from polio, cerebral palsy, or muscular dystrophy
- idiopathic (most common), may be transmitted as an autosomal dominant or multifactorial trait (appears in a previously straight spine during the growing years).

Idiopathic scoliosis can be further classified according to age at onset:
- infantile (affects mostly boys between birth and age 3 and causes left thoracic and right lumbar curves)
- juvenile (affects both sexes between ages 4 and 10 and causes varying types of curvature)
- adolescent (generally affects girls from age 10 until skeletal maturity and causes varying types of curvature).

CAUSES
Possible causes include:
- functional: poor posture or a discrepancy in leg lengths (postural scoliosis), not fixed deformity of the spinal column
- structural: deformity of the vertebral bodies, leading to curvature.

PATHOPHYSIOLOGY
Differential stress on vertebral bone causes an imbalance of osteoblastic activity; the curve progresses rapidly during the adolescent growth spurt. Without treatment, the imbalance continues into adulthood.

SIGNS AND SYMPTOMS
Scoliosis rarely produces subjective symptoms until it's well established. When symptoms occur, they include:
- backache from stress on the vertebrae
- fatigue
- dyspnea.

The most common curve in functional or structural scoliosis arises in the thoracic segment, with convexity to the right and compensatory curves (S curves) in the cervical and lumbar segments, both with convexity to the left. As the spine curves later-ally, compensatory curves develop to maintain body balance. Subtle signs are related to the curvature and include:
- uneven hemlines or pant legs that appear unequal in length
- one hip that appears higher than the other.

Physical examination shows:
- unequal shoulder heights, elbow levels, and heights of iliac crests
- asymmetric thoracic cage and misalignment of the spinal vertebrae when the patient bends over
- asymmetric paraspinal muscles, rounded on the convex side of the curve and flattened on the concave side
- asymmetric gait.

COMPLICATIONS
Without treatment, curves greater than 40 degrees progress. Untreated scoliosis may result in:
- pulmonary insufficiency (curvature may decrease lung capacity)
- back pain
- degenerative arthritis of the spine
- vertebral disk disease
- sciatica.

DIAGNOSIS
Diagnosis of scoliosis includes:
- anterior, posterior, and lateral spinal X-rays, taken with the patient standing upright and bending (confirm scoliosis and determine the degree of curvature [Cobb method] and flexibility of the spine)
- scoliometer to measure the angle of trunk rotation.

TREATMENT
The severity of the deformity and potential spine growth determine appropriate treatment, which may include:
- close observation
- exercise
- brace
- surgery
- a combination of these.

To be most effective, treatment should begin early, when spinal deformity is still subtle. For a curve less than 25 degrees, or mild scoliosis, treatment includes:
- X-rays to monitor curve

- examination every 3 months
- exercise program to strengthen torso muscles and prevent curve progression.

For a curve of 30 to 50 degrees:
- spinal exercises and a brace (may halt progression but doesn't reverse the established curvature); braces can be adjusted as the patient grows and worn until bone growth is complete)
- transcutaneous electrical stimulation (alternative therapy).

A lateral curve continues to progress at the rate of 1 degree per year even after skeletal maturity. For a curve of 40 degrees or more, treatment includes:
- surgery (supportive instrumentation, with spinal fusion in severe cases)
- periodic postoperative checkups for several months to monitor stability of the correction.

AGE ALERT
Scoliosis commonly affects adolescent girls, who are likely to be distressed by limitations on their activities and treatment with orthopedic appliances. Therefore, emotional support is crucial in addition to meticulous skin and cast care and patient teaching.

Sprains
A sprain is a complete or incomplete tear of the supporting ligaments surrounding a joint. It usually follows a sharp twist. An immobilized sprain may heal in 2 to 3 weeks without surgical repair, after which the patient can gradually resume normal activities. A sprained ankle is the most common joint injury, followed by sprains of the wrist, elbow, and knee.

CAUSES
Causes of sprains include:
- sharply twisting with force stronger than that of the ligament, inducing joint movement beyond normal range of motion
- fractures or dislocations.

PATHOPHYSIOLOGY
When a ligament is torn, an inflammatory exudate develops in the hematoma between the torn ends. Granulation tissue grows inward from the surrounding soft

tissue and cartilage. Collagen formation begins 4 to 5 days after the injury, eventually organizing fibers parallel to the lines of stress. With the aid of vascular fibrous tissue, the new tissue eventually fuses with surrounding tissues. As further reorganization takes place, the new ligament separates from the surrounding tissue and eventually becomes strong enough to withstand normal muscle tension.

SIGNS AND SYMPTOMS
Possible signs and symptoms of sprain include:
- localized pain (especially during joint movement) caused by trauma and exudate
- swelling and heat caused by inflammation
- loss of mobility because of pain (may not occur until several hours after the injury)
- skin discoloration from blood escaping into surrounding tissues.

COMPLICATIONS
Possible complications of sprain include:
- recurring dislocation caused by torn ligaments that don't heal properly, requiring surgical repair (occasionally)
- loss of function in a ligament (if a strong muscle pull occurs and stretches the ligament before it heals, it may heal in a lengthened shape with an excessive amount of scar tissue).

DIAGNOSIS
Sprain may be diagnosed by:
- history of recent injury or chronic overuse
- X-ray to rule out fracture
- stress radiography to visualize the injury in motion
- arthroscopy
- arthrography.

TREATMENT
Treatment to control pain and swelling includes:
- immobilizing the injured joint to promote healing
- intermittently applying ice for 12 to 48 hours to control swelling (place a towel

Muscle-tendon ruptures

Perhaps the most serious muscle-tendon injury is a rupture of the muscle-tendon junction. This type of rupture may occur at any such junction, but it's most common at the Achilles' tendon, which extends from the back of the calf muscle to the foot. An Achilles' tendon rupture produces a sudden, sharp pain and, until swelling begins, a palpable defect. This rupture typically occurs in men between ages 35 and 40, especially during physical activities such as jogging or tennis.

To distinguish an Achilles' tendon rupture from other ankle injuries, perform this simple test: With the patient prone and his feet hanging off the foot of the table, squeeze the calf muscle. The response establishes the diagnosis:

◆ Plantar flexion — The tendon is intact.
◆ Ankle dorsiflexion — The tendon is partially intact.
◆ No flexion of any kind — The tendon is ruptured.

An Achilles' tendon rupture usually requires surgical repair, followed by a long leg cast for 4 weeks, and then a short cast for 4 more weeks.

■ prevention: tape wrists or ankles before sports activities to prevent sprains (athletes).

Strains

Strain is a general term for muscle or tendon damage that commonly results from sudden, forced motion causing it to be stretched beyond normal capacity. Typically, it is seen in traumatic or sports injuries. Injury ranges from excessive stretch (muscle pull) to muscle rupture. (See *Muscle-tendon ruptures.*) If the muscle ruptures, the body of the muscle protrudes through the fascia. A strained muscle can usually heal without complications.

 AGE ALERT
Tendon rupture is more common in elderly people; muscle rupture, in younger people.

CAUSES
Possible causes of strain include:
■ vigorous muscle overuse or overstress, causing the muscle to become stretched beyond normal capacity, especially when the muscle isn't adequately stretched before the activity (acute strain)
■ knife or gunshot wound causing a traumatic rupture (acute strain)
■ repeated overuse (chronic strain).

PATHOPHYSIOLOGY
Bleeding into the muscle and surrounding tissue occurs if the muscle is torn. When a tendon or muscle is torn, an inflammatory exudate develops between the torn ends. Granulation tissue grows inward from the surrounding soft tissue and cartilage. Collagen formation begins 4 to 5 days after the injury, eventually organizing fibers parallel to the lines of stress. With the aid of vascular fibrous tissue, the new tissue eventually fuses with surrounding tissues. As further reorganization takes place, the new tendon or muscle separates from the surrounding tissue and eventually becomes strong enough to withstand normal muscle strain. If a muscle is chronically strained, calcium may deposit into a muscle, limiting movement by causing stiffness and muscle fatigue.

between the ice pack and the skin to prevent a cold injury)
■ an elastic bandage or cast, or if the sprain is severe, a soft cast or splint to immobilize the joint
■ elevating the joint above the level of the heart for 48 to 72 hours (immediately after the injury) (Remember the "RICE" acronym — **R**est, **I**ce, **C**ompression, **E**levation, page 367.)
■ codeine or another analgesic (if injury is severe)
■ crutch and gait training (for sprained ankle)
■ immediate surgical repair to hasten healing, including suturing the ligament ends in close approximation (for some athletes)

SIGNS AND SYMPTOMS

Signs and symptoms of acute strain include:

- sharp, transient pain (myalgia) caused by trauma and inflammatory exudate
- snapping noise from the tearing of the muscle
- rapid swelling that may continue for 72 hours because of the inflammatory process
- limited function because of pain and inflammation
- tender muscle (when severe pain subsides) caused by the injury
- ecchymoses (after several days) because of bleeding into the tissue and muscle.

Signs and symptoms of chronic strain include:

- stiffness
- soreness
- generalized tenderness.

COMPLICATIONS

Possible complications of strain include:

- complete muscle rupture requiring surgical repair
- myositis ossificans (chronic inflammation with bony deposits) caused by scar tissue calcification (late complication).

DIAGNOSIS

Diagnosis of strain may include:

- history of a recent injury or chronic overuse
- X-ray to rule out fracture
- stress radiography to visualize the injury in motion
- biopsy showing muscle regeneration and connective tissue repair (rarely done).

TREATMENT

Possible treatments for acute strain includes:

- compression wrap to immobilize the affected area
- elevating the injured part above the level of the heart to reduce swelling
- analgesics
- application of ice for up to 48 hours, then application of heat to enhance blood flow, reduce cramping, and promote healing
- surgery to suture the tendon or muscle ends.

Tendinitis and bursitis

Tendinitis is a painful inflammation of tendons and of tendon-muscle attachments to bone, usually in the shoulder rotator cuff, hip, Achilles' tendon, or hamstring. Bursitis is a painful inflammation of one or more of the bursae — closed sacs lubricated with small amounts of synovial fluid that ease the movement of muscles and tendons over bony areas (as in the shoulder, elbow, or heel). Bursitis usually occurs in the subdeltoid, olecranon, trochanteric, calcaneal, or prepatellar bursae.

CAUSES

Tendinitis commonly results from:

- overuse (such as strain during sports activity)
- another musculoskeletal disorder (rheumatic diseases, congenital defects)
- postural misalignment
- abnormal body development
- hypermobility.

Bursitis usually occurs in middle age from:

- recurring trauma that stresses or pressures a joint
- an inflammatory joint disease (rheumatoid arthritis, gout).

▲ AGE ALERT
A common form of tendinitis in adolescents is patellar tendinitis linked to inflammation of the tibial epiphysis in Osgood-Schlatter disease.

Chronic bursitis follows attacks of acute bursitis or repeated trauma and infection. Septic bursitis can result from wound infection or from bacterial invasion of skin over the bursa.

PATHOPHYSIOLOGY

A tendon is a band of dense, fibrous connective tissue that attaches muscle to bone. Tendons are extremely strong, flexible, and inelastic. Tendinitis is an inflammation of the tendon, usually resulting from a strain.

The role of the bursa, a fibrous sac lined with synovial fluid, is to act as a cushion and allow the tendon to move smoothly over bone. Bursitis is an inflammation of the bursa. The inflammation leads to excessive production of fluid in the sac, which becomes distended and presses on

Anatomy of tendons and bursae

Tendons, like stiff rubberbands, hold the muscles in place and enable them to move the bones. Bursae are located at friction points around joints and between tendons, cartilage, or bone. Bursae keep these body parts cushioned so they move freely.

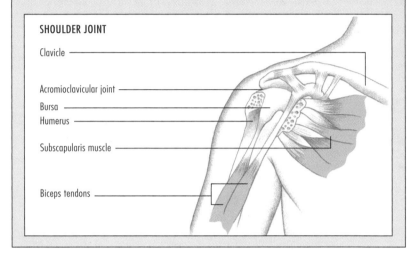

SHOULDER JOINT

Clavicle

Acromioclavicular joint

Bursa

Humerus

Subscapularis muscle

Biceps tendons

sensory nerve endings, causing pain. (See *Anatomy of tendons and bursae*.)

SIGNS AND SYMPTOMS
The patient with tendinitis of the shoulder complains of restricted shoulder movement, especially abduction, and localized pain, which is most severe at night and usually interferes with sleep. The pain, the result of inflammation, extends from the acromion (the shoulder's highest point) to the deltoid muscle insertion, predominantly in the so-called painful arc — that is, when the patient abducts his arm between 50 and 130 degrees. Fluid accumulation causes swelling. In calcific tendinitis, calcium deposits in the tendon cause proximal weakness and, if calcium erodes into adjacent bursae, acute calcific bursitis.

In bursitis, fluid accumulation in the bursae causes irritation, inflammation, sudden or gradual pain, and limited movement. Other symptoms vary according to the affected site. Subdeltoid bursitis impairs arm abduction, prepatellar bursitis

("housemaid's knee") produces pain when the patient climbs stairs, and hip bursitis makes crossing the legs painful.

COMPLICATIONS
Complications may include:
■ scar tissue and subsequent disability, if tendinitis is left untreated
■ acute calcific bursitis, if calcium erodes into adjacent tissue
■ extreme pain and restricted joint movement, if bursitis is left untreated.

DIAGNOSIS
Diagnosis of tendonitis is based on:
■ X-rays that appear normal at first but later show bony fragments, osteophyte sclerosis, or calcium deposits
■ arthrographic results that are usually normal, with occasional small irregularities on the undersurface of the tendon.

Computed tomography scan and magnetic resonance imaging (MRI) have replaced X-ray and even arthrography of the shoulder as diagnostic tools.

- MRI identifies tears, partial tears, inflammation, or tumor but not irregularities of the tendon sheath itself.

Diagnosis of shoulder tendinitis must rule out other causes of shoulder pain, such as myocardial infarction, cervical spondylosis, and tendon tear or rupture. Significantly, in tendinitis, heat aggravates pain; in other painful joint disorders, heat usually provides relief.

Diagnosis of bursitis is based on:
- localized pain and inflammation
- history of unusual strain or injury 2 to 3 days before onset of pain
- normal X-ray findings in early stages, except for calcific bursitis, in which X-rays may show calcium deposits.

TREATMENT

Treatment to relieve pain includes resting the joint (by immobilization with a sling, splint, or cast), systemic analgesics, application of cold, ultrasound, or local injection of an anesthetic and corticosteroids to reduce inflammation. A mixture of a corticosteroid and an anesthetic such as lidocaine usually provides immediate pain relief. Extended-release injections of a corticosteroid, such as triamcinolone or prednisolone, offer longer-term pain relief. Until the patient is free from pain and able to perform range-of-motion (ROM) exercises easily, treatment also includes oral nonsteroidal anti-inflammatory drugs such as ibuprofen, naproxen, indomethacin, or oxaprozin. Short-term analgesics include propoxyphene, codeine, acetaminophen with codeine and, occasionally, oxycodone.

Supplementary treatment includes fluid removal by aspiration and heat therapy; for calcific tendinitis, ice packs, physical therapy, ultrasonography, or hydrotherapy generally helps maintain or regain range of motion. It may be necessary to delay treatment until the acute attack is over to ensure maximum patient adherence. Rarely, calcific tendinitis requires surgical removal of calcium deposits. Long-term control of chronic bursitis and tendinitis may require changes in lifestyle to prevent recurring joint irritation.

11

Hematologic system

Blood, although a fluid, is one of the body's major tissues. It continuously circulates through the heart and blood vessels, carrying vital elements to every part of the body.

Blood performs several vital functions through its special components: the liquid protein (plasma) and the formed constituents (erythrocytes, leukocytes, and thrombocytes) suspended in it. Erythrocytes (red blood cells) carry oxygen to the tissues and remove carbon dioxide. Leukocytes (white blood cells) act in inflammatory and immune responses. Plasma (a clear, straw-colored fluid) carries antibodies and nutrients to tissues and carries waste away. Plasma coagulation factors and thrombocytes (platelets) control clotting.

Hematopoiesis, the process of blood formation, occurs primarily in the marrow. There primitive blood cells (stem cells) differentiate into the precursors of erythrocytes (normoblasts), leukocytes, and thrombocytes. (See *Mapping out blood cell formation*, pages 398 and 399.)

The average person has 5 to 6 L of circulating blood, which constitutes 5% to 7% of body weight (as much as 10% in premature neonates). The viscosity of blood is three to five times that of water. Blood has an arterial pH of 7.35 to 7.45 and is either bright red (arterial blood) or dark red (venous blood), depending on the degree of oxygen saturation and the hemoglobin level.

Pathophysiologic changes

Bone marrow cells reproduce rapidly and have a short life span, and the storage of circulating cells in the marrow is minimal. Thus, bone marrow cells and their precursors are particularly vulnerable to physiologic changes that affect cell production. Disease can affect the structure or concentration of any hematologic cell.

Hemoglobin

The protein hemoglobin is the major component of the red blood cell. Hemoglobin consists of an iron-containing molecule (heme) bound to the protein globulin. Oxygen binds to the heme component and is carried throughout the body and released to the cells. The hemoglobin picks up carbon dioxide and hydrogen ions from the cells and delivers them to the lungs, where they're released.

A variety of mutations or abnormalities in the hemoglobin protein can cause abnormal oxygen transport.

Red blood cells

Red blood cell (RBC) disorders may be quantitative or qualitative. A deficiency of RBCs (anemia) can follow a condition that destroys or inhibits the formation of these cells. (See *Erythropoiesis*.)

Common factors leading to anemia include:

- drugs, toxins, ionizing radiation
- congenital or acquired defects that cause bone marrow to stop producing new RBCs cells and generally suppress production of all blood cells
- metabolic abnormalities (sideroblastic anemia)
- deficiency of vitamins (vitamin B_{12} deficiency, or pernicious anemia) or minerals (iron, folic acid, copper, and cobalt deficiency anemias) leading to inadequate erythropoiesis
- excessive chronic or acute blood loss (posthemorrhagic anemia)
- chronic illnesses, such as renal disease, cancer, and chronic infections
- intrinsically defective RBCs (as in sickle cell anemia) or extrinsically defective RBCs (as in hemolytic transfusion reaction).

Decreased plasma volume can cause a relative excess of RBCs. The few conditions characterized by excessive production of RBCs include:

- abnormal proliferation of all bone marrow cells (polycythemia vera)
- abnormality of a single element (such as erythropoietin excess caused by hypoxemia or pulmonary disease).

Leukocytosis

Leukocytosis is an elevation in the number of white blood cells (WBCs). All types, or only one type, of WBCs may be increased. (See *WBC types and functions,* page 400.) Leukocytosis is a normal physiologic response to infection or inflammation. Other factors, such as temperature changes, emotional disturbances, anesthesia, surgery, strenuous exercise, pregnancy, and some drugs, hormones, and toxins can also cause leukocytosis. Abnormal leukocytosis occurs in malignancies and bone marrow disorders.

Leukopenia

Leukopenia is a deficiency of WBCs — all types or only one type. It can be caused by a number of conditions or diseases, such as human immunodeficiency virus infection, prolonged stress, bone marrow disease or destruction, radiation or chemotherapy, lupus erythematosus, leukemia, thyroid disease, or Cushing's syndrome.

Erythropoiesis

The tissues' demand for oxygen and the blood cells' ability to deliver it regulate red blood cell (RBC), or erythrocyte, production, which is known as *erythropoiesis.* Lack of oxygen in the tissues (hypoxia) stimulates RBC production, which triggers the formation and release of the hormone erythropoietin. In turn, erythropoietin, 90% of which is produced by the kidneys and 10% by the liver, activates bone marrow to produce RBCs. Androgens may also stimulate erythropoiesis, which accounts for higher RBC counts in men.

The formation of an RBC begins with an uncommitted stem cell that may eventually develop into a red or white blood cell. Such formation requires certain vitamins — B_{12} and folic acid — and minerals — copper, cobalt, and especially iron, which is vital to hemoglobin's oxygen-carrying capacity. Iron is obtained from various foods and absorbed in the duodenum and jejunum. An excess of iron is temporarily stored in reticuloendothelial cells, especially those in the liver, as ferritin and hemosiderin until it's released for use in the bone marrow to form new RBCs.

Because WBCs fight infection, leukopenia increases the risk of infectious illness.

Thrombocytosis

Thrombocytosis is an excess of circulating platelets than greater than 400,000/μl. Thrombocytosis may be primary or secondary.

PRIMARY THROMBOCYTOSIS

In primary thrombocytosis, the number of platelet precursor cells, called *megakaryocytes,* is increased and the platelet count is greater than 1 million/μl. The condition may result from an intrinsic abnormality of platelet function and increased platelet mass. It may accompany polycythemia vera or chronic granulocytic leukemia. In the presence of thrombocytosis, both he-

(Text continues on page 400.)

Mapping out blood cell formation

Blood cell formation and development in the bone marrow is called *hematopoiesis*. This chart breaks down the process from the time the five unipotential stem cells are "born" from the multipotential stem cell until they each reach "adulthood" as fully formed cells — erythrocytes, granulocytes, agranulocytes, or platelets.

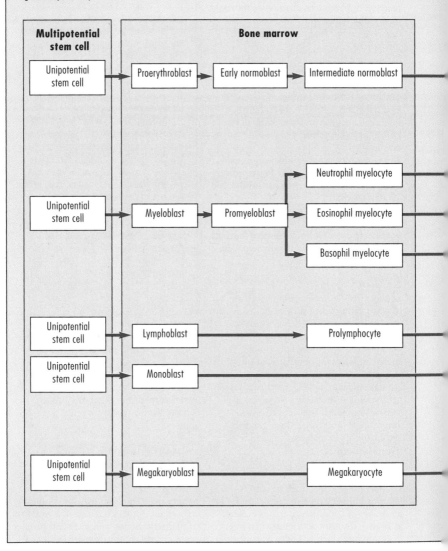

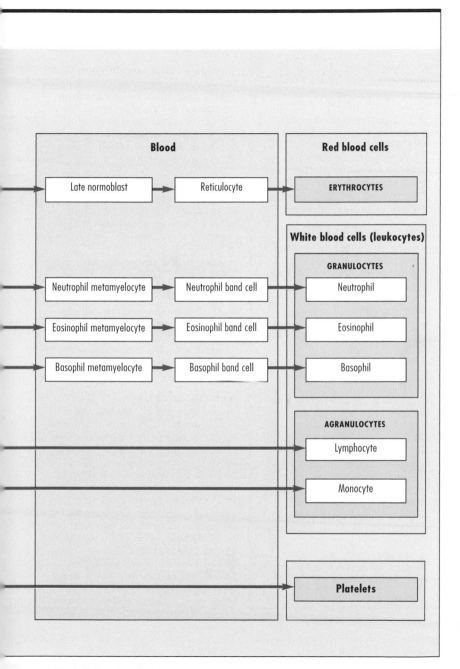

WBC types and functions

White blood cells (WBCs), or leukocytes, protect the body against harmful bacteria and infection. WBCs are classified as *granular* leukocytes (neutrophils, eosinophils, and basophils) or *nongranular* leukocytes (lymphocytes, monocytes, and plasma cells). WBCs are usually produced in bone marrow; lymphocytes and plasma cells are produced in lymphoid tissue as well. Neutrophils have a circulating half-life of less than 6 hours, and some lymphocytes may survive for weeks or months. Normally, WBCs number between 5,000 and 10,000/µl. The five types of WBCs are:

◆ Neutrophils — The predominant form of granulocyte, they make up about 60% of WBCs and help devour invading organisms by phagocytosis.

◆ Eosinophils — Minor granulocytes, they may defend against parasites and lung and skin infections and act in allergic reactions. They account for 1% to 5% of the total WBC count.

◆ Basophils — Minor granulocytes, they may release heparin and histamine into the blood and participate in delayed hypersensitivity reactions. They account for up to 1% of the total WBC count.

◆ Lymphocytes — They appear as B cells and T cells. B cells form lymphoid follicles, produce humoral antibodies, and help T-cell-mediated delayed hypersensitivity reactions and the rejection of foreign cells or cell products. Lymphocytes account for 20% to 40% of the total WBC count.

◆ Monocytes — Along with neutrophils, they help devour invading organisms by phagocytosis. Monocytes help process antigens for lymphocytes and form macrophages in the tissues. They account for 1% to 6% of the total WBC count.

This process consumes exorbitant amounts of coagulation factors and thereby increases the risk of hemorrhage.

SECONDARY THROMBOCYTOSIS

Secondary thrombocytosis is a result of an underlying cause, such as stress, exercise, hemorrhage, or hemolytic anemia. Stress and exercise release stored platelets from the spleen. Hemorrhage or hemolytic anemia signals the bone marrow to produce more megakaryocytes.

Thrombocytosis may also occur after a splenectomy. Because the spleen is the primary site of platelet storage and destruction, platelet count may rise after its removal until the bone marrow begins producing fewer platelets.

*D*ISORDERS

Specific causes of hematologic disorders include trauma, chronic disease, surgery, malnutrition, drugs, exposure to toxins or radiation, and genetic or congenital defects that disrupt production or function of blood cells.

Aplastic anemias

Aplastic or hypoplastic anemias result from injury to or destruction of stem cells in bone marrow or the bone marrow matrix, causing pancytopenia (anemia, leukopenia, and thrombocytopenia) and bone marrow hypoplasia. Although commonly used interchangeably with other terms for bone marrow failure, aplastic anemia properly refers to pancytopenia resulting from the decreased functional capacity of a hypoplastic, fatty bone marrow.

CLINICAL ALERT
These disorders generally produce fatal bleeding or infection, especially when they're idiopathic or caused by chloramphenicol use or infectious hepatitis. The death rate for severe aplastic anemia is 80% to 90%.

CAUSES

Possible causes of aplastic anemia are:
■ radiation (about half of such anemias)

morrhage and thrombosis may occur. This paradox occurs because accelerated clotting results in a generalized activation of prothrombin and a consequent excess of thrombin clots in the microcirculation.

- drugs (antibiotics, anticonvulsants) or toxic agents (such as benzene or chloramphenicol)
- autoimmune reactions (unconfirmed), severe disease (especially hepatitis), or preleukemic and neoplastic infiltration of bone marrow
- congenital (idiopathic anemias). Two identified forms of aplastic anemia are congenital: hypoplastic or Blackfan-Diamond anemia (develops between ages 2 and 3 months) and Fanconi's syndrome (develops between birth and age 10).

PATHOPHYSIOLOGY

Aplastic anemia usually develops when damaged or destroyed stem cells inhibit blood cell production. Less commonly, they develop when damaged bone marrow microvasculature creates an unfavorable environment for cell growth and maturation.

SIGNS AND SYMPTOMS

Signs and symptoms of aplastic anemia vary with the severity of pancytopenia but develop insidiously in many cases. They may include:

- progressive weakness and fatigue, shortness of breath, headache, pallor, and ultimately tachycardia and heart failure caused by hypoxia and increased venous return
- ecchymosis, petechiae, and hemorrhage, especially from the mucous membranes (nose, gums, rectum, vagina) or into the retina or central nervous system because of thrombocytopenia
- infection (fever, oral and rectal ulcers, sore throat) without characteristic inflammation because of neutropenia (neutrophil deficiency).

COMPLICATIONS

A possible complication of aplastic anemia is:

- life-threatening hemorrhage from the mucous membranes.

DIAGNOSIS

The following test results help diagnose aplastic anemia:

- 1 million/µl or fewer red blood cells (RBCs) of normal color and size (normochromic and normocytic).

RBCs may be macrocytic (larger than normal) and anisocytotic (of excessive variation in size), with:

- very low absolute reticulocyte count
- elevated serum iron level (unless bleeding occurs), normal or slightly reduced total iron-binding capacity, presence of hemosiderin (a derivative of hemoglobin), and microscopically visible tissue iron storage
- decreased platelet, neutrophil, and lymphocyte counts
- abnormal coagulation test results (bleeding time) reflecting decreased platelet count
- "dry tap" (no cells) from bone marrow aspiration at several sites
- biopsy showing severely hypocellular or aplastic marrow, with varied amounts of fat, fibrous tissue, or gelatinous replacement; absence of tagged iron (because iron is deposited in the liver rather than in the bone marrow) and megakaryocytes (platelet precursors); and depression of RBCs and precursors (erythroid elements).

Differential diagnosis must rule out paroxysmal nocturnal hemoglobinuria and other diseases in which pancytopenia is common.

TREATMENT

Effective treatment must eliminate an identifiable cause and provide vigorous supportive measures, including:

- packed RBC or platelet transfusion; experimental histocompatibility locus antigen-matched leukocyte transfusions
- bone marrow transplantation (treatment of choice for anemia caused by severe aplasia and for patients who need constant RBC transfusions)
- for patients with leukopenia, special measures to prevent infection (avoidance of exposure to communicable diseases, diligent hand washing, and so forth)
- specific antibiotics for infection (not given prophylactically because they encourage resistant strains of organisms)
- respiratory support with oxygen in addition to blood transfusions (for patients with low hemoglobin levels)

Foods high in folic acid

FOOD	MCG/100 G
Asparagus spears	109
Beef liver	294
Broccoli spears	54
Collards (cooked)	102
Mushrooms	24
Oatmeal	33
Peanut butter	57
Red beans	180
Wheat germ	305

- corticosteroids to stimulate erythro-poiesis; marrow-stimulating agents such as androgens (controversial); antilympho-cyte globulin (experimental); immunosup-pressive agents (if other therapy isn't effec-tive); and colony-stimulating factors to encourage growth of specific cellular components.

Folic acid deficiency anemia

Folic acid deficiency anemia is a common, slowly progressive, megaloblastic anemia. It usually occurs in infants, adolescents, pregnant and lactating women, people with alcoholism, elderly people, and peo-ple with malignant or intestinal diseases.

CAUSES

Folic acid deficiency anemia may result from:
- alcohol abuse (alcohol may suppress metabolic effects of folate)
- poor diet (common in people with al-coholism, elderly people living alone, and infants, especially those with infections or diarrhea)
- impaired absorption (because of intesti-nal dysfunction from bowel resection and

such disorders as celiac disease, tropical sprue, and regional jejunitis)
- bacteria competing for available folic acid
- overcooking of food, which can destroy a high percentage of folic acid in foods (see *Foods high in folic acid*)
- limited capacity to store folic acid (in infants)
- prolonged drug therapy (anticonvul-sants and estrogens, including oral contra-ceptives)
- increased folic acid requirements during pregnancy, during rapid growth in infancy (common because of recent increase in survival of premature neonates), during childhood and adolescence (because of general use of folate-poor cow's milk), and in patients with neoplastic diseases and some skin diseases (chronic exfoliative dermatitis).

PATHOPHYSIOLOGY

Folic acid (pteroylglutamic acid, folacin) is found in most body tissues, where it acts as a coenzyme in metabolic processes in-volving one carbon transfer. It's essential for formation and maturation of red blood cells (RBCs) and for synthesis of deoxyri-bonucleic acid. Although folic acid is stored in the body in relatively small amounts (about 70 mg), this vitamin is plentiful in most well-balanced diets.

Even so, because folic acid is water-soluble and unstable when exposed to heat, cooking easily destroys it. Also, about 20% of folic acid intake is excreted unabsorbed. Insufficient daily folic acid intake (less than 50 mcg/day) usually in-duces folic acid deficiency within 4 months as the amount stored in the liver is depleted. This deficiency inhibits cell growth, particularly of RBCs, leading to production of few, deformed RBCs. These enlarged red cells characteristic of the megaloblastic anemias have a shortened life span of weeks rather than months.

SIGNS AND SYMPTOMS

Folic acid deficiency anemia gradually pro-duces clinical features characteristic of oth-er megaloblastic anemias, without the neurologic manifestations: progressive fa-tigue, shortness of breath, palpitations, weakness, glossitis, nausea, anorexia, headache, fainting, irritability, forgetfulness, pallor, and slight jaundice. Folic acid deficiency anemia doesn't cause neurologic impairment unless it's linked to vitamin B_{12} deficiency, as in pernicious anemia.

COMPLICATIONS

Folic acid deficiency anemia produces no complications.

DIAGNOSIS

The Schilling test and a therapeutic trial of vitamin B_{12} injections distinguish between folic acid deficiency anemia and pernicious anemia. Significant findings include macrocytosis, decreased reticulocyte count, abnormal platelets, and serum folate level less than 4 mg/ml.

TREATMENT

Treatment consists primarily of folic acid supplements and elimination of contributing causes. Folic acid supplements may be given orally (usually 400 mcg/day) or parenterally (to patients who are severely ill, have malabsorption, or are unable to take oral medication). Many patients respond favorably to a well-balanced diet. If the patient has a combined B_{12} and folate deficiency, folic acid replenishment alone may aggravate neurologic dysfunction.

Iron deficiency anemia

Iron deficiency anemia is a disorder of oxygen transport in which hemoglobin synthesis is deficient. A common disease worldwide, iron deficiency anemia affects 10% to 30% of the adult population in the United States. Iron deficiency anemia occurs most commonly in premenopausal women, infants (particularly premature or low-birth-weight neonates), children, and adolescents (especially girls). The prognosis after replacement therapy is favorable.

CAUSES

Possible causes of iron deficiency anemia are:

■ inadequate dietary intake of iron (less than 1 mg/day), as in prolonged non-supplemented breast-feeding or bottle-feeding of infants or during periods of stress, such as rapid growth, in children and adolescents

■ iron malabsorption, as in chronic diarrhea, partial or total gastrectomy, and malabsorption syndromes, such as celiac disease and pernicious anemia

■ blood loss caused by drug-induced GI bleeding (from anticoagulants, aspirin, steroids), heavy menses, hemorrhage from trauma, peptic ulcers, cancer, increased laboratory blood samples in chronically ill patients, sequestration (increased amount of blood within a limited vascular space) in patients on dialysis, or varices

■ pregnancy, which diverts maternal iron to the fetus for erythropoiesis

■ intravascular hemolysis-induced hemoglobinuria or paroxysmal nocturnal hemoglobinuria

■ mechanical trauma to red blood cells (RBCs) caused by a prosthetic heart valve or vena cava filters.

PATHOPHYSIOLOGY

Iron deficiency anemia occurs when the supply of iron is inadequate for optimal formation of RBCs, resulting in smaller than normal (microcytic) cells with less color (hypochromic) on staining. Body stores of iron, including plasma iron, become depleted, and the concentration of serum transferrin, which binds with and carries iron, decreases. Insufficient iron stores lead to a depleted RBC mass with subnormal hemoglobin concentration and, in turn, subnormal oxygen-carrying capacity of the blood.

SIGNS AND SYMPTOMS

Because iron deficiency anemia progresses gradually, many people show only symptoms of an underlying condition. They tend not to seek medical treatment until anemia is severe.

At advanced stages, signs and symptoms include:

■ dyspnea on exertion, fatigue, listlessness, pallor, inability to concentrate, irritability, headache, and a susceptibility to infection caused by decreased oxygen-carrying capacity of the blood because of decreased hemoglobin levels

■ increased cardiac output and tachycardia caused by decreased oxygen perfusion

- coarsely ridged, spoon-shaped (koilonychia), brittle, and thin nails caused by decreased capillary circulation
- sore, red, and burning tongue caused by papillae atrophy
- sore, dry skin in the corners of the mouth caused by epithelial changes.

COMPLICATIONS
Possible complications include:
- infection and pneumonia
- pica (compulsive eating of nonfood materials, such as starch or dirt)
- bleeding
- overdosage of oral or I.M. iron supplements.

DIAGNOSIS
Blood studies (serum iron, total iron-binding capacity, ferritin levels) and iron stores in bone marrow may confirm iron deficiency anemia. The results of these tests can be misleading because of complicating factors, such as infection, pneumonia, blood transfusion, or iron supplements. Characteristic blood test results include:
- low hemoglobin level (males, less than 12 g/dl; females, less than 10 g/dl)
- low hematocrit (males, less than 47%; females, less than 42%)
- low serum iron with high binding capacity level
- low serum ferritin level
- low RBC count, with microcytic and hypochromic cells (in early stages, RBC count is possibly normal, except in infants and children)
- decreased mean corpuscular hemoglobin level in severe anemia
- depleted or absent iron stores (by specific staining) and hyperplasia of normal precursor cells (by bone marrow studies).

Diagnosis must also include:
- exclusion of other causes of anemia, such as thalassemia minor, cancer, and chronic inflammatory, hepatic, or renal disease.

TREATMENT
The first priority of treatment is to determine the underlying cause of anemia. Only then can iron replacement therapy begin. Possible treatments are:

- oral preparation of iron (treatment of choice) or a combination of iron and ascorbic acid (enhances iron absorption)
- parenteral iron (for a maximum rate of hemoglobin regeneration, or for patients nonadherent to oral dosing, those who need more iron than can be given orally, or who have malabsorption that prevents adequate iron absorption).

Because total-dose I.V. infusion of supplemental iron is painless and requires fewer injections, it's usually preferred to I.M. administration. Considerations include:
- total-dose infusion of iron dextran in normal saline solution given over 1 to 8 hours (pregnant patients and geriatric patients with severe anemia)
- I.V. test dose of 0.5 ml given first (to minimize the risk of an allergic reaction).

Pernicious anemia
Pernicious anemia, the most common type of megaloblastic anemia, is caused by malabsorption of vitamin B_{12}.

AGE ALERT
Onset typically occurs between ages 50 and 60, and incidence increases with age.

If not treated, pernicious anemia is fatal. Its manifestations subside with treatment, but some neurologic deficits may be permanent.

CAUSES
Possible causes of pernicious anemia include:
- genetic predisposition (suggested by familial incidence)
- immunologically related diseases, such as thyroiditis, myxedema, and Graves' disease (significantly higher incidence in these people)
- partial gastrectomy (iatrogenic induction)
- advanced age (progressive loss of vitamin B_{12} absorption).

AGE ALERT
Elderly people typically have a dietary deficiency of vitamin B_{12} in addition to, or instead of, poor absorption.

PATHOPHYSIOLOGY
Pernicious anemia is characterized by decreased production of hydrochloric acid in

the stomach and a deficiency of *intrinsic factor*, which is normally secreted by the parietal cells of the gastric mucosa and is essential for vitamin B_{12} absorption in the ileum. The resulting vitamin B_{12} deficiency inhibits cell growth, particularly of red blood cells (RBCs), leading to production of few, deformed RBCs with poor oxygen-carrying capacity. It also causes neurologic damage by impairing myelin formation.

SIGNS AND SYMPTOMS

Characteristically, pernicious anemia has an insidious onset but eventually causes an unmistakable triad of symptoms, including:

- weakness caused by tissue hypoxia
- sore tongue caused by atrophy of the papillae
- numbness and tingling in the extremities as a result of interference with impulse transmission because of demyelination.

Other common manifestations include:

- pale appearance of lips and gums because of hypoxemia
- faintly jaundiced sclera and pale to bright yellow skin caused by hemolysis-induced hyperbilirubinemia
- high susceptibility to infection, especially of the genitourinary tract.

Pernicious anemia may also have GI, neurologic, and cardiovascular effects.

GI symptoms include:

- nausea, vomiting, anorexia, weight loss, flatulence, diarrhea, and constipation because of disturbed digestion caused by gastric mucosal atrophy and decreased hydrochloric acid production
- gingival bleeding and tongue inflammation (may hinder eating and intensify anorexia).

Neurologic symptoms are related to impaired myelin formation and subsequent interference with neuron transmission and may include:

- neuritis; weakness in extremities
- peripheral numbness and paresthesia
- disturbed position sense
- lack of coordination; ataxia; impaired fine finger movement
- positive Babinski's and Romberg's signs
- light-headedness

- altered vision (diplopia, blurred vision), taste, and hearing (tinnitus); optic muscle atrophy
- loss of bowel and bladder control; and, in males, impotence, because of demyelination (initially affects peripheral nerves but gradually extends to the spinal cord) caused by vitamin B_{12} deficiency
- irritability, poor memory, headache, depression, and delirium (some symptoms are temporary, but irreversible central nervous system [CNS] changes may have occurred before treatment).

Cardiovascular symptoms include:

- low hemoglobin levels because of widespread destruction of RBCs caused by increasingly fragile cell membranes
- palpitations, wide pulse pressure, dyspnea, orthopnea, tachycardia, premature beats and, eventually, heart failure caused by compensatory increased cardiac output.

COMPLICATIONS

Possible complications include:

- hypokalemia (first week of treatment)
- permanent CNS symptoms (if the patient isn't treated within 6 months of appearance of symptoms)
- gastric polyps
- stomach cancer.

DIAGNOSIS

Laboratory screening must rule out other anemias with similar symptoms but different treatments, such as:

- folic acid deficiency anemia
- vitamin B_{12} deficiency resulting from malabsorption caused by GI disorders, gastric surgery, radiation, or drug therapy.

Decreased hemoglobin levels by 1 g/dl in elderly men and slightly decreased hematocrit in both men and women reflect decreased bone marrow function and decreased hematopoiesis and, in men, decreased androgen levels; they aren't an indicator of pernicious anemia. Diagnosis of pernicious anemia is established by:

- family history of this disorder
- hemoglobin level 4 to 5 g/μl
- low RBC count
- mean corpuscular volume greater than 120 μl because of increased amounts of hemoglobin in larger-than-normal RBCs

- serum vitamin B_{12} less than 0.1 mcg/ml
- bone marrow aspiration showing erythroid hyperplasia (crowded red bone marrow), with increased numbers of megaloblasts but few normally developing RBCs
- gastric analysis showing absence of free hydrochloric acid after histamine or pentagastrin injection
- Schilling test for excretion of radiolabeled vitamin B_{12} (definitive test for pernicious anemia)
- serologic findings including intrinsic factor antibodies and antiparietal cell antibodies.

TREATMENT

Treatment for pernicious anemia includes:
- early parenteral vitamin B_{12} replacement (can reverse pernicious anemia, minimize complications, and possibly prevent permanent neurologic damage)
- concomitant iron and folic acid replacement to prevent iron deficiency anemia (rapid cell regeneration increasing the patient's iron and folate requirements)
- after initial response, decreasing vitamin B_{12} dosage to monthly self-administered maintenance dose (must be taken for life)
- bed rest for extreme fatigue until hemoglobin level rises
- blood transfusions for dangerously low hemoglobin level
- digoxin, diuretic, low-sodium diet (if patient is in heart failure)
- antibiotics to combat infections.

Sideroblastic anemias

Sideroblastic anemias are a group of heterogenous disorders with a common defect: Iron isn't used in hemoglobin synthesis, despite the availability of adequate iron stores. These anemias may be hereditary or acquired. The acquired form can be primary or secondary. Hereditary sideroblastic anemia commonly responds to treatment with pyridoxine (vitamin B_6). The primary acquired (idiopathic) form, known as *refractory anemia with ringed sideroblasts,* resists treatment and is usually fatal within 10 years of the onset of complications or of a concomitant disease. This form is most common in elderly people. It's commonly linked to thrombocytopenia or leukopenia as part of a myelodysplastic syndrome. Correction of the secondary acquired form depends on the cause.

CAUSES

Hereditary sideroblastic anemia appears to be transmitted by:
- X-linked inheritance, occurring mostly in young males (female carriers usually show no signs of this disorder).

The acquired form may be caused by:
- ingestion of or exposure to toxins (such as alcohol and lead) or drugs (such as isoniazid and chloramphenicol)
- other diseases, such as rheumatoid arthritis, lupus erythematosus, multiple myeloma, tuberculosis, and severe infections.

PATHOPHYSIOLOGY

In sideroblastic anemia, normoblasts fail to use iron to synthesize hemoglobin. As a result, iron is deposited in the mitochondria of normoblasts, which are then called ringed sideroblasts. Iron toxicity can cause organ damage; untreated, it can damage the nuclei of red blood cell (RBC) precursors.

SIGNS AND SYMPTOMS

Possible signs and symptoms of sideroblastic anemia include:
- anorexia, fatigue, weakness, dizziness, pale skin and mucous membranes and, occasionally, enlarged lymph nodes because of iron toxicity
- dyspnea, exertional angina, slight jaundice, and hepatosplenomegaly because of heart and liver failure caused by excessive iron accumulation in these organs
- increased GI absorption of iron, causing signs of hemosiderosis (hereditary sideroblastic anemia)
- other symptoms depending on the underlying cause (secondary sideroblastic anemia).

COMPLICATIONS

Possible complications are:
- heart, liver, and pancreatic disease
- respiratory complications
- acute myelogenous leukemia.

DIAGNOSIS
Diagnosis is confirmed by:
- ringed sideroblasts on microscopic examination of bone marrow aspirate stained with Prussian blue or alizarin red dye (see *Ringed sideroblast*)
- hypochromic or normochromic and slightly macrocytic RBCs on microscopic examination; RBC precursors may be megaloblastic, with anisocytosis and poikilocytosis (abnormal variation in shape)
- low hemoglobin level with high serum iron, transferrin, urobilinogen, and bilirubin levels because of RBC lysis
- normal platelet and leukocyte counts (occasional thrombocytopenia or leukopenia).

TREATMENT
Treatment of sideroblastic anemias depends on the underlying cause and includes:
- several weeks of treatment with high doses of pyridoxine for hereditary form
- removal of the causative drug or toxin or treatment of the underlying condition (symptoms usually subside in acquired secondary form)
- folic acid supplements (may be beneficial when megaloblastic nuclear changes in RBC precursors are present)
- deferoxamine to treat chronic iron overload as needed
- blood transfusions (providing hemoglobin) or high doses of androgens (effective palliative measures for some patients with primary acquired form)
- phlebotomy to prevent hemochromatosis (the accumulation of iron in body tissues) increases the rate of erythropoiesis and uses up excess iron stores, reducing serum and total-body iron levels.

Allergic purpura
Allergic purpura, a nonthrombocytopenic purpura, is an acute or chronic vascular inflammation affecting the skin, joints, and GI and genitourinary tracts, in association with allergy symptoms. When allergic purpura primarily affects the GI tract, with accompanying joint pain, it's called *Henoch-Schönlein syndrome,* or *anaphylactoid purpura.* The term *allergic purpura* applies to purpura linked to many other

CLOSER LOOK
Ringed sideroblast

Electron microscopy shows large iron deposits in the mitochondria that surround the nucleus, forming the characteristic ringed sideroblast of hemochromatosis.

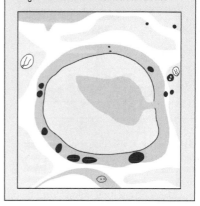

conditions, such as erythema nodosum. An acute attack of allergic purpura can last for several weeks and is potentially fatal (usually from renal failure), but most patients do recover.

Fully developed allergic purpura is persistent and debilitating, possibly leading to chronic glomerulonephritis (especially if caused by a streptococcal infection). Allergic purpura affects more males than females and is most prevalent in children ages 3 to 7. The prognosis is more favorable for children than for adults.

CAUSES
Causes may include:
- a bacterial infection (particularly streptococcal infection)
- allergic reactions to some drugs and vaccines, insect bites, and some foods (such as wheat, eggs, milk, and chocolate).

PATHOPHYSIOLOGY
Although the mechanism of allergic purpura isn't completely understood, it's probably an autoimmune reaction directed against vascular walls, triggered by a bacte-

Purpuric lesions

Lesions of allergic purpura, such as those on the foot and leg pictured below, typically vary in size.

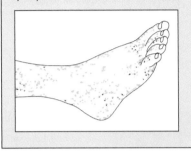

rial infection. Typically, upper respiratory tract infection occurs 1 to 3 weeks before the onset of symptoms. An inflammation of the veins and capillaries disrupts the vascular wall, resulting in loss of red blood cells and bleeding.

SIGNS AND SYMPTOMS
Characteristic skin lesions of allergic purpura are purple, macular, ecchymotic, and of varying size and are caused by vascular leakage into the skin and mucous membranes. (See *Purpuric lesions.*) The lesions usually appear in symmetric patterns on the arms, legs, and buttocks and are accompanied by pruritus, paresthesia and, occasionally, angioneurotic edema.

 AGE ALERT
In children, skin lesions are generally urticarial and expand and become hemorrhagic. Scattered petechiae may appear on the legs, buttocks, and perineum.

Henoch-Schönlein syndrome commonly produces transient or severe colic, tenesmus (spasmodic contraction of the anal sphincter) and constipation, vomiting, and edema or hemorrhage of the mucous membranes of the bowel, resulting in GI bleeding, occult blood in the stool and, possibly, intussusception. Such GI abnormalities may precede overt, cutaneous signs of purpura. Musculoskeletal symptoms, such as rheumatoid pains and peri-

articular effusions, usually affect the legs and feet.

In 25% to 50% of patients, allergic purpura is linked to genitourinary signs and symptoms: nephritis; renal hemorrhages that may cause microscopic hematuria and disturb renal function; bleeding from the mucosal surfaces of the ureters, bladder, or urethra; and, occasionally, glomerulonephritis. Also possible are moderate and irregular fever, headache, anorexia, and localized edema of the hands, feet, or scalp.

COMPLICATIONS
Complications, which may appear many years after the episode of allergic purpura, may include:
■ renal disease (renal failure and acute glomerulonephritis), which may be fatal
■ hypertension and resulting blood loss from renal damage.

DIAGNOSIS
No laboratory test clearly identifies allergic purpura (although white blood cell count and erythrocyte sedimentation rate are elevated). Diagnosis therefore necessitates careful clinical observation, in many cases during the second or third attack. Except for a positive tourniquet test (a test to assess the ability of capillaries to withstand increased pressure), coagulation and platelet function tests are usually normal. Small bowel X-rays may reveal areas of transient edema; in many cases tests for blood in the urine and stool are positive. Increased blood urea nitrogen and creatinine levels may indicate renal involvement. Diagnosis must rule out other forms of nonthrombocytopenic purpura.

TREATMENT
Treatment is generally symptomatic; for example, severe allergic purpura may require steroids to relieve edema and analgesics to relieve joint and abdominal pain. Some patients with chronic renal disease may benefit from immunosuppression with azathioprine along with identification of the provocative allergen. An accurate allergy history is essential.

Disseminated intravascular coagulation

Disseminated intravascular coagulation (DIC) occurs as a complication of diseases and conditions that accelerate clotting, causing occlusion of small blood vessels, organ necrosis, depletion of circulating clotting factors and platelets, activation of the fibrinolytic system, and consequent severe hemorrhage. Clotting in the microcirculation usually affects the kidneys and extremities but may occur in the brain, lungs, pituitary and adrenal glands, and GI mucosa. DIC, also called *consumption coagulopathy* or *defibrination syndrome,* is generally an acute condition but may be chronic in cancer patients. Prognosis depends on early detection and treatment, the severity of the hemorrhage, and treatment of the underlying disease. (See *Understanding DIC and its treatment,* page 410.)

CAUSES

Causes of DIC include:
- infection, including gram-negative or gram-positive septicemia and viral, fungal, rickettsial, and protozoal infection
- obstetric complications, including abruptio placentae, amniotic fluid embolism, retained dead fetus, septic abortion, and eclampsia
- neoplastic disease, including acute leukemia, metastatic carcinoma, and aplastic anemia
- disorders that produce necrosis, including extensive burns or trauma, brain tissue destruction, transplant rejection, and hepatic necrosis
- other conditions, including heatstroke, shock, poisonous snakebite, cirrhosis, fat embolism, incompatible blood transfusion, cardiac arrest, surgery requiring cardiopulmonary bypass, giant hemangioma, severe venous thrombosis, and purpura fulminans.

PATHOPHYSIOLOGY

It isn't clear why certain disorders lead to DIC or whether they use a common mechanism. In many people, the triggering mechanisms may be the entrance of foreign protein into the circulation and vascular endothelial injury.

Regardless of how DIC begins, the typical accelerated clotting results in generalized activation of prothrombin and a consequent excess of thrombin. The thrombin converts fibrinogen to fibrin, producing fibrin clots in the microcirculation. This process uses huge amounts of coagulation factors (especially fibrinogen, prothrombin, platelets, and factors V and VIII), causing hypofibrinogenemia, hypoprothrombinemia, thrombocytopenia, and deficiencies in factors V and VIII. Circulating thrombin also activates the fibrinolytic system, which dissolves fibrin clots into fibrin degradation products. Hemorrhage may be mostly the result of the anticoagulant activity of fibrin degradation products as well as depletion of plasma coagulation factors.

SIGNS AND SYMPTOMS

Signs and symptoms of DIC caused by the anticoagulant activity of fibrin degradation products and depletion of plasma coagulation factors include:
- abnormal bleeding
- cutaneous oozing of serum
- petechiae or blood blisters
- bleeding from surgical or I.V. sites
- bleeding from the GI tract
- epistaxis (nosebleed)
- hemoptysis (spitting of blood, blood-stained sputum).

Other signs and symptoms include:
- cyanotic, cold, mottled fingers and toes, caused by fibrin clots in the microcirculation resulting in tissue ischemia
- severe muscle, back, abdominal, and chest pain from tissue hypoxia
- nausea and vomiting (may be a manifestation of GI bleeding)
- shock caused by hemorrhage
- confusion, possibly caused by cerebral thrombus and decreased cerebral perfusion
- dyspnea caused by poor tissue perfusion and oxygenation
- oliguria because of decreased renal perfusion.

COMPLICATIONS

Complications of DIC include:

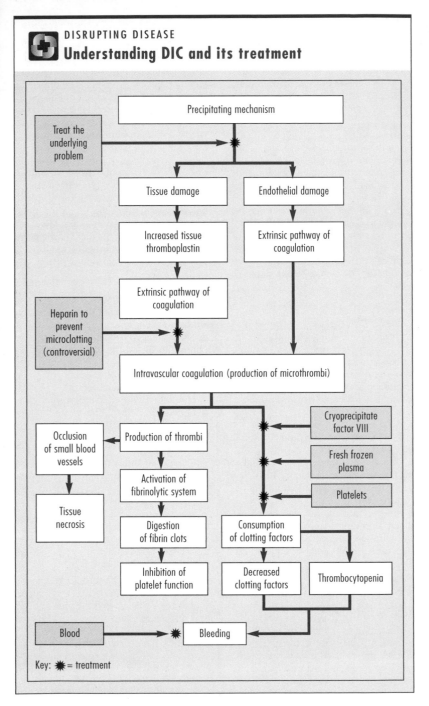

DISRUPTING DISEASE
Understanding DIC and its treatment

- acute tubular necrosis
- shock
- multiple organ failure.

DIAGNOSIS

Diagnosis of DIC is based on:
- decreased platelet count, usually less than 100,000/µl, because platelets are consumed during thrombosis
- fibrinogen level less than 150 mg/dl because fibrinogen is consumed in clot formation (levels may be normal if elevated by hepatitis or pregnancy)
- prothrombin time greater than 15 seconds
- partial thromboplastin time greater than 60 seconds
- increased fibrin degradation products, typically greater than 45 mcg/ml, because of excess fibrinolysis by plasmin
- D-dimer test (presence of an asymmetrical carbon compound fragment formed in the presence of fibrin split products) positive at less than 1:8 dilution
- positive fibrin monomers, diminished levels of factors V and VIII, fragmentation of red blood cells (RBCs), and hemoglobin level less than 10 g/dl
- reduced urine output (less than 30 ml/ hour), elevated blood urea nitrogen (greater than 25 mg/dl), and elevated serum creatinine (greater than 1.3 mg/dl).

TREATMENT

Treatment includes:
- prompt recognition and treatment of underlying disorder
- blood, fresh frozen plasma, platelet, or packed RBC transfusions to support hemostasis in active bleeding
- heparin in early stages to prevent microclotting and as a last resort in hemorrhage (controversial in acute DIC after sepsis). (See *Understanding DIC and its treatment*.)

Erythroblastosis fetalis

Erythroblastosis fetalis, a hemolytic disease of the fetus and neonate, stems from an incompatibility of fetal and maternal blood; that is, mother and fetus have different ABO blood groups or the fetus is Rh-positive and the mother is Rh-negative. In these cases, the mother's immune system generates antibodies against fetal red cells.

The effects of hemolytic disease are more severe in Rh incompatibility than in ABO incompatibility. ABO incompatibility may resolve after birth without life-threatening complications. ABO incompatibility occurs in about 25% of all pregnancies, but only 1 in 10 cases results in hemolytic disease. Rh incompatibility occurs in less than 10% of pregnancies and rarely causes hemolytic disease in the first pregnancy.

In severe, untreated erythroblastosis fetalis, the prognosis is poor, especially if the fetus's or the neonate's brain and spinal cord become infiltrated with bilirubin (a condition called *kernicterus*). About 70% of these neonates die, usually within the first week of life; survivors inevitably have severe neurologic damage, including sensory impairment, mental deficiencies, and cerebral palsy. Most fetuses with hydrops fetalis (the most severe form of this disorder, linked to profound anemia and edema) are stillborn; the few who are delivered alive rarely survive longer than a few hours.

CAUSES

Erythroblastosis fetalis is caused by:
- ABO incompatibility
- Rh factor isoimmunization. (See *What happens in Rh isoimmunization*, page 412.)

PATHOPHYSIOLOGY

The pathophysiologies of ABO and Rh incompatibility are different.

ABO incompatibility. Each blood group has specific antigens on red blood cells (RBCs) and specific antibodies in the serum. As in transfusion, the maternal immune system forms antibodies against fetal cells when blood groups differ. Most commonly, the mother has group O blood and the fetus has group A or B blood. Of course, a mother with group A or B blood won't form antibodies against a group O fetus, who has no fetal blood group antigens. Because the blood of most adults already contains anti-A or anti-B antibodies, ABO incompatibility can cause hemolytic

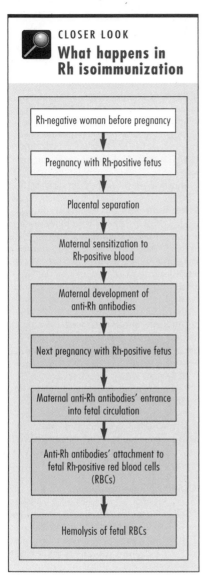

CLOSER LOOK

What happens in Rh isoimmunization

Rh-negative woman before pregnancy

↓

Pregnancy with Rh-positive fetus

↓

Placental separation

↓

Maternal sensitization to Rh-positive blood

↓

Maternal development of anti-Rh antibodies

↓

Next pregnancy with Rh-positive fetus

↓

Maternal anti-Rh antibodies' entrance into fetal circulation

↓

Anti-Rh antibodies' attachment to fetal Rh-positive red blood cells (RBCs)

↓

Hemolysis of fetal RBCs

---

tal blood antigens inherited from the father. A woman with Rh-negative blood may also become sensitized from receiving blood transfusions with Rh antigens; from inadequate doses of Rh$_o$(D); or from failure to receive Rh$_o$(D) after significant blood leakage from fetus to mother in abruptio placentae (premature detachment of the placenta).

A subsequent pregnancy with a fetus with Rh-positive blood provokes maternal production of agglutinating antibodies, which cross the placental barrier, attach to Rh-positive RBCs in the fetus, and cause hemolysis and anemia. To compensate, the fetal blood-forming organs step up the production of RBCs, and erythroblasts (immature RBCs) appear in the fetal circulation. Extensive hemolysis releases more unconjugated bilirubin than the liver can conjugate and excrete, causing hyperbilirubinemia and hemolytic anemia.

SIGNS AND SYMPTOMS
Signs and symptoms of erythroblastosis fetalis include:
■ jaundice caused by large amounts of unconjugated bilirubin released by hemolysis
■ anemia caused by hemolysis
■ hepatosplenomegaly.

COMPLICATIONS
Complications of erythroblastosis fetalis include:
■ fetal death in utero
■ severe anemia
■ heart failure
■ kernicterus.

DIAGNOSIS
Diagnosis can involve both prenatal and neonatal findings. Prenatal findings include:
■ maternal history (of erythroblastotic stillbirths, abortions, previously affected children, previous anti-Rh titers)
■ blood typing and screening (should be done frequently to determine changes in the degree of maternal immunization)
■ paternal blood typing for ABO and Rh blood groups
■ maternal history of blood transfusion

---

disease even if fetal erythrocytes don't escape into the maternal circulation during pregnancy.

Rh incompatibility. During her first pregnancy, a woman with Rh-negative blood becomes sensitized (during delivery or abortion) by exposure to Rh-positive fe-

- amniotic fluid analysis showing increased bilirubin and anti-Rh titers
- radiologic studies showing edema and, in hydrops fetalis, the "halo" sign (edematous, elevated, subcutaneous fat layers) and the "Buddha" position (fetus's legs are crossed).

Neonatal findings indicating erythroblastosis fetalis include:

- direct Coombs' test of umbilical cord blood to measure RBC (Rh-positive) antibodies in the neonate (positive only when the mother is Rh-negative and the fetus is Rh-positive)
- cord hemoglobin level less than 10 g/dl, indicating severe disease
- many nucleated RBCs on a peripheral blood smear.

TREATMENT

Treatment depends on the degree of maternal sensitization and the effects of hemolytic disease on the fetus or neonate. It may include:

- intrauterine-intraperitoneal transfusion of fetus (if amniotic fluid analysis suggests the fetus is severely affected and isn't mature enough to deliver)
- planned delivery (usually 2 to 4 weeks before term date, depending on maternal history, serologic test results, and amniocentesis findings)
- exchange transfusion of the neonate to remove antibody-coated RBCs and prevent hyperbilirubinemia by replacing the infant's blood with fresh type O, Rh-negative blood
- albumin infusion to bind bilirubin
- phototherapy (exposure to ultraviolet light to reduce bilirubin levels)
- gamma globulin containing anti-Rh antibody ($Rh_o[D]$) to prevent Rh isoimmunization in Rh-negative females (ineffective if a previous pregnancy, abortion, or transfusion has already sensitized the mother).

Neonatal therapy for hydrops fetalis includes:

- intubation to maintain ventilation
- removal of excess fluid to relieve ascites and respiratory distress
- exchange transfusion
- maintaining body temperature.

Hypersplenism

Hypersplenism is a syndrome marked by exaggerated activity of the spleen and, possibly, splenomegaly (enlarged spleen). This disorder results in peripheral blood cell deficiency as the spleen traps and destroys peripheral blood cells.

CAUSES

Hypersplenism may be idiopathic (if primary) or caused by a disorder outside the spleen, such as:

- *infectious disorders* — acute (abscesses, subacute infective endocarditis) or chronic (tuberculosis, malaria, Felty's syndrome)
- *congestive disorders* — cirrhosis, thrombosis
- *hyperplastic disorders* — hemolytic anemia, polycythemia vera
- *infiltrative disorders* — Gaucher's disease, Niemann-Pick disease
- *cystic or neoplastic disorders* — cysts, leukemia, lymphoma, myelofibrosis.

PATHOPHYSIOLOGY

In hypersplenism, the spleen's normal filtering and phagocytic functions accelerate indiscriminately, automatically removing antibody-coated, aging, and abnormal cells, even though some cells may be functionally normal. The spleen may also temporarily sequester normal platelets and RBCs, withholding them from circulation. In this manner, the enlarged spleen may trap as much as 90% of the body's platelets and up to 45% of its RBC mass.

SIGNS AND SYMPTOMS

Most patients with hypersplenism develop anemia, leukopenia, or thrombocytopenia, in many cases with splenomegaly. They may contract bacterial infections frequently (from leukopenia), bruise easily, hemorrhage spontaneously from the mucous membranes and GI or genitourinary tract (from thrombocytopenia), and have ulcerations of the mouth, legs, and feet (probably because of leukopenia). They commonly develop fever, weakness, and palpitations. Patients with secondary hypersplenism may have other clinical abnormalities, depending on the underlying disease.

COMPLICATIONS

Complications may include:
- anemia
- leukopenia
- thrombocytopenia.

DIAGNOSIS

Diagnosis requires evidence of abnormal splenic destruction of RBCs or platelets (or their sequestration) and splenomegaly.

The most definitive test measures erythrocytes in the spleen and liver after I.V. infusion of chromium-labeled RBCs or platelets. A high spleen-liver ratio of radioactivity indicates splenic destruction or sequestration.

Complete blood count shows decreased hemoglobin level (as low as 4 g/dl), white blood cell count (less than 4,000/µl), and platelet count (less than 125,000/µl), and an elevated reticulocyte count (more than 75,000/µl). Spleen biopsy, scan, and angiography may be useful, although biopsy is hazardous and should be avoided, if possible. In sequestration, the spleen is palpable. Abdominal palpation should be used cautiously because it can cause injury, bleeding, or rupture.

TREATMENT

Splenectomy is indicated only in transfusion-dependent patients whose condition is refractory to medical therapy. Splenectomy seldom cures the patient but does correct the effects of cytopenia. Postoperative complications may include infection and thromboembolic disease. Occasionally, splenectomy may result in accelerated blood cell destruction in the bone marrow and liver. Secondary hypersplenism calls for treatment of the underlying disease.

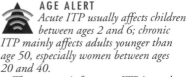

AGE ALERT
Older adults may be at higher risk for infection because of decreased leukocyte and lymphocyte production. Fewer and weaker lymphocytes and changes in the immune system lessen the antigenantibody response in older adults.

Idiopathic thrombocytopenic purpura

Idiopathic thrombocytopenic purpura (ITP) is a deficiency of platelets that occurs when the immune system destroys the body's own platelets. ITP may be acute, as in postviral thrombocytopenia, or chronic, as in essential thrombocytopenia or autoimmune thrombocytopenia.

AGE ALERT
Acute ITP usually affects children between ages 2 and 6; chronic ITP mainly affects adults younger than age 50, especially women between ages 20 and 40.

The prognosis for acute ITP is excellent; nearly four of five patients recover without treatment. The prognosis for chronic ITP is good; remissions lasting weeks or years are common, especially among women.

CAUSES

Causes of ITP include:
- viral infection
- immunization with a live virus vaccine
- immunologic disorders
- drug reactions.

PATHOPHYSIOLOGY

ITP occurs when circulating immunoglobulin (Ig) G molecules react with host platelets, which are then destroyed in the spleen and, to a lesser degree, in the liver. Normally, the life span of platelets in circulation is 7 to 10 days. In ITP, platelets survive 1 to 3 days or less.

SIGNS AND SYMPTOMS

Signs and symptoms of ITP are caused by decreased levels of platelets and may include:
- nose bleeds
- oral bleeding
- hemorrhages into the skin, mucous membranes, and other tissues, causing red discoloration of skin (purpura)
- small purplish hemorrhagic spots on skin (petechiae)
- excessive menstrual bleeding.

COMPLICATIONS

Possible complications of ITP are:
- hemorrhage
- cerebral hemorrhage
- purpuric lesions of vital organs (such as the brain and kidney).

DIAGNOSIS

Diagnosis of ITP includes:

- platelet count less than 20,000/µl
- prolonged bleeding time
- abnormal size and appearance of platelets
- decreased hemoglobin level (if bleeding occurred)
- bone marrow studies showing abundant megakaryocytes (platelet precursor cells) and a circulating platelet survival time of only several hours to a few days
- humoral tests that measure platelet-linked IgG.

TREATMENT

Treatment for acute ITP includes:

- glucocorticoids to prevent further platelet destruction
- immunoglobulin to prevent platelet destruction
- plasmapheresis
- platelet pheresis.

Treatment for chronic ITP includes:

- corticosteroids to suppress phagocytic activity and help platelet production
- splenectomy (when splenomegaly accompanies the initial thrombocytopenia)
- blood and blood component transfusions and vitamin K to correct anemia and coagulation defects.

Alternative treatments include:

- immunosuppressants to help stop platelet destruction
- high-dose I.V. immunoglobulin.

Polycythemia vera

Polycythemia vera is a chronic disorder characterized by increased red blood cell (RBC) mass, erythrocytosis, leukocytosis, thrombocytosis, and increased hemoglobin level, with normal or increased plasma volume. This disease is also known as *primary polycythemia, erythremia, polycythemia rubra vera, splenomegalic polycythemia,* or *Vaquez-Osler disease.* It typically occurs between ages 40 and 60, most commonly among Jewish males of European ancestry. It seldom affects children and doesn't appear to be familial.

The prognosis depends on age at diagnosis, the type of treatment used, and complications. Mortality is high if polycythemia is untreated, linked to leukemia, or associated with myeloid metaplasia (presence of marrow-like tissue and ectopic hematopoiesis in extramedullary sites, such as liver and spleen, and nucleated erythrocytes in blood).

CAUSES

The cause of polycythemia vera is unknown, but it's probably related to:

- multipotential stem cell defect.

PATHOPHYSIOLOGY

In polycythemia vera, uncontrolled and rapid cellular reproduction and maturation cause proliferation or hyperplasia of all bone marrow cells (panmyelosis).

Increased RBC mass makes the blood abnormally viscous and inhibits blood flow to the microcirculation. Decreased blood flow and thrombocytosis set the stage for intravascular thrombosis.

SIGNS AND SYMPTOMS

Possible signs and symptoms of polycythemia vera include:

- feeling of fullness in the head or headache caused by altered blood volume, as in hypervolemia and hyperviscosity
- dizziness caused by hypervolemia and hyperviscosity
- ruddy cyanosis (plethora) of the nose and clubbing of the fingers or toes caused by thrombosis in smaller vessels
- painful pruritus (itching) caused by abnormally high concentrations of mast cells in the skin and their releases of heparin and histamine.

COMPLICATIONS

Possible complications include:

- hemorrhage
- vascular thromboses
- uric acid stones.

DIAGNOSIS

These test results help diagnose polycythemia vera:

- increased RBC mass
- normal arterial oxygen saturation linked to splenomegaly
- increased uric acid level
- increased blood histamine levels
- decreased serum iron concentration

- decreased or absent urinary erythropoietin
- bone marrow biopsy showing excess production of myeloid stem cells.

TREATMENT
Treatment may include:
- phlebotomy to reduce RBC mass
- myelosuppressive therapy with radioactive phosphorus (32P) to suppress erythropoiesis (may increase the risk of leukemia), or hydroxyurea.

Secondary polycythemia
Secondary polycythemia, also called *reactive polycythemia,* is excessive production of circulating red blood cells (RBCs) caused by hypoxia, tumor, or disease. It occurs in about 2 of every 100,000 people living at or near sea level; the incidence increases among those living at high altitudes.

CAUSES
Secondary polycythemia may be caused by:
- increased production of erythropoietin
- conditions that cause prolonged tissue hypoxia, such as shock or compression of major blood vessels.

PATHOPHYSIOLOGY
Secondary polycythemia may result from increased production of the hormone erythropoietin—which stimulates bone marrow to produce RBCs—in a compensatory response to several conditions. These include hypoxemia caused by such conditions as chronic obstructive pulmonary disease, hemoglobin abnormalities (such as carboxyhemoglobinemia in heavy smokers), heart failure (causing a decreased ventilation-perfusion ratio), right-to-left shunting of blood in the heart (as in transposition of the great vessels), central or peripheral alveolar hypoventilation (as in barbiturate intoxication), and low air oxygen content at high altitudes.

Increased production of erythropoietin may also be an inappropriate (pathologic) response to renal, central nervous system, or endocrine disorders or to certain neoplasms (such as renal tumors, uterine myoma, or cerebellar hemangiomas).

SIGNS AND SYMPTOMS
Possible signs and symptoms are:
- ruddy cyanotic skin, emphysema, and hypoxemia without hepatomegaly or hypertension (in the hypoxic patient)
- clubbing of the fingers (when the underlying cause is cardiovascular).

COMPLICATIONS
Complications may include:
- hemorrhage
- thromboemboli caused by hemoconcentration.

DIAGNOSIS
Diagnosis of secondary polycythemia is based on these test results:
- high hematocrit and hemoglobin level
- high mean corpuscular volume and mean corpuscular hemoglobin
- high urinary erythropoietin level
- high blood histamine level
- normal or low arterial oxygen saturation
- bone marrow biopsy showing hyperplasia or erythroid precursors.

TREATMENT
The goal of treatment is to correct the underlying disease or environmental condition, and may include:
- phlebotomy or pheresis to reduce blood volume (to correct hazardous hyperviscosity or if treatment of the primary disease isn't effective)
- continuous low-flow oxygen therapy to correct severe hypoxia.

Spurious polycythemia
Spurious polycythemia is characterized by an increased hematocrit and a normal or low red blood cell (RBC) total mass. It results from lowered plasma volume and subsequent hemoconcentration. It's also known as *relative polycythemia, stress erythrocytosis, stress polycythemia, benign polycythemia, Gaisböck's disease,* or *pseudopolycythemia.* It usually affects middle-aged people and is more common in men than in women.

CAUSES
Causes of spurious polycythemia include:
- dehydration

- hemoconcentration caused by stress
- high-normal RBC mass and low-normal plasma volume
- hypertension
- thromboembolic disease
- elevated serum cholesterol and uric acid
- familial tendency.

PATHOPHYSIOLOGY

Conditions that promote severe fluid loss decrease plasma volume and lead to hemoconcentration. Such conditions include persistent vomiting or diarrhea, burns, adrenocortical insufficiency, aggressive diuretic therapy, decreased fluid intake, diabetic acidosis, and renal disease.

Nervous stress causes hemoconcentration by some unknown mechanism. This form of erythrocytosis (chronically elevated hematocrit) is particularly common in the middle-aged man who is a chronic smoker and has a type A personality (tense, hard driving, and anxious).

In many people, an increased hematocrit merely reflects a normally high RBC mass and low plasma volume. This situation is particularly common in people who don't smoke, aren't obese, and have no history of hypertension.

SIGNS AND SYMPTOMS

Signs and symptoms of spurious polycythemia may include:

- headaches or dizziness because of altered circulation caused by hypervolemia and hyperviscosity
- ruddy appearance caused by cyanosis
- slight hypertension from increased blood volume
- tendency to hyperventilate when recumbent
- cardiac or pulmonary disease.

COMPLICATIONS

A potential complication of spurious polycythemia is:

- thromboemboli.

DIAGNOSIS

These test results help diagnose spurious polycythemia:

- high hemoglobin level and hematocrit
- high RBC count
- normal RBC mass

- normal arterial oxygen saturation
- normal bone marrow
- low or normal plasma volume
- possibly hyperlipidemia
- possibly uricosuria.

TREATMENT

Treatment includes:

- appropriate fluids and electrolytes to correct dehydration
- measures to prevent further fluid loss, such as antidiarrheal medication if needed, avoiding dietary diuretics (such as caffeine), preventing excessive perspiration, and remaining hydrated.

Thalassemia

Thalassemia, a hereditary group of hemolytic anemias, is characterized by defective synthesis in the polypeptide chains of the protein component of hemoglobin. Consequently, red blood cell (RBC) synthesis is also impaired.

CULTURAL DIVERSITY
Thalassemia is most common in people of Mediterranean ancestry (especially Italian and Greek) but also occurs in people whose ancestors originated in Africa, southern China, southeast Asia, and India.

In b-thalassemia, the most common form of this disorder, synthesis of the beta polypeptide chain is defective. It occurs in three clinical forms: major, intermedia, and minor. The severity of the resulting anemia depends on whether the patient is homozygous or heterozygous for the thalassemic trait. The prognosis varies:

- *Thalassemia major*—Patients seldom survive to adulthood.
- *Thalassemia intermedia*—Children develop normally into adulthood, although puberty is usually delayed.
- *Thalassemia minor*—Patients have normal life span.

CAUSES

Causes of thalassemia are:

- homozygous inheritance of the partially dominant autosomal gene (thalassemia major or thalassemia intermedia)
- heterozygous inheritance of the same gene (thalassemia minor).

PATHOPHYSIOLOGY

Total or partial deficiency of beta polypeptide chain production impairs hemoglobin synthesis and results in continual production of fetal hemoglobin, lasting even past the neonatal period. Normally, immunoglobulin synthesis switches from gamma-to beta-polypeptides at the time of birth. This conversion doesn't happen in thalassemic neonates. Their RBCs are hypochromic and microcytic.

SIGNS AND SYMPTOMS

Possible signs and symptoms of thalassemia major (also known as *Cooley's anemia, Mediterranean disease,* and *erythroblastic anemia* are related to the development of hypochromic and microcytic RBCs subsequently impairing oxygenation that lead to:

- development, during the second 6 months of life, of severe anemia, bone abnormalities, failure to thrive, and life-threatening complications (infant healthy at birth)
- pallor and yellow skin and sclera in infants ages 3 to 6 months
- splenomegaly or hepatomegaly, with abdominal enlargement; frequent infections; bleeding tendencies (especially nose bleeds); anorexia
- small body, large head (characteristic features), and possible mental retardation
- possible features similar to Down syndrome in infants, because of thickened bone at the base of the nose caused by bone marrow hyperactivity.

Signs and symptoms of thalassemia intermedia are:

- some degree of anemia, jaundice, and splenomegaly
- possibly signs of hemosiderosis caused by increased intestinal absorption of iron.

A sign of thalassemia minor is:

- mild anemia (usually produces no symptoms and is often overlooked; it should be differentiated from iron deficiency anemia).

COMPLICATIONS

Possible complications of thalassemia include:

- pathologic fractures because of expansion of the marrow cavities with thinning of the long bones
- cardiac arrhythmias
- heart failure.

DIAGNOSIS

Diagnosis of thalassemia major includes:

- low RBC and hemoglobin level, microcytosis, and high reticulocyte count
- elevated bilirubin and urinary and fecal urobilinogen levels
- low serum folate level reflects increased folate use by hypertrophied bone marrow
- peripheral blood smear showing target cells, microcytes, pale nucleated RBCs, and marked anisocytosis
- thinning and widening of the marrow space of skull and long bone, seen on X-ray, because of overactive bone marrow
- granular appearance of bones of skull and vertebrae, areas of osteoporosis in long bones shown on X-ray, deformed (rectangular or biconvex) fingers or toes
- significantly increased fetal hemoglobin level and slightly increased hemoglobin A_2 level on quantitative hemoglobin studies
- exclusion of iron deficiency anemia (which also produces hypochromic microcytic RBCs).

Diagnosis of thalassemia intermedia includes:

- hypochromic microcytic RBCs (less severe than in thalassemia major).

Diagnosis of thalassemia minor includes:

- hypochromic microcytic RBCs
- significantly increased hemoglobin A_2 level and moderately increased fetal hemoglobin level on quantitative hemoglobin studies.

TREATMENT

Treatment of thalassemia major is essentially supportive and includes:

- prompt treatment with appropriate antibiotics for infections
- folic acid supplements to help maintain folic acid levels despite increased requirements
- transfusions of packed RBCs to increase hemoglobin levels (used judiciously to minimize iron overload)

- splenectomy and bone marrow transplantation (effectiveness hasn't been confirmed)
- no treatment for thalassemia intermedia and thalassemia minor
- no iron supplements (contraindicated in all forms of thalassemia).

Thrombocytopenia

Thrombocytopenia, the most common cause of hemorrhagic disorders, is a deficiency of circulating platelets. It may be congenital or acquired; the acquired form is more common. Because platelets are needed for coagulation, this disease poses a serious threat to hemostasis. The prognosis is excellent in drug-induced thrombocytopenia if the offending drug — usually carbamazepine or heparin — is withdrawn; in such cases, recovery may be immediate. In other types, the prognosis depends on the patient's response to treatment of the underlying cause.

CAUSES
Possible causes of thrombocytopenia include:
- decreased or defective platelet production in the bone marrow (as in leukemia, aplastic anemia, or drug toxicity)
- increased platelet destruction outside the marrow caused by an underlying disorder (such as cirrhosis of the liver, disseminated intravascular coagulation, or severe infection)
- sequestration (increased amount of blood in a limited vascular area such as the spleen)
- blood loss.

PATHOPHYSIOLOGY
In thrombocytopenia, lack of platelets can cause inadequate hemostasis. Four mechanisms are responsible: decreased platelet production, decreased platelet survival, pooling of blood in the spleen, and intravascular dilution of circulating platelets. Megakaryocytes, giant cells in the bone marrow, produce platelets. Platelet production decreases when the number of megakaryocytes is reduced or when platelet production becomes dysfunctional. (See *What happens in thrombocytopenia*, pages 420 and 421.)

SIGNS AND SYMPTOMS
Possible signs and symptoms of thrombocytopenia are:
- petechiae or blood blisters caused by bleeding into the skin
- bleeding into mucous membrane
- malaise, fatigue, and general weakness related to blood loss and decreased tissue oxygenation
- large blood-filled blisters in the mouth (in adults).

COMPLICATIONS
Complications include:
- hemorrhage
- death.

DIAGNOSIS
These tests help diagnose thrombocytopenia:
- platelet count usually less than 100,000/µl in adults
- prolonged bleeding time
- platelet antibody studies to help determine why the platelet count is low (also used to select treatment)
- platelet survival studies to help differentiate between ineffective platelet production and platelet destruction as causes of thrombocytopenia
- bone marrow studies to determine the number, size, and maturity of megakaryocytes in severe disease, helping identify ineffective platelet production as the cause and ruling out malignant disease.

TREATMENT
Treatment of thrombocytopenia may include:
- withdrawal of the offending drug or treatment of the underlying cause
- corticosteroids to increase platelet production
- lithium carbonate or folate to stimulate bone marrow production
- I.V. gamma globulin to increase platelet production
- platelet transfusion to treat complications of severe hemorrhage
- splenectomy to correct disease caused by platelet destruction (because the spleen is the primary site of platelet removal and antibody production).

CLOSER LOOK
What happens in thrombocytopenia

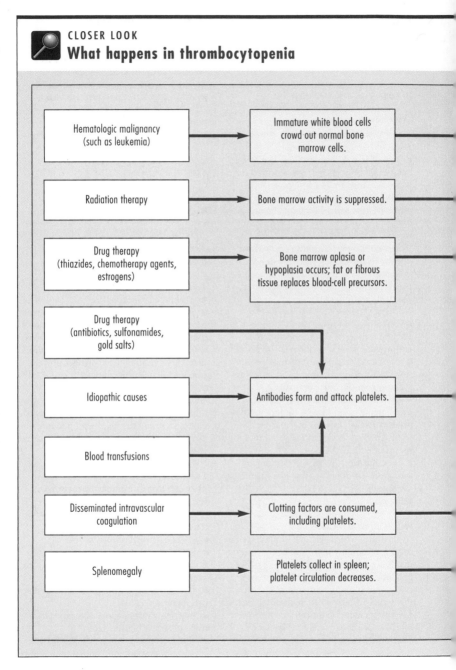

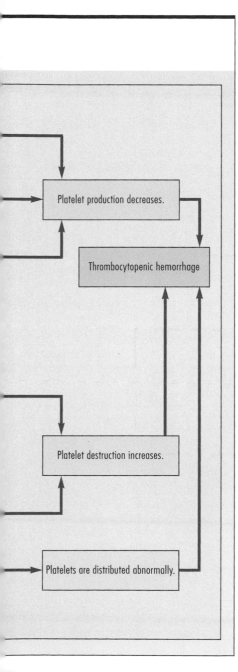

Platelet production decreases.

Thrombocytopenic hemorrhage

Platelet destruction increases.

Platelets are distributed abnormally.

Von Willebrand's disease

Von Willebrand's disease is a hereditary bleeding disorder, occurring more often in females and characterized by prolonged bleeding time, moderate deficiency of coagulation factor VIII (antihemophilic factor A), and impaired platelet function. This disease commonly causes bleeding from the skin or mucosal surfaces and, in females, excessive uterine bleeding. Bleeding may range from mild and asymptomatic to severe, potentially fatal, hemorrhage. The prognosis is usually good.

CAUSES
Von Willebrand's disease is caused by:
- inherited autosomal dominant trait.
  Recently, an acquired form has been identified in patients with cancer and immune disorders.

PATHOPHYSIOLOGY
Von Willebrand's disease results from a deficiency or abnormality of von Willebrand's factor (vWF). This factor acts as a carrier for the factor VIII molecule and is needed for proper platelet function. As a result of this deficiency, platelet adhesion is defective and coagulation factor VIII becomes deficient. Subsequently, coagulation time is prolonged.

Defective platelet function is characterized in vivo by decreased agglutination and adhesion at the bleeding site and in vitro by reduced platelet retention.

SIGNS AND SYMPTOMS
The signs and symptoms associated with von Willebrand's disease are related to prolonged coagulation time, which may cause:
- easy bruising
- epistaxis (nose bleed)
- bleeding from the gums
- petechiae (rarely)
- hemorrhage after laceration or surgery (in severe forms)
- menorrhagia (in severe forms)
- GI bleeding (in severe forms)
- excessive postpartum bleeding (uncommon)

- massive soft tissue hemorrhage and bleeding into joints (rare).

COMPLICATIONS
A complication of von Willebrand's disease is:
- hemorrhage.

DIAGNOSIS
These test results help diagnose von Willebrand's disease:
- prolonged bleeding time (longer than 6 minutes)
- slightly prolonged partial thromboplastin time (longer than 45 seconds)
- absent or low factor VIII
- absent or low factor VIII–related antigens
- low factor VIII activity
- coagulation factor assay, using ristocetin, shows defective in vitro platelet aggregation
- normal platelet count and clot retraction.

TREATMENT
Treatment includes:
- infusion of cryoprecipitate or blood fractions rich in factor VIII to shorten bleeding time and replenish factor VIII
- parenteral or intranasal desmopressin (DDAVP) to increase serum levels of vWF.

12

Immune system

The immune system is responsible for safeguarding the body from disease-causing microorganisms. It's part of a complex system of host defenses.

Host defenses may be innate or acquired. Innate defenses include physical and chemical barriers, the complement complex, and cells such as phagocytes (cells programmed to destroy foreign cells, such as bacteria) and natural killer lymphocytes.

Physical barriers, such as the skin and mucous membranes, prevent invasion by most organisms. Chemical barriers include lysozymes (found in such body secretions as tears, mucus, and saliva) and hydrochloric acid in the stomach. Lysozymes destroy bacteria by removing cell walls. Hydrochloric acid breaks down foods and destroys pathogens carried by food or swallowed mucus.

Organisms that penetrate this first line of defense simultaneously trigger the inflammatory and immune responses, some innate and others acquired.

Acquired immunity comes into play when the body encounters a cell or cell product that it recognizes as foreign, such as a bacterium or a virus. The two types of immunity provided by cells are humoral (provided by B lymphocytes) and cell-mediated (provided by T lymphocytes). All cells involved in the inflammatory and immune responses arrive from a single type of stem cell in the bone marrow. B cells mature in the marrow, and

T cells migrate to the thymus, where they mature.

The inflammatory response is the immediate local response to tissue injury, whether from trauma or infection. Primarily, it involves the action of polymorphonuclear leukocytes, basophils, and mast cells. Platelets monocytes, and macrophages also are involved to varying degrees.

IMMUNE RESPONSE

The immune response primarily involves the interaction of antigens (foreign proteins), B lymphocytes, T lymphocytes, macrophages, cytokines, complement, and polymorphonuclear leukocytes. Some immunoactive cells circulate constantly; others remain in the tissues and organs of the immune system, such as the thymus, lymph nodes, bone marrow, spleen, and tonsils. In the thymus, the T lymphocytes, which are involved in cell-mediated immunity, become able to differentiate self (host) from nonself (foreign) substances (antigens). In contrast, B lymphocytes, which are involved in humoral immunity, mature in the bone marrow. The key mechanism in humoral immunity is the production of immunoglobulin by B cells and the subsequent activation of the complement cascade. The lymph nodes, spleen, liver, and intestinal lym-

Structure of the immunoglobulin molecule

The immunoglobulin molecule consists of four polypeptide chains: two heavy (H) and two light (L) chains, held together by disulfide bonds. The H chain has one variable (V) and at least three constant (C) regions. The L chain has one V and one C region. Together, the V regions form a pocket known as the *antigen-binding site*. This site is located within the antigen-binding fragment (Fab) region of the molecule. Part of the C region of the H chains forms the crystallizable fragment (Fc) region of the molecule. This region mediates effector mechanisms, such as complement activation, and is the portion of the immunoglobulin molecule bound by Fc receptors on phagocytic cells, mast cells, and basophils. Each immunoglobulin molecule also has two-antibody-combining sites (except for the immunoglobulin [Ig] M molecule, which has 10, and IgA, which may have two or more).

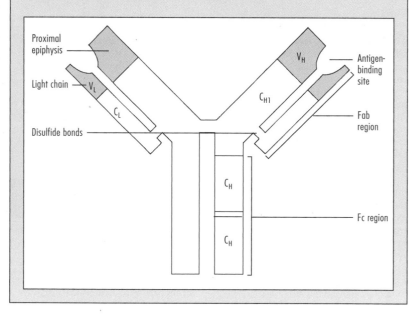

phoid tissue help remove and destroy circulating antigens in the blood and lymph.

Antigens

An antigen is a substance that can induce an immune response. T and B lymphocytes have specific receptors that respond to specific antigen molecular shapes, called *epitopes*. In B cells, this receptor is an immunoglobulin, also called an *antibody*.

MAJOR HISTOCOMPATIBILITY COMPLEX

The T-cell antigen receptor recognizes antigens only in association with specific cell-surface molecules known as the *major histocompatibility complex* (MHC).

The MHC, also known as the *human leukocyte antigen* (HLA) *locus,* is a cluster of genes on human chromosome 6 that has a pivotal role in the immune response. Every person receives one set of MHC genes from each parent, and both sets of genes are expressed on the individual's cells. These genes produce MHC molecules, which participate in:

- the recognition of self versus nonself
- the interaction of immunologically active cells by coding for cell-surface proteins.

MHC molecules differ among individuals. Slightly different antigen receptors can recognize a large number of distinct antigens by their specific genetic coding.

Groups or clones of lymphocytes exist that have identical receptors for a specific antigen. The clone of a lymphocyte rapidly proliferates when exposed to the specific antigen. Some lymphocytes further differentiate, while others become memory cells, which allow a more rapid response—the memory or anamnestic response—to subsequent challenge by the antigen.

HAPTENS

Most antigens are large molecules, such as proteins or polysaccharides. Smaller molecules, such as drugs that aren't antigenic by themselves, are known as *haptens*. They can bind with larger molecules, or carriers, and become antigenic or immunogenic.

ANTIGENICITY

Many factors influence the intensity of a foreign substance's interaction with the host's immune system (antigenicity):

- physical and chemical characteristics of the antigen
- its relative foreignness; for example, little or no immune response may follow the transfusion of serum proteins between humans, but a vigorous immune response (serum sickness) commonly follows transfusion of horse serum proteins to a human
- the host's genetic makeup, especially the MHC molecules.

Humoral immunity

The humoral immune response is one of two types of immune responses that can occur when foreign substances invade the body. The other is the cell-mediated response. The humoral response is also called an *antibody-mediated* response.

B LYMPHOCYTES

B lymphocytes and their products, *immunoglobulins*, are the basis of humoral immunity. A soluble antigen binds with the B-cell antigen receptor, initiating the humoral immune response. The activated B cells differentiate into plasma cells, which secrete immunoglobulins, also called *antibodies*. This response is regulated by T lymphocytes and their products—lymphokines, such as interleukin-2 (IL-2), IL-4, IL-5, and interferon-8—which determine which class of immunoglobulins a B cell will manufacture.

IMMUNOGLOBULINS

The immunoglobulins secreted by plasma cells are four-chain molecules with two heavy and two light chains. Each chain has a variable (V) region and one or more constant (C) regions, which are coded by separate genes. The V regions of both light and heavy chains participate in antigen binding. The C regions of the heavy chain provide a binding site for crystallizable fragment (Fc) receptors on cells and govern other mechanisms. (See *Structure of the immunoglobulin molecule*.)

There are five known classes of immunoglobulins (Igs): IgG, IgM, IgA, IgE, and IgD. These are distinguished by the constant portions of their heavy chains, but each class has a kappa or lambda light chain, which gives rise to many subtypes and provides almost limitless combinations of light and heavy chains that give immunoglobulins their specificity. (See *Classification of immunoglobulins*, page 426.)

A clone of B cells is specific for only one antigen, and the V regions of its Ig light chains determine that specificity. The class of immunoglobulin can change if the association between the cell's V region genes and heavy chain C region genes changes through a process known as isotype switching. For example, a clone of B cells genetically programmed to recognize tetanus toxoid will first make an IgM antibody against tetanus toxoid and later an IgG or other antibody against it.

Classification of immunoglobulins

This table shows the five classifications of immunoglobulins (Igs).

CLASSIFICATION	DESCRIPTION
IgA	◆ Secretory immunoglobulin (monomer in serum, dimer in secretory form) ◆ Found in colostrum, saliva, tears, nasal fluids, and respiratory, GI, and genitourinary secretions ◆ Accounts for 20% of total serum immunoglobulins ◆ Important role in preventing antigenic agents from attaching to epithelial surfaces
IgD	◆ Minute amounts found in serum (monomer) ◆ Predominant on surface of B lymphocytes ◆ Primarily an antigen receptor ◆ Possible function in controlling lymphocyte activation or suppression
IgE	◆ Found only in trace amounts ◆ Involved in release of vasoactive amines stored in basophils and tissue mast cell granules that cause the allergic effects
IgG	◆ Smallest immunoglobulin (monomer) ◆ Found in all body fluids ◆ Can cross membranes as a single structural unit ◆ Accounts for 75% of total serum immunoglobulins ◆ Produced mainly in secondary immune response ◆ Classic antibody reactions, including precipitation, agglutination, neutralization, and complement fixation ◆ Major antibacterial and antiviral antibody
IgM	◆ Largest immunoglobulin (pentamer) ◆ Usually found only in the vascular system ◆ Cannot readily cross membrane barriers because of its size ◆ Accounts for 5% of total serum immunoglobulins ◆ Dominant activity in primary or initial immune response ◆ Classic antibody reactions, including precipitation, agglutination, neutralization, and complement fixation

Cell-mediated immunity

The cell-mediated immune response protects the body against bacterial, viral, and fungal infections and defends against transplanted cells and tumor cells. T lymphocytes and macrophages are the chief participants in the cell-mediated immune response. A macrophage processes the antigen and then presents it to T lymphocytes.

MACROPHAGES

Macrophages influence both immune and inflammatory responses. Macrophage precursors circulate in the blood. When they collect in various tissues and organs, they differentiate into different types of macrophages. Unlike B and T lymphocytes, macrophages lack surface receptors for specific antigens. Instead, they have receptors for the C region of the heavy chain (Fc region) of immunoglobulin, for fragments of the third component of complement (C3), and for nonimmunologic substances such as carbohydrate molecules.

One of the most important functions of macrophages is presentation of antigen to T lymphocytes. Macrophages ingest and process the antigen, then deposit it on their own surfaces in association with human leukocyte antigen (HLA). T lymphocytes become activated when they recognize the antigen-HLA complex. Macrophages also function in the inflammatory response by producing IL-1, which generates fever, and by synthesizing complement proteins and other mediators that have phagocytic, microbicidal, and tumoricidal effects.

T LYMPHOCYTES

Immature T lymphocytes are derived from the bone marrow and migrate to the thymus, where they mature. In maturation, the products of the major histocompatibility complex (MHC) genes "teach" T cells to distinguish between self and nonself.

Five types of T cells exist with specific functions:

- memory cells — sensitized cells, remain dormant until second exposure to antigen (also known as *secondary immune response*)
- lymphokine-producing cells — mediate delayed hypersensitivity reactions
- cytotoxic T cells — carry out direct destruction of antigen or the cells carrying the antigen
- helper T cells — also known as *T4 cells*, facilitate the humoral and cell-mediated responses
- suppressor T cells — also known as *T8 cells*, inhibit humoral and cell-mediated responses.

T cells acquire specific surface molecules (markers) that identify their potential role when needed in the immune response. These markers and the T-cell antigen receptor together promote the particular activation of each type of T cell. T-cell activation requires presentation of antigens in the context of a specific HLA antigen: class II HLA for helper T cells; class I for cytotoxic T cells. T-cell activation also requires IL-1, produced by macrophages, and IL-2, produced by T cells.

NATURAL KILLER CELLS

This group is a discrete population of large lymphocytes. Natural killer cells recognize surface changes on body cells infected with a virus. They bind to and, in many cases, kill the infected cells.

CYTOKINES

Cytokines are low-molecular-weight proteins involved in the communication among macrophages and the lymphocytes. They induce or regulate a variety of immune or inflammatory responses. Cytokines, which are produced in a cascadelike pattern, include colony-stimulating factors, interferons, interleukins, tumor necrosis factors, and transforming growth factor.

Complement system

The chief humoral effector of the inflammatory response, the complement system includes more than 20 serum proteins. When activated, these proteins interact in a cascadelike process that has profound biological effects. Complement activation takes place through one of two pathways.

CLASSIC PATHWAY

In the classic pathway, IgM or IgG binds with the antigen to form antigen-antibody complexes that activate the first complement component, C_1. This in turn activates C_4, then C_2, and finally, C_3.

ALTERNATE PATHWAY

In the alternate pathway, activating surfaces such as bacterial cell membranes directly amplify spontaneous cleavage of C_3. Once C_3 is activated in either pathway, activation of the terminal components, C_5 to C_9, follows.

The major biological effects of complement activation include chemotaxis (phagocyte attraction), phagocyte activation, histamine release, viral neutralization, promotion of phagocytosis by opsonization (making the bacteria susceptible to phagocytosis), and lysis of cells and bacteria. Kinins are peptides that cause vasodilation and enhance vascular permeability and smooth muscle contraction. Kinins and other mediators of inflammation derived from the kinin and coagulation pathways interact with the complement system.

Polymorphonuclear leukocytes

Other key factors in the inflammatory response are the polymorphonuclear leukocytes: neutrophils, eosinophils, basophils, and mast cells.

NEUTROPHILS

Neutrophils, the most numerous of these leukocytes, derived from bone marrow, increase dramatically in number in response to infection and inflammation. They're the first to respond to acute infection. Neutrophils are highly mobile cells attracted to areas of inflammation and are the main constituent of pus.

Neutrophils have surface receptors for immunoglobulins and complement fragments, and they avidly ingest bacteria or other particles that are coated with target-identifying antibodies (*opsonins*). Toxic oxygen metabolites and enzymes such as lysozyme promptly kill the ingested organisms. Unfortunately, in addition to killing invading organisms, neutrophils also damage host tissues.

EOSINOPHILS

Eosinophils, also derived from bone marrow, multiply in allergic and parasitic disorders. Although their phagocytic function isn't clearly understood, evidence suggests that they participate in host defense against parasites. Their products may also lessen inflammatory response in allergic disorders.

BASOPHILS AND MAST CELLS

Basophils and mast cells also function in immune disorders. Mast cells, unlike basophils, aren't blood cells. Basophils circulate in peripheral blood, whereas mast cells accumulate in connective tissue, particularly in the lungs, intestines, and skin. Both types of cells have surface receptors for IgE. When their receptors are cross-linked by an IgE antigen complex, they release mediators characteristic of the allergic response.

$\mathcal{P}$ATHOPHYSIOLOGIC CHANGES

The host defense system and the immune response are highly complex processes, subject to malfunction at any point along the sequence of events. This malfunction may involve exaggeration, misdirection, or an absence or depression of activity, leading to an immune disorder.

Immune response malfunction

When the immune system responds inappropriately, three basic categories of reactions may occur: hypersensitivity, autoimmune response, and alloimmune response. The type of reaction is determined by the source of the antigen, such as environment, self, or other person, to which the immune system is responding.

HYPERSENSITIVITY

Hypersensitivity is an exaggerated or inappropriate response that occurs on second exposure to an antigen. The result is inflammation and the destruction of healthy tissue. *Allergy* refers to the harmful effects resulting from a hypersensitivity to antigens, also called *allergens*.

Hypersensitivity reactions may be immediate, occurring within minutes to hours of reexposure, or delayed, occurring several hours after reexposure. A delayed hypersensitivity reaction typically is most severe days after the reexposure.

Generally, hypersensitivity reactions are classified as one of four types: type I (mediated by IgE), type II (tissue-specific), type III (immune complex–mediated), type IV (cell-mediated). (See *Classification of hypersensitivity reactions*, pages 430 and 431.)

Type I hypersensitivity

Allergens activate T cells, which induce B-cell production of IgE, which binds to the Fc receptors on the surface of mast cells. Repeated exposure to relatively large doses of the allergen is usually necessary to cause this response. When enough IgE has been produced, the person is sensitized to the allergen. At the next exposure to the same antigen, the antigen binds with the surface IgE, cross-links the Fc receptors, and causes mast cells to degranulate and release various mediators. Degranulation also may be triggered by complement-driven anaphylatoxins—C3a and C5a—or by certain drugs such as morphine.

Some of the mediators released are preformed, whereas others are newly synthesized on activation of the mast cells. Preformed mediators include heparin, histamine, proteolytic (protein-splitting) and other enzymes, and chemotactic factors for eosinophils and neutrophils. Newly synthesized mediators include prostaglandins and leukotrienes. Mast cells also produce a variety of cytokines, which initiate smooth muscle contraction, vasodilation, bronchospasm, edema, increased vascular permeability, mucus secretion, and cellular infiltration by eosinophils and neutrophils. These effects result in some of the classic associated signs and symptoms, such as hypotension, wheezing, swelling, urticaria, and rhinorrhea.

Type II hypersensitivity
Type II hypersensitivity, a tissue-specific reaction, generally involves the destruction of a target cell by an antibody directed against cell-surface antigens. Alternatively, the antibody may be directed against small molecules adsorbed (attracted to and retained on the surface) to cells or against cell-surface receptors, rather than against the cell constituents themselves. Tissue damage occurs through several mechanisms:

■ binding of antigen and antibody activates complement, which ultimately disrupts cellular membranes—complement-mediated lysis

■ various phagocytic cells with receptors for immunoglobulin (Fc region) and complement fragments envelop and destroy opsonized targets, such as red blood cells, leukocytes, and platelets

■ cytotoxic T cells and natural killer cells, although not antigen specific, also contribute to tissue damage by releasing toxic substances that destroy the cells

■ antibody binding causes the target cell to malfunction rather than causing its destruction.

Type III hypersensitivity
Circulating antigen-antibody complexes (immune complexes) accumulate and are deposited in the tissues. The most common tissues involved are the kidneys, joints, skin, and blood vessels. Normally, the tissues clear excess immune complexes from the circulation, but immune complexes deposited in the tissues activate the complement cascade, causing local inflammation, and trigger platelet release of vasoactive amines that increase vascular permeability, so that more immune complexes accumulate in the vessel walls.

Probably the most harmful effects of this process result from the creation of complement fragments that attract neutrophils. The neutrophils try to ingest the immune complexes. They're generally unsuccessful, but in the attempt, the neutrophils release lysosomal enzymes that add to the tissue damage.

The formation of immune complexes is dynamic and ever-changing. The complexes that form in us as children may be totally different from those formed in later years. Also, more than one type of immune complex may be present at one time.

Type IV hypersensitivity
These cell-mediated reactions involve the processing of the antigen by the macrophages. Once processed, the antigen is presented to the T cells. Cytotoxic T cells, if activated, attack and destroy the target cells directly. When lymphokine T cells are activated, they release lymphokines, which recruit and activate other lymphocytes, monocytes, macrophages, and polymorphonuclear leukocytes. The coagulation, cytokine, and complement cascades also contribute to tissue damage in this type of reaction.

AUTOIMMUNE REACTIONS
In autoimmune reactions, the body's normal defenses become self-destructive, recognizing self-antigens as foreign. What

(Text continues on page 432.)

CLOSER LOOK
Classification of hypersensitivity reactions

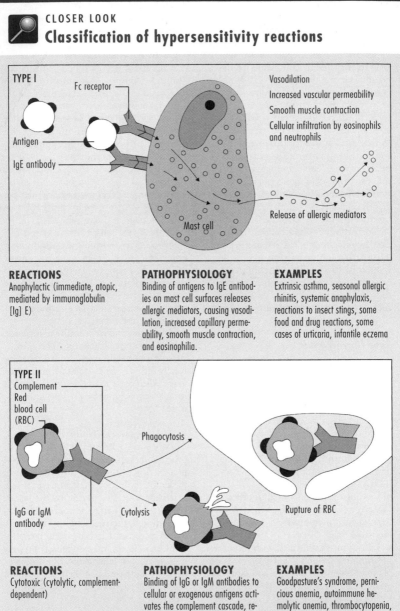

TYPE I

Fc receptor

Antigen

IgE antibody

Mast cell

Vasodilation

Increased vascular permeability

Smooth muscle contraction

Cellular infiltration by eosinophils and neutrophils

Release of allergic mediators

REACTIONS
Anaphylactic (immediate, atopic, mediated by immunoglobulin [Ig] E)

PATHOPHYSIOLOGY
Binding of antigens to IgE antibodies on mast cell surfaces releases allergic mediators, causing vasodilation, increased capillary permeability, smooth muscle contraction, and eosinophilia.

EXAMPLES
Extrinsic asthma, seasonal allergic rhinitis, systemic anaphylaxis, reactions to insect stings, some food and drug reactions, some cases of urticaria, infantile eczema

TYPE II

Complement
Red
blood cell
(RBC)

Phagocytosis

IgG or IgM
antibody

Cytolysis

Rupture of RBC

REACTIONS
Cytotoxic (cytolytic, complement-dependent)

PATHOPHYSIOLOGY
Binding of IgG or IgM antibodies to cellular or exogenous antigens activates the complement cascade, resulting in phagocytosis or cytolysis.

EXAMPLES
Goodpasture's syndrome, pernicious anemia, autoimmune hemolytic anemia, thrombocytopenia, some drug reactions, hyperacute renal allograft rejection, hemolytic disease of the neonate

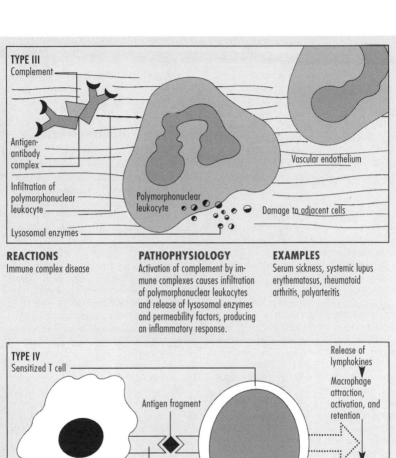

TYPE III
Complement
Antigen-antibody complex
Infiltration of polymorphonuclear leukocyte
Lysosomal enzymes
Polymorphonuclear leukocyte
Vascular endothelium
Damage to adjacent cells

REACTIONS
Immune complex disease

PATHOPHYSIOLOGY
Activation of complement by immune complexes causes infiltration of polymorphonuclear leukocytes and release of lysosomal enzymes and permeability factors, producing an inflammatory response.

EXAMPLES
Serum sickness, systemic lupus erythematosus, rheumatoid arthritis, polyarteritis

TYPE IV
Sensitized T cell
Antigen fragment
Antigen-presenting cell
MHC molecule
Release of lymphokines
Macrophage attraction, activation, and retention
Lysozyme release
Damage to surrounding tissue

REACTIONS
Delayed (cell-mediated)

PATHOPHYSIOLOGY
Antigen-presenting cells give antigen to T cells in association with major histocompatibility complex (MHC). The sensitized T cells release lymphokines that stimulate macrophages. Lysozymes are released, and surrounding tissue is damaged.

EXAMPLES
Contact dermatitis, graft-versus-host disease, allograft rejection, some drug sensitivities, Hashimoto's thyroiditis, sarcoidosis

causes this misdirected response isn't clearly understood. For example, drugs or viruses have been implicated as causing some autoimmune reactions, but in diseases such as rheumatoid arthritis and systemic lupus erythematosus, the mechanism for misdirection is unclear.

Autoimmune reactions are believed to result from a combination of factors, including genetic, hormonal, and environmental influences. Many are characterized by B-cell hyperactivity and by hypergammaglobulinemia. B-cell hyperactivity may be related to T-cell abnormalities. Hormonal and genetic factors strongly influence the onset of some autoimmune disorders.

AGE ALERT
Immune function starts declining at sexual maturity and continues declining with age. During this decline, the immune system begins losing its ability to differentiate between self and nonself, leading to an increase in the incidence of autoimmune disorders.

ALLOIMMUNE REACTIONS
Alloimmune reactions are directed at antigens from the tissues of others of the same species. Alloimmune reactions commonly occur in transplant and transfusion reactions, in which the recipient reacts to antigens, primarily human leukocyte antigen (HLA), on the donor cells. This immune response is also seen in neonates with erythroblastosis fetalis. (See chapter 11, Hematologic system.) This type of response is commonly linked to a type II hypersensitivity reaction.

IMMUNODEFICIENCY
An absent or depressed immune response increases susceptibility to infection. Immunodeficiency may be primary, reflecting a defect involving T cells, B cells, or lymphoid tissues, or secondary, resulting from an underlying disease or factor that depresses or blocks the immune response. The most common forms of immunodeficiency are caused by viral infection or are iatrogenic reactions to therapeutic drugs.

DISORDERS

The environment contains thousands of pathogenic microorganisms. Normally, our host defense system protects us from these harmful invaders, but when this network of safeguards breaks down, the result is an altered immune response or immune system failure.

Acquired immunodeficiency syndrome
Human immunodeficiency virus (HIV) infection may cause acquired immunodeficiency syndrome (AIDS). Although it's characterized by gradual destruction of cell-mediated (T-cell) immunity, it also affects humoral immunity and even autoimmunity because of the central role of the $CD4^+$ (helper) T lymphocyte in immune reactions. The resulting immunodeficiency makes the patient susceptible to opportunistic infections, cancers, and other abnormalities that define AIDS.

This syndrome was first described by the Centers for Disease Control and Prevention (CDC) in 1981. Because transmission is similar, AIDS shares epidemiologic patterns with hepatitis B and sexually transmitted diseases.

Depending on individual variations and the presence of cofactors that influence disease progression, the time from acute HIV infection to the appearance of symptoms (mild to severe) to the diagnosis of AIDS and, eventually, to death varies greatly. Current combination drug therapy in conjunction with treatment and prophylaxis of common opportunistic infections can delay the disease progression and prolong survival.

CAUSES
The HIV-I retrovirus is the primary cause. Transmission occurs by contact with infected blood or body fluids and is linked to identifiable high-risk behaviors. It's disproportionately represented in:
- homosexual and bisexual men
- I.V. drug users
- neonates of infected women

- recipients of contaminated blood or blood products (dramatically decreased since mid-1985)
- heterosexual partners of people in these above groups

PATHOPHYSIOLOGY

The natural history of AIDS begins with infection by the HIV retrovirus and ends with death. The virus is detectable only by laboratory tests. Twenty years of data strongly suggest that HIV isn't transmitted by casual household or social contact. The HIV virus may enter the body by any of several routes involving the transmission of blood or body fluids, for example:

- direct inoculation during intimate sexual contact, especially linked to the mucosal trauma of receptive rectal intercourse
- transfusion of contaminated blood or blood products (a risk lessened by routine testing of all blood products)
- sharing of contaminated injection needles
- transplacental or postpartum transmission from infected mother to fetus (by cervical or blood contact at delivery and in breast milk).

HIV strikes helper T cells bearing the CD4+ antigen. Normally a receptor for major histocompatibility complex molecules, the antigen serves as a receptor for the retrovirus and allows it to enter the cell. Viral binding also requires the presence of a coreceptor (believed to be the chemokine receptor CCR5) on the cell surface. The virus also may infect CD4+ antigen–bearing cells of the GI tract, uterine cervix, and neuroglia.

Like other retroviruses, HIV copies its genetic material in a reversed manner compared with other viruses and cells. Through the action of reverse transcriptase, HIV produces deoxyribonucleic acid (DNA) from its viral ribonucleic acid (RNA). Transcription is usually poor, leading to mutations, some of which make HIV resistant to antiviral drugs. The viral DNA enters the nucleus of the cell and is incorporated into the host cell's DNA, where it's transcribed into more viral RNA. If the host cell reproduces, it duplicates the HIV DNA along with its own

and passes it on to the daughter cells. Thus, if activated, the host cell carries this information and, if activated, replicates the virus. Viral enzymes, proteases, arrange the structural components and RNA into viral particles that move out to the periphery of the host cell, where the virus buds and emerges from the host cell. Thus, the virus is now free to travel and infect other cells. (See *How HIV replicates,* page 434.)

HIV replication may lead to cell death or it may become latent. HIV infection leads to profound pathologic changes, either directly through destruction of CD4+ cells, other immune cells, and neuroglial cells, or indirectly through the secondary effects of CD4+ T-cell dysfunction and resulting immunosuppression.

The HIV infectious process takes three forms:

- immunodeficiency (opportunistic infections and unusual cancers)
- autoimmunity (lymphoid interstitial pneumonitis, arthritis, hypergammaglobulinemia, and production of autoimmune antibodies)
- neurologic dysfunction (AIDS dementia complex, HIV encephalopathy, and peripheral neuropathies).

SIGNS AND SYMPTOMS

HIV infection shows itself in many ways. After a high-risk exposure and inoculation, the infected person usually experiences a mononucleosis-like syndrome, which may be attributed to flu or another virus and then may remain asymptomatic for years. In this latent stage, the only sign of HIV infection is laboratory evidence of seroconversion.

When symptoms appear, they may take many forms, including:

- persistent generalized lymphadenopathy caused by impaired function of CD4+ cells
- nonspecific symptoms, including weight loss, fatigue, night sweats, fevers related to altered function of CD4+ cells, immunodeficiency, and infection of other CD4+ antigen–bearing cells
- neurologic symptoms resulting from HIV encephalopathy and infection of neuroglial cells

CLOSER LOOK
How HIV replicates

Human immunodeficiency virus (HIV), like other viruses, requires a host cell to reproduce. However, because HIV is a retrovirus, it carries its genetic material in ribonucleic acid (RNA), rather than in deoxyribonucleic (DNA). During replication, this genetic material in the RNA must be converted into DNA. The flowchart below shows the steps in HIV replication needed to create a new virus cell.

HIV enters the blood stream.

↓

HIV attaches to the surface of the CD4⁺ T lymphocyte.

↓

Proteins on the HIV cell surface bind to the protein receptors on the host cell's surface.

↓

HIV penetrates the host cell membrane and injects its protein coat into host cell's cytoplasm.

↓

HIV's genetic information, RNA, is released into the cell after its protective coat is partially dissolved.

↓

The single stranded viral RNA, via the action of reverse transcriptase, is converted (transcribed) into double-stranded DNA.

↓

Viral DNA integrates itself into the host cell's nucleus.

↓

Integrase, an enzyme, inserts HIV's double-stranded DNA into the host cell's DNA.

↓

When the host cell is activated, the viral DNA takes over, telling the host cell to produce RNA (now viral RNA).

↓

Two strands of RNA are produced and transported out of the nucleus.

↓

One strand becomes the subunits of the HIV (that is, enzymes and structural proteins); the other becomes the genetic material for new viruses.

↓

Cleavage occurs (viral subunits are separated) through the action of protease, a viral enzyme.

↓

HIV subunits combine to make up new viral particles and begin to break down the host cell membrane.

↓

The genetic material in the new viral particles merges with the cell membrane that has been changed, forming a new viral envelope (outer covering).

↓

Viral budding occurs, in which the new HIV is released to enter the circulation.

Opportunistic infections in AIDS

This table shows the complicating infections that may occur in acquired immunodeficiency syndrome (AIDS). Opportunistic conditions not shown in the table include Kaposi's sarcoma, wasting disease, and AIDS dementia complex.

MICROBIOLOGICAL AGENT	ORGANISM	CONDITION
Protozoa	*Pneumocystis carinii* *Cryptosporidium* *Toxoplasma gondii* *Histoplasma*	*Pneumocystis carinii* pneumonia Cryptosporidiosis Toxoplasmosis Histoplasmosis
Fungi	*Candida albicans* *Cryptococcus neoformans*	Candidiasis Cryptococcosis
Viruses	Herpes Cytomegalovirus	Herpes simplex 1 and 2 Cytomegalovirus retinitis
Bacteria	*Mycobacterium tuberculosis* *M. avium-intracellulare*	Tuberculosis Mycobacteriosis

■ opportunistic infection or cancer related to immunodeficiency.

▲ **AGE ALERT**
In children, HIV infection has a mean incubation time of 17 months. Signs and symptoms resemble those in adults, except for findings related to sexually transmitted diseases. Children have a high incidence of opportunistic bacterial infections: otitis media, sepsis, chronic salivary gland enlargement, lymphoid interstitial pneumonia, Mycobacterium avium-intracellulare *complex function, and pneumonias, including* Pneumocystis carinii.

COMPLICATIONS
Complications of AIDS are:
■ repeated opportunistic infections. (See *Opportunistic infections in AIDS.*)

DIAGNOSIS
■ laboratory criteria:
– positive screening test for HIV antibody (confirmed by a positive result with a more sensitive and specific HIV antibody test, such as Western blot or immunofluorescence antibody test).
– positive result of a detectable quantity on HIV virologic tests, such as HIV nucleic acid detection, HIV p24 antigen test, or HIV isolation (culture).
■ clinical criteria:
– the presence of one or more conditions specified by the CDC as Categories A, B, or C. (See *Conditions associated with AIDS.*)

TREATMENT
No cure has yet been found for AIDS. Primary therapy includes the use of various combinations of three different types of antiretrovirals to try to gain the maximum benefit of inhibiting HIV viral replication with the fewest adverse reactions. Current recommendations include the use of two nucleosides plus one protease inhibitor, or two nucleosides and one nonnucleoside to help inhibit the production of resistant, mutant strains. The drugs include:

Conditions associated with AIDS

The Centers for Disease Control and Prevention (CDC) lists AIDS-associated diseases under three categories. From time to time the CDC adds to these lists.

CATEGORY A
◆ Persistent generalized lymph node enlargement
◆ Acute primary human immunodeficiency virus (HIV) infection with accompanying illness
◆ History of acute HIV infection

CATEGORY B
◆ Bacillary angiomatosis
◆ Oropharyngeal or persistent vulvovaginal candidiasis, fever, or diarrhea lasting longer than 1 month
◆ Idiopathic thrombocytopenic purpura
◆ Pelvic inflammatory disease (PID), especially with a tubulo-ovarian abscess
◆ Peripheral neuropathy

CATEGORY C
◆ Candidiasis of the bronchi, trachea, lungs, or esophagus
◆ Invasive cervical cancer
◆ Disseminated or extrapulmonary coccidioidomycosis
◆ Extrapulmonary cryptococcosis

◆ Chronic interstitial cryptosporidiosis
◆ Cytomegalovirus (CMV) disease affecting organs other than the liver, spleen, or lymph nodes
◆ CMV retinitis with vision loss
◆ Encephalopathy related to HIV
◆ Herpes simplex infection with chronic ulcers or herpetic bronchitis, pneumonitis, or esophagitis
◆ Disseminated or extrapulmonary histoplasmosis
◆ Chronic intestinal isopsoriasis
◆ Kaposi's sarcoma
◆ Burkitt's lymphoma or its equivalent
◆ Immunoblastic lymphoma or its equivalent
◆ Primary brain lymphoma
◆ Disseminated or extrapulmonary *Mycobacterium avium complex or M. kansasii*
◆ Pulmonary or extrapulmonary *M. tuberculosis*
◆ Disseminated or extrapulmonary infection with any other species of *Mycobacterium*
◆ *Pneumocystis carinii* pneumonia
◆ Recurrent pneumonia
◆ Progressive multifocal leukoencephalopathy
◆ Recurrent *Salmonella* septicemia
◆ Toxoplasmosis of the brain
◆ Wasting disease caused by HIV

■ protease inhibitors to block replication of virus particles formed through the action of viral protease (reducing the number of new virus particles produced)
■ nucleoside reverse-transcriptase inhibitors to interfere with the copying of viral RNA into DNA by the enzyme reverse transcriptase
■ nonnucleoside reverse-transcriptase inhibitors to interfere with the action of reverse transcriptase.
Additional treatment may include:
■ immunomodulators to boost the immune system weakened by AIDS and retroviral therapy
■ human granulocyte colony-stimulating growth factor to stimulate neutrophil pro-

duction (retroviral therapy causes anemia, so patients may receive epoetin alfa)
■ anti-infective and antineoplastics to combat opportunistic infections and associated cancers (some prophylactically to help resist opportunistic infections)
■ supportive therapy, including nutritional support, fluid and electrolyte replacement therapy, pain relief, and psychological support.

Allergic rhinitis
Allergic rhinitis is a reaction to airborne (inhaled) allergens. Depending on the allergen, the resulting rhinitis and conjunctivitis may occur seasonally (as in "hay fever") or year-round (as in perennial aller-

gic rhinitis). Allergic rhinitis is the most common atopic allergic reaction, affecting more than 20 million people in the United States. It's most prevalent in young children and adolescents but can occur in all age-groups.

CAUSES

Allergic rhinitis is caused by an immunoglobulin (Ig) E–mediated type I hypersensitivity response to an environmental antigen (allergen) in a genetically susceptible person. Common triggers include:

- windborne pollens
- spring — alder, birch, cottonwood, elm, maple, oak
- summer — grasses, sheep sorrel, and English plantain
- autumn — ragweed, other weeds
- perennial allergens and irritants
- dust mite excreta, fungal spores, molds
- feather pillows
- cigarette smoke
- animal dander.

PATHOPHYSIOLOGY

During primary exposure to an allergen, T cells recognize the foreign allergens and release chemicals that instruct B cells to produce specific antibodies, IgE. IgE antibodies attach themselves to mast cells. Mast cells with attached IgE can remain in the body for years, ready to react when they next encounter the same allergen.

The second time the allergen enters the body, it comes into direct contact with the IgE antibodies attached to the mast cells. This stimulates the mast cells to release chemicals, such as histamine, which initiate a response that causes tightening of the smooth muscles in the airways; dilation of small blood vessels; increased mucus secretion in the nasal cavity and airways; and itching.

SIGNS AND SYMPTOMS

In seasonal allergic rhinitis, the key signs and symptoms are related to the effects of the chemical mediators released. These include: paroxysmal sneezing, profuse watery rhinorrhea, nasal obstruction or congestion, and pruritus of the nose and eyes caused by histamine release. These reactions are usually accompanied by pale,

cyanotic, edematous nasal mucosa; red and edematous eyelids and conjunctivae; excessive lacrimation (tears); and headache or sinus pain. Some patients also complain of itching in the throat and malaise.

In perennial allergic rhinitis, conjunctivitis and other extranasal effects are rare, but chronic nasal obstruction is common. In many cases, this obstruction extends to eustachian tube obstruction, particularly in children.

In both types of allergic rhinitis, dark circles may appear under the patient's eyes ("allergic shiners") because of venous congestion in the maxillary sinuses. The severity of signs and symptoms may vary from season to season and from year to year.

COMPLICATIONS

Complications may include:

- sinus and middle ear infections caused by swelling of the turbinates and mucous membranes
- nasal polyps, which may result from edema and infection and can increase nasal obstruction.

DIAGNOSIS

Microscopic examination of sputum and nasal secretions reveals large numbers of eosinophils. Blood chemistry shows normal or elevated IgE. A definitive diagnosis is based on the patient's personal and family history of allergies as well as physical findings during a symptomatic phase. Skin testing paired with tested responses to environmental stimuli can pinpoint the responsible allergens given the patient's history.

To distinguish between allergic rhinitis and other disorders of the nasal mucosa, the practitioner should remember these differences:

- In chronic vasomotor rhinitis, eye symptoms are absent, rhinorrhea is mucoid, and seasonal variation is absent.
- In infectious rhinitis (the common cold), the nasal mucosa is beet red; nasal secretions contain polymorphonuclear, not eosinophilic, exudate; and signs and symptoms include fever and sore throat. This condition isn't a recurrent seasonal phenomenon.

■ In rhinitis medicamentosa, which results from excessive use of nasal sprays or drops, nasal drainage and mucosal redness and swelling disappear when such medication is withheld.
■ In children, differential diagnosis should rule out a nasal foreign body, such as a bean or a button.

TREATMENT

Treatment goals are to control symptoms by eliminating the environmental antigen, if possible, and providing drug therapy and immunotherapy.
■ Antihistamines block histamine effects but commonly produce anticholinergic adverse effects (sedation, dry mouth, nausea, dizziness, blurred vision, and nervousness). Newer antihistamines, such as fexofenadine, produce fewer adverse effects and are less likely to cause sedation.
■ Inhaled intranasal corticosteroids produce local anti-inflammatory effects with minimal systemic adverse effects. The most commonly used intranasal corticosteroids are beclomethasone, flunisolide, and fluticasone. These drugs usually aren't effective for acute exacerbations; nasal decongestants and oral antihistamines may be needed instead.
■ Advise the patient to use intranasal corticosteroids regularly, as prescribed, for optimal effectiveness. Cromolyn may help prevent allergic rhinitis. However, this drug may take up to 4 weeks to produce a satisfactory effect and must be taken regularly during allergy season.
■ Long-term management includes immunotherapy, or desensitization with injections of extracted allergens, administered before or during allergy season or perennially. Seasonal allergies require particularly close dosage regulation.

Anaphylaxis

Anaphylaxis is an acute, potentially life-threatening type I (immediate) hypersensitivity reaction marked by the sudden onset of rapidly progressive urticaria (vascular swelling in skin accompanied by itching) and respiratory distress. With prompt recognition and treatment, the prognosis is good, but a severe reaction may precipitate vascular collapse, leading to systemic shock and, possibly, death. The reaction typically occurs within minutes but can occur up to 1 hour after reexposure to the antigen.

CAUSES

The cause of anaphylaxis is usually the ingestion of or other systemic exposure to sensitizing drugs or other substances. Such substances may include:
■ serums (usually horse serum)
■ vaccines
■ allergen extracts
■ enzymes such as L-asparaginase
■ hormones
■ penicillin or other antibiotics (these induce anaphylaxis in 1 to 4 of every 10,000 patients treated; most likely after parenteral administration or prolonged therapy and in patients with an inherited tendency to food or drug allergy, or atopy)
■ sulfonamides
■ local anesthetics
■ salicylates
■ polysaccharides
■ diagnostic chemicals, such as sulfobromophthalein sodium, sodium dehydrocholate, and radiographic contrast media
■ food proteins, such as those in legumes, nuts, berries, seafood, and egg albumin
■ food additives containing sulfite
■ insect venom.

PATHOPHYSIOLOGY

Anaphylaxis requires previous sensitization or exposure to the specific antigen, resulting in immunoglobulin (Ig) E production by plasma cells in the lymph nodes and enhancement by helper T cells. IgE antibodies then bind to membrane receptors on mast cells in connective tissue and to basophils.

On reexposure, the antigen binds to adjacent IgE antibodies or cross-linked IgE receptors, activating a series of cellular reactions that trigger mast cell degranulation. With degranulation, powerful chemical mediators, such as serotonin, histamine, eosinophil chemotactic factor of anaphylaxis, and platelet-activating factor, are released from the mast cells. IgG or IgM enters into the reaction and activates the complement cascade, leading to the release of the complement fractions.

At the same time, two other chemical mediators, bradykinin and leukotrienes, induce vascular collapse by stimulating contraction of certain groups of smooth muscles and increasing vascular permeability. These substances, together with the other chemical mediators, cause vasodilation, smooth muscle contraction, enhanced vascular permeability, and increased mucus production. Continued release, along with the spread of these mediators through the body by way of the basophils in the circulation, triggers the systemic responses. Also, increased vascular permeability leads to decreased peripheral resistance and plasma leakage from the circulation to the extravascular tissues. Consequent reduction of blood volume causes hypotension, hypovolemic shock, and cardiac dysfunction. (See *Understanding anaphylaxis*, pages 440 and 441.)

SIGNS AND SYMPTOMS

An anaphylactic reaction produces sudden physical distress within seconds or minutes after exposure to the specific allergen. A delayed or persistent reaction may occur up to 24 hours later. The shorter the time interval between exposure and the onset of symptoms, the more severe the reaction usually is. The first symptoms include:
- feeling of impending doom or fright caused by activation of IgE and subsequent release of chemical mediators
- sweating caused by release of histamine and vasodilation
- sneezing, shortness of breath, nasal pruritus, urticaria, and angioedema (swelling of nerves and blood vessels) caused by histamine release and increased capillary permeability.

Systemic manifestations may include:
- hypotension, shock, and sometimes cardiac arrhythmias caused by increased vascular permeability and subsequent decrease in peripheral resistance and leakage of plasma fluids
- nasal mucosal edema, profuse watery rhinorrhea, itching, nasal congestion, and sudden sneezing attacks caused by histamine release, vasodilation, and increased capillary permeability
- edema of the upper respiratory tract, resulting in hypopharyngeal and laryngeal

obstruction, caused by increased capillary permeability and mast cell degranulation
- hoarseness, stridor, wheezing, and accessory muscle use caused by bronchiole smooth muscle contraction and increased mucus production
- severe stomach cramps, nausea, diarrhea, and urinary urgency and incontinence resulting from smooth muscle contraction of the intestines and bladder.

COMPLICATIONS

Complications of anaphylaxis include:
- respiratory obstruction
- systemic vascular collapse
- death.

DIAGNOSIS

No single diagnostic test can identify anaphylaxis. Anaphylaxis can be diagnosed by the rapid onset of severe respiratory or cardiovascular symptoms after ingestion or injection of a drug, vaccine, diagnostic agent, food, or food additive, or after an insect sting. If these symptoms occur without a known allergic stimulus, other possible causes of shock (such as acute myocardial infarction, status asthmaticus, or heart failure) must be ruled out.

These test results may provide some clues to the patient's risk for anaphylaxis:
- skin tests showing hypersensitivity to a specific allergen
- elevated serum IgE levels.

TREATMENT

Treatment includes:
- immediate administration of epinephrine 1:1,000 aqueous solution to reverse bronchoconstriction and cause vasoconstriction, I.M. or subcutaneously if the patient hasn't lost consciousness and is normotensive, or I.V. if the reaction is severe (repeating dosage every 5 to 20 minutes as needed)
- tracheostomy or endotracheal intubation and mechanical ventilation to maintain a patent airway
- oxygen therapy to increase tissue perfusion

(Text continues on page 442.)

CLOSER LOOK
Understanding anaphylaxis

An anaphylactic reaction requires previous sensitization or exposure to the specific antigen. What happens next in anaphylaxis is described here.

1. RESPONSE TO THE ANTIGEN
Immunoglobulin (Ig)M and IgG recognize the antigen as a foreign substance and attach to it.

Destruction of the antigen by the complement cascade begins but remains unfinished, either because of insufficient amounts of the protein catalyst or because the antigen inhibits certain complement enzymes. The patient has no signs and symptoms at this stage.

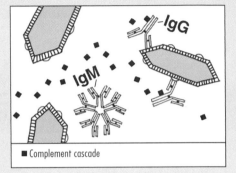

■ Complement cascade

2. RELEASED CHEMICAL MEDIATORS
The antigen's continued presence activates IgE on basophils. The activated IgE promotes the release of mediators, including histamine, serotonin, and leukotrienes. The sudden release of histamine causes vasodilation and increases capillary permeability. The patient begins to have signs and symptoms, including sudden nasal congestion, itchy and watery eyes, flushing, sweating, weakness, and anxiety.

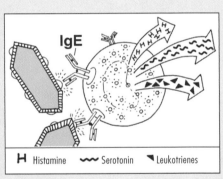

H Histamine   ~~~ Serotonin   ◀ Leukotrienes

3. INTENSIFIED RESPONSE
The activated IgE also stimulates mast cells in connective tissue along the venule walls to release more histamine and eosinophil chemotactic factor of anaphylaxis (ECF-A). These substances produce disruptive lesions that weaken the venules. Now, red and itchy skin, wheals, and swelling appear, and signs and symptoms worsen.

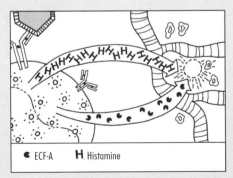

◀ ECF-A   **H** Histamine

4. DISTRESS
In the lungs, histamine causes endothelial cells to burst and endothelial tissue to tear away from surrounding tissue. Fluids leak into the alveoli, and leukotrienes prevent the alveoli from expanding, thus reducing pulmonary compliance. Tachypnea, crowing, use of accessory muscles, and cyanosis signal respiratory distress. Resulting neurologic signs and symptoms include changes in level of consciousness, severe anxiety, and possibly seizures.

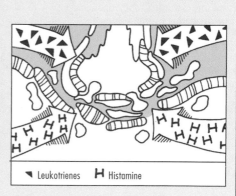

◄ Leukotrienes   H Histamine

5. DETERIORATION
Meanwhile, basophils and mast cells begin to release prostaglandins and bradykinin along with histamine and serotonin. These substances increase vascular permeability, causing fluids to leak from the vessels. Shock, confusion, cool and pale skin, generalized edema, tachycardia, and hypotension signal rapid vascular collapse.

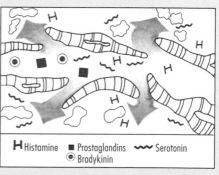

H Histamine   ■ Prostaglandins   ∿ Serotonin
⊙ Bradykinin

6. FAILED COMPENSATORY MECHANISMS
Damage to the endothelial cells causes basophils and mast cells to release heparin. Additional substances are also released to neutralize the other mediators. Eosinophils release arylsulfatase B to neutralize the leukotrienes, phospholipase D to neutralize heparin, and cyclic adenosine monophosphate (AMP) and the prostaglandins E_1 and E_2 to increase the metabolic rate. But these events can't reverse anaphylaxis. Hemorrhage, disseminated intravascular coagulation, and cardiopulmonary arrest result.

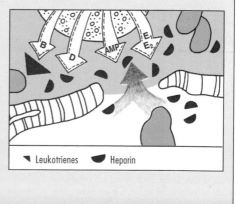

◄ Leukotrienes   ◆ Heparin

- longer-acting epinephrine, corticosteroids, and diphenhydramine to reduce the allergic response (long-term management)
- albuterol aerosolized (mini-nebulizer) treatment
- cimetidine or other histamine-2 blocker
- aminophylline to reverse bronchospasm
- volume expanders to maintain and restore circulating plasma volume
- I.V. vasopressors, such as norepinephrine and dopamine, to stabilize blood pressure
- cardiopulmonary resuscitation to treat cardiac arrest.

Atopic dermatitis

Atopic dermatitis is a chronic skin disorder characterized by superficial skin inflammation and intense itching. Although this disorder may appear at any age, it typically begins during infancy or early childhood. It may then subside spontaneously, followed by exacerbations in late childhood, adolescence, or early adulthood. Atopic dermatitis affects less than 1% of the population.

CAUSES

The exact etiology of atopic dermatitis is unknown, but a genetic predisposition is likely.

Possible contributing factors include:
- food allergy
- infection
- chemical irritants
- extremes of temperature and humidity
- psychological stress or strong emotions.

▲ **AGE ALERT**
About 10% of childhood cases of atopic dermatitis are caused by allergy to certain foods, especially eggs, peanuts, milk, or wheat.

PATHOPHYSIOLOGY

The allergic mechanism of hypersensitivity results in a release of inflammatory mediators through sensitized antibodies of the immunoglobulin (Ig) E class. Histamine and other cytokines induce acute inflammation. Abnormally dry skin and a decreased threshold for itching set up the "itch-scratch-itch" cycle, which eventually causes lesions (excoriations, lichenification).

SIGNS AND SYMPTOMS

Scratching the skin causes vasoconstriction and intensifies pruritus, resulting in erythematous, weeping lesions. Eventually, the lesions become scaly and lichenified. Usually, they're located in areas of flexion and extension, such as the neck, antecubital fossa, popliteal folds, and behind the ears. In children with atopic dermatitis, severe pruritus leads to characteristic pink pigmentation and swelling of the upper eyelid and a double fold under the lower lid (Morgan's line or Dennie's sign).

COMPLICATIONS

Complications may include:
- scarring
- severe viral infections
- bacterial and fungal skin infections
- ocular disorders
- allergic contact dermatitis.

DIAGNOSIS

Typically, the patient has a history of atopy, such as asthma, hay fever, or urticaria; family members may have a similar history. Laboratory tests reveal eosinophilia and elevated serum IgE levels.

TREATMENT

Measures to ease this chronic disorder include meticulous skin care, environmental control of offending allergens, and drug therapy. Because dry skin aggravates itching, frequent application of nonirritating topical lubricants is important, especially after bathing or showering. Minimizing exposure to allergens and irritants, such as wools and harsh detergents, also helps control symptoms.

Drug therapy involves corticosteroids and antipruritics. Active dermatitis responds well to topical corticosteroids such as fluocinolone and flurandrenolide. These drugs should be applied immediately after bathing for optimal penetration. Oral antihistamines are commonly used, especially hydroxyzine and the phenothiazine derivatives, such as methdilazine and trimeprazine, to help control itching. A bedtime dose may reduce involuntary scratching during sleep. If secondary infection develops, antibiotics are necessary.

Because this disorder may frustrate the patient and caregiver, counseling may play a role in treatment.

Latex allergy

Latex allergy is a hypersensitivity reaction to products that contain natural latex, a substance that's derived from the sap of the rubber tree (not synthetic latex). This substance is found in an increasing number of products at home and at work. The hypersensitivity reactions can range from local dermatitis to life-threatening anaphylactic reaction.

CAUSES

Exposure to latex proteins found in natural rubber products produces a true latex allergy. Those in frequent contact with latex-containing products are at risk for developing a latex allergy. More frequent exposure leads to a higher risk.

The populations at highest risk are:
- medical and dental professionals
- workers in latex companies
- patients with spina bifida, or other conditions that require multiple surgeries involving latex material.

Other people at risk include patients with a history of:
- asthma or other allergies, especially to bananas, avocados, tropical fruits, or chestnuts
- multiple intra-abdominal or genitourinary surgeries
- frequent intermittent urinary catheterization.

PATHOPHYSIOLOGY

A true latex allergy is an immunoglobulin (Ig) E–mediated immediate hypersensitivity reaction. Mast cells release histamine and other secretory products. Vascular permeability increases and vasodilation and bronchoconstriction occur.

Chemical sensitivity dermatitis is a type IV delayed hypersensitivity reaction to the chemicals used in processing rather than to the latex itself. In a cell-mediated allergic reaction, sensitized T lymphocytes are triggered, stimulating the proliferation of other lymphocytes and mononuclear cells. This results in tissue inflammation and contact dermatitis.

SIGNS AND SYMPTOMS

With a true latex allergy, the patient shows signs and symptoms of anaphylaxis, including:
- hypotension caused by vasodilation and increased vascular permeability
- tachycardia caused by hypotension
- urticaria and pruritus caused by histamine release
- difficulty breathing, bronchospasm, wheezing, and stridor caused by bronchoconstriction
- angioedema from increased vascular permeability and loss of water to tissues.

COMPLICATIONS

Like anaphylaxis, a true latex allergy may lead to:
- respiratory obstruction
- systemic vascular collapse
- death.

DIAGNOSIS

Diagnosis of latex allergy is based mainly on history and physical assessment. The following tests are also useful:
- radioallergosorbent test showing specific IgE antibodies to latex (safest for use in patients with history of type I hypersensitivity)
- patch test resulting in hives with itching or redness as a positive response.

TREATMENT

Treatment includes:
- prevention of exposure, including use of latex-free products to decrease possible exacerbation of hypersensitivity
- drug therapy, such as corticosteroids, antihistamines, and histamine-2 receptor blockers before and after possible exposure to latex to depress immune response and block histamine release.

If the patient is experiencing an acute emergency, treatment includes:
- immediate administration of epinephrine 1:1,000 aqueous solution to reverse bronchoconstriction and cause vasoconstriction, I.M. or subcutaneously if the patient hasn't lost consciousness and is normotensive, or I.V. if the reaction is severe (repeating dosage every 5 to 20 minutes as needed)

- tracheostomy or endotracheal intubation and mechanical ventilation to maintain a patent airway
- oxygen therapy to increase tissue perfusion
- volume expanders to maintain and restore circulating plasma volume
- I.V. vasopressors, such as norepinephrine and dopamine, to stabilize blood pressure
- cardiopulmonary resuscitation to treat cardiac arrest
- longer-acting epinephrine, corticosteroids, and diphenhydramine to reduce the allergic response (long-term management)
- drugs to reverse bronchospasm, including aminophylline and albuterol.

Lupus erythematosus

Lupus erythematosus is a chronic inflammatory disorder of the connective tissues that appears in two forms: discoid lupus erythematosus, which affects only the skin, and systemic lupus erythematosus (SLE), which affects multiple organ systems as well as the skin and can be fatal. SLE is characterized by recurring remissions and exacerbations, which are especially common during the spring and summer.

The prognosis improves with early detection and treatment but remains poor for patients who develop cardiovascular, renal, or neurologic complications, or severe bacterial infections.

CAUSES

The exact cause of SLE remains a mystery, but available evidence points to interrelated immunologic, environmental, hormonal, and genetic factors. These may include:
- physical or mental stress
- streptococcal or viral infections
- exposure to sunlight or ultraviolet light
- immunization
- pregnancy
- abnormal estrogen metabolism
- treatment with certain drugs, such as procainamide, hydralazine, anticonvulsants and, less frequently, penicillins, sulfa drugs, and hormonal contraceptives.

PATHOPHYSIOLOGY

Autoimmunity is believed to be the prime mechanism linked to SLE. The body produces antibodies against components of its own cells, such as the antinuclear antibody (ANA), and immune complex disease follows. Patients with SLE may produce antibodies against many different tissue components, such as red blood cells (RBCs), neutrophils, platelets, lymphocytes, or almost any organ or tissue in the body.

SIGNS AND SYMPTOMS

The onset of SLE may be acute or insidious and produces no characteristic clinical pattern. (See *Signs of systemic lupus erythematosus.*)

Although SLE may involve any organ system, signs and symptoms all relate to tissue injury and subsequent inflammation and necrosis resulting from the invasion by immune complexes. They commonly include:
- fever
- weight loss
- malaise
- fatigue
- rashes
- polyarthralgia.

Additional signs and symptoms may include:
- joint involvement, similar to rheumatoid arthritis (although the arthritis of lupus is usually nonerosive)
- skin lesions, most commonly an erythematous rash in areas exposed to light (the classic butterfly rash over the nose and cheeks occurs in less than 50% of the patients) or a scaly, papular rash (mimics psoriasis), especially in sun-exposed areas of the skin
- vasculitis (especially in the digits), possibly leading to infarctive lesions, necrotic leg ulcers, or digital gangrene
- Raynaud's phenomenon (about 20% of patients)
- patchy alopecia and painless ulcers of the mucous membranes
- pulmonary abnormalities, such as pleurisy, pleural effusions, pneumonitis, pulmonary hypertension and, rarely, pulmonary hemorrhage

■ cardiac involvement, such as pericarditis, myocarditis, endocarditis, and early coronary atherosclerosis

■ microscopic hematuria, pyuria, and urine sediment with cellular casts caused by glomerulonephritis, possibly progressing to kidney failure (particularly when untreated)

■ urinary tract infections, possibly because of heightened susceptibility to infection

■ seizure disorders and mental dysfunction

■ central nervous system (CNS) involvement, such as emotional instability, psychosis, and organic brain syndrome

■ headaches, irritability, and depression (common).

Constitutional symptoms of SLE include:

■ aching, malaise, fatigue

■ low-grade or spiking fever and chills

■ anorexia and weight loss

■ lymph node enlargement (diffuse or local, and nontender)

■ abdominal pain

■ nausea, vomiting, diarrhea, constipation

■ irregular menstrual periods or amenorrhea during the active phase of SLE.

COMPLICATIONS

Possible complications of SLE include:

■ concomitant infections

■ urinary tract infections

■ renal failure

■ osteonecrosis of hip from long-term corticosteroid use.

DIAGNOSIS

Test results that may indicate SLE include:

■ complete blood count with differential possibly showing anemia and a decreased white blood cell (WBC) count

■ platelet count, which may be decreased

■ erythrocyte sedimentation rate, which is often elevated

■ serum electrophoresis, which may show hypergammaglobulinemia.

Other diagnostic tests include:

■ ANA and lupus erythematosus cell tests showing positive results in active SLE

■ anti–double-stranded deoxyribonucleic acid (anti-dsDNA) antibody; most specific

---

Signs of systemic lupus erythematosus

Diagnosing systemic lupus erythematosus (SLE) is difficult because it often mimics other diseases; symptoms may be vague and vary greatly among patients.

For these reasons, the American Rheumatism Association issued a list of criteria for classifying SLE, to be used primarily for consistency in epidemiologic surveys. Usually, four or more of these signs are present at some time during the course of the disease:

◆ malar or discoid rash

◆ photosensitivity

◆ oral or nasopharyngeal ulcerations

◆ nonerosive arthritis (of two or more peripheral joints)

◆ pleuritis or pericarditis

◆ profuse proteinuria (more than 0.5 g/day) or excessive cellular casts in the urine

◆ seizures or psychoses

◆ hemolytic anemia, leukopenia, lymphopenia, or thrombocytopenia

◆ anti–double-stranded DNA or positive findings of antiphospholipid antibodies (elevated immunoglobulin [Ig]G or IgM anticardiolipin antibodies, positive test result for lupus anticoagulant, or false-positive serologic test results for syphilis)

◆ abnormal antinuclear antibody titer.

---

test for SLE, correlates with disease activity, especially renal involvement, and helps monitor response to therapy; may be low or absent in remission

■ urine studies that may show RBCs and WBCs, urine casts and sediment, and protein loss of more than 0.5 g/24 hours

■ serum complement blood studies showing decreased serum complement (C3 and C4) levels indicating active disease

■ chest X-ray possibly showing pleurisy or lupus pneumonitis

■ electrocardiography possibly showing a conduction defect with cardiac involvement or pericarditis

- kidney biopsy to determine disease stage and extent of renal involvement
- lupus anticoagulant and anticardiolipin tests possibly positive in some patients (usually in patients prone to antiphospholipid syndrome of thrombosis, abortion, and thrombocytopenia).

TREATMENT
Treatment for SLE may include:
- nonsteroidal anti-inflammatory drugs, including aspirin, to control arthritis symptoms
- topical corticosteroid creams such as hydrocortisone or triamcinolone for acute skin lesions
- intralesional corticosteroids or antimalarials such as hydroxychloroquine to treat refractory skin lesions
- systemic corticosteroids to reduce systemic symptoms of SLE, for acute generalized exacerbations, or for serious disease related to vital organ systems, such as pleuritis, pericarditis, lupus nephritis, vasculitis, and CNS involvement
- high-dose corticosteroids and cytotoxic therapy (such as cyclophosphamide) to treat diffuse proliferative glomerulonephritis
- dialysis or kidney transplant for renal failure
- antihypertensive drugs and dietary changes to minimize effects of renal involvement.

Rheumatoid arthritis

Rheumatoid arthritis (RA) is a chronic, systemic inflammatory disease that primarily attacks peripheral joints and the surrounding muscles, tendons, ligaments, and blood vessels. Partial remissions and unpredictable exacerbations mark the course of this potentially disabling disease. RA strikes women three times more commonly as it does men.

RA occurs worldwide, affecting more than 6.5 million people in the United States alone.

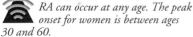

AGE ALERT
RA can occur at any age. The peak onset for women is between ages 30 and 60.

This disease usually requires lifelong treatment and, sometimes, surgery. (See

Drug therapy for rheumatoid arthritis, pages 448 and 449.)

In most patients, it follows an intermittent course and allows normal activity between flares, although 10% of affected people have total disability from severe joint deformity, associated extra-articular symptoms, such as vasculitis, or both. The prognosis worsens with the development of nodules, vasculitis, and high titers of rheumatoid factor (RF).

CAUSES
The cause of the chronic inflammation characteristic of RA isn't known. Possible theories include:
- abnormal immune activation (occurring in a genetically susceptible individual) leading to inflammation, complement activation, and cell proliferation within joints and tendon sheaths
- possible infection (viral or bacterial), hormone action, or lifestyle factors influencing onset
- RF development of an antibody against the body's own IgG; RF aggregates into complexes, generates inflammation, causing eventual cartilage damage and triggering other immune responses.

PATHOPHYSIOLOGY
If not stopped, the inflammatory process in the joints occurs in four stages:
- synovitis develops from congestion and edema of the synovial membrane and joint capsule. Infiltration by lymphocytes, macrophages, and neutrophils continues the local inflammatory response. These cells, as well as fibroblast-like synovial cells, produce enzymes that help to degrade bone and cartilage
- pannus — thickened layers of granulation tissue — covers and invades cartilage and eventually destroys the joint capsule and bone
- fibrous ankylosis — fibrous invasion of the pannus and scar formation — occludes the joint space; bone atrophy and misalignment causing visible deformities and disrupting the articulation of opposing bones, which cause muscle atrophy and imbalance and, possibly, partial dislocations (subluxations)

- fibrous tissue calcifies, resulting in bony ankylosis and total immobility.

SIGNS AND SYMPTOMS

RA usually develops insidiously and at first causes nonspecific signs and symptoms, most likely related to the initial inflammatory reactions before the inflammation of the synovium, including:

- fatigue
- malaise
- anorexia and weight loss
- persistent low-grade fever
- lymphadenopathy
- vague articular symptoms.

As the disease progresses, signs and symptoms include:

- specific localized, bilateral, and symmetric articular symptoms, frequently in the fingers at the proximal interphalangeal, metacarpophalangeal, and metatarsophalangeal joints, possibly extending to the wrists, knees, elbows, and ankles from inflammation of the synovium
- stiffening of affected joints after inactivity, especially on arising in the morning, caused by progressive synovial inflammation and destruction
- spindle-shaped fingers from marked edema and congestion in the joints
- joint pain and tenderness, at first only with movement but eventually even at rest, caused by prostaglandin release, edema, and synovial inflammation and destruction
- feeling of warmth at joint from inflammation
- diminished joint function and deformities as synovial destruction continues
- flexion deformities or hyperextension of metacarpophalangeal joints, subluxation of the wrist, and stretching of tendons pulling the fingers to the ulnar side (ulnar drift), or characteristic swan-neck or boutonnière deformity from joint swelling and loss of joint space
- carpal tunnel syndrome from synovial pressure on the median nerve causing paresthesia in the fingers.

Extra-articular findings may include:

- gradual appearance of rheumatoid nodules—subcutaneous, round or oval, nontender masses (20% of RF-positive patients), usually on elbows, hands, or Achilles tendon from destruction of the synovium
- vasculitis possibly leading to skin lesions, leg ulcers, and multiple systemic complications from infiltration of immune complexes and subsequent tissue damage and necrosis in the vasculature
- pericarditis, pulmonary nodules or fibrosis, pleuritis, or inflammation of the sclera and overlying tissues of the eye from immune-complex invasion and subsequent tissue damage and necrosis
- peripheral neuropathy with numbness or tingling in the feet or weakness and loss of sensation in the fingers from infiltration of the nerve fibers
- stiff, weak, or painful muscles caused by limited mobility and decreased use.

COMPLICATIONS

Complications of RA include:

- fibrosis and ankylosis
- soft tissue contractures
- pain
- joint deformities
- Sjögren's syndrome
- destruction of second cervical vertebra
- spinal cord compression
- temporomandibular joint disease
- infection
- osteoporosis
- myositis (inflammation of voluntary muscles)
- cardiopulmonary lesions
- lymphadenopathy
- peripheral neuritis.

DIAGNOSIS

Test results indicating RA include:

- X-rays showing bone demineralization and soft-tissue swelling (early stages), cartilage loss and narrowed joint spaces, and, finally, cartilage and bone destruction and erosion, subluxations, and deformities (later stages)
- RF titer positive in 75% to 80% of patients (titer of 1:160 or higher)
- synovial fluid analysis showing increased volume and turbidity but decreased viscosity and elevated white blood cell counts (usually greater than 10,000/µl)
- serum protein electrophoresis possibly showing elevated serum globulin levels

DISRUPTING DISEASE
Drug therapy for rheumatoid arthritis

The flowchart below identifies the major pathophysiologic events in rheumatoid arthritis and shows where in this chain of events the major drug therapies act to control the disease.

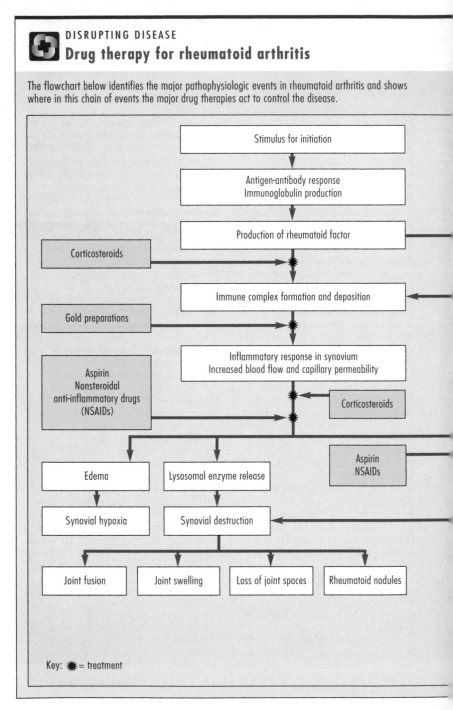

Key: ✸ = treatment

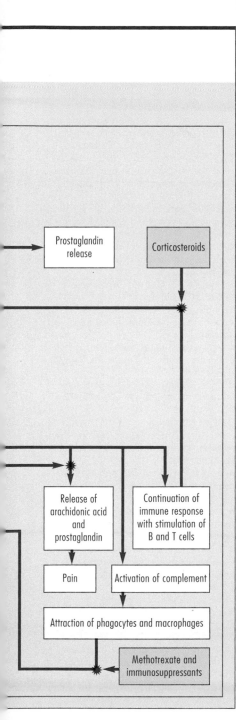

■ erythrocyte sedimentation rate and C-reactive protein levels showing elevations in 85% to 90% of patients (may be useful to monitor response to therapy because elevation frequently parallels disease activity)
■ complete blood count usually showing moderate anemia, slight leukocytosis, and slight thrombocytosis.

TREATMENT
Treatment for RA involves pharmacologic therapy and supportive measures, including:
■ salicylates, particularly aspirin (mainstay of therapy) to decrease inflammation and relieve joint pain
■ nonsteroidal anti-inflammatory drugs, such as fenoprofen, ibuprofen, and indomethacin, to relieve inflammation and pain
■ antimalarials such as hydroxychloroquine, sulfasalazine, gold salts, and penicillamine to reduce acute and chronic inflammation
■ corticosteroids such as prednisone in low doses for anti-inflammatory effects, in higher doses for immunosuppressive effect on T cells
■ azathioprine, cyclosporine, and methotrexate in early disease for immunosuppression by suppressing T and B lymphocyte proliferation causing destruction of the synovium
■ synovectomy (removal of destructive, proliferating synovium, usually in the wrists, knees, and fingers) to possibly halt or delay the course of the disease
■ osteotomy (cutting of bone or excision of a wedge of bone) to realign joint surfaces and redistribute stress
■ tendon transfers to prevent deformities or relieve contractures
■ joint reconstruction or total joint arthroplasty, including metatarsal head and distal ulnar resectional arthroplasty, insertion of a Silastic prosthesis between metacarpophalangeal and proximal interphalangeal joints (severe disease)
■ arthrodesis (joint fusion) for stability and relief from pain (sacrifices joint mobility).

Urticaria and angioedema

Urticaria, commonly known as *hives*, is an episodic, usually self-limited skin reaction characterized by local dermal wheals surrounded by an erythematous flare. Angioedema is a subcutaneous and dermal eruption that produces deeper, larger wheals (usually on the hands, feet, lips, genitals, and eyelids) and a more diffuse swelling of loose subcutaneous tissue. Urticaria and angioedema can occur simultaneously, but angioedema may last longer.

Urticaria and angioedema are common allergic reactions that may occur in 20% of the general population.

CAUSES

The causes of these reactions may include:
■ allergy to drugs, foods, insect stings and, occasionally, inhalant allergens (animal dander and cosmetics) that provoke an immunoglobulin (Ig) E–mediated response to protein allergens (although certain drugs may cause urticaria without an IgE response)
■ external physical stimuli, such as cold (usually in young adults), heat, water, or sunlight.

PATHOPHYSIOLOGY

Several mechanisms and underlying disorders may provoke urticaria and angioedema, including IgE-induced release of mediators from cutaneous mast cells; binding of IgG or IgM to an antigen, resulting in complement activation; and such disorders as localized or secondary infections (such as respiratory infection), neoplastic diseases (for example, Hodgkin's disease), connective tissue diseases (for example, systemic lupus erythematosus), collagen vascular diseases, and psychogenic diseases.

When urticaria and angioedema are part of an anaphylactic reaction, they almost always persist long after the systemic response has subsided. This occurs because circulation to the skin is the last to be restored after an allergic reaction, which results in slow histamine reabsorption at the reaction site.

Nonallergic urticaria and angioedema are probably also related to histamine release by some still-unknown mechanism. Dermographism urticaria, which develops after stroking or scratching the skin, occurs in as much as 20% of the population. Such urticaria develops with varying pressure, usually under tight clothing, and is aggravated by scratching.

SIGNS AND SYMPTOMS

The characteristic features of urticaria are distinct, raised, evanescent dermal wheals surrounded by an erythematous flare. These lesions may vary in size. In cholinergic urticaria, the wheals may be tiny and blanched, surrounded by erythematous flares.

Angioedema characteristically produces nonpitted swelling of deep subcutaneous tissue, usually on the eyelids, lips, genitalia, and mucous membranes. These swellings don't usually itch but may burn and tingle.

COMPLICATIONS

Complications may include:
■ skin abrasion and infection caused by scratching
■ life-threatening laryngeal edema, if angioedema involves the upper respiratory tract
■ severe abdominal colic, with possible GI involvement that can lead to surgery.

DIAGNOSIS

An accurate patient history can help determine the cause of urticaria. Such a history should include:
■ drug history, including over-the-counter preparations (vitamins, aspirin, and antacids)
■ frequent ingestion of highly allergenic foods (strawberries, milk products, fish, eggs, wheat, nuts)
■ environmental influences (pets, carpet, clothing, soap, inhalants, cosmetics, hair dye, and insect bites and stings).

Diagnosis also requires physical assessment to rule out similar conditions as well as a complete blood count, urinalysis, erythrocyte sedimentation rate, and a chest X-ray to rule out inflammatory infections. Skin testing, an elimination diet, and a food diary (recording time and amount of food eaten and circumstances) can pinpoint provoking allergens. The food diary may also suggest other allergies. For instance, a patient allergic to fish may also be allergic to iodine contrast materials.

Recurrent angioedema without urticaria, along with a familial history, points to hereditary angioedema. (See *Hereditary angioedema*.) Decreased serum levels of complement 4 and complement 1 esterase inhibitors confirm this diagnosis.

TREATMENT

Treatment aims are to prevent or limit contact with triggering factors or, if this is impossible, to desensitize the patient to them and to relieve symptoms. During desensitization, progressively larger doses of specific antigens (determined by skin testing) are injected intradermally.

Hydroxyzine or another antihistamine can ease itching and swelling in every kind of urticaria. Corticosteroid therapy may be necessary for some patients.

Vasculitis

Vasculitis includes a broad spectrum of disorders characterized by inflammation and necrosis of blood vessels. Its clinical effects depend on the vessels involved and reflect tissue ischemia caused by blood flow obstruction. The prognosis is also variable. For example, hypersensitivity vasculitis is usually a benign disorder limited to the skin, but more extensive polyarteritis nodosa can be rapidly fatal. Vasculitis can occur at any age, except for mucocutaneous lymph node syndrome, which occurs only during childhood. Vasculitis may be a primary disorder or occur because of other disorders, such as rheumatoid arthritis or systemic lupus erythematosus.

CAUSES

Vasculitis has been linked to a history of serious infectious disease, such as hepatitis B or bacterial endocarditis, and high-dose antibiotic therapy.

PATHOPHYSIOLOGY

How vascular damage develops in vasculitis isn't well understood. Current theory holds that it's initiated by excessive circulating antigen, which triggers the formation of soluble antigen–antibody complexes. These complexes can't be cleared effectively by the reticuloendothelial system, so

---

Hereditary angioedema

A nonallergenic type of angioedema, hereditary angioedema results from an autosomal dominant trait — a hereditary deficiency of an alpha globulin, the normal inhibitor of C1 esterase (a component of the complement system). This deficiency allows uninhibited C1 esterase release, resulting in the vascular changes common to angioedema.

The clinical effects of hereditary angioedema usually appear in childhood with recurrent episodes of subcutaneous or submucosal edema at irregular intervals of weeks, months, or years — in many cases after trauma or stress. Hereditary angioedema is unifocal, without urticarial pruritus but linked to recurrent edema of the skin and mucosa (especially of the GI and respiratory tracts). GI tract involvement may cause nausea, vomiting, and severe abdominal pain. Laryngeal angioedema may cause fatal airway obstruction.

Treatment of acute hereditary angioedema may require androgens such as danazol. Tracheotomy may be necessary to relieve airway obstruction resulting from laryngeal angioedema.

---

they're deposited in blood vessel walls (type III hypersensitivity). Increased vascular permeability linked to release of vasoactive amines by platelets and basophils exacerbates this process. The deposited complexes activate the complement cascade, resulting in chemotaxis of neutrophils, which release lysosomal enzymes. In turn, these enzymes cause vessel damage and necrosis, which may precipitate thrombosis, occlusion, hemorrhage, and ischemia.

Another mechanism that may contribute to vascular damage is the cell-mediated (T-cell) immune response. In this response, circulating antigen triggers lymphocytes to release soluble mediators, which attracts macrophages. The macrophages release intracellular enzymes, which cause vascular damage. Macro-

Types of vasculitis

TYPE	VESSELS INVOLVED	SIGNS AND SYMPTOMS
Polyarteritis nodosa	Small to medium arteries throughout body, with lesions that tend to be segmental, occur at bifurcations and branchings of arteries, spread distally to arterioles and, in severe cases, circumferentially involve adjacent veins	Hypertension, abdominal pain, myalgias, headache, joint pain, and weakness
Allergic granulomatosis angiitis (Churg-Strauss syndrome)	Small to medium arteries (including arterioles, capillaries, and venules), mainly of the lungs but also other organs	Resemblance to polyarteritis nodosa with hallmark of severe pulmonary involvement
Polyangiitis overlap syndrome	Small to medium arteries (including arterioles, capillaries, and venules) of the lungs and other organs	Combined symptoms of polyarteritis nodosa, allergic angiitis, and granulomatosis
Wegener's granulomatosis	Small to medium vessels of the respiratory tract and kidney	Fever, pulmonary congestion, cough, malaise, anorexia, weight loss, and mild to severe hematuria
Temporal arteritis	Medium to large arteries, most commonly branches of the carotid artery	Fever, myalgia, jaw claudication, visual changes, and headache (linked to polymyalgia rheumatica syndrome)
Takayasu's arteritis (aortic arch syndrome)	Medium to large arteries, particularly the aortic arch, its branches, and, possibly, the pulmonary artery	Malaise, pallor, nausea, night sweats, arthralgias, anorexia, weight loss, pain or paresthesia distal to affected area, bruits, loss of distal pulses, syncope, and, if a carotid artery is involved, diplopia and transient blindness; may progress to heart failure or stroke
Hypersensitivity vasculitis	Small vessels, especially of the skin	Palpable purpura, papules, nodules, vesicles, bullae, ulcers, or chronic or recurrent urticaria
Mucocutaneous lymph node syndrome (Kawasaki disease)	Small to medium vessels, primarily of the lymph nodes; may progress to involve coronary arteries	Fever; nonsuppurative cervical adenitis; edema; congested conjunctivae; erythema of oral cavity, lips, and palms; and desquamation of fingertips; may progress to arthritis, myocarditis, pericarditis, myocardial infarction, and cardiomegaly
Behçet's syndrome	Small vessels, primarily of the mouth and genitalia, but also of the eyes, skin, joints, GI tract, and central nervous system	Recurrent oral ulcers, eye lesions, genital lesions, and cutaneous lesions

phages can also transform into the epithelioid and multinucleated giant cells that typify the granulomatous vasculitides. Phagocytosis of immune complexes by macrophages aids granuloma formation.

DIAGNOSIS

History of symptoms; elevated erythrocyte sedimentation rate (ESR); leukocytosis; anemia; thrombocytosis; depressed C3 complement; rheumatoid factor greater than 1:60; circulating immune complexes; tissue biopsy showing necrotizing vasculitis

History of asthma; eosinophilia; tissue biopsy showing granulomatous inflammation with eosinophilic infiltration

Possible history of allergy; eosinophilia; tissue biopsy showing granulomatous inflammation with eosinophilic infiltration

Tissue biopsy showing necrotizing vasculitis with granulomatous inflammation; leukocytosis; elevated ESR and immunoglobulin (Ig) A and IgG levels; low titer rheumatoid factor; circulating immune complexes; antineutrophil cytoplasmic antibody in more than 90% of patients

Decreased hemoglobin; elevated ESR; tissue biopsy showing panarteritis with infiltration of mononuclear cells, giant cells within vessel wall, fragmentation of internal elastic lamina, and proliferation of intima

Decreased hemoglobin; leukocytosis; positive lupus erythematosus cell preparation and elevated ESR; arteriography showing calcification and obstruction of affected vessels; tissue biopsy showing inflammation of adventitia and intima of vessels, and thickening of vessel walls

History of exposure to antigen, such as a microorganism or drug; tissue biopsy showing leukocytoclastic angiitis, usually in postcapillary venules, with infiltration of polymorphonuclear leukocytes, fibrinoid necrosis, and extravasation of erythrocytes

History of symptoms; elevated ESR; tissue biopsy showing intimal proliferation and infiltration of vessel walls with mononuclear cells; echocardiography necessary

History of symptoms

SIGNS AND SYMPTOMS AND DIAGNOSIS

Clinical effects of vasculitis and diagnosis confirming laboratory procedures depend on the blood vessels involved. (See *Types of vasculitis.*)

Complications may include:
- renal, cardiac, and hepatic involvement that may be fatal if vasculitis is left untreated
- renal failure, renal hypertension, glomerulitis
- fibrous scarring of the lung tissue
- stroke
- GI bleeding.

TREATMENT

Treatment of vasculitis aims to minimize irreversible tissue damage associated with ischemia.

- In primary vasculitis, treatment may involve removal of an offending antigen or use of anti-inflammatory or immunosuppressant drugs. For example, antigenic drugs, food, and other environmental substances should be identified and eliminated, if possible.
- Drug therapy in primary vasculitis commonly involves low-dose cyclophosphamide with daily corticosteroids. In rapidly fulminant vasculitis, cyclophosphamide dosage may be increased daily for the first 2 to 3 days, followed by the regular dose. Prednisone should be given in divided doses for 7 to 10 days, with consolidation to a single morning dose by 2 to 3 weeks. When the vasculitis appears to be in remission or when prescribed cytotoxic drugs take full effect, corticosteroids are tapered down to a single daily dose. Finally, an alternate-day schedule of steroids may continue for 3 to 6 months before slow discontinuation of steroids.
- In secondary vasculitis, treatment focuses on the underlying disorder.

13

Endocrine system

The endocrine system consists of glands, specialized cell clusters, hormones, and target tissues. The glands and cell clusters secrete hormones and chemical transmitters in response to stimulation from the nervous system and other sites. Together with the nervous system, the endocrine system regulates and integrates the body's metabolic activities and maintains internal homeostasis. Each target tissue has receptors for specific hormones. Hormones connect with the receptors, and the resulting hormone-receptor complex triggers the target cell's response.

HORMONAL REGULATION

The hypothalamus, the main integrative center for the endocrine and autonomic nervous systems, helps control some endocrine glands by neural and hormonal pathways. Neural pathways connect the hypothalamus to the posterior pituitary gland, or neurohypophysis. Neural stimulation of the posterior pituitary causes the secretion of two *effector hormones*: antidiuretic hormone (ADH, also known as *vasopressin*) and oxytocin.

The hypothalamus also exerts hormonal control at the anterior pituitary gland, or adenohypophysis, by releasing and inhibiting hormones and factors, which arrive by a portal system. Hypothalamic hormones stimulate the pituitary gland to synthesize and release *trophic* (nourishment and growth controlling) *hormones*, such as corticotropin (also called *adrenocorticotropic hormone*), thyroid-stimulating hormone (TSH), and gonadotropins, such as luteinizing hormone (LH) and follicle-stimulating hormone (FSH). Secretion of trophic hormones stimulates the adrenal cortex, thyroid gland, and gonads. Hypothalamic hormones also stimulate the pituitary gland to release or inhibit the release of effector hormones, such as growth hormone (GH) and prolactin.

In a patient with a possible endocrine disorder, this complex hormonal sequence requires careful assessment to identify the dysfunction, which may result from defects in the gland; defects of effector, releasing, or trophic hormones; or defects of the target tissue. Hyperthyroidism, for example, may result from excessive thyrotropin-releasing hormone, TSH, or thyroid hormones or from excessive response of the thyroid gland.

Besides hormonal and neural controls, a negative feedback system regulates the endocrine system. (See *Feedback mechanism of the endocrine system.*) The feedback mechanism may be simple or complex. Simple feedback occurs when the level of one substance regulates secretion of a hormone. For example, a low calcium level stimulates the parathyroid glands to secrete parathyroid hormone (PTH),

CLOSER LOOK
Feedback mechanism of the endocrine system

The hypothalamus receives regulatory information (feedback) from its own circulating hormones (simple loop) and also from target glands (complex loop).

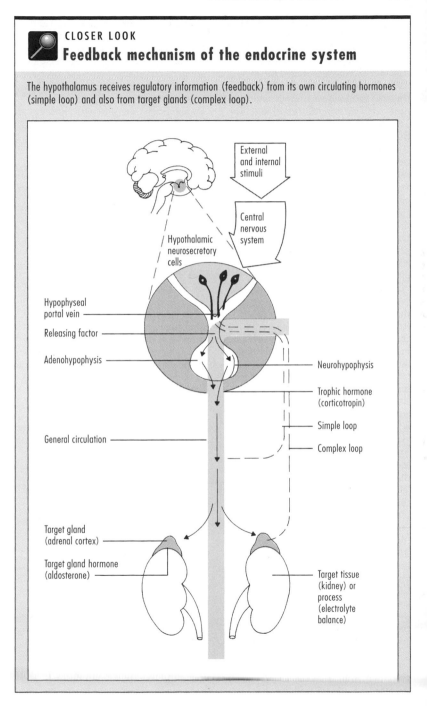

and a high calcium level inhibits PTH secretion.

One example of complex feedback occurs through the hypothalamic-pituitary target organ axis. Secretion of the hypothalamic corticotropin-releasing hormone releases pituitary corticotropin, which in turn stimulates adrenal cortisol secretion. Then, an increased cortisol level inhibits corticotropin by decreasing corticotropin-releasing hormone secretion or corticotropin directly. Corticosteroid therapy disrupts the hypothalamic-pituitary-adrenal axis by suppressing the hypothalamic-pituitary secretion mechanism. Because abrupt withdrawal of steroids doesn't allow time for recovery of the hypothalamic-pituitary-adrenal axis to stimulate cortisol secretion, it can induce life-threatening adrenal crisis.

Rhythms

The endocrine system is also controlled by rhythms, many of which last 24 hours (*circadian*). Circadian rhythm controls corticotropin and cortisol levels — increasing levels of these hormones in the early morning hours and decreasing them in the late afternoon. Stress, caused by pyrogens, surgery, hypoglycemia, exercise, severe emotional trauma, and other conditions, enhances corticotropin release and abolishes corticotropin circadian rhythmicity. High-dose glucocorticoid administration suppresses stress-related corticotropin release. An *infradian* rhythm is a biorhythm that repeats in patterns greater than 24-hour periods. The menstrual cycle is an example of an infradian rhythm — in this case, 28 days.

HORMONAL EFFECTS

The posterior pituitary gland secretes oxytocin and ADH. Oxytocin stimulates contraction of the uterus and causes the milk-letdown reflex in lactating women. ADH controls the concentration of body fluids by altering the permeability of the distal and collecting tubules of the kidneys to conserve water. ADH secretion depends on plasma osmolality (the characteristic of a solution determined by the ionic concentration of the dissolved substance and the solution), which is monitored by hypothalamic neurons. Hypovolemia and hypotension are the most powerful stimulators of ADH release. Other stimulators include trauma, nausea, morphine, tranquilizers, certain anesthetics, positive-pressure breathing, pain, and stress.

In addition to the trophic hormones, the anterior pituitary secretes prolactin, which stimulates milk secretion, and GH. GH affects most body tissues. It triggers growth by stimulating protein synthesis and fat mobilization, and by decreasing carbohydrate use by muscle and fat tissue. The thyroid gland synthesizes and secretes the iodinated hormones, thyroxine (T_4) and triiodothyronine (T_3). Thyroid hormones are necessary for normal growth and development, and act on many tissues to increase metabolic activity and protein synthesis.

The parathyroid glands secrete PTH, which regulates calcium and phosphate metabolism. PTH elevates serum calcium levels by stimulating resorption (removal) of calcium and excretion of phosphate from bone and — by stimulating the conversion of vitamin D to its most active form — enhances absorption of calcium from the GI tract. Calcitonin, another hormone secreted by the thyroid gland, affects calcium metabolism, although its precise role in humans is unknown.

The pancreas produces glucagon from the alpha cells and insulin from the beta cells. Glucagon, the hormone of the fasting state, releases stored glucose from the liver to increase blood glucose levels. Insulin, the hormone of the postprandial (occurring after a meal) state, helps move glucose into the cells, promotes glucose storage, stimulates protein synthesis, and enhances free fatty acid uptake and storage.

The adrenal cortex secretes mineralocorticoids, glucocorticoids, and sex steroid hormones (androgens). Aldosterone, a mineralocorticoid, regulates the reabsorption of sodium and the excretion of potassium by the kidneys. Although affected by corticotropin, aldosterone is mainly regulated by the renin-angiotensin system. Together, aldosterone, angiotensin II, and renin may be implicated in the pathogenesis of hypertension.

Cortisol, a glucocorticoid, stimulates gluconeogenesis (the formation of glucose from molecules that aren't carbohydrates), increases protein breakdown and free fatty acid mobilization, suppresses the immune response, and facilitates an appropriate response to stress.

The adrenal medulla is an aggregate of nervous tissue that produces the catecholamines epinephrine and norepinephrine, which cause vasoconstriction. In addition, epinephrine stimulates the fight-or-flight response — dilation of bronchioles and increased blood pressure, blood glucose level, and heart rate. The adrenal cortex as well as the gonads secretes androgens, which are steroid sex hormones. In males and premenopausal females, the contribution of adrenal androgens is very small, but in postmenopausal females, the adrenals are the major source of sex hormones.

The testes synthesize and secrete testosterone in response to gonadotropic hormones, especially LH, from the anterior pituitary gland; spermatogenesis occurs in response to FSH. The ovaries produce steroid hormones (primarily estrogen and progesterone) in response to anterior pituitary trophic hormones.

PATHOPHYSIOLOGIC CHANGES

Alterations in hormone levels, either significantly high or low, may result from various causes. Feedback systems may fail to function properly or may respond to the wrong signals. Dysfunction of an endocrine gland may show as either failure to produce adequate amounts of active hormone or excessive synthesis or release. After hormones are released, they may be degraded at an altered rate or inactivated by antibodies before reaching the target cell. Abnormal target cell responses include receptor-associated alterations and intracellular alterations.

Receptor-associated alterations

Receptor-associated alterations have been linked to water-soluble hormones (peptides) and involve:
- fewer receptors, resulting in reduced or defective hormone-receptor binding
- impaired receptor function, resulting in insensitivity to the hormone
- presence of antibodies against specific receptors, either reducing available binding sites or mimicking hormone action and suppressing or exaggerating target cell response
- unusual expression of receptor function.

Intracellular alterations

Intracellular alterations involve the inadequate synthesis of the second messenger (intracellular substance) needed to convert the hormonal signal into intracellular events. The two different mechanisms that may be involved include:
- faulty response of target cells for water-soluble hormones to hormone-receptor binding and failure to generate the required second messenger
- abnormal response of the target cell to the second messenger and failure to express the usual hormonal effect.

Pathophysiologic aberrations affecting target cells for lipid-soluble (steroid) hormones occur less frequently or may be recognized less frequently.

DISORDERS

Common dysfunctions of the endocrine system are classified as hypofunction and hyperfunction, inflammation, and tumor.

Adrenal hypofunction

Adrenal hypofunction is classified as primary or secondary. Primary adrenal hypofunction or insufficiency (Addison's disease) originates within the adrenal gland and is characterized by the decreased secretion of mineralocorticoids, glucocorticoids, and androgens. Secondary adrenal hypofunction is caused by a disorder outside the gland such as impaired pituitary secretion of corticotropin. It's characterized by decreased glucocorticoid secretion. The secretion of aldosterone, the major mineralocorticoid, is commonly unaffected.

Addison's disease is relatively uncommon and can occur at any age and in both sexes. Secondary adrenal hypofunction occurs when a patient abruptly stops long-term exogenous steroid therapy or when the pituitary is injured by a tumor or by infiltrative or autoimmune processes—these occur when circulating antibodies react specifically against adrenal tissue, causing inflammation and infiltration of the cells by lymphocytes. With early diagnosis and adequate replacement therapy, the prognosis for both primary and secondary adrenal hypofunction is good.

Adrenal crisis (addisonian crisis), a critical deficiency of mineralocorticoids and glucocorticoids, generally follows acute stress, sepsis, trauma, surgery, or the omission of steroid therapy in patients who have chronic adrenal insufficiency. Adrenal crisis is a medical emergency that needs immediate, vigorous treatment.

Autoimmune Addison's disease is most common in white females, and a genetic predisposition is likely. It's more common in patients with a familial predisposition to autoimmune endocrine diseases. Most cases of Addison's disease are diagnosed in people from their 20s through their 40s.

CAUSES

Primary and secondary adrenal hypofunction and adrenal crisis have different causes. The most common cause of primary hypofunction is:

■ destruction of more than 90% of both adrenal glands, usually by an autoimmune process in which circulating antibodies react specifically against the adrenal tissue; called *Addison's disease.*

Other causes include:

■ tuberculosis (once the chief cause, now responsible for fewer than 20% of adult cases)
■ bilateral adrenalectomy
■ hemorrhage into the adrenal gland
■ neoplasms
■ infections (histoplasmosis, cytomegalovirus [CMV])

■ family history of autoimmune disease (may predispose the patient to Addison's disease and other endocrinopathies).

Causes of secondary hypofunction (glucocorticoid deficiency) include:

■ hypopituitarism (causing decreased corticotropin secretion)
■ abrupt withdrawal of long-term corticosteroid therapy (long-term exogenous corticosteroid stimulation suppresses pituitary corticotropin secretion, resulting in adrenal gland atrophy)
■ removal of a corticotropin-secreting tumor.

Adrenal crisis is usually caused by:

■ exhausted body stores of glucocorticoids in a person with adrenal hypofunction after trauma, surgery, or other physiologic stress.

PATHOPHYSIOLOGY

Addison's disease is a chronic condition that results from the partial or complete destruction of the adrenal cortex. It manifests as a clinical syndrome in which the symptoms are associated with deficient production of the adrenocortical hormones, cortisol, aldosterone, and androgens. High levels of corticotropin and corticotropin-releasing hormone accompany the low glucocorticoid levels.

Corticotropin acts primarily to regulate the adrenal release of glucocorticoids (primarily cortisol); mineralocorticoids, including aldosterone; and sex steroids that supplement those produced by the gonads. Corticotropin secretion is controlled by corticotropin-releasing hormone from the hypothalamus and by negative feedback control by the glucocorticoids.

Addison's disease involves all zones of the cortex, causing deficiencies of the adrenocortical secretions, glucocorticoids, androgens, and mineralocorticoids.

Manifestations of adrenocortical hormone deficiency become apparent when 90% of the functional cells in both glands are lost. Usually, cellular atrophy is limited to the cortex, although medullary involvement may occur, resulting in catecholamine deficiency. Cortisol deficiency causes decreased liver gluconeogenesis (the formation of glucose from molecules that aren't carbohydrates). The resulting low blood glucose levels can become dangerously low in patients who take insulin routinely.

Aldosterone deficiency causes increased renal sodium loss and enhances potassium reabsorption. Sodium excretion causes a reduction in water volume that leads to hypotension. Patients with Addison's disease may have normal blood pressure when supine, but show marked hypotension and tachycardia after standing for several minutes. Low plasma volume and arteriolar pressure stimulate renin release and a resulting increased production of angiotensin II.

Androgen deficiency may decrease hair growth in axillary and pubic areas as well as on the extremities of women. The metabolic effects of testicular androgens make such hair growth less noticeable in men.

Addison's disease is a decrease in the biosynthesis, storage, or release of adrenocortical hormones. In about 80% of the patients, an autoimmune process causes partial or complete destruction of both adrenal glands. Autoimmune antibodies can block the corticotropin receptor or bind with corticotropin, preventing it from stimulating adrenal cells.

Infection is the second most common cause of Addison's disease, specifically tuberculosis, which causes about 20% of the cases. Other diseases that can cause Addison's disease include acquired immunodeficiency syndrome, systemic fungal infections, CMV, adrenal tumor, and metastatic cancers. Infection can impair cellular function and affect corticotropin at any stage of regulation.

SIGNS AND SYMPTOMS

Clinical features vary with the type of adrenal hypofunction. Signs and symptoms of primary hypofunction include:
- weakness, fatigue caused by alterations in adrenal hormone balance
- weight loss, nausea, vomiting, and anorexia resulting from glucocorticoid deficiency
- conspicuous bronze color of the skin, especially in the creases of the hands and over the metacarpophalangeal joints (hand

and finger), elbows, and knees caused by elevated levels of corticotropin
- darkening of scars, areas of vitiligo (absence of pigmentation), and increased pigmentation of the mucous membranes, especially the buccal mucosa, from decreased secretion of cortisol (causing simultaneous secretion of excessive amounts of corticotropin and melanocyte-stimulating hormone by the pituitary gland)
- associated cardiovascular abnormalities, including orthostatic hypotension, decreased cardiac size and output, and weak, irregular pulse caused by mineralocorticoid deficiency
- decreased tolerance for even minor stress, because of glucocorticoid deficiency
- fasting hypoglycemia caused by decreased gluconeogenesis
- craving for salty food caused by decreased mineralocorticoid secretion (which normally causes salt retention).

Signs and symptoms of secondary hypofunction include:
- signs and symptoms similar to those of primary hypofunction, but without hyperpigmentation caused by low corticotropin and melanocyte-stimulating hormone levels
- possibly no hypotension and electrolyte abnormalities because of fairly normal aldosterone secretion
- usually normal androgen secretion.

Signs and symptoms of addisonian crisis are related to the severe deficiencies of adrenal hormones and may include:
- profound weakness and fatigue
- nausea, vomiting, and dehydration
- hypotension
- high fever followed by hypothermia (occasionally).

COMPLICATIONS

Possible complications of adrenal hypofunction include:
- hyperpyrexia
- psychotic reactions
- results from deficient or excessive steroid treatment
- shock
- profound hypoglycemia
- ultimate vascular collapse, renal shutdown, coma, and death (if untreated).

DIAGNOSIS

Diagnosis of adrenal hypofunction is based on:

■ plasma cortisol levels confirming adrenal insufficiency (corticotropin stimulation test to differentiate between primary and secondary adrenal hypofunction)

■ metyrapone test for suspicion of secondary adrenal hypofunction (oral or I.V. metyrapone blocks cortisol production and should stimulate the release of corticotropin from the hypothalamic-pituitary system; in Addison's disease, the hypothalamic-pituitary system responds normally and plasma corticotropin levels are high, but because the adrenal glands are destroyed, plasma concentrations of the cortisol precursor 11-deoxycortisol increase, as do urinary 17-hydroxycorticosteroids)

■ rapid corticotropin stimulation test by I.V. or I.M. administration of cosyntropin, a synthetic form of corticotropin, after baseline sampling for cortisol and corticotropin (samples drawn for cortisol 30 and 60 minutes after injection), to differentiate between primary and secondary adrenal hypofunction. An elevated level is indicative of a primary disorder. A low corticotropin level indicates a secondary disorder.

In a patient with typical addisonian symptoms, the following laboratory findings strongly suggest acute adrenal insufficiency:

■ decreased plasma cortisol level (less than 10 mcg/dl in the morning; less in the evening)

■ decreased serum sodium and fasting blood glucose levels

■ increased serum potassium, calcium, and blood urea nitrogen levels

■ elevated hematocrit; increased lymphocyte and eosinophil counts

■ X-rays showing adrenal calcification if the cause is infectious.

TREATMENT

Treatment for adrenal hypofunction may include:

■ lifelong corticosteroid replacement, usually with cortisone or hydrocortisone, both of which have a mineralocorticoid effect (primary or secondary adrenal hypofunction)

CLINICAL ALERT

If the patient also has diabetes and is receiving corticosteroid therapy, blood glucose levels need to be monitored because steroid replacement may require adjustment of insulin dosage.

■ oral fludrocortisone, a synthetic mineralocorticoid, to prevent dangerous dehydration, hypotension, hyponatremia, and hyperkalemia (in Addison's disease)

■ I.V. bolus of hydrocortisone, 100 mg every 6 hours for 24 hours; then, 50 to 100 mg I.M. or diluted with dextrose in saline solution and given I.V. until the patient's condition stabilizes; up to 300 mg/day of hydrocortisone (by any route) and 3 to 5 L of I.V. saline and glucose solutions combined may be needed (adrenal crisis).

With proper treatment, adrenal crisis usually subsides quickly; blood pressure stabilizes, and water and sodium levels return to normal. After the crisis, maintenance doses of hydrocortisone preserve physiologic stability.

Congenital adrenal hyperplasia

Congenital adrenal hyperplasia (CAH) encompasses a group of genetic disorders resulting in the deficiency or absence of one of five enzymes needed for the biosynthesis of glucocorticoids and mineralocorticoids. Manifestations are usually present at birth or during early childhood, but symptoms may appear later in life in nonclassic CAH. CAH is uncommon and typically has an autosomal recessive mode of inheritance. When successfully treated, sexual functioning and fertility aren't affected.

The most common adrenal disorder in infants and children is CAH. There are two common forms: simple virilizing CAH and salt-losing CAH. Acquired adrenal virilism, usually the result of an adrenal tumor, is rare and affects twice as many females as males. With successful treatment, a normal quality of life and life span are expected. In older patients, androgen excess may be part of the syndrome of polycystic ovaries or may be caused by an adrenal carcinoma.

AGE ALERT
Salt-losing CAH may cause fatal adrenal crisis in neonates.

CAUSES

The cause of CAH is genetic, as an autosomal recessive trait.

PATHOPHYSIOLOGY

Cortisol levels are regulated by a negative-feedback mechanism. Corticotropin in the blood stimulates the release of cortisol precursors and, consequently, of cortisol, aldosterone, and androgens. In turn, cortisol suppresses corticotropin secretion. With a deficiency of the enzyme 21-hydroxylase, cortical secretion of cortisol is impaired and pituitary secretion of corticotropin is increased. Corticotropin stimulates the adrenal cortex, which in turn stimulates aldosterone and androgen biosynthesis and release.

In salt-losing CAH, 21-hydroxylase is almost absent. Corticotropin secretion increases, causing excessive production of cortisol precursors, including salt-wasting compounds. Plasma, cortisol, and aldosterone levels — all dependent on 21-hydroxylase — fall precipitously; these reductions, combined with the excessive production of salt-wasting compounds, cause acute renal crisis. Corticotropin hypersecretion stimulates adrenal androgens possibly even more than in simple virilizing CAH, and produces masculinization.

SIGNS AND SYMPTOMS

Signs and symptoms of CAH may include:
■ ambiguous genitalia (enlarged clitoris with urethral opening at the base and a combination of the labia and scrotum) caused by virilization from increased androgens; otherwise, normal genital tract and gonads
■ pubic and axillary hair at an earlier age, a deep voice, acne, and facial hair, but no menarche (female approaching puberty)
■ no apparent manifestations (male neonates)
■ accentuated masculine characteristics, including a deepened voice, acne, enlarged phallus with small testes, and frequent erections (male approaching puberty) resulting from increased androgen biosynthesis and release
■ high androgen levels causing rapid bone and muscle growth (children)
■ short stature caused by premature epiphyseal closure and high androgen levels (adults)
■ more severe changes, including development of a penis in female neonates (salt-losing CAH).

Because males with CAH have no external abnormalities, diagnosis is more difficult and is usually delayed until other symptoms occur. In the second week of life, symptoms of a salt-wasting crisis include apathy, failure to eat, diarrhea, and adrenal crisis (vomiting, dehydration from hyponatremia, and hyperkalemia). If adrenal crisis isn't treated promptly, dehydration and electrolyte imbalance cause cardiovascular collapse and cardiac arrest.

COMPLICATIONS

Possible complications of CAH include:
■ death (salt-wasting crisis), caused by dehydration and hyperkalemia
■ precocious puberty
■ menstrual irregularities
■ sexual dysfunction, infertility, and altered external genitalia
■ adrenal crisis
■ altered growth.

DIAGNOSIS

Diagnosis of CAH may include:
■ elevated urine 17-ketosteroid levels (can be suppressed by dexamethasone [Decadron])
■ elevated serum 17-hydroxyprogesterone level after I.V. bolus of corticotropin
■ serum hyperkalemia, hyponatremia, and hypochloremia (present but not diagnostic)
■ elevated 24-hour urine pregnanetriol level
■ normal or decreased 24-hour urine 17-hydroxycorticosteroid levels.

TREATMENT

Treatment of CAH includes:
■ daily cortisone or hydrocortisone to stop the excessive output of corticotropin and subsequent excessive androgen production (initial and subsequent doses

guided by urinary 17-ketosteroids levels)
given I.M. until the infant is old enough
to tolerate pills (usually about 18 months)
■ I.V. sodium chloride and glucose to
reestablish and maintain fluid and electrolyte balance, with desoxycorticosterone
I.M. and hydrocortisone I.V. as needed
(adrenal crisis); glucocorticoid (cortisone
or hydrocortisone) and perhaps mineralocorticoids (desoxycorticosterone, fludrocortisone, or both after stabilization)
■ sex chromatin and karyotype studies to
determine genetic sex (with ambiguous external genitalia); possible reconstructive
surgery for females between ages 1 and 3.

Cushing's syndrome

Cushing's syndrome is a cluster of clinical
abnormalities caused by excessive adrenocortical hormones (particularly cortisol)
or related corticosteroids and, to a lesser
extent, androgens and aldosterone. Cushing's disease (pituitary corticotropin excess) accounts for about 80% of endogenous cases of Cushing's syndrome.
Cushing's disease occurs most commonly
between ages 20 and 40 and is three to
eight times more common in females.

AGE ALERT
*Cushing's syndrome caused by
ectopic corticotropin secretion is
more common in adult men, with peak incidence between ages 40 and 60. In 20%
of patients, Cushing's syndrome results from
a cortisol-secreting tumor. Adrenal tumors,
rather than pituitary tumors, are more
common in children, especially girls.*

The annual incidence of endogenous
cortisol excess in the United States is two
to four cases per 1 million people per year.
The incidence of Cushing's syndrome resulting from exogenous administration of
cortisol is uncertain, but it's known to be
much greater than that of endogenous
types. The prognosis for endogenous
Cushing's syndrome is guardedly favorable
with surgery, but morbidity and mortality
are high without treatment. About 50% of
those with untreated Cushing's syndrome
die within 5 years of onset as a result of
overwhelming infection, suicide, complications from generalized arteriosclerosis
(coronary artery disease), and severe
hypertensive disease.

CAUSES

Causes of Cushing's syndrome include:
■ anterior pituitary hormone (corticotropin) excess
■ autonomous, ectopic corticotropin secretion by a tumor outside the pituitary
(usually malignant, frequently oat cell
carcinoma of the lung)
■ excessive glucocorticoid administration,
including prolonged use.

PATHOPHYSIOLOGY

Cushing's syndrome is caused by prolonged exposure to excess glucocorticoids.
Cushing's syndrome can be *exogenous*,
resulting from chronic glucocorticoid or
corticotropin administration, or *endogenous*, resulting from increased cortisol or
corticotropin secretion. Cortisol excess
results in anti-inflammatory effects and
excessive catabolism of protein and peripheral fat to support hepatic glucose
production. The mechanism may be
corticotropin-dependent (elevated plasma
corticotropin levels stimulate the adrenal
cortex to produce excess cortisol), or
corticotropin-independent (excess cortisol
is produced by the adrenal cortex or ex-
ogenously administered). Excess cortisol
suppresses the hypothalamic-pituitary-
adrenal axis.

SIGNS AND SYMPTOMS

As with other endocrine disorders, Cushing's syndrome induces changes in many
body systems. Signs and symptoms depend on the degree and duration of hypercortisolism, the presence or absence of
androgen excess, and any additional
tumor-related effects (adrenal carcinoma
or ectopic corticotropin syndrome). Specific clinical effects vary with the system
affected and include:
■ diabetes mellitus, with decreased glucose tolerance, fasting hyperglycemia, and
glucosuria caused by cortisol-induced insulin resistance and increased gluconeogenesis in the liver (endocrine and
metabolic systems)
■ muscle weakness caused by hypokalemia or loss of muscle mass from increased
catabolism, pathologic fractures because of
decreased bone mineral ionization, osteopenia, osteoporosis, and skeletal growth

retardation in children (musculoskeletal system)

■ purple striae; facial plethora (edema and blood vessel distention); acne; fat pads above the clavicles, over the upper back (buffalo hump), on the face (moon facies), and throughout the trunk (truncal obesity) with slender arms and legs; little or no scar formation; poor wound healing because of decreased collagen and weakened tissues; spontaneous ecchymosis; hyperpigmentation; fungal skin infections (skin)

■ peptic ulcer caused by increased gastric secretions and pepsin production and decreased gastric mucus, abdominal pain, increased appetite, weight gain (GI system)

■ irritability and emotional lability, ranging from euphoric behavior to depression or psychosis; insomnia caused by the cortisol's role in neurotransmission; headache (central nervous system)

■ hypertension caused by sodium and secondary fluid retention; heart failure; left ventricular hypertrophy; capillary weakness from protein loss, which leads to bleeding and ecchymosis; dyslipidemia; ankle edema (cardiovascular system)

■ increased susceptibility to infection because of decreased lymphocyte production and suppressed antibody formation; decreased resistance to stress; suppressed inflammatory response masking even severe infection (immunologic system)

■ fluid retention, increased potassium excretion, ureteral calculi from increased bone demineralization with hypercalciuria (renal and urologic systems)

■ increased androgen production with clitoral hypertrophy, mild virilism, hirsutism, and amenorrhea or oligomenorrhea in women; sexual dysfunction; decreased libido; impotence (reproductive system).

COMPLICATIONS

Complications of Cushing's syndrome include:

■ osteoporosis
■ increased susceptibility to infections
■ hirsutism
■ ureteral calculi
■ metastasis of malignant tumors.

DIAGNOSIS

Diagnosis is based on the following laboratory test results:

■ hyperglycemia, hypernatremia, glucosuria, hypokalemia, and metabolic alkalosis

■ urinary free cortisol levels greater than 150 mcg/24 hours

■ dexamethasone suppression test to confirm the diagnosis and determine the cause, possibly an adrenal tumor or a nonendocrine, corticotropin-secreting tumor

■ blood levels of corticotropin-releasing hormone, corticotropin, and different glucocorticoids to diagnose and localize cause to pituitary or adrenal gland.

TREATMENT

Differentiation among pituitary, adrenal, and ectopic causes of hypercortisolism is essential for effective treatment, which is specific for the cause of cortisol excess and includes medication, radiation, and surgery. Possible treatments include:

■ surgery for tumors of the adrenal and pituitary glands or other tissue (such as the lung)

■ radiation therapy (tumor)

■ drug therapy, which may include ketoconazole, metyrapone, and aminoglutethimide to inhibit cortisol synthesis; mitotane to destroy the adrenocortical cells that secret cortisol; and bromocriptine and cyproheptadine to inhibit corticotropin secretion.

Diabetes insipidus

A disorder of water metabolism, diabetes insipidus results from a deficiency of circulating vasopressin (also called *antidiuretic hormone* [ADH]) or from renal resistance to this hormone. *Pituitary diabetes insipidus* is caused by a deficiency of vasopressin, and *nephrogenic diabetes insipidus* is caused by the resistance of renal tubules to vasopressin. Diabetes insipidus is characterized by excessive fluid intake and hypotonic polyuria. A decrease in ADH levels leads to altered intracellular and extracellular fluid control, causing renal excretion of a large amount of urine.

The disorder may start at any age and is slightly more common in men than in women. The incidence is slightly greater today than in the past.

In uncomplicated diabetes insipidus, the prognosis is good with adequate water replacement, and patients usually lead normal lives.

CAUSES

The cause of diabetes insipidus may be:
- acquired, familial, idiopathic, neurogenic, or nephrogenic
- associated with stroke, hypothalamic or pituitary tumors, and cranial trauma or surgery (neurogenic diabetes insipidus)
- X-linked recessive trait or end-stage renal failure (nephrogenic diabetes insipidus, less common)
- caused by certain drugs, such as lithium, phenytoin, or alcohol (transient diabetes insipidus).

PATHOPHYSIOLOGY

Diabetes insipidus is related to an insufficiency of ADH, leading to polyuria and polydipsia. The three forms of diabetes insipidus are neurogenic, nephrogenic, and psychogenic.

Neurogenic, or central, diabetes insipidus is an inadequate response of ADH to plasma osmolarity, which occurs when an organic lesion of the hypothalamus, infundibular stem, or posterior pituitary partially or completely blocks ADH synthesis, transport, or release. The many organic lesions that can cause diabetes insipidus include brain tumors, hypophysectomy, aneurysms, thrombosis, skull fractures, infections, and immunologic disorders. Neurogenic diabetes insipidus has an acute onset. A three-phase syndrome can occur, which involves:
- progressive loss of nerve tissue and increased diuresis
- normal diuresis
- polyuria and polydipsia, the manifestation of permanent loss of the ability to secrete adequate ADH.

Nephrogenic diabetes insipidus is caused by an inadequate renal response to ADH. The collecting duct permeability to water doesn't increase in response to ADH. Nephrogenic diabetes insipidus is generally related to disorders and drugs that damage the renal tubules or inhibit the genera-

tion of cyclic adenosine monophosphate in the tubules, preventing activation of the second messenger. Causative disorders include pyelonephritis, amyloidosis, destructive uropathies, polycystic disease, and intrinsic renal disease. Drugs include lithium, general anesthetics such as methoxyflurane, and demeclocycline. In addition, hypokalemia or hypercalcemia impairs the renal response to ADH. A rare genetic form of nephrogenic diabetes insipidus is an X-linked recessive trait.

Psychogenic diabetes insipidus is caused by an extremely large fluid intake, which may be idiopathic or related to psychosis or sarcoidosis. The polydipsia and resultant polyuria wash out ADH more quickly than it can be replaced. Chronic polyuria may overwhelm the renal medullary concentration gradient, rendering patients partially or totally unable to concentrate urine.

Regardless of the cause, insufficient ADH causes the immediate excretion of large volumes of dilute urine and leads to plasma hyperosmolality. In conscious people, the thirst mechanism is stimulated, usually for cold liquids. With severe ADH deficiency, urine output may be greater than 12 L/day, with a low specific gravity. Dehydration develops rapidly if fluids aren't replaced.

SIGNS AND SYMPTOMS

Signs and symptoms of diabetes insipidus include:
- polydipsia (cardinal symptom) — fluid intake of 5 to 20 L/day caused by stimulation of thirst mechanism
- polyuria (cardinal symptom) — urine output of 2 to 20 L/24-hour period of dilute urine caused by insufficient ADH
- nocturia, leading to sleep disturbance and fatigue
- low urine specific gravity — less than 1.006 caused by polyuria
- fever
- changes in level of consciousness caused by central nervous system cellular dehydration
- hypotension caused by a decrease in vascular volume related to fluid loss
- tachycardia in response to depleted vascular volume

- headache and vision disturbances caused by electrolyte disturbance and dehydration
- abdominal fullness, anorexia, and weight loss caused by almost continuous fluid consumption.

COMPLICATIONS
Possible complications of diabetes insipidus include:
- dilation of the urinary tract
- severe dehydration
- shock and renal failure if dehydration is severe.

DIAGNOSIS
Diagnosis is based on:
- urinalysis showing almost colorless urine of low osmolality (50 to 200 mOsm/kg, less than that of plasma) and low specific gravity (less than 1.005)
- water deprivation test to identify vasopressin deficiency, resulting in renal inability to concentrate urine.

TREATMENT
Until the cause of diabetes insipidus can be identified and eliminated, the administration of vasopressin can control fluid balance and prevent dehydration. Medications include:
- hydrochlorothiazide with potassium supplement for central and nephrogenic diabetes insipidus
- vasopressin aqueous preparation subcutaneously several times daily, effective for only 2 to 6 hours (used as a diagnostic agent and, rarely, in acute disease)
- desmopressin acetate orally, by nasal spray absorbed through the mucous membranes, or subcutaneous or I.V. injection, effective for 8 to 20 hours depending on the dosage
- chlorpropamide to decrease thirst sensation in patients with continued hypernatremia.

Diabetes mellitus
Diabetes mellitus is a metabolic disorder characterized by hyperglycemia (elevated glucose level) resulting from lack of insulin, lack of insulin effect, or both. Three general classifications are recognized:
- type 1, absolute insulin insufficiency

- type 2, insulin resistance with varying degrees of insulin secretory defects
- gestational diabetes, which emerges during pregnancy.

Onset of type 1 diabetes mellitus usually occurs before age 30 (although it may occur at any age); the patient is usually thin and requires exogenous insulin and dietary management to achieve control. In contrast, type 2 diabetes mellitus usually occurs in obese adults after age 40 and is treated with diet and exercise in combination with various oral antidiabetic drugs, although treatment may include insulin therapy.

Medical advances permit increased longevity and improved quality of life if the patient carefully monitors blood glucose levels, uses the data to make pharmacologic and lifestyle changes, and uses new insulin delivery systems such as subcutaneous insulin pumps. In addition, medications now available enhance the body's own glucose metabolism and insulin sensitivity to optimize glycemic control and prevent progression to long-term complications.

CAUSES
Evidence indicates that diabetes mellitus has diverse causes, including:
- heredity
- environment (infection, diet, toxins, stress)
- lifestyle changes in genetically susceptible people
- pregnancy.

PATHOPHYSIOLOGY
In people genetically susceptible to type 1 diabetes mellitus, a triggering event, possibly a viral infection, causes production of autoantibodies against the beta cells of the pancreas. The resultant destruction of the beta cells leads to a decline in and ultimate lack of insulin secretion. Insulin deficiency leads to hyperglycemia, enhanced lipolysis (decomposition of fat), and protein catabolism. These characteristics occur when more than 90% of the beta cells have been destroyed.

Type 2 diabetes mellitus is a chronic disease caused by one or more of the following factors: impaired insulin secretion, inappropriate hepatic glucose production, or peripheral insulin receptor insensitivity. Genetic factors are significant, and onset is accelerated by obesity and a sedentary lifestyle. Again, added stress can be a pivotal factor.

Gestational diabetes mellitus occurs when a woman in whom diabetes hasn't previously been diagnosed shows glucose intolerance during pregnancy. This may occur if placental hormones counteract insulin, causing insulin resistance. Gestational diabetes mellitus is a significant risk factor for the future occurrence of type 2 diabetes mellitus.

SIGNS AND SYMPTOMS

CLINICAL ALERT
Type 1 diabetes usually has a rapid onset, typically with polydipsia, polyuria, polyphagia, weakness, weight loss, dry skin, and ketoacidosis. Type 2 diabetes is typically slow and insidious in onset and usually unaccompanied by symptoms.

Signs and symptoms of diabetes mellitus include:
■ polyuria and polydipsia because of high serum osmolality caused by high glucose levels
■ anorexia (common) resulting from elevated glucose levels, or polyphagia (occasional) most likely caused by cellular starvation and cellular depletion of nutrient stores
■ weight loss (usually 10% to 30%; people with type 1 diabetes typically have almost no body fat at time of diagnosis) caused by prevention of normal metabolism of carbohydrates, fats, and proteins because of impaired or absent insulin function
■ headaches, fatigue, lethargy, reduced energy levels, and impaired school and work performance because of low intracellular glucose levels
■ muscle cramps, irritability, and emotional lability caused by electrolyte imbalance
■ vision changes, such as blurring, caused by glucose-induced swelling
■ numbness and tingling caused by neural tissue damage

■ abdominal discomfort and pain caused by autonomic neuropathy, causing gastroparesis and constipation
■ nausea, diarrhea, or constipation caused by dehydration and electrolyte imbalances or autonomic neuropathy
■ abnormally slow healing of skin infections or wounds; itching of skin
■ recurrent monilial infections of the vagina or anus.

COMPLICATIONS
Complications of diabetes mellitus include:
■ microvascular disease, including retinopathy, nephropathy, and neuropathy
■ dyslipidemia
■ macrovascular disease, including coronary, peripheral, and cerebral artery disease
■ diabetic ketoacidosis
■ hyperosmolar hyperglycemic nonketotic syndrome
■ excessive weight gain
■ skin ulcerations
■ chronic renal failure.

DIAGNOSIS
In adult men and nonpregnant women, diabetes mellitus is diagnosed by two of the following criteria obtained more than 24 hours apart, using the same test twice or any combination:
■ fasting plasma glucose level of 126 mg/dl or more on at least two occasions
■ typical symptoms of uncontrolled diabetes and random blood glucose level of 200 mg/dl or more
■ blood glucose level of 200 mg/dl or more 2 hours after ingesting 75 g of oral dextrose.

Diagnosis may also be based on:
■ diabetic retinopathy on ophthalmologic examination
■ other diagnostic and monitoring tests, including urinalysis for acetone and test for glycosylated hemoglobin (reflects glycemic control over the past 2 to 3 months).

TREATMENT
Effective treatment of all types of diabetes optimizes blood glucose control and decreases complications. Treatment for type 1 diabetes mellitus includes:

- insulin replacement, meal planning, and exercise (current forms of insulin replacement include mixeddose, split mixed-dose, and multiple daily injection regimens, and continuous subcutaneous insulin infusions)
- pancreas transplantation (currently requires chronic immunosuppression). (See *Treatment of type 1 diabetes mellitus,* pages 468 and 469.)

Treatment of type 2 diabetes mellitus includes:

- oral antidiabetic drugs to stimulate endogenous insulin production, increase insulin sensitivity at the cellular level, suppress hepatic gluconeogenesis, and delay GI absorption of carbohydrates (drug combinations may be used).

Treatment of both types of diabetes mellitus includes:

- careful monitoring of blood glucose levels
- individualized meal plan designed to meet nutritional needs, control blood glucose and lipid levels, and reach and maintain appropriate body weight (plan to be followed consistently with meals eaten at regular times)
- weight reduction (obese patient with type 2 diabetes mellitus) or high calorie allotment, depending on growth stage and activity level (type 1 diabetes mellitus).

Treatment of gestational diabetes involves:

- medical nutrition therapy
- injectable insulin if blood glucose control isn't achieved with diet alone (because oral antidiabetic agents are teratogenic and, therefore, are contraindicated during pregnancy)
- postpartum counseling to address the high risk of gestational diabetes in subsequent pregnancies and type 2 diabetes later in life
- regular exercise and prevention of weight gain to help prevent type 2 diabetes.

Gonadotropin deficiency

Gonadotropin deficiency is a lack of hormones (follicle-stimulating hormone [FSH] and luteinizing hormone [LH]) that stimulate the sex glands, primarily the testes and ovaries. Chronic gonadotropin deficiency, if not treated, can cause infertility and osteopenia (decreased bone mass). A decrease in testosterone results in decreased bone cell formation.

CAUSES

Causes of gonadotropin deficiency include:

- pituitary tumor or hemorrhage
- oversecretion of target gland hormone, such as estrogen, progesterone, or testosterone
- prolactin-secreting tumor
- hypothalamic suppression of gonadotropin-releasing hormone (Gn-RH) during periods of physical or emotional stress, obesity, or starvation
- genetics.

PATHOPHYSIOLOGY

Gn-RH is secreted by the hypothalamus and causes the anterior pituitary to secrete the gonadotropins — testosterone, estrogen, FSH, and LH. In males and females, estrogen, progesterone, and testosterone (typically called *androgen* or *male sex hormone*), produced by the gonads, function in a negative-feedback loop that regulates Gn-RH secretion.

Testosterone, which is responsible for masculine sex characteristics and sperm production, also functions in bone, muscle, and red blood cell formation and has a role in neural signaling. Estrogen serves many functions, among them cognitive, bone, and vaginal maintenance. FSH and LH maintain the corpus luteum and pregnancy.

Several mechanisms can cause Gn-RH deficiency, including:

- pituitary tumor producing another hormone that impinges on the gonadotropin-producing cells and physically impairs Gn-RH biosynthesis
- medical treatments such as radiation (impairs Gn-RH–producing cells)
- oversecretion of estrogen, progesterone, or testosterone by dysfunctional target glands, causing Gn-RH inhibition through the negative-feedback loop
- action of prolactin (inhibits pituitary secretion of Gn-RH; prolactin-secreting tumors can cause Gn-RH deficiency)

(Text continues on page 470.)

DISRUPTING DISEASE
Treatment of type 1 diabetes mellitus

The following algorithm shows the pathophysiologic process of diabetes and points for treatment intervention.

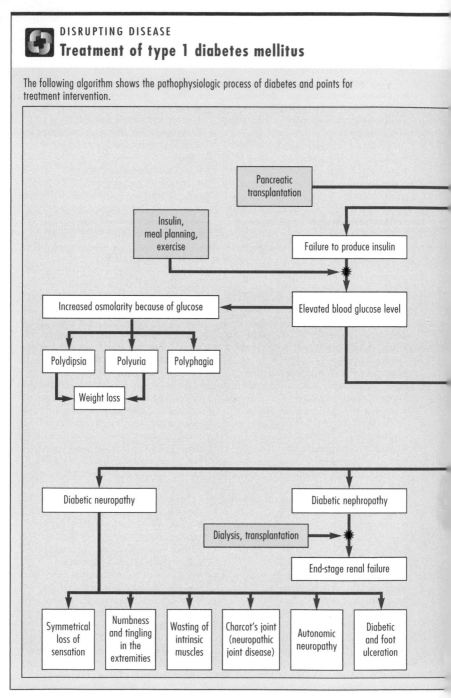

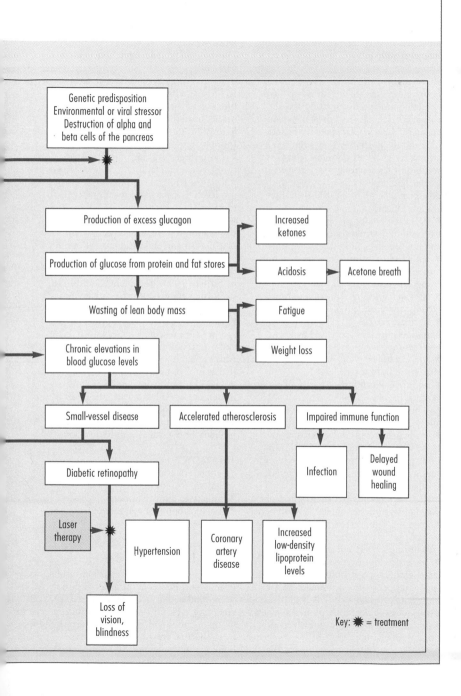

■ reduced Gn-RH secretion caused by response of hypothalamus to physical stress, obesity, or starvation (for example, females in competitive athletics may not enter menarche or may cease menstruation for extended periods).

SIGNS AND SYMPTOMS

Many symptoms are directly related to a reduction in the differentiating sexual characteristics that are caused and maintained by the gonadotropins (FSH and LH) and the hormones they stimulate, androgens (male sex hormone, most commonly testosterone) and estrogen. These signs and symptoms vary with the degree and length of Gn-RH deficiency, and may include:
■ decreased libido, strength, and body hair, and fine wrinkles around the eyes and lips (adults)
■ amenorrhea; vaginal, uterine, and breast atrophy; clitoral enlargement; voice deepening; and beard growth (women)
■ testicular atrophy, reduction in beard growth, and erectile dysfunction (men)
■ decreased red blood cells and loss of bone and muscle mass caused by low testosterone levels
■ mood and behavior changes caused by changes in testosterone levels
■ anosmia, which is the absence of a sense of smell (genetic cases).

The age at onset of Gn-RH deficiency affects the presentation in children:
■ inadequate sexual differentiation shown by ambiguity, pseudohermaphroditism (individual shows one or more contraindications of the morphologic sex criteria), or normal-appearing female genitalia with male genetic coding (if deficiency occurs during first trimester of fetal development)
■ microphallus and partial or complete lack of testicular descent (if deficiency occurs during second and third trimesters)
■ underdevelopment of secondary sex characteristics, poor muscle development, lack of deepening voice in males, sparse body hair, gynecomastia (enlarged breast tissue), delayed fusion of epiphyseal plates, and continued long-bone growth (childhood through puberty).

COMPLICATIONS

A complication of gonadotropin deficiency is infertility.

DIAGNOSIS

Diagnosis of gonadotropin deficiency is based on:
■ serum estrogen, testosterone, and Gn-RH levels to differentiate between dysfunction of the hypothalamus or of the ovaries or testicles
■ low testosterone and high Gn-RH levels (primary testicular failure)
■ low estrogen and high Gn-RH levels (primary ovarian failure)
■ low Gn-RH and testosterone or estrogen levels (hypothalamic or pituitary dysfunction)
■ human chorionic gonadotropin (hCG) stimulation test (hCG, 500 IU/1.7 m^2 or 100 IU/kg in children, given after measuring baseline testosterone; after 3 to 4 days, testosterone levels should increase by 50% to 200% because hCG and LH stimulate Leydig's cells to stimulate testicular function)
■ clomiphene citrate test (normal response, 30% to 200% increase in FSH and 0% to 65% increase in testosterone) with impaired or absent increase in hypothalamic or pituitary disorders
■ Gn-RH stimulation test (rapid I.V. injection of Gn-RH stimulates the pituitary to secrete LH and FSH), with insufficient elevation of LH or FSH levels indicating pituitary or hypothalamus dysfunction.

TREATMENT

Treatment of gonadotropin deficiency includes:
■ surgery to remove tumors
■ gonadotropin, estrogen, or testosterone replacement
■ stress reduction and weight gain or loss.

Growth hormone deficiency

Growth hormone (GH) deficiency results from hypofunction of the anterior pituitary gland with a resulting decreased secretion of GH. GH deficiency includes a group of childhood disorders characterized by subnormal growth velocity, delayed bone age, and a subnormal response to

Ulcers

Ulcers result from three main causes: infection with *Helicobacter pylori,* use of nonsteroidal anti-inflammatory drugs, and pathologic hypersecretion of gastric acids.

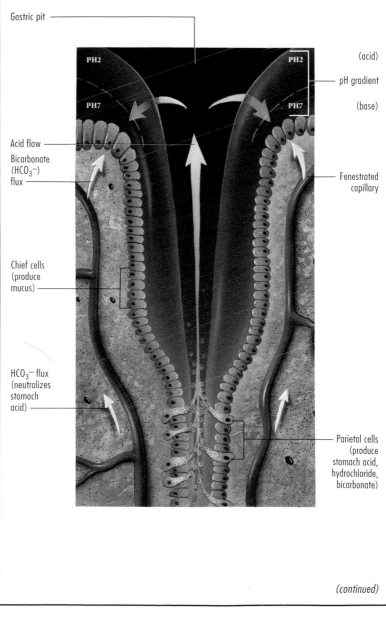

Gastric pit

(acid)

pH gradient

(base)

Acid flow

Bicarbonate (HCO_3^-) flux

Fenestrated capillary

Chief cells (produce mucus)

HCO_3^- flux (neutralizes stomach acid)

Parietal cells (produce stomach acid, hydrochloride, bicarbonate)

(continued)

lcers *(continued)*

TYPES OF ULCERS

Ulcers may occur anywhere in the esophagus, stomach, pylorus, duodenum, or jejunum, with the crater of the ulcer penetrating through one or more layers of tissue. If damage recurs or if healing doesn't take place, the crater may penetrate the wall and extend to adjacent tissues and organs such as the pancreas.

Erosion
Penetration of only the superficial layer

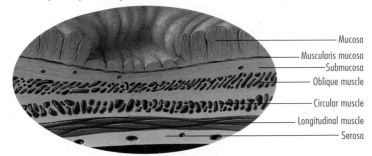

- Mucosa
- Muscularis mucosa
- Submucosa
- Oblique muscle
- Circular muscle
- Longitudinal muscle
- Serosa

Acute ulcer
Penetration into the muscular layer

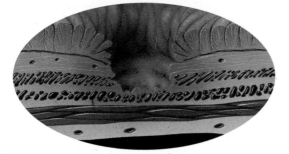

Perforating ulcer
Penetration of the wall, creating a passage for gastric acids, other fluids, and air to enter adjacent spaces

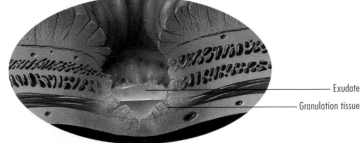

- Exudate
- Granulation tissue

A CLOSER LOOK AT *H. PYLORI*

H. pylori is a contributing factor in chronic gastritis (chronic inflammation of stomach mucosa) and in ulcer formation. It's typically seen within the muscular layers and between the cells that line the gastric pits. These bacteria cause tissue inflammation, which can lead to ulcers.

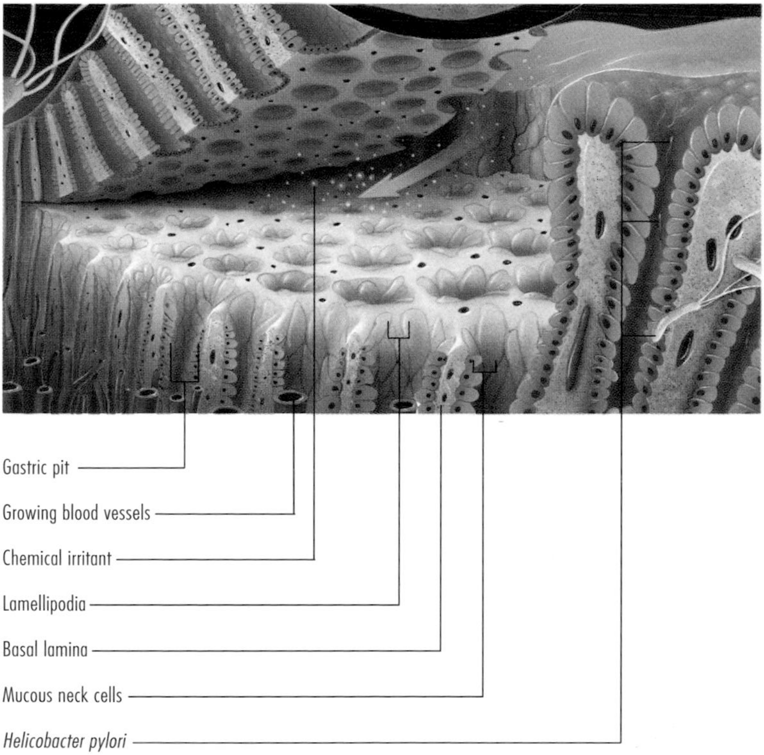

Gastric pit

Growing blood vessels

Chemical irritant

Lamellipodia

Basal lamina

Mucous neck cells

Helicobacter pylori

Carpal tunnel syndrome

Carpal tunnel syndrome is a disorder involving pain, numbness, and weakness resulting from compression of the median nerve against the inelastic transverse carpal ligament. Usually, this syndrome is caused by pressure from the swollen synovium of the flexor tendons. If left untreated, carpal tunnel syndrome can lead to discomfort, impaired function of the hands, and permanent disability.

THE CARPAL TUNNEL

The carpal tunnel is a narrow, rigid passage formed by the carpal bones of the wrist and the tough, inelastic transverse carpal ligament. Traveling through the tunnel are nine flexor tendons and the median nerve. The flexor muscles originate in the forearm and attach as tendons to bones of the fingers and thumb. As these muscles contract to bend the fingers, the tendons slide through the carpal tunnel. The median nerve travels through the carpal tunnel and then divides into a motor branch that controls the thumb muscles, and sensory branches that provide more than half of the hand with its sense of touch.

Any factor that increases the pressure within the carpal tunnel can contribute to development of the syndrome. Typically, several factors are present, including:
◆ systemic disorders, such as diabetes, rheumatoid arthritis, hypothyroidism, and amyloidosis
◆ repetitive trauma; repetitive movements that expose the nerve to compression forces and stretching
◆ edema (increased fluid within the tunnel), resulting from tissue injury, heart failure, or pregnancy
◆ trauma such as fractures or dislocations of the wrist
◆ inherited small bone structure.

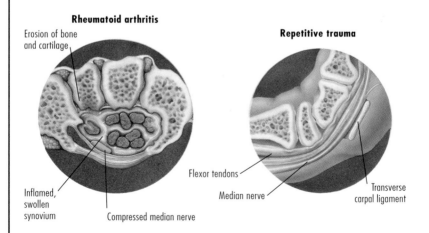

Rheumatoid arthritis

Erosion of bone and cartilage

Repetitive trauma

Flexor tendons

Median nerve

Transverse carpal ligament

Inflamed, swollen synovium

Compressed median nerve

WHAT HAPPENS IN CARPAL TUNNEL SYNDROME

When pressure increases in the tunnel, the median nerve is compressed, decreasing blood flow. The resulting lack of oxygen and nutrients to the area interferes with nerve conduction. If the compression persists, the nerve begins to swell. The myelin sheath begins to thin and degenerate. In addition, tenosynovitis occurs, leading to a thickening of the tendon synovium caused by mechanical stress applied to the sliding tendons during repetitive movements.

Cross section of wrist with carpal tunnel syndrome

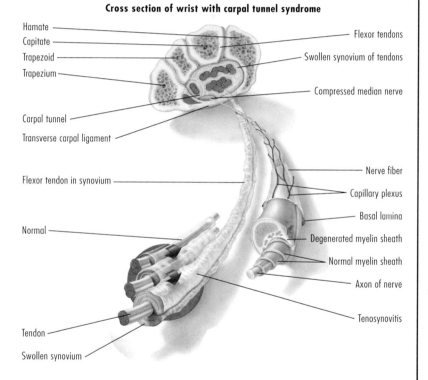

Hamate
Capitate
Trapezoid
Trapezium

Carpal tunnel

Transverse carpal ligament

Flexor tendon in synovium

Normal

Tendon

Swollen synovium

Flexor tendons
Swollen synovium of tendons

Compressed median nerve

Nerve fiber
Capillary plexus
Basal lamina
Degenerated myelin sheath
Normal myelin sheath
Axon of nerve
Tenosynovitis

Allergic rhinitis

Allergic rhinitis is a reaction to airborne (inhaled) allergens. Depending on the allergen, the resulting rhinitis and conjunctivitis may occur seasonally (hay fever) or year-round (perennial allergic rhinitis).

WHAT HAPPENS IN ALLERGIC RHINITIS

During primary exposure to an allergen, T cells recognize the foreign allergens and release chemicals that instruct B cells to produce specific antibodies called immunoglobulin (Ig) E. IgE antibodies attach themselves to mast cells. Mast cells with attached IgE can remain in the body for years, ready to react when they next encounter the same allergen.

Primary exposure

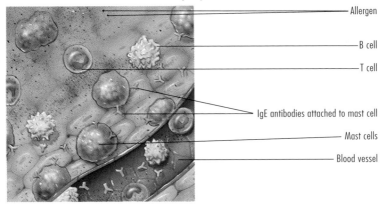

Allergen

B cell

T cell

IgE antibodies attached to mast cell

Mast cells

Blood vessel

The second time the allergen enters the body (reexposure), it comes into direct contact with the IgE antibodies attached to the mast cells. This stimulates the mast cells to release chemicals, such as histamine, which initiate a response that causes tightening of the smooth muscles in the airways; dilation of small blood vessels; increased mucus secretion in the nasal cavity and airways; and itching.

Reexposure

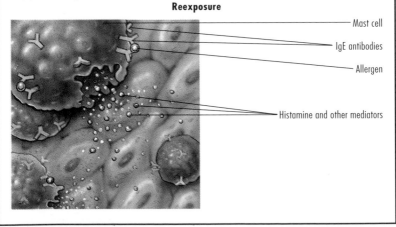

Mast cell

IgE antibodies

Allergen

Histamine and other mediators

Osteoporosis

Osteoporosis is a metabolic disease of the skeleton that reduces the amount of bone tissue. Bones weaken as local cells resorb or take up bone tissue. Trabecular bone at the core becomes less dense, and cortical bone on the perimeter loses thickness.

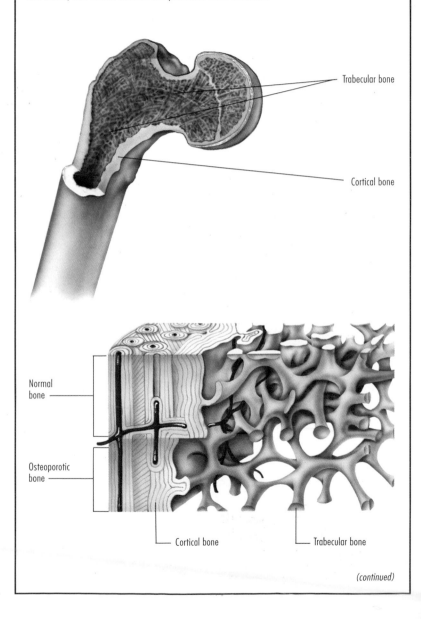

Trabecular bone

Cortical bone

Normal bone

Osteoporotic bone

Cortical bone

Trabecular bone

(continued)

Osteoporosis *(continued)*

CONTROLLING MINERAL BALANCE
Normally, the blood absorbs calcium from the digestive system and deposits it in the bones. In osteoporosis, blood levels of calcium are reduced because of dietary calcium deficiency, inability of the intestines to absorb calcium, or postmenopausal estrogen deficiency. To maintain the blood calcium level as close to normal as possible, resorption from the bones increases, causing osteoporosis.

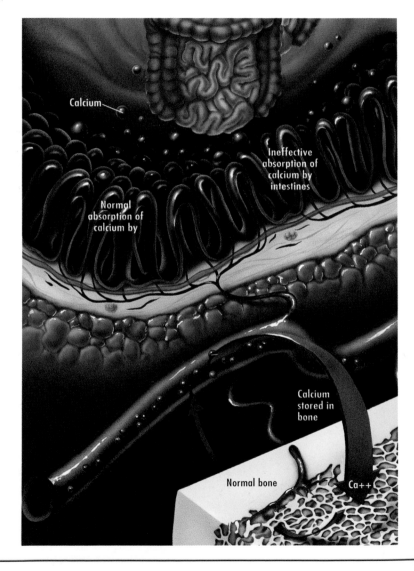

Calcium

Ineffective absorption of calcium by intestines

Normal absorption of calcium by

Calcium stored in bone

Normal bone

Ca++

In addition to enhancing bone resorption, low calcium enhances the effects of two other factors: parathyroid hormone (PTH) and vitamin D. PTH is produced by the parathyroid glands, which are buried in the thyroid gland. Vitamin D is supplied by the diet, produced in the skin as a reaction to sunlight, and processed into a very potent form in the liver and kidneys. Both substances stimulate calcium absorption from the intestine and increase resorption from the bone. This results in an increased sacrifice of bone calcium to maintain normal levels of calcium in the blood.

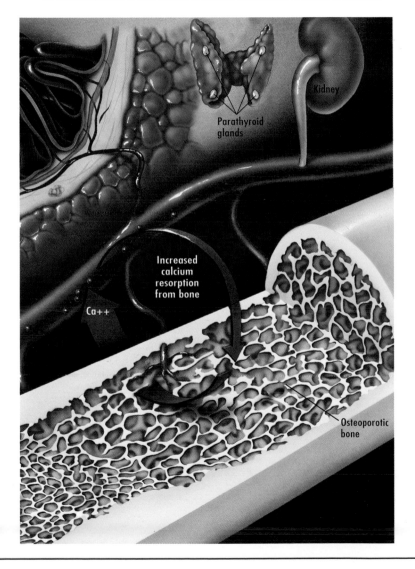

Sexually transmitted diseases

Sexually transmitted diseases (STDs) are illnesses easily spread through sexual or intimate physical contact. STDs are caused by bacteria, viruses, protozoa, or parasites. Of the 20 known STDs, chlamydial infection, trichomoniasis, gonorrhea, and acquired immunodeficiency syndrome (AIDS) (caused by human immunodeficiency virus [HIV]) are the most common. If untreated, STDs can cause serious health problems for men and women.

CHLAMYDIAL INFECTION

Chlamydia trachomatis is the bacterium responsible for causing the most common STD infection in the United States. It's commonly termed the silent STD because the symptoms are mild and many women are asymptomatic.

Chlamydia trachomatis

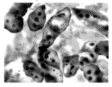

TRICHOMONIASIS

Trichomoniasis, commonly called trich, is one of the most common STDs. It's caused by the protozoan *Trichomonas vaginalis*. Evidence of the infection varies from no symptoms to those of vaginal inflammation, frothy vaginal discharge, white penile discharge, and offensive odor.

Trichomonas vaginalis

GONORRHEA

Gonorrhea, commonly called the hidden STD, is caused by the bacterium *Neisseria gonorrhoeae*. It's transmitted almost exclusively by sexual intercourse. Initially, there may be no signs of infection. However, if left untreated, gonorrhea can lead to pelvic inflammatory disease, arthritis, prostatitis, sterility, heart problems, neurologic disorders, and blindness.

Neisseria gonorrhoeae

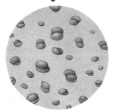

SYPHILIS

Syphilis is called the latent STD because major symptoms don't appear until 6 to 12 weeks after infection. Syphilis is caused by the spirochete Treponema palladium, which causes painless sores and swollen lymph nodes. If left untreated, symptoms may disappear altogether or return irregularly. A more serious condition occurs 10 to 25 years later as organs and tissues are destroyed by the infestation of spirochetes.

Treponema pallidum

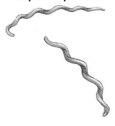

AIDS

The most dangerous STD is AIDS, which is caused by HIV. As a result of the infection, a person's immune system is dramatically weakened, placing him at risk for the development of opportunistic diseases.

HIV

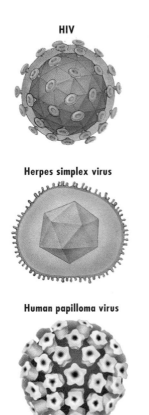

HERPES

Herpes is caused by the herpes simplex virus (HSV), which has two forms. HSV-1 affects mostly the upper body, causing cold sores, fevers, and blisters on the lips. HSV-2 affects the genitals, causing tingling and burning sensations and the formation of blisters that burst into painful ulcers. It's called the manageable STD because, although it can't be cured, it can be easily treated and controlled.

Herpes simplex virus

GENITAL WARTS

Genital warts, caused by the human papilloma virus (HPV), and considered the growing STD because the number of cases is on the rise. Like many STDs, the person may be asymptomatic. Small hard spots may grow 3 weeks to 3 months after the infection. Genital warts are suspected as a contributing factor in cervical, vulvar, and penile cancers.

Human papilloma virus

MITES AND LICE

Pubic lice and scabies mites are two of the most widespread STDs. Pubic lice are visible to the naked eye and are found anchored to the base of pubic hairs. They survive by feeding on blood. Scabies mites are highly contagious and move easily from host to host. They cause tiny gray scaly swellings between the fingers and on wrists, genitals, and axillae. Reddish lumps may appear later on the limbs and trunk. Both infections cause skin irritation and intense itching.

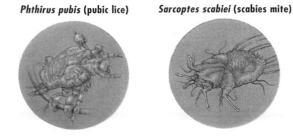

Phthirus pubis (pubic lice)   *Sarcoptes scabiei* (scabies mite)

Diabetes mellitus

WHAT IS DIABETES?
Diabetes is a group of chronic or life-long diseases that affect the way the body uses food to make the energy necessary for life. Primarily, diabetes is a disruption of carbohydrate (sugar and starch) metabolism that also affects fats and proteins. There are two main forms of diabetes (type 1 and type 2) as well as conditions of glucose intolerance, gestational diabetes, and diabetes caused by pancreatic disorders. Regardless of the form, metabolic control under a physician's care is essential for good health.

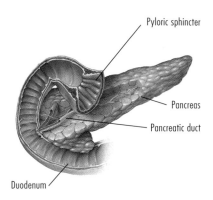

WHAT IS INSULIN?
Insulin is an essential hormone produced in the pancreas and released into the bloodstream. Insulin attaches itself to cells at places called insulin receptors. When attached, insulin allows sugar or glucose from the foods we eat to enter the liver, fat, and muscle cells, where it's used for energy.

Type 1 diabetes
Pancreas with no insulin production

TYPE 1 DIABETES MELLITUS
In type 1 diabetes, the pancreas produces little or no insulin. Without insulin, sugar can't enter the cells to be used for energy. The body's tissues are starved, and blood glucose levels grow dangerously high. The disorder usually begins in youth, but it may also occur in older adults. Type 1 diabetes accounts for 5% to 10% of patients with diabetes; these patients require insulin therapy.

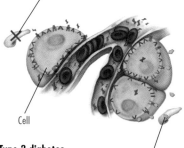

Cell

Type 2 diabetes
Pancreas producing little or ineffective insulin

TYPE 2 DIABETES MELLITUS
In type 2 diabetes, the pancreas produces insufficient or ineffective amounts of insulin and defective or insufficient insulin receptors, which control the transport of sugar into the cells. Type 2 diabetes typically develops in people over age 40. Most newly diagnosed patients with type 2 diabetes are overweight but can control their diabetes through diet and weight loss. Some patients may require oral medications or insulin injections to achieve glucose control.

Glucose
Closed glucose channel
Open glucose channel

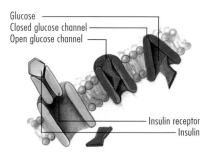

Insulin receptor
Insulin

GLUCOSE METABOLISM
1. Carbohydrates (sugars and starches) from the food we eat are broken down in the stomach and intestines into glucose.

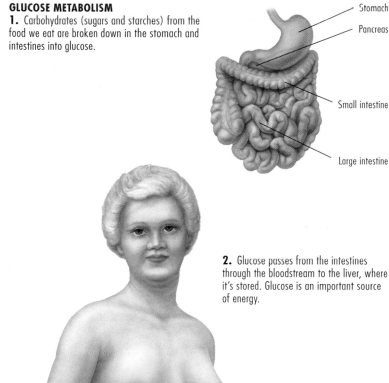

Stomach

Pancreas

Small intestine

Large intestine

2. Glucose passes from the intestines through the bloodstream to the liver, where it's stored. Glucose is an important source of energy.

Liver

Pancreas

3. The pancreas, through insulin, controls the amount of sugar stored in and released from the liver for use throughout the body.

(continued)

Diabetes mellitus (continued)

4. Insulin also controls the cells in the muscle fibers, fat, kidneys, and other organs. Without proper insulin levels, these cells don't absorb sugar from the bloodstream and don't receive enough nutrition.

Brain

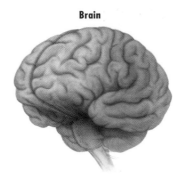

Kidney

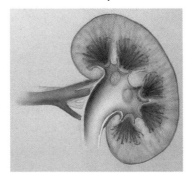

Muscle fiber

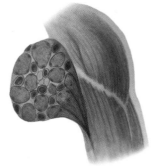

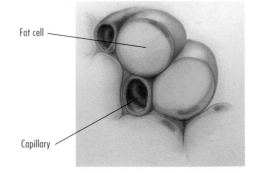

Fat cell

Capillary

LONG-TERM HEALTH PROBLEMS

High plasma glucose levels caused by diabetes may damage small and large blood vessels and nerves. Diabetes may also lower the body's ability to fight infection. As a result, people with diabetes are more likely to have serious eye problems, kidney disease, heart attacks, strokes, high blood pressure, poor circulation, tingling in hands and feet, sexual problems, amputations, and infections. Good diabetes control may help prevent these problems or make them less serious.

Loss of vision

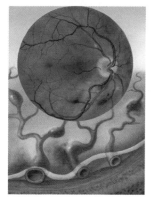

Nerve damage

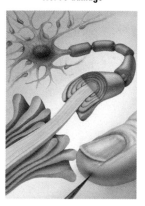

Kidney failure

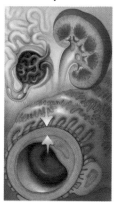

Heart disease

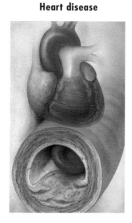

Poor circulation

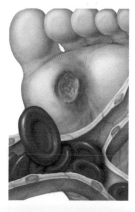

Metabolic syndrome

Metabolic syndrome is a group of conditions that occur as a cluster in one person. The cluster of conditions places the person at risk for developing coronary artery disease, stroke, and diabetes. About 25% of the population in the United States is believed to be affected by this syndrome.

The exact mechanism for this syndrome isn't known. Some studies suggest the syndrome is closely associated with a person's metabolism. Normally, food is absorbed into the bloodstream in the form of glucose and other substances. When glucose levels rise, the pancreas releases insulin. Insulin attaches to the body's cells allowing glucose to enter where it is used for energy. In some people, the body's cells are insulin resistant (don't respond). This insulin resistance is thought to be behind the development of metabolic syndrome.

COMPONENTS OF METABOLIC SYNDROME

Metabolic syndrome involves four conditions: obesity, high blood pressure, high blood glucose level, and an abnormal cholesterol profile. To be diagnosed with metabolic syndrome, a person must have at least three of the four conditions.

Brain

— Stroke

Heart

— Coronary artery disease

Pancreas

— Diabetes

High blood glucose level
Sugar builds up in the bloodstream causing organ system degeneration

High blood pressure
If untreated, damages the lining of the arteries

Fibrous plaque
Elevated cholesterol levels lead to fibrous plaque deposits in the · blood vessels

GH deficiency in children

SYNDROME	DESCRIPTION
Isolated growth hormone (GH) deficiency	Genetic disorder causing dwarfism if not treated with GH replacement
Neurosecretory failure	Idiopathic disorder with subnormal growth velocity and delayed bone age, but GH levels that exceed the limits for deficiency; variable response to GH replacement
Panhypopituitarism	GH and other trophic hormones deficient; all requiring replacement
Turner's syndrome	Chromosomal defect causing multiple abnormalities, decreased GH response to provocative stimuli and, possibly, increased target-organ resistance to GH or insulin-like growth factors; modest increases in height achieved with high doses of GH
Down syndrome	Chromosomal defect causing multiple abnormalities, including short stature; growth stimulated by GH replacement but quality of life isn't improved
Intrauterine growth retardation	Low birth weight; catch-up growth (usually occurring during the first year) to within acceptable standards; short stature in adults if absence of catch-up growth during the first year; growth stimulation possible with GH
Growth retardation	Short children with normal growth velocity and bone age; adult height at least 4" (10 cm) less than predicted from parents' heights; modest and inconsistent response to GH therapy
Familial short stature	Short children with normal growth velocity and bone age; adult height within range predicted from parents' heights; modest and inconsistent response to GH therapy
Constitutional delay of growth and development	Short children with delayed bone age but normal growth velocity and rates of bone age advancement
Chronic renal failure and renal transplantation	Children with slow growth but normal GH response and levels of insulin-like growth factor 1; height increases possible with GH therapy; however, increased risk of malignancy in patients taking immunosuppressive drugs

Adapted with permission from a report by the Drug and Therapeutics Committee of the Lawson Wilkins Pediatric Endocrine Society. "Guidelines for the Use of Growth Hormone in Children with Short Stature," *Journal of Pediatrics* 127(6):857-67, December 1995.

at least two stimuli for release of the hormone. (See *GH deficiency in children*.) GH deficiency in adults is characterized by general weakness and increased mortality.

CAUSES

Possible causes of GH deficiency include:
■ autosomal recessive, autosomal dominant, or X-linked trait

- pituitary or central nervous system tumor
- pituitary hypoxic necrosis
- pituitary inflammation
- hypothalamic failure
- GH receptor insensitivity
- biologically inactive GH
- hematologic disorders
- idiopathic causes
- trauma
- pituitary irradiation.

PATHOPHYSIOLOGY

The absence or deficiency of GH synthesis causes growth failure in children. In adults, metabolic derangements decrease GH response to stimulation.

SIGNS AND SYMPTOMS

Signs and symptoms of GH deficiency are related to the lack of the hormone production and include:

- short stature (two standard deviations less than the predicted mean for age and sex)
- reduced muscle mass and increased subcutaneous fat caused by decreased protein synthesis and insufficient muscle anabolism
- hypoglycemia (usually in neonates)
- delayed or lack of sexual development.

COMPLICATIONS

Complications of GH deficiency may include:

- short stature and possible related psychosocial difficulties (if untreated)
- fatal seizures, especially during periods of stress, caused by fasting hypoglycemia
- gonadotropin deficiency
- multiple pituitary hormone deficiencies
- increased cardiovascular mortality (adults).

DIAGNOSIS

Diagnosis of GH deficiency is based on:

- decreased levels of serum GH and somatomedin C (a metabolite of GH).

TREATMENT

Treatment of GH deficiency includes:

- exogenous GH given subcutaneously up to several times weekly during puberty.

Growth hormone excess

Growth hormone (GH) excess that begins in adulthood (after epiphyseal closure) is called *acromegaly*. GH excess that's present before closure of the epiphyseal growth plates of the long bones causes *pituitary gigantism*. In both cases, the result is increased growth of bone, cartilage, and other tissues as well as increased catabolism of carbohydrates and protein synthesis. Acromegaly is rare, with a prevalence of about 70 people per million in the United States. Most cases are diagnosed in people in their 30s and 40s, but acromegaly is usually present for years before diagnosis. GH excess is a slow but progressive disease that decreases longevity if untreated. Morbidity and mortality tend to be related to coronary artery disease and hypertension.

The earliest clinical sign of acromegaly is soft-tissue swelling of the extremities, which causes coarsening and hypertrophy of the facial features.

In gigantism, a proportional overgrowth of all body tissues starts before epiphyseal closure. This causes remarkable height increases — as much as 6" (15.2 cm) per year. Gigantism affects infants and children, causing them to reach as much as three times the normal height for their age. As adults, they may reach a height of more than 7′ 6″ (228.6 cm).

CAUSES

GH excess is caused by:

- eosinophilic or mixed-cell adenomas of the anterior pituitary gland.

PATHOPHYSIOLOGY

A GH-secreting tumor creates an unpredictable GH secretion pattern, which replaces the usual peaks that occur 1 to 4 hours after the onset of sleep. Elevated GH and somatomedin levels stimulate tissue growth. In pituitary gigantism, because the epiphyseal plates aren't closed, the excess GH stimulates linear growth. It also increases the bulk of bones and joints and causes enlargement of internal organs and metabolic abnormalities. In acromegaly, the excess GH increases bone density and width, and the proliferation of connective and soft tissues.

SIGNS AND SYMPTOMS

Acromegaly develops slowly, and gigantism is characterized by rapid growth. Signs and symptoms of acromegaly include:

- diaphoresis, oily skin, hypermetabolism, hypertrichosis (excessive hair growth), weakness, arthralgias, malocclusion of the teeth, and new skin tags (typical)
- severe headache, central nervous system impairment, bitemporal hemianopsia (defective vision), loss of visual acuity, and blindness (if the tumor compresses the optic chiasm or nerves)
- cartilaginous and connective tissue overgrowth, causing a characteristic hulking appearance, with an enlarged supraorbital ridge and thickened ears and nose
- marked prognathism (projection of the jaw) that may interfere with chewing
- laryngeal hypertrophy, paranasal sinus enlargement, and thickening of the tongue causing the voice to sound deep and hollow
- arrowhead appearance of distal phalanges on X-rays, thickened fingers
- irritability, hostility, and various psychological disturbances
- bowlegs, barrel chest, arthritis, osteoporosis, kyphosis, hypertension, and arteriosclerosis (prolonged effects of excessive GH secretion)
- glucose intolerance and clinical diabetes mellitus caused by action of GH as an insulin antagonist.

Signs and symptoms of gigantism include:

- backache, arthralgia, and arthritis caused by rapid bone growth
- excessive height caused by rapid growth before epiphyseal plate closure
- headache, vomiting, seizure activity, vision disturbances, and papilledema (edema where the optic nerve enters the eye chamber) caused by tumor compressing nerves and tissue in surrounding structures
- deficiencies of other hormone systems (if GH-producing tumor destroys other hormone-secreting cells)
- glucose intolerance and diabetes mellitus caused by insulin-antagonistic actions of GH.

COMPLICATIONS

Possible complications of GH excess are:

- cardiomegaly
- hypertension
- diabetes mellitus.

DIAGNOSIS

Diagnosis of GH excess is based on:

- elevated plasma GH level measured by radioimmunoassay (results of random blood sampling may be misleading owing to pulsatile GH secretion)
- somatomedin C, a metabolite of GH (a better diagnostic alternative)
- glucose suppression test (glucose normally suppresses GH secretion; if glucose infusion doesn't suppress GH to less than 2 ng/ml and the patient has characteristic clinical features, hyperpituitarism is likely)
- skull X-rays, computed tomography scan, or magnetic resonance imaging to show the presence and extent of pituitary lesion
- bone X-rays showing a thickening of the cranium (especially frontal, occipital, and parietal bones) and long bones, and osteoarthritis in the spine (support the diagnosis)
- elevated blood glucose levels.

TREATMENT

Treatment may involve:

- tumor removal by cranial or transsphenoidal hypophysectomy or pituitary radiation therapy
- mandatory surgery for a tumor causing blindness or other severe neurologic disturbances (acromegaly)
- replacement of thyroid, cortisone, and gonadal hormones (postoperative therapy)
- bromocriptine and octreotide to inhibit GH synthesis (adjunctive treatment).

Hyperaldosteronism

In hyperaldosteronism, hypersecretion of the mineralocorticoid aldosterone by the adrenal cortex causes excessive reabsorption of sodium and water and excessive renal excretion of potassium.

Incidence of hyperaldosteronism is three times as high in women as in men and is highest between ages 30 and 50.

CAUSES

Causes of hyperaldosteronism may include:

- benign aldosterone-producing adrenal adenoma, in 70% of patients
- bilateral adrenocortical hyperplasia (in children) or carcinoma (rarely).

In 15% to 30% of patients, the cause is unknown.

PATHOPHYSIOLOGY

Hyperaldosteronism may be primary (uncommon) or secondary. In primary hyperaldosteronism (Conn's syndrome), chronic excessive secretion of aldosterone is independent of the renin-angiotensin system and, in fact, suppresses plasma renin activity. This aldosterone excess enhances sodium and water reabsorption and potassium loss by the kidneys, which leads to mild hypernatremia and, simultaneously, hypokalemia and increased extracellular fluid volume. Expansion of intravascular fluid volume also occurs and results in volume-dependent hypertension and increased cardiac output. Excessive ingestion of English black licorice or licorice-like substances can produce a syndrome similar to primary hyperaldosteronism caused by the mineralocorticoid action of glycyrrhizic acid.

Secondary hyperaldosteronism results from an extra-adrenal abnormality that stimulates the adrenal gland to increase aldosterone production. For example, conditions that reduce renal blood flow (renal artery stenosis) and extracellular fluid volume or that produce a sodium deficit activate the renin-angiotensin system and, subsequently, increase aldosterone secretion. Thus, secondary hyperaldosteronism can result from conditions that induce hypertension through increased renin production (such as Wilms' tumor), ingestion of oral contraceptives, and pregnancy.

Secondary hyperaldosteronism may also result from disorders unrelated to edema, such as Bartter's syndrome and salt-losing nephritis; or those that induce edema, such as nephrotic syndrome, hepatic cirrhosis with ascites, and heart failure.

SIGNS AND SYMPTOMS

Most clinical effects of hyperaldosteronism result from hypokalemia, which increases neuromuscular irritability and produces:

- muscle weakness
- intermittent, flaccid paralysis
- fatigue
- headaches
- paresthesia
- possibly, tetany (resulting from metabolic alkalosis), which can lead to hypocalcemia.

Other characteristic findings include:

- vision disturbances
- loss of renal concentrating ability, resulting in nocturnal polyuria and polydipsia
- azotemia (an excess of urea or other nitrogenous compounds in the blood), indicating chronic potassium depletion nephropathy.

Diabetes mellitus is common, perhaps because hypokalemia interferes with normal insulin secretion. Hypertension and its accompanying complications are also common.

COMPLICATIONS

Complications of hyperaldosteronism include:

- neuromuscular irritability, tetany, paresthesia
- seizures
- left ventricular hypertrophy, heart failure, death
- metabolic alkalosis, nephropathy, azotemia.

DIAGNOSIS

In a nonedematous patient who isn't taking diuretics, doesn't have obvious GI losses (from vomiting or diarrhea), and has a normal sodium intake, persistently low serum potassium levels suggest hyperaldosteronism. If hypokalemia develops in a hypertensive patient shortly after starting treatment with potassium-wasting diuretics (such as thiazides), and if it persists after the diuretic has been discontinued and potassium replacement therapy has been instituted, evaluation for hyperaldosteronism is necessary.

- A low plasma renin level that fails to increase appropriately during volume depletion (upright posture, sodium depletion) and a high plasma aldosterone level during volume expansion by salt loading confirm primary hyperaldosteronism in a hypertensive patient without edema.

■ Serum bicarbonate level is usually elevated, with ensuing alkalosis caused by hydrogen and potassium ion loss in the distal renal tubules.

■ Other tests show markedly increased urine aldosterone levels, increased plasma aldosterone levels and, in secondary hyperaldosteronism, increased plasma renin levels.

■ A suppression test is useful to differentiate between primary and secondary hyperaldosteronism. During this test, the patient receives oral desoxycorticosterone for 3 days while plasma aldosterone levels and urine metabolites are continuously measured. These levels decrease in secondary hyperaldosteronism but remain the same in primary hyperaldosteronism. Simultaneously, renin levels are low in primary hyperaldosteronism and high in secondary hyperaldosteronism.

■ Other helpful diagnostic evidence includes an increase in plasma volume of 30% to 50% above normal, electrocardiogram signs of hypokalemia (ST-segment depression and U waves), chest X-ray showing left ventricular hypertrophy from chronic hypertension, and localization of the tumor by adrenal angiography or computed tomography scan.

TREATMENT

Although treatment of primary hyperaldosteronism may include unilateral adrenalectomy, administration of a potassium-sparing diuretic—spironolactone—and sodium restriction may control hyperaldosteronism without surgery. For bilateral adrenal hyperplasia, spironolactone is the drug of choice. Treatment of secondary hyperaldosteronism must include correction of the underlying cause.

Hyperparathyroidism

Hyperparathyroidism results from excessive secretion of parathyroid hormone (PTH) from one or more of the four parathyroid glands. PTH promotes bone resorption, and hypersecretion leads to hy-

percalcemia and hypophosphatemia. Renal and GI absorption of calcium increase.

Primary hyperparathyroidism is usually diagnosed based on elevated calcium levels found on laboratory test results in asymptomatic patients. It's two to three times more common in women than in men.

CAUSES

Hyperparathyroidism may be primary or secondary. In primary hyperparathyroidism:

■ one or more parathyroid glands enlarge and increase PTH secretion and serum calcium levels, most commonly caused by a single adenoma, but this may be a component of multiple endocrine neoplasia (all four glands usually involved).

In secondary hyperparathyroidism, a hypocalcemia-producing abnormality outside the parathyroids causes excessive compensatory production of PTH. Causes include:

■ rickets, vitamin D deficiency, chronic renal failure, and osteomalacia (inadequate mineralization of bone) caused by phenytoin.

PATHOPHYSIOLOGY

Overproduction of PTH by a tumor or hyperplastic tissue increases intestinal calcium absorption, reduces renal calcium clearance, and increases bone calcium release. Response to this excess varies for each patient for an unknown reason.

Hypophosphatemia results when excessive PTH inhibits renal tubular phosphate reabsorption. The hypophosphatemia aggravates hypercalcemia by increasing the sensitivity of the bone to PTH.

SIGNS AND SYMPTOMS

Signs and symptoms of primary hyperparathyroidism result from hypercalcemia and are typically present in several body systems. Signs and symptoms may include:

■ polyuria, nephrocalcinosis, nocturia, polydipsia, dehydration, uremia symptoms, renal colic pain, nephrolithiasis, and renal insufficiency

■ vague aches and pains, arthralgias, localized swellings

■ chronic lower back pain and easy fracturing caused by bone degeneration; bone tenderness; chondrocalcinosis (decreased bone mass); osteopenia and osteoporosis, especially on the vertebrae; erosions of the adjoining joint surface; subchondral fractures; traumatic synovitis; and pseudogout (skeletal and articular systems)

■ pancreatitis causing constant, severe epigastric pain that radiates to the back; peptic ulcers, causing abdominal pain, anorexia, nausea, and vomiting (GI system)

■ muscle weakness and atrophy, particularly in the legs (neuromuscular system)

■ psychomotor and personality disturbances, emotional lability, depression, slow mentation (mental activity), poor memory, drowsiness, ataxia, overt psychosis, stupor and, possibly, coma

■ pruritus caused by ectopic calcifications in the skin

■ skin necrosis, cataracts, calcium microthrombi to lungs and pancreas, anemia, and subcutaneous calcification (other systems).

Secondary hyperparathyroidism may produce the same features of calcium imbalance with skeletal deformities of the long bones (such as rickets) as well as symptoms of the underlying disease.

COMPLICATIONS

Complications of hyperparathyroidism include:

■ pathologic fractures
■ renal damage
■ urinary tract infections
■ hypertension
■ cardiac arrhythmias
■ insulin hypersecretion, decreased insulin sensitivity
■ pseudogout.

DIAGNOSIS

Findings differ in primary and secondary disease. In primary disease, diagnosis is based on:

■ hypercalcemia and high concentrations of serum PTH on radioimmunoassay (confirms the diagnosis)

■ X-rays showing diffuse demineralization of bones, bone cysts, outer cortical bone

absorption, and subperiosteal erosion of the phalanges and distal clavicles

■ microscopic bone examination by X-ray spectrophotometry typically showing increased bone turnover

■ elevated urine and serum calcium, chloride, and alkaline phosphatase levels; decreased serum phosphorus levels

■ elevated uric acid and creatinine levels, which may also increase basal gastric acid secretion and serum immunoreactive gastrin

■ increased serum amylase levels (may indicate acute pancreatitis).

Diagnosis of *secondary* disease is based on:

■ normal or slightly decreased serum calcium level, variable serum phosphorus level, especially when the cause is rickets, osteomalacia, or kidney disease

■ patient history possibly showing familial kidney disease, seizure disorders, or drug ingestion.

TREATMENT

Effective treatment varies, depending on the cause of the disease. In primary hyperparathyroidism, surgery is the only definitive therapy. The only effective long-term medical therapy is maintaining hydration in mild hyperparathyroidism.

Treatment of primary disease includes:

■ surgery to remove the adenoma or, depending on the extent of hyperplasia, all but one-half of one gland, to provide normal PTH levels (may relieve bone pain within 3 days, but renal damage may be irreversible)

CLINICAL ALERT
After a parathyroidectomy, calcium gluconate or calcium chloride I.V. should be readily available at the bedside for emergency administration should tetany occur.

■ treatments to decrease calcium levels, such as forcing fluids, limiting dietary intake of calcium, and promoting sodium and calcium excretion through forced diuresis, and use of furosemide or ethacrynic acid (preoperatively or if surgery isn't feasible or necessary)

■ oral sodium or potassium phosphate; subcutaneous calcitonin; I.V. plicamycin

- I.V. magnesium and phosphate or sodium phosphate solution by mouth or retention enema (for potential postoperative magnesium and phosphate deficiencies), possibly supplemental calcium, vitamin D, or calcitriol (serum calcium level decreases to low-normal range during the first 4 to 5 days after surgery).

Treatment of secondary disease includes:
- vitamin D to correct the underlying cause of parathyroid hyperplasia; aluminum hydroxide preparation to correct hyperphosphatemia in the patient with kidney disease
- dialysis in the patient with renal failure to decrease phosphorus levels (may be lifelong)
- enlarged glands may not revert to normal size and function even after calcium levels have been controlled in the patient with chronic secondary hyperparathyroidism
- for severe hypercalcemia (serum calcium greater than 14 mg/dl) or for the patient with severe symptoms, administration of calcitonin, a rapid-acting agent, along with hydration; possible initiation of pamidronate, a slower-acting agent, to provide a longer-lasting effect.

Hyperthyroidism

Hyperthyroidism, or thyrotoxicosis, is a metabolic imbalance that results from the overproduction of thyroid hormone. The most common form is Graves' disease, which increases thyroxine (T_4) production, enlarges the thyroid gland (goiter), and causes multiple system changes. (See *Other forms of hyperthyroidism.*)

AGE ALERT
The incidence of Graves' disease is highest in women between ages 30 and 60, especially those with a family history of thyroid abnormalities; only 5% of the patients are younger than age 15.

With treatment, most patients can lead normal lives, but thyroid storm — an acute, severe exacerbation of thyrotoxicosis — is a medical emergency that may have life-threatening cardiac, hepatic, or renal consequences.

Other forms of hyperthyroidism

◆ *Toxic adenoma,* a small, benign nodule in the thyroid gland that secretes thyroid hormone, is the second most common cause of hyperthyroidism. The cause of toxic adenoma is unknown; incidence is highest in elderly persons. Clinical effects are essentially similar to those of Graves' disease, except that toxic adenoma doesn't induce ophthalmopathy, pretibial myxedema, or acropachy. Presence of adenoma is confirmed by radioactive iodine (^{131}I) uptake and thyroid scan, which show a single hyperfunctioning nodule suppressing the rest of the gland. Treatment includes ^{131}I therapy, or surgery to remove adenoma after antithyroid drugs achieve a euthyroid (normal functioning) state.

◆ *Thyrotoxicosis factitia* results from chronic ingestion of thyroid hormone for thyrotropin suppression in patients with thyroid carcinoma, or from thyroid hormone abuse by people who are trying to lose weight.

◆ *Functioning metastatic thyroid carcinoma* is a rare disease that causes excess production of thyroid hormone.

◆ *Thyroid-stimulating hormone-secreting pituitary tumor* causes overproduction of thyroid hormone.

◆ *Subacute thyroiditis* is a virus-induced granulomatous inflammation of the thyroid, producing transient hyperthyroidism with fever, pain, pharyngitis, and tenderness in the thyroid gland.

◆ *Silent thyroiditis* is a self-limiting, transient form of hyperthyroidism, with histologic thyroiditis but no inflammatory symptoms.

CAUSES
Thyrotoxicosis may result from both genetic and immunologic factors, including:
- increased incidence in monozygotic twins, pointing to an inherited factor, probably autosomal recessive gene

- occasional coexistence with other endocrine abnormalities, such as type 1 diabetes mellitus, thyroiditis, and hyperparathyroidism
- defect in suppressor T-lymphocyte function permitting production of autoantibodies (thyroid-stimulating immunoglobulin and thyroidd-stimulating hormone [TSH]-binding inhibitory immunoglobulin)
- clinical thyrotoxicosis precipitated by excessive dietary intake of iodine or possibly stress (patients with latent disease)
- stress, such as surgery, infection, toxemia of pregnancy, or diabetic ketoacidosis, can precipitate thyroid storm (inadequately treated thyrotoxicosis)
- medications, such as lithium and amiodarone
- toxic nodules or tumors.

PATHOPHYSIOLOGY
The thyroid gland secretes thyroxine (T_4) or triiodothyronine (T_3), and calcitonin. T_4 and T_3 stimulate protein, lipid, and carbohydrate metabolism primarily through catabolic pathways. Calcitonin removes calcium from the blood and incorporates it into bone.

Biosynthesis, storage, and release of thyroid hormones are controlled by the hypothalamic-pituitary axis through a negative-feedback loop. Thyrotropin-releasing hormone (TRH) from the hypothalamus stimulates the release of TSH by the pituitary. Circulating T_3 levels provide negative feedback through the hypothalamus to decrease TRH levels, and through the pituitary to decrease TSH levels.

Although the exact mechanism isn't understood, hyperthyroidism has a hereditary component, and it's usually associated with other autoimmune endocrinopathies.

Graves' disease is an autoimmune disorder characterized by the production of autoantibodies that attach to and then stimulate TSH receptors on the thyroid gland. A goiter is an enlarged thyroid gland, either the result of increased stimulation or a response to increased metabolic demand. The latter occurs in iodine-deficient areas of the world, where the incidence of goiter increases during puberty (a time of increased metabolic demand). These goiters often regress to normal size after puberty in males, but not in females. Sporadic goiter in non-iodine-deficient areas is of unknown origin. Endemic and sporadic goiters are nontoxic and may be diffuse or nodular. Toxic goiters may be uninodular or multinodular and may secrete excess thyroid hormone.

Pituitary tumors with TSH-producing cells are rare, as is hypothalamic disease causing TRH excess.

SIGNS AND SYMPTOMS
Signs and symptoms of hyperthyroidism include:
- enlarged thyroid (goiter) resulting from of increased stimulation or a response to increased metabolic demand
- nervousness caused by hypermetabolic state
- heat intolerance and sweating caused by hypermetabolic state and subsequent increase in vasodilation
- weight loss, despite increased appetite, resulting from hypermetabolic state
- frequent bowel movements resulting from sympathetic nervous system stimulation and stimulation of gastrointestinal motility
- tremor and palpitations caused by increased sympathetic nervous system activity and possible increased sensitivity of neural synapses
- exophthalmos (characteristic, but absent in many patients with thyrotoxicosis).

Other signs and symptoms, common because thyrotoxicosis profoundly affects virtually every body system, include:
- difficulty concentrating caused by accelerated cerebral function; excitability or nervousness caused by increased basal metabolic rate from T_4; fine tremor, shaky handwriting, and clumsiness from increased activity in the spinal cord area that controls muscle tone; emotional instability and mood swings ranging from occasional outbursts to overt psychosis (central nervous system)
- moist, smooth, warm, flushed skin (patient sleeps with minimal covers and little clothing); fine, soft hair; premature patchy graying and increased hair loss in both sexes; friable nails and onycholysis (distal nail separated from the bed); pretibial myxede-

ma (nonpitting edema of the anterior surface of the legs, dermopathy), producing thickened skin; accentuated hair follicles; sometimes itchy or painful raised red patches of skin with occasional nodule formation; microscopic examination showing increased mucin deposits (skin, hair, and nails)
■ systolic hypertension, tachycardia, full bounding pulse, wide pulse pressure, cardiomegaly, increased cardiac output and blood volume, visible point of maximal impulse, paroxysmal supraventricular tachycardia and atrial fibrillation (especially in elderly people), and occasional systolic murmur at the left sternal border (cardiovascular)
■ increased respiratory rate, dyspnea on exertion and at rest, possibly caused by cardiac decompensation and increased cellular oxygen use (respiratory)
■ excessive oral intake with weight loss; nausea and vomiting caused by increased GI motility and peristalsis; increased defecation; soft stools or, in severe disease, diarrhea; liver enlargement (GI)
■ weakness, fatigue, and muscle atrophy; rare coexistence with myasthenia gravis; possibly generalized or localized paralysis associated with hypokalemia; and, rarely, acropachy (softt-tissue swelling accompanied by underlying bone changes where new bone formation occurs) (musculoskeletal)
■ oligomenorrhea or amenorrhea, decreased fertility, increased incidence of spontaneous abortion (women), gynecomastia caused by increased estrogen levels (men), diminished libido (both sexes) (reproductive)
■ exophthalmos caused by combined effects of accumulated mucopolysaccharides and fluids in the retro-orbital tissues, forcing the eyeball outward and lid retraction, thereby producing characteristic staring gaze; occasional inflammation of conjunctivae, corneas, or eye muscles; diplopia; and increased tearing (eyes).
Thyrotoxicosis can escalate to thyroid storm, a life-threatening medical emergency. Thyroid storm may present these symptoms:
■ extreme irritability, hypertension
■ high fever (up to 106° F [41.1° C])

■ tachycardia, pulmonary edema, shock
■ tremors, emotional lability, extreme irritability, confusion, delirium, psychosis, apathy, stupor, coma
■ diarrhea, abdominal pain, nausea and vomiting, jaundice, hyperglycemia.

AGE ALERT
Consider apathetic thyrotoxicosis, a morbid condition resulting from overactive thyroid, in elderly patients with atrial fibrillation or depression.

COMPLICATIONS
Possible complications include:
■ muscle wasting, atrophy, and paralysis
■ visual loss or diplopia
■ heart failure, arrhythmias
■ hypoparathyroidism after surgical removal of thyroid
■ hypothyroidism after radioiodine treatment.

DIAGNOSIS
Diagnosis of thyrotoxicosis is usually straightforward. It depends on a careful clinical history and physical examination, a high index of suspicion, and routine hormone determinations. The following tests confirm the disorder:
■ radioimmunoassay showing increased serum T_4 and T_3 levels
■ low TSH levels
■ thyroid scan showing increased uptake of radioactive iodine (^{131}I) in Graves' disease and, usually, in toxic multinodular goiter and toxic adenoma; low radioactive uptake in thyroiditis and thyrotoxic factitia (test contraindicated in pregnancy)
■ ultrasonography confirming subclinical ophthalmopathy.

TREATMENT
The primary forms of therapy include:
■ antithyroid drugs
■ single oral dose of ^{131}I (radioactive iodine) — treatment of choice for patients not planning to have children; patients of reproductive age must give informed consent for this treatment, because ^{131}I concentrates in the gonads)
■ surgery.
Appropriate treatment depends on:
■ severity of thyrotoxicosis
■ causes

- patient's age and parity
- how long surgery will be delayed (if patient is appropriate candidate for surgery).

Antithyroid therapy includes antithyroid drugs for children, young adults, pregnant women, and patients who refuse surgery or ^{131}I treatment. Antithyroid drugs are preferred in patients with new-onset Graves' disease because of spontaneous remission in many of these patients; these drugs are also used to correct the thyrotoxic state in preparation for ^{131}I treatment or surgery. Treatment options include:

- thyroid hormone antagonists, including propylthiouracil (PTU) and methimazole, to block thyroid hormone synthesis (hypermetabolic symptoms subside within 4 to 8 weeks after therapy begins, but remission of Graves' disease requires continued therapy for 6 months to 2 years)
- propranolol until antithyroid drugs reach their full effect, to manage tachycardia and other peripheral effects of excessive hypersympathetic activity resulting from blocking the conversion of T_4 to the active T_3 hormone
- minimum dosage needed to keep maternal thyroid function within the high-normal range until delivery, and to minimize the risk of fetal hypothyroidism; PTU is the preferred agent (during pregnancy)
- possibly antithyroid medications and propranolol for neonates for 2 to 3 months because most infants of hyperthyroid mothers are born with mild and transient thyrotoxicosis caused by placental transfer of thyroid-stimulating immunoglobulins (neonatal thyrotoxicosis)
- continuous control of maternal thyroid function because thyrotoxicosis is sometimes exacerbated in the puerperal period; antithyroid drugs gradually tapered and thyroid function reassessed after 3 to 6 months postpartum
- periodic checks of infant's thyroid function with a breast-feeding mother who is taking low-dose antithyroid treatment because of possible presence of small amounts of the drug in breast milk, which can rapidly lead to thyrotoxicity in the neonate

- single oral dose of ^{131}I (treatment of choice for patients not planning to have children; patients of reproductive age must give informed consent for this treatment, because ^{131}I concentrates in the gonads).

During treatment with ^{131}I, the thyroid gland picks up the radioactive element as it would regular iodine. The radioactivity destroys some of the cells that normally concentrate iodine and produce T_4, thus decreasing thyroid hormone production and normalizing thyroid size and function.

In most patients, hypermetabolic symptoms diminish 6 to 8 weeks after such treatment, but some patients may require a second dose. Almost all patients treated with ^{131}I eventually become hypothyroid.

Treatment with surgery includes:

- subtotal thyroidectomy to decrease the thyroid gland's capacity for hormone production (patients who refuse or aren't candidates for ^{131}I treatment)
- iodides (Lugol's solution or saturated solution of potassium iodide), antithyroid drugs, and propranolol to relieve hyperthyroidism preoperatively (if patient doesn't become euthyroid, surgery should be delayed, and antithyroid drugs and propranolol given to decrease the systemic effects [cardiac arrhythmias] of thyrotoxicosis)
- lifelong regular medical supervision because most patients become hypothyroid, sometimes as long as several years after surgery.

Treatment of ophthalmopathy includes:

- local application of topical medications, such as prednisone acetate suspension, but may require high doses of corticosteroids
- calcium channel blockers, such as diltiazem and verapamil, to block the peripheral effects of thyroid hormones
- external-beam radiation therapy or surgical decompression (severe exophthalmos causing pressure on optic nerve and orbital contents).

Emergency treatment of thyroid storm includes:

- antithyroid drug to stop conversion of T_4 to T_3 and to block sympathetic effect; corticosteroids to inhibit the conversion of T_4 to T_3; and iodide to block the release of thyroid hormone

- supportive measures, including the administration of nutrients, vitamins, fluids, oxygen, hypothermia blankets, and sedatives.

Hypoparathyroidism

Hypoparathyroidism is caused by disease, injury, or congenital malfunction of the parathyroid glands. Because the parathyroid glands primarily regulate calcium balance, hypoparathyroidism causes hypocalcemia and consequent neuromuscular symptoms ranging from paresthesia to tetany.

Parathyroid hormone (PTH) is regulated directly by serum calcium levels, not by the pituitary or hypothalamus. PTH normally maintains normocalcemia by regulating bone resorption and GI absorption of calcium. It also maintains an inverse relationship between serum calcium and phosphate levels by inhibiting phosphate reabsorption in the renal tubules.

The clinical effects of hypoparathyroidism are usually correctable with replacement therapy. Some complications of long-term hypocalcemia, such as cataracts and basal ganglion calcifications, are irreversible.

CAUSES
Hypoparathyroidism may be acute or chronic and is classified as idiopathic or acquired. Possible causes include:
- acute pancreatitis or malabsorption
- renal failure
- osteomalacia
- autoimmune genetic disorder or congenital absence of the parathyroid glands (idiopathic)
- accidental removal of or injury to the parathyroid glands during thyroidectomy or other neck surgery or, rarely, from massive thyroid irradiation (acquired)
- ischemic infarction of the parathyroid glands during surgery, amyloidosis, neoplasms, or trauma (acquired)
- impairment of hormone synthesis and release caused by hypomagnesemia, suppression of normal gland function caused by hypercalcemia, and delayed maturation of parathyroid function (acquired, reversible).

AGE ALERT
The incidence of the idiopathic and reversible forms of hypoparathyroidism is greatest in children; the incidence of the irreversible acquired form is greatest in adults who have undergone surgery for hyperthyroidism or other head and neck conditions.

PATHOPHYSIOLOGY
Underproduction of PTH causes hypocalcemia and hyperphosphatemia. Surgical manipulation of the neck may damage the parathyroid glands, possibly by causing ischemia. The degree of hypoparathyroidism can vary from decreased PTH reserve to frank tetany. Hypomagnesemia can prevent PTH secretion in patients with chronic GI magnesium losses, nutritional deficiencies, and renal magnesium wasting.

SIGNS AND SYMPTOMS
Mild hypoparathyroidism may be asymptomatic but usually causes:
- hypocalcemia and high serum phosphate levels affecting the central nervous system (CNS) and other systems.

Signs and symptoms of chronic hypoparathyroidism include:
- neuromuscular irritability, increased deep tendon reflexes, Chvostek's sign (spasm of the hyperirritable facial nerve when it's tapped), dysphagia, organic brain syndrome, psychosis, mental deficiency in children, and tetany caused by hypocalcemia and hyperphosphatemia
- difficulty walking and a tendency to fall (chronic tetany).

Signs and symptoms of acute hypoparathyroidism include:
- tingling in the fingertips, around the mouth, and occasionally in the feet (first symptom); spreading and becoming more severe, producing muscle tension and spasms and consequent adduction of the thumbs, wrists, and elbows; pain varying with the degree of muscle tension but seldom affecting the face, legs, and feet (acute overt tetany)
- laryngospasm, stridor, cyanosis, and seizures (CNS abnormalities); worst during hyperventilation, pregnancy, infection, withdrawal of thyroid hormone, or ad-

ministration of diuretics, and before menstruation (acute tetany)

■ abdominal pain; intestinal malabsorption with steatorrhea (excessive amounts of fat in the feces); dry, lusterless hair; spontaneous hair loss; brittle fingernails developing ridges or falling out; dry, scaly skin; exfoliative dermatitis; candidal infections; cataracts; and weakened tooth enamel, causing teeth to stain, crack, and decay easily (effects of hypocalcemia).

COMPLICATIONS

Possible complications include:
■ cardiac arrhythmias, heart failure
■ cataracts
■ basal ganglia calcifications
■ stunted growth, teeth malformation, and mental retardation
■ parkinsonian symptoms
■ hypothyroidism.

DIAGNOSIS

The following test results confirm the diagnosis of hypoparathyroidism:
■ radioimmunoassay for PTH showing decreased serum PTH level
■ decreased serum and urine calcium level
■ increased serum phosphorus level
■ reduced serum creatinine level
■ electrocardiography showing prolonged QT and ST intervals caused by hypocalcemia
■ inflating a blood pressure cuff on the upper arm to between diastolic and systolic blood pressure and maintaining this inflation for 3 minutes, eliciting Trousseau's sign (carpal spasm), to show clinical evidence of hypoparathyroidism.

TREATMENT

Treatment of hypoparathyroidism includes:
■ immediate I.V. calcium salts, such as 10% calcium gluconate, to increase ionized serum calcium levels (acute, life-threatening tetany)
■ breathing into a paper bag and inhaling one's own carbon dioxide causes a mild respiratory acidosis that increases serum calcium levels (awake patient can cooperate)
■ sedatives and anticonvulsants to control spasms until calcium levels increase

■ increased dietary intake of calcium
■ maintenance therapy with oral calcium and vitamin D supplements (chronic tetany)
■ vitamin D and calcium supplements because of calcium absorption from the small intestine requiring the presence of vitamin D (treatment of reversible disease, usually lifelong)
■ calcitriol if hepatic or renal problems make the patient unable to tolerate vitamin D.

Hypopituitarism

Hypopituitarism, also known as *panhypopituitarism,* is a complex syndrome marked by metabolic dysfunction, sexual immaturity, and growth retardation (when it occurs in childhood). The cause is a deficiency of the hormones secreted by the anterior pituitary gland. Panhypopituitarism is a partial or total failure of all six of this gland's vital hormones — corticotropin, thyroid-stimulating hormone (TSH), luteinizing hormone (LH), follicle-stimulating hormone (FSH), human growth hormone, and prolactin. Partial and complete forms of hypopituitarism affect adults and children; in children, these diseases may cause dwarfism and delayed puberty. The prognosis may be good with adequate replacement therapy and correction of the underlying causes.

Primary hypopituitarism usually develops in a predictable pattern. It generally starts with decreased gonadotropin (FSH and LH) levels and consequent hypogonadism. Growth hormone deficiency causes short stature, delayed growth, and delayed puberty in children. Decreased TSH levels cause hypothyroidism and, finally, decreased corticotropin levels result in adrenal insufficiency. When hypopituitarism follows surgical ablation or trauma, the pattern of hormonal events may not necessarily follow that sequence. Damage to the hypothalamus or neurohypophysis may cause diabetes insipidus.

CAUSES

Hypopituitarism may be primary or secondary. Primary hypopituitarism may be caused by:
■ tumor of the pituitary gland

■ congenital defects (hypoplasia or aplasia of the pituitary gland)
■ pituitary infarction (in women most commonly from postpartum hemorrhage)
■ partial or total hypophysectomy by surgery, irradiation, or chemical agents
■ granulomatous disease such as tuberculosis (rare)
■ idiopathic or autoimmune origin (occasionally).

Secondary hypopituitarism is caused by:
■ deficiency of releasing hormones produced by the hypothalamus, either idiopathic or resulting from infection, trauma, or a tumor.

PATHOPHYSIOLOGY
Hypopituitarism describes the abnormally low secretion of an anterior pituitary hormone, and panhypopituitarism describes the abnormally low secretion of all anterior pituitary hormones. Both can result from malfunction of the pituitary gland or the hypothalamus. The result is a lack of stimulation of target endocrine organs and some degree of deficiency of the target organ hormone, which may not be discovered until the body is stressed and the expected increases in secretions from the target organs don't occur.

SIGNS AND SYMPTOMS
Signs and symptoms of hypopituitarism include:
■ corticotropin deficiency, causing weakness, fatigue, weight loss, fasting hypoglycemia, altered mental function, and depigmentation of skin caused by hypercortisolism; loss of axillary and pubic hair caused by androgen deficiency in females; orthostatic hypotension and hyponatremia caused by aldosterone deficiency
■ TSH deficiency, causing weight gain, constipation, cold intolerance, fatigue, coarse hair, and slow thought process; growth retardation in children
■ gonadotropin (FSH and LH) deficiency, causing sexual dysfunction and infertility
■ antidiuretic hormone deficiency, causing diabetes insipidus
■ prolactin deficiency, causing lactation dysfunction or gynecomastia.

COMPLICATIONS
Possible complications include:
■ blindness due to pressure on optic nerve from invading tumor
■ adrenal crisis.

DIAGNOSIS
Diagnosis of hypopituitarism includes:
■ hormonal deficiency of the tropic and target organ hormones affected, chosen after evaluation of clinical picture
■ hypoglycemia (caused by insulin administration) stimulating secretion of corticotropin (consistently low levels of corticotropin indicate pituitary and hypothalamic failure)
■ computed tomography or magnetic resonance imaging of pituitary and target glands, showing destruction of the anterior pituitary or atrophy of target glands (adrenal cortex, thyroid, or gonads).

TREATMENT
The most effective treatment of hypopituitarism is:
■ replacement of hormones secreted by the target glands (cortisol, thyroxine, and androgen or cyclic estrogen); prolactin not replaced
■ clomiphene or cyclic gonadotropin-releasing hormone to induce ovulation in the patient of reproductive age.

Hypothyroidism in adults
Hypothyroidism results from hypothalamic, pituitary, or thyroid insufficiency or resistance to thyroid hormone. The disorder can progress to life-threatening myxedema coma. Hypothyroidism is more prevalent in women than men; in the United States, the incidence is increasing significantly in people ages 40 to 50.

▲ **AGE ALERT**
Hypothyroidism occurs primarily after age 40. After age 65, the prevalence increases to as much as 10% in women and 3% in men.

CAUSES
Causes of hypothyroidism in adults include:
■ inadequate production of thyroid hormone, usually after thyroidectomy or radiation therapy (particularly with

Clinical findings in acquired hypothyroidism

Typical findings in acquired hypothyroidism are listed below:

HISTORY
◆ Arthritis
◆ Cold intolerance
◆ Constipation
◆ Decreased sociability
◆ Drowsiness
◆ Dry skin
◆ Fatigue
◆ Lethargy
◆ Memory impairment
◆ Menstrual disorders
◆ Muscle cramps
◆ Psychosis
◆ Somnolence
◆ Weakness

PHYSICAL EXAMINATION
◆ Anemia
◆ Bradycardia
◆ Brittle hair
◆ Cool skin
◆ Delayed relaxation of reflexes
◆ Dementia
◆ Dry skin
◆ Gravelly voice
◆ Hypothermia
◆ Large tongue
◆ Loss of lateral third of eyebrow
◆ Puffy face and hands
◆ Slow speech
◆ Weight changes

Adapted with permission from Martinez, M., et al. "Making Sense of Hypothyroidism: An Approach to Testing and Treatment," *Postgraduate Medicine* 93(6):143, May 1993.

ciency (usually dietary), or use of such antithyroid medications as propylthiouracil.

PATHOPHYSIOLOGY
Hypothyroidism may reflect a malfunction of the hypothalamus, pituitary, or thyroid gland, all of which are part of the same negative-feedback mechanism, but disorders of the hypothalamus and pituitary rarely cause hypothyroidism. Primary hypothyroidism, a disorder of the gland itself, is most common.

Chronic autoimmune thyroiditis, also called *chronic lymphocytic thyroiditis,* occurs when autoantibodies destroy thyroid gland tissue. Chronic autoimmune thyroiditis associated with goiter is called *Hashimoto's thyroiditis.* The cause of this autoimmune process is unknown, although heredity has a role, and specific human leukocyte antigen subtypes are associated with greater risk.

Outside the thyroid, antibodies can reduce the effect of thyroid hormone in two ways. First, antibodies can block the thyroid-stimulating hormone (TSH) receptor and prevent the production of TSH. Second, cytotoxic antithyroid antibodies may attack thyroid cells.

SIGNS AND SYMPTOMS
Signs and symptoms of hypothyroidism include:
■ weakness, fatigue, forgetfulness, sensitivity to cold, unexplained weight gain, and constipation (typical, vague, early clinical features) (see *Clinical findings in acquired hypothyroidism*)
■ characteristic signs and symptoms of myxedema: coarse, dry, flaky, inelastic skin; puffy face, hands, and feet; hoarseness; periorbital edema; upper eyelid droop; dry, sparse hair; and thick, brittle nails
■ cardiovascular involvement, including decreased cardiac output, slow pulse rate, signs of poor peripheral circulation and, occasionally, an enlarged heart.

Other common effects include:
■ anorexia, abdominal distention, menorrhagia, decreased libido, infertility, ataxia, and nystagmus; reflexes with delayed relaxation time (especially in the Achilles tendon)

iodine 131 [^{131}I]), or caused by inflammation, chronic autoimmune thyroiditis (Hashimoto's disease), or such conditions as amyloidosis and sarcoidosis (rare)
■ pituitary failure to produce TSH, hypothalamic failure to produce thyrotropin-releasing hormone (TRH), inborn errors of thyroid hormone synthesis, iodine defi-

Thyroid test results in hypothyroidism

DYSFUNCTION INVOLVES	THYROTROPIN-RELEASING HORMONE	THYROID-STIMULATING HORMONE	TH (T_3 AND T_4)
Hypothalamus	Low	Low	Low
Pituitary gland	High	Low	Low
Thyroid gland	High	High	Low
Peripheral conversion of thyroid hormone (TH)	High	Low or normal	T_3 and T_4 low, but reverse T_3 elevated

■ progression to myxedema coma, which is usually gradual but may develop abruptly, with stress aggravating severe or prolonged hypothyroidism, including progressive stupor, hypoventilation, hypoglycemia, hyponatremia, hypotension, and hypothermia.

COMPLICATIONS
Possible complications include:
■ heart failure
■ myxedema coma
■ infection
■ megacolon
■ organic psychosis
■ infertility.

DIAGNOSIS
Diagnosis of hypothyroidism is based on:
■ radioimmunoassay showing low triiodothyronine (T_3) and thyroxine (T_4) levels
■ increased TSH level with the cause of thyroid disorder; decreased level with hypothalamic or pituitary disorder cause
■ thyroid panel differentiating primary hypothyroidism (thyroid gland hypofunction), secondary hypothyroidism (pituitary hyposecretion of TSH), tertiary hypothyroidism (hypothalamic hyposecretion of TRH), and euthyroid sick syndrome (impaired peripheral conversion of thyroid hormone caused by a suprathy-

roidal illness such as severe infection) (see *Thyroid test results in hypothyroidism*)
■ elevated serum cholesterol, alkaline phosphatase, and triglyceride levels
■ normocytic, normochromic anemia
■ low serum sodium levels, decreased blood pH, and increased partial pressure of carbon dioxide, indicating respiratory acidosis (myxedema coma).

TREATMENT
Treatment includes:
■ gradual thyroid hormone replacement with synthetic T_4 and, occasionally, T_3

▲ **AGE ALERT**
Elderly patients should initially be given a very low dose of T_4 to avoid cardiac problems; TSH levels guide gradual increases in dosage.

■ surgical excision, chemotherapy, or radiation
■ supportive care if the patient develops myxedema coma.

Hypothyroidism in children

A deficiency of thyroid hormone secretion during fetal development and early infancy results in infantile cretinism (congenital hypothyroidism). Hypothyroidism in infants is seen as respiratory difficulties, cyanosis, persistent jaundice, lethargy, somnolence, large tongue, abdominal distention, poor feeding, and hoarse crying. Prompt treatment of hypothyroidism in infants prevents physical and mental retardation. Older children who become hypothyroid have similar symptoms to those of adults, plus poor skeletal growth and late epiphyseal maturation and dental development. Sexual maturation may be accelerated in younger children and delayed in older children.

Cretinism is three times more common in girls than boys. Early diagnosis and treatment allow the best prognosis; infants treated before age 3 months usually grow and develop normally. Athyroid children who remain untreated beyond age 3 months, and children with acquired hypothyroidism who remain untreated beyond age 2 years, have irreversible mental retardation; their skeletal abnormalities are reversible with treatment. Mental retardation can be prevented by appropriate treatment if child acquires hypothyroidism after age 2 years.

CAUSES
Causes include:
- defective embryonic development (most common cause), causing congenital absence or underdevelopment of the thyroid gland (cretinism in infants)
- inherited autosomal recessive defect in the synthesis of thyroxine (next most common cause)
- antithyroid drugs taken during pregnancy, causing cretinism in infants (less common)
- chronic autoimmune thyroiditis (cretinism after age 2 years)
- iodine deficiency during pregnancy.

PATHOPHYSIOLOGY
Hypothyroidism in infants and children is related to decreased thyroid hormone production or secretion. Loss of functional thyroid tissue can be caused by an autoimmune process. Defective thyroid synthesis may be related to congenital defects, with thyroid dysgenesis (defective development) the most common. Iodine deficiency or antithyroid drugs used by the mother during pregnancy can also contribute. Hypothyroidism may also be related to decreased thyroid-stimulating hormone (TSH) secretion or resistance to TSH.

SIGNS AND SYMPTOMS
Signs and symptoms include:
- infant with infantile cretinism will have normal weight and length at birth, with characteristic signs developing within 3 to 6 months; delayed onset of most symptoms until weaning from breast-feeding because of small amounts of thyroid hormone in breast milk
- typically, an infant with cretinism sleeps excessively, seldom cries (except for occasional hoarse crying), and is inactive; parents may describe the infant as a "good baby—no trouble at all" (behavior actually caused by reduced metabolism and progressive mental impairment)
- abnormal deep tendon reflexes, hypotonic abdominal muscles, protruding abdomen, and slow, awkward movements
- feeding difficulties; constipation; jaundice because the immature liver can't conjugate bilirubin
- large, protruding tongue obstructing respiration; loud and noisy breathing through open mouth; dyspnea on exertion; anemia; abnormal facial features, such as a short forehead, puffy wide-set eyes (periorbital edema), wrinkled eyelids, a broad short and upturned nose, and a dull expression reflecting mental retardation
- cold, mottled skin caused by poor circulation; and dry, brittle, and dull hair
- teeth erupting late and decaying early, below-normal body temperature, and slow pulse rate
- growth retardation shown as short stature, caused by delayed epiphyseal maturation, particularly in the legs; obesity; head appearing abnormally large because of stunted arms and legs; delayed or accelerated sexual development.

COMPLICATIONS
Complications include:
- skeletal malformations and irreversible mental retardation (for hypothyroid infant not treated by age 3 months; early treatment helps prevent retardation)
- learning disabilities
- accelerated or delayed sexual maturation.

DIAGNOSIS
Diagnosis is based on:

- elevated TSH level linked to low T_3 and T_4 levels pointing to cretinism (because early detection and treatment can minimize the effects of cretinism, many states require measurement of infant thyroid hormone levels at birth)
- thyroid scan and ^{131}I uptake tests showing decreased uptake and confirming the absence of thyroid tissue in athyroid children
- increased gonadotropin levels compatible with sexual precocity in older children may coexist with hypothyroidism
- electrocardiogram showing bradycardia and flat or inverted T waves in untreated infants
- hip, knee, and thigh X-rays showing absence of the femoral or tibial epiphyseal line and markedly delayed skeletal development relative to chronological age
- low T_4 and normal TSH levels suggesting hypothyroidism caused by hypothalamic or pituitary disease (rare).

TREATMENT
Early detection is mandatory to prevent irreversible mental retardation and permit normal physical development. Treatment includes:

- oral levothyroxine, beginning with moderate doses and gradually increasing to levels sufficient for lifelong maintenance (rapid increase in dosage may precipitate thyrotoxicity); children require proportionately higher doses than adults because children metabolize thyroid hormone more quickly.

Simple goiter
Simple (or nontoxic) goiter is a thyroid gland enlargement that isn't caused by inflammation or a neoplasm and is commonly classified as endemic or sporadic. Inherited defects may be responsible for insufficient thyroxine (T_4) synthesis or impaired iodine metabolism. Because families tend to congregate in a single geographic area, this familial factor may contribute to the incidence of endemic and sporadic goiters.

Simple goiter affects more females than males, especially during adolescence, pregnancy, and menopause, when the body's demand for thyroid hormone increases. Sporadic goiter affects no particular population segment. With appropriate treatment, the prognosis is good.

CAUSES
Causes of endemic goiter include inadequate dietary iodine. Causes of sporadic goiter include:

- ingestion of large amounts of foods containing agents that inhibit T_4 production, such as rutabagas, cabbage, soybeans, peanuts, peaches, peas, strawberries, spinach, and radishes
- ingestion by a pregnant woman of certain drugs, such as propylthiouracil, iodides, para-aminosalicylic acid, phenylbutazone, cobalt, and lithium, which may cross the placenta and affect the fetus.

PATHOPHYSIOLOGY
Goiters can occur in the presence of hypothyroidism, hyperthyroidism, or normal levels of thyroid hormone. In the presence of a severe underlying disorder, compensatory responses may cause both thyroid enlargement (goiter) and hypothyroidism. Simple goiter occurs when the thyroid gland can't secrete enough thyroid hormone to meet metabolic requirements. As a result, the thyroid gland enlarges to compensate for inadequate hormone synthesis, a compensation that usually overcomes mild to moderate hormonal impairment.

Endemic goiter usually results from inadequate secretion of thyroid hormone caused by inadequate dietary intake of iodine associated with such factors as iodine-depleted soil or malnutrition. Since the introduction of iodized salt in the United States, cases of endemic goiter have virtually disappeared.

Sporadic goiter is triggered by certain drugs or foods that inhibit or block production of thyroid hormones.

SIGNS AND SYMPTOMS
Thyroid enlargement may range from a mildly enlarged gland to a massive, multinodular goiter. (See *Massive goiter,* page 488.)

Massive goiter

Massive multinodular goiter causes gross distention and swelling of the neck.

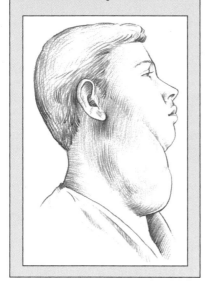

COMPLICATIONS

Because simple goiter doesn't alter the patient's metabolic state, complications arise solely from enlargement of the thyroid gland compressing adjacent tissues, and include:
- respiratory distress
- dysphagia
- venous engorgement; development of collateral venous circulation in the chest
- congestion of the face, some cyanosis and, lastly, distress when the patient raises her arms until they touch the side of her head.

DIAGNOSIS

Diagnosis of simple goiter requires a thorough patient history and physical examination to rule out disorders with similar clinical effects, such as Graves' disease, Hashimoto's thyroiditis, and thyroid carcinoma. A detailed patient history may also reveal goitrogenic medications or foods or endemic influence. The results of diagnostic laboratory tests include the following:

- serum thyroid levels — normal
- TSH — high or normal levels
- serum T_4 concentrations — low-normal or normal
- ^{131}I uptake — normal or increased (50% of the dose at 24 hours).

TREATMENT

The goal of treatment is to reduce thyroid hyperplasia.
- Exogenous thyroid hormone replacement with levothyroxine (treatment of choice) inhibits TSH secretion and allows the gland to rest.
- Small doses of iodide (Lugol's iodine or potassium iodide solution) commonly relieves goiter caused by iodine deficiency.
- Avoidance of known goitrogenic drugs and foods is recommended.
- For large goiter that's unresponsive to treatment, subtotal thyroidectomy may be necessary.

Syndrome of inappropriate antidiuretic hormone

Syndrome of inappropriate antidiuretic hormone (SIADH) results when excessive ADH secretion is triggered by stimuli other than increased extracellular fluid osmolarity and decreased extracellular fluid volume, reflected by hypotension. SIADH is a relatively common complication of surgery or critical illness. The prognosis varies with the degree of disease and the speed at which it develops. SIADH usually resolves within 3 days of effective treatment.

CAUSES

The most common cause of SIADH is oat cell carcinoma of the lung, which secretes excessive levels of ADH or vasopressin-like substances. Other neoplastic diseases — such as pancreatic and prostatic cancer, Hodgkin's disease, thymoma (tumor on the thymus), and renal carcinoma — may also trigger SIADH.

Less common causes include:
- central nervous system disorders, including brain tumor or abscess, stroke, head injury, and Guillain-Barré syndrome
- pulmonary disorders, including pneumonia, tuberculosis, lung abscess, asper-

gillosis, bronchiectasis, and positive-pressure ventilation
- drugs that either increase ADH production or potentiate ADH action, such as antidepressants, nonsteroidal anti-inflammatory drugs, chlorpropamide, vincristine, cyclophosphamide, carbamazepine, clofibrate, metoclopramide, and morphine
- other conditions, including psychosis, myxedema, acquired immunodeficiency syndrome, physiologic stress, and pain.

PATHOPHYSIOLOGY
In the presence of excessive ADH, excessive water reabsorption from the distal convoluted tubule and collecting ducts causes hyponatremia and normal to slightly increased extracellular fluid volume.

SIGNS AND SYMPTOMS
Signs and symptoms of SIADH include:
- thirst, anorexia, fatigue, and lethargy (first signs), followed by vomiting and intestinal cramping caused by hyponatremia and electrolyte imbalance manifestations
- weight gain, edema, water retention and decreased urine output caused by hyponatremia
- additional neurologic symptoms, such as restlessness, confusion, anorexia, headache, irritability, decreasing reflexes, seizures, and coma, caused by electrolyte imbalances, worsening with the degree of water intoxication
- decreased deep tendon reflexes resulting from central nervous system effects of water and electrolyte imbalances.

COMPLICATIONS
Complications of SIADH include:
- cerebral edema
- brain herniation
- central pontine myelinosis.

DIAGNOSIS
SIADH is diagnosed by the following laboratory results:
- serum osmolality less than 280 mOsm/kg of water
- hyponatremia (serum sodium less than 135 mEq/L [135 mmol/L]); lower values indicating worse condition

- elevated urinary sodium level (more than 20 mEq/L [20 mmol/L]) and increased osmolality (greater than 150 mOsm/kg)
- elevated serum ADH level
- normal blood urea nitrogen levels.

TREATMENT
Treatment of SIADH includes:
- restricted water intake (500 to 1,000 ml/day) (symptomatic treatment)
- administration of 200 to 300 ml of 3% saline solution to slowly and steadily increase serum sodium level (severe water intoxication); if too rapid a rise, cerebral edema may result
- correction of underlying cause of SIADH when possible
- surgical resection, irradiation, or chemotherapy to alleviate water retention for SIADH resulting from cancer
- demeclocycline to block the renal response to ADH (if fluid restriction is ineffective)
- furosemide with normal or hypertonic saline to maintain urine output and block ADH secretion.

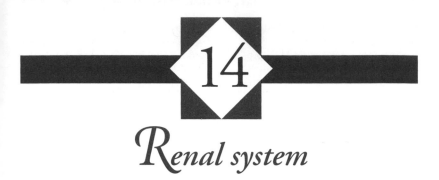

Renal system

The components of the renal system are the kidneys, ureters, bladder, and urethra. The kidneys, located retroperitoneally (behind the peritoneum) in the lumbar area, produce and excrete urine to maintain homeostasis. They regulate the volume, electrolyte concentration, and acid-base balance of body fluids; detoxify the blood and eliminate wastes; regulate blood pressure; and support red blood cell production (erythropoiesis). The ureters are tubes that extend from the kidneys to the bladder; their only function is to carry urine to the bladder. The bladder is a muscular bag that serves as reservoir for urine until it leaves the body through the urethra.

PATHOPHYSIOLOGIC CHANGES

Wastes are eliminated from the body by urine formation—glomerular filtration, tubular reabsorption, and tubular secretion—and excretion. Glomerular filtration is the process of filtering the blood as it flows through the kidneys. The glomerulus of the renal tubule filters plasma and then reabsorbs the filtrate. Glomerular function depends on the permeability of the capillary walls, vascular pressure, and filtration pressure. The normal glomerular filtration rate (GFR) is about 120 ml/minute. To prevent too much fluid from leaving the vascular system, tubular reabsorption opposes capillary filtration. Reab-

sorption takes place as capillary filtration progresses. When fluid filters through the capillaries, albumin, which doesn't pass through capillary walls, remains behind. As the albumin concentration inside the capillaries increases, the capillaries begin to draw water back in by osmosis. This osmotic force controls the quantities of water and diffusible solutes that enter and leave the capillaries.

Anything that affects filtration or reabsorption affects total filtration effort. Capillary pressure and interstitial fluid colloid osmotic pressure affect filtration. Interstitial fluid pressure and plasma colloid osmotic pressure affect reabsorption.

Altered renal perfusion; renal disease affecting the vessels, glomeruli, or tubules; or obstruction to urine flow can slow the GFR. The results are retention of nitrogenous wastes (azotemia), such as blood urea nitrogen (BUN) and creatinine, which can lead to acute renal failure.

Capillary pressure

The renal arteries branch into five segmental arteries, which supply different areas of the kidneys. The segmental arteries then branch into several divisions from which the afferent arterioles and vasa recta arise. Renal veins follow a similar branching pattern—characterized by stellate vessels and segmental branches—and empty into the inferior vena cava. The tubular system receives its blood supply from a peritubular capillary network. The ureteral veins follow the arteries and drain into the renal vein. The bladder receives blood through vesical arteries. Vesical veins unite to form the pudendal plexus, which empties into the iliac veins. A rich lymphatic system drains the renal cortex, kidneys, ureters, and bladder.

Capillary pressure reflects mean arterial pressure (MAP). Increased MAP increases capillary pressure, which in turn increases the GFR. When MAP decreases, so do capillary pressure and GFR. Autoregulation of afferent and efferent arterioles minimizes and controls changes in capillary pressure, unless MAP exceeds 180 mm Hg or is less than 80 mm Hg.

The kidneys are innervated by sympathetic branches from the celiac plexus, upper lumbar splanchnic and thoracic nerves, and the intermesenteric and superior hypogastric plexuses, which surround the kidneys. Similar numbers of sympathetic and parasympathetic nerves from the renal plexus, superior hypogastric plexus, and intermesenteric plexus innervate the ureters. Nerves that arise from the inferior hypogastric plexus innervate the bladder. The parasympathetic nerve supply to the bladder controls urination.

Increased sympathetic activity and angiotensin II constrict afferent and efferent arterioles, decreasing the capillary pressure. Because these changes affect both the afferent and efferent arterioles, they have no net effect on GFR.

Inadequate renal perfusion accounts for 40% to 80% of acute renal failure. Volume loss (as with GI hemorrhage, burns, diarrhea, and diuretic use), volume sequestration (as in pancreatitis, peritonitis, and rhabdomyolysis), or decreased effective circulating volume (as in cardiogenic shock and sepsis) may reduce circulating blood volume. Decreased cardiac output caused by peripheral vasodilatation (by sepsis or drugs) or profound renal vasoconstriction (as in severe heart failure, hepatorenal syndrome, or with such drugs as nonsteroidal anti-inflammatory drugs [NSAIDs]) also lessen renal perfusion.

Hypovolemia causes a decrease in MAP that triggers a series of neural and humoral responses: activation of the sympathetic nervous system and renin-angiotensin-aldosterone system, and release of arginine vasopressin. Prostaglandin-mediated relax-

ation of afferent arterioles and angiotensin II–mediated constriction of efferent arterioles maintain GFR. GFR decreases steeply if MAP decreases to less than 80 mm Hg. Drugs that block prostaglandin production (such as NSAIDs) can cause severe vasoconstriction and acute renal failure during hypotension.

Prolonged renal hypoperfusion causes acute tubular necrosis. Processes involving large renal vessels, microvasculature, glomeruli, or tubular interstitium cause intrinsic renal disease. Emboli or thrombi, aortic dissection, or vasculitis can occlude renal arteries. Cholesterol-rich atheroemboli can occur spontaneously or follow aortic instrumentation. If they lodge in medium and small renal arteries, they trigger an eosinophil-rich inflammatory reaction.

AGE ALERT
After age 40, a person's renal function begins to diminish. If he lives to age 90, it may have decreased by as much as 50%. This change is reflected in a decreased GFR and is caused by age-related changes in the renal vasculature that disturb glomerular hemodynamics as well as by reduced cardiac output and atherosclerotic changes that reduce renal blood flow by more than 50%.

Interstitial fluid colloid osmotic pressure

Few plasma proteins and red blood cells are filtered out of the glomeruli, so interstitial fluid colloid osmotic pressure (the force of albumin in the interstitial fluid) remains low. Large quantities of plasma protein flow through glomerular capillaries. Size and surface charge keep albumin, globulin, and other large proteins from crossing the glomerular wall. Smaller proteins leave the glomerulus but are absorbed by the proximal tubule.

Injury to the glomeruli or peritubular capillaries can increase interstitial fluid colloid osmotic pressure, drawing fluid out of the glomerulus and the peritubular capillaries. Swelling and edema occur in Bowman's space and the interstitial space surrounding the tubule. Increased interstitial fluid pressure opposes glomerular filtration, causes collapse of the surrounding

CLOSER LOOK
The glomerulus

The normal internal structures separating the capillary lumen and the urinary space in the glomerulus are shown here.

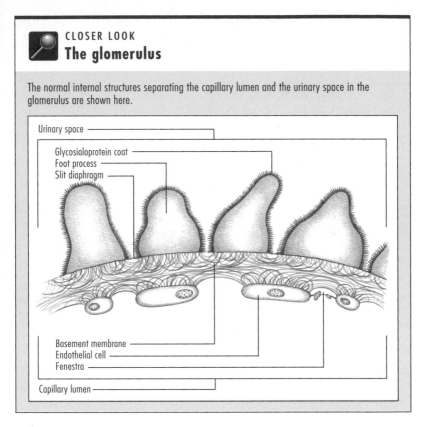

Urinary space

Glycosialoprotein coat
Foot process
Slit diaphragm

Basement membrane
Endothelial cell
Fenestra

Capillary lumen

nephrons (functional unit of the kidneys) and peritubular capillaries, and leads to hypoxia and renal cell injury or death. When cells die, intracellular enzymes are released that stimulate immune and inflammatory reactions. This further contributes to swelling and edema.

The resulting increase in interstitial fluid pressure can interfere with glomerular filtration and tubular reabsorption. Loss of glomerular filtration renders the kidney incapable of regulating blood volume and electrolyte composition. Diseases that damage the tubules alter their permeability, causing tubular proteinuria because small proteins can move from capillaries into tubules.

Normal glomerular cells, which are endothelial in nature, form a barrier that prevents cells and other particles from crossing the membrane. The basement

membrane typically traps larger proteins. The channels of the basement membrane are coated with glycoproteins that are rich in glutamate, aspartate, and sialic acid. This coating of the membrane produces a negatively charged barrier that impedes the passage of such anionic molecules as albumin. (See *The glomerulus*.)

Glomerular disease disrupts the basement membrane, allowing large proteins to leak out. Damage to epithelial cells permits albumin leakage. Hypoalbuminemia, as in nephrotic syndrome, is the result of excessive loss of albumin in the urine, increased renal catabolism, and inadequate hepatic synthesis of albumin. Plasma oncotic pressure (the osmotic pressure due to colloids in the plasma that tend to counterbalance hydrostatic capillary pressure) decreases and edema results as fluid moves from capillaries into the interstitium. Consequent activation of the renin-angiotensin system, arginine-vasopressin, and sympathetic nervous system increases renal salt and water reabsorption, which further contributes to edema. The severity of edema is directly related to the degree of hypoalbuminemia, and is exacerbated by heart disease or peripheral vascular disease.

Plasma colloid pressure

Protein concentration of the plasma determines the plasma colloid pressure (the pulling force of albumin in the intravascular fluid), the major force influencing reabsorption of fluid into the capillaries. Plasma protein levels can decrease as a result of liver disease, protein loss in the urine, and protein malnutrition.

As oncotic pressure decreases, less fluid moves back into the capillaries and fluid begins to accumulate in the tubular and peritubular areas. Swelling around the tubule causes collapse of the tubule and peritubular capillaries, hypoxia, and death of the nephrons.

Diminished plasma oncotic pressure and urine protein loss stimulate hepatic lipoprotein synthesis, and the resulting hyperlipidemia appears as lipid bodies (fatty casts, oval fat bodies) in the urine. Metabolic disturbances result as other proteins are lost in the urine, including thyroxine-binding globulin, cholecalciferol-binding protein, transferrin, and metal-binding proteins. Urine losses of antithrombin III, decreased serum levels of proteins S and C, hyperfibrinogenemia, and enhanced platelet aggregation lead to a hypercoagulable state, as in nephrotic syndrome. Some patients also develop severe immunoglobulin G deficiency, which increases susceptibility to infection.

Structural variations

Variations in normal anatomic structure of the urinary tract occur in 10% to 15% of the total population and range from minor and easily correctable to lethal. Ectopic kidneys, which result if the embryonic kidneys don't ascend from the pelvis to the abdomen, function normally. If the embryonic kidneys fuse as they ascend, a single U-shaped kidney results, causing no symptoms in about one-third of affected

---

Congenital nephropathies and uropathies

The following congenital conditions can affect kidney function:

◆ *Renal hypoplasia* — the kidney is small because of a reduced number of normally developed nephrons; the hypoplasia may be unilateral or bilateral

◆ *Renal dysplasia* — the kidney is abnormally shaped, and the involved areas are nonfunctional.

◆ *Renal malrotation* — the kidney is positioned abnormally

◆ *Ectopic kidney* — the kidney is located in the pelvis or thorax, causing reflux from the bladder into the ureters

◆ *Horseshoe kidney* — the lower poles of the kidneys are fused by an isthmus

◆ *Obstructive uropathy* — a pathological condition (abnormal vasculature, adhesions, kinks, or masses) that blocks the flow of urine, usually causing hydronephrosis.

◆ *Ureterocele* — a prolapse of the end portion of the ureter into the bladder leading to an obstruction in urine flow.

---

people. The most common problems linked to "horseshoe" kidneys include hydronephrosis, infection, and calculus formation.

AGE ALERT
Structural abnormalities of the renal system account for about 45% of renal failure in children.

Urinary tract malformations are commonly linked to certain nonrenal anomalies. These characteristics include low-set and malformed ears, chromosomal disorders (especially trisomies 13 and 18), absent abdominal muscles, spinal cord and lower extremity anomalies, imperforate anus or genital deviation, Wilms' tumor, congenital ascites, and cystic disease of the liver. Urinary tract malformations may also be linked to a positive family history of renal disease (hereditary nephritis or cystic disease). (See *Congenital nephropathies and uropathies*.)

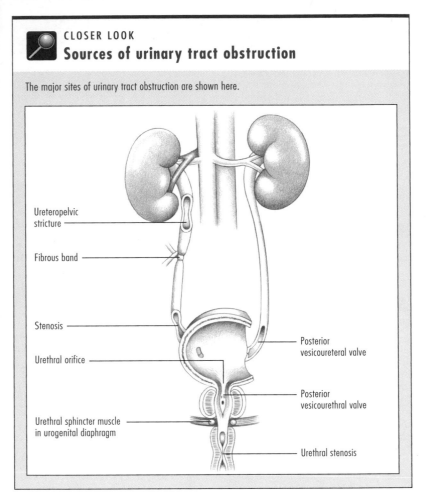

CLOSER LOOK
Sources of urinary tract obstruction

The major sites of urinary tract obstruction are shown here.

Ureteropelvic stricture

Fibrous band

Stenosis

Urethral orifice

Urethral sphincter muscle in urogenital diaphragm

Posterior vesicoureteral valve

Posterior vesicourethral valve

Urethral stenosis

Obstruction

Obstruction along the urinary tract causes urine to accumulate behind the source of obstruction, leading to infection or damage. (See *Sources of urinary tract obstruction.*) Obstructions may be congenital or acquired. Causes include tumors, calculi (stones), trauma, strictures (from surgical intervention and scarring), edema, pregnancy, benign prostatic hyperplasia or carcinoma, inflammation of the GI tract, and loss of ureteral peristaltic activity or bladder muscle function.

Consequences of obstruction depend on the location and whether it's unilateral or bilateral, partial or complete, acute or chronic, and on the cause. For example, obstruction of a ureter causes hydroureter, or an accumulation of urine within the ureter, which increases retrograde pressure to the renal pelvis and calyces. As urine accumulates in the renal collection system, hydronephrosis results. If the obstruction is complete and acute, increasing pressure transmitted to the proximal tubule inhibits glomerular filtration. If GFR declines to zero, the result is renal failure.

Chronic partial obstruction compresses structures as urine accumulates, and the result is papillary and medullary infarct.

The kidneys initially increase in size, but progressive atrophy follows, with eventual loss of renal mass. The underlying tubular damage decreases the kidney's ability to conserve sodium and water and excrete hydrogen ions and potassium; sodium and bicarbonate are wasted. Urine volume is excessive, even though GFR has declined. The result is an increased risk of dehydration and metabolic acidosis.

Tubular obstruction, from renal calculi or scarring from repeated infection, can increase interstitial fluid pressure. As fluid accumulates in the nephron, it backs up into Bowman's capsule and space. If the obstruction is unrelieved, nephrons and capillaries collapse, and renal damage is irreversible. The papillae, which are the final site of urine concentration, are particularly affected.

Relief of the obstruction is usually followed by copious diuresis of sodium and water retained during the period of obstruction, and a return to normal GFR. Excessive loss of sodium and water (more than 10 L/day) is uncommon. If GFR doesn't recover quickly, diuresis may not be significant after relief of the obstruction.

Unresolved obstruction can result in infection or even renal failure. Obstructions below the bladder cause urine to accumulate, forming a medium for bacterial growth.

AGE ALERT
Urinary tract infections are most common in girls ages 7 to 11. This is a result of bacteria ascending the urethra.

Cystitis is an infection of the bladder that results in mucosal inflammation and congestion. The detrusor muscle becomes hyperactive, decreasing bladder capacity and leading to reflux of urine into the ureters. This transient reflux can cause acute or chronic pyelonephritis if bacteria ascend to the kidney.

Bilateral obstruction of the ureters not relieved within 1 week of onset causes acute or chronic renal failure. Chronic renal failure progresses over weeks to months without symptoms until 90% of renal function is lost.

DISORDERS

Renal disorders include acute pyelonephritis, acute and chronic renal failure, acute tubular necrosis, congenital anomalies, glomerulonephritis, nephrotic syndrome, neurogenic bladder, polycystic kidney, renal agenesis, renal calculi, and vesicoureteral reflux.

Acute pyelonephritis

Acute pyelonephritis, also known as *acute infective tubulointerstitial nephritis,* is a sudden inflammation caused by bacteria that mainly affects the interstitial area and the renal pelvis or, less commonly, the renal tubules. It's one of the most common renal diseases and may affect one or both kidneys. With treatment and continued follow-up care, the prognosis is good, and extensive permanent damage is rare.

Pyelonephritis is more common in females, probably because of a shorter urethra and the short distance from the urinary meatus to the vagina and the rectum — both conditions allow bacteria to reach the bladder more easily — and a lack of the antibacterial prostatic secretions produced in males. Incidence increases with age and is higher in the following groups:
- sexually active women — intercourse increases the risk of bacterial contamination
- pregnant women — about 5% develop asymptomatic bacteriuria; if untreated, about 40% develop pyelonephritis
- people with diabetes — neurogenic bladder causes incomplete emptying and urinary stasis; glycosuria may support bacterial growth in the urine
- people with other renal diseases — compromised renal function increases susceptibility.

CAUSES
Acute pyelonephritis results from bacterial infection of the kidneys. Infecting bacteria usually are normal intestinal and fecal flora that grow readily in urine. The most common causative organism is *Escherichia coli,* but *Klebsiella, Proteus, Pseudomonas, Staphylococcus aureus,* and *Enterococcus fae-*

calis (formerly *Streptococcus faecalis*) may also cause this infection.

PATHOPHYSIOLOGY

Typically, the infection spreads from the bladder to the ureters, then to the kidneys, as in vesicoureteral reflux. Vesicoureteral reflux may result from congenital weakness at the junction of the ureter and the bladder. Bacteria refluxed to intrarenal tissues may create colonies of infection within 24 to 48 hours. Infection can also result from instrumentation (such as catheterization, cystoscopy, or urologic surgery), from a hematogenic infection (as in septicemia or endocarditis), or possibly from lymphatic infection.

Pyelonephritis can also result from an inability to empty the bladder (for example, in persons with neurogenic bladder), urinary stasis, or urinary obstruction from tumors, strictures, or benign prostatic hyperplasia.

SIGNS AND SYMPTOMS

Typical clinical features of pyelonephritis include:
- urinary urgency and frequency, burning during urination, dysuria, nocturia, and hematuria (usually microscopic but may be gross) caused by urinary tract irritation
- cloudy urine that has an ammonia-like or fishy odor resulting from bacteria in the urine and subsequent leukocyte response
- a temperature of 102° F (38.9° C) or higher, shaking chills, nausea and vomiting, flank pain, anorexia, and general fatigue caused by infectious process

These symptoms characteristically develop rapidly over a few hours or a few days. Although these symptoms may disappear within days, even without treatment, residual bacterial infection is likely and may cause symptoms to recur later.

AGE ALERT
Elderly patients may exhibit GI or pulmonary symptoms rather than the usual febrile responses to pyelonephritis. In children younger than age 2, fever, vomiting, nonspecific abdominal complaints, or failure to thrive may be the only signs of acute pyelonephritis.

COMPLICATIONS

Complications may include:
- septic shock
- chronic pyelonephritis
- chronic renal insufficiency.

DIAGNOSIS

Diagnosis requires urinalysis and culture. Typical findings include:
- *pyuria (pus in urine)* — Urine sediment reveals the presence of leukocytes singly, in clumps, and in casts and, possibly, a few red blood cells.
- *significant bacteriuria* — Urine culture reveals more than 100,000 organisms/μl of urine.
- *low specific gravity and osmolality* — These findings result from a temporarily decreased ability to concentrate urine.
- *slightly alkaline urine pH* — This finding results from a temporarily decreased ability to concentrate urine.
- *proteinuria, glycosuria, and ketonuria* — These conditions are less common.

Computed tomography (CT) scan also helps in the evaluation of acute pyelonephritis. CT scan of the kidneys, ureters, and bladder may reveal calculi, tumors, or cysts in the kidneys and the urinary tract. Excretory urography may show asymmetrical kidneys.

TREATMENT

Treatment centers on antibiotic therapy appropriate to the specific infecting organism after identification by urine culture and sensitivity studies. For example:
- *Enterococcus* requires treatment with ampicillin, penicillin G, or vancomycin.
- *Staphylococcus* requires penicillin G or, if resistance develops, a semisynthetic penicillin such as nafcillin or a cephalosporin.
- *Escherichia coli* may be treated with sulfisoxazole, nalidixic acid, and nitrofurantoin.
- *Proteus* may be treated with ampicillin, sulfisoxazole, nalidixic acid, and a cephalosporin.
- *Pseudomonas* requires gentamicin, tobramycin, or carbenicillin.

When the infecting organism can't be identified, therapy usually consists of a broad-spectrum antibiotic, such as ampicillin or cephalexin. If the patient is pregnant or elderly, antibiotics must be prescribed cautiously. Urinary analgesics, such as phenazopyridine, are also appropriate.

Symptoms may disappear after several days of antibiotic therapy. Although urine usually becomes sterile within 48 to 72 hours, the course of such therapy as that listed is 10 to 14 days. Follow-up treatment includes culturing urine 1 week after drug therapy stops, then periodically for the next year to detect residual or recurring infection. Most patients with uncomplicated infections respond well to therapy and don't suffer reinfection.

If infection is caused by an obstruction or a vesicoureteral reflux, antibiotics may be less effective; surgery may then be necessary to relieve the obstruction or correct the anomaly. Patients at high risk for recurring urinary tract and kidney infections, such as those with prolonged use of an indwelling catheter or maintenance antibiotic therapy, require long-term follow-up. Recurrent episodes of acute pyelonephritis can eventually result in chronic pyelonephritis. (See *Chronic pyelonephritis.*)

Acute renal failure

Acute renal failure, the sudden interruption of renal function, can be caused by obstruction, poor circulation, or underlying kidney disease. Whether prerenal, intrarenal, or postrenal, it usually passes through three distinct phases: oliguric, diuretic, and recovery. About 5% of all hospitalized patients develop acute renal failure. The condition is usually reversible with treatment, but if not treated, it may progress to end-stage renal disease, prerenal azotemia, and death.

CAUSES

Acute renal failure may be prerenal, intrarenal, or postrenal. Causes of prerenal failure include:

■ arrhythmias that cause reduced cardiac output
■ cardiac tamponade
■ cardiogenic shock
■ heart failure
■ myocardial infarction
■ burns
■ dehydration

> # Chronic pyelonephritis
>
> Chronic pyelonephritis is a persistent kidney inflammation that can scar the kidneys and may lead to chronic renal failure. Its cause may be bacterial, metastatic, or urogenous. This disease is most common in patients who are predisposed to recurrent acute pyelonephritis, such as those with urinary obstructions or vesicoureteral reflux.
>
> Patients with chronic pyelonephritis may have a childhood history of unexplained fevers or bed-wetting. Clinical effects may include flank pain, anemia, low urine specific gravity, proteinuria, leukocytes in urine and, especially in late stages, hypertension. Uremia rarely develops from chronic pyelonephritis unless structural abnormalities exist in the excretory system. Bacteriuria may be intermittent. When no bacteria are found in the urine, diagnosis depends on excretory urography (renal pelvis may appear small and flattened) and renal biopsy.
>
> Effective treatment of chronic pyelonephritis requires control of hypertension, elimination of the existing obstruction (when possible), and long-term antimicrobial therapy.

■ overuse of diuretic drugs
■ hemorrhage
■ hypovolemic shock
■ trauma
■ antihypertensive drugs
■ sepsis
■ arterial embolism
■ arterial or venous thrombosis
■ tumor
■ disseminated intravascular coagulation
■ eclampsia
■ malignant hypertension
■ vasculitis.
Causes of intrarenal failure include:
■ poorly treated prerenal failure
■ nephrotoxins
■ obstetric complications
■ crush injuries
■ myopathy
■ transfusion reaction

- acute glomerulonephritis
- acute interstitial nephritis
- acute pyelonephritis
- bilateral renal vein thrombosis
- malignant nephrosclerosis
- papillary necrosis
- polyarteritis nodosa
- renal myeloma
- sickle cell disease
- systemic lupus erythematosus
- vasculitis.

Causes of postrenal failure include:

- bladder obstruction
- ureteral obstruction
- urethral obstruction.

PATHOPHYSIOLOGY

The pathophysiology of prerenal, intrarenal, and postrenal failure differs.

Prerenal failure. Prerenal failure ensues when a condition that lessens blood flow to the kidneys leads to hypoperfusion. Examples include hypovolemia, hypotension, vasoconstriction, or inadequate cardiac output. Azotemia (excess nitrogenous waste products in the blood) develops in 40% to 80% of cases of acute renal failure.

When renal blood flow is interrupted, so is oxygen delivery. The ensuing hypoxemia and ischemia can rapidly and irreversibly damage the kidney. The tubules are most susceptible to hypoxemia's effects.

Azotemia is a consequence of renal hypoperfusion. The impaired blood flow results in decreased glomerular filtration rate (GFR) and increased tubular reabsorption of sodium and water. A decrease in GFR causes electrolyte imbalance and metabolic acidosis. Usually, restoring renal blood flow and glomerular filtration reverses azotemia.

Intrarenal failure. Intrarenal failure, also called *intrinsic* or *parenchymal renal failure,* results from damage to the filtering structures of the kidneys. Causes of intrarenal failure are classified as nephrotoxic, inflammatory, or ischemic. When the damage is caused by nephrotoxicity or inflammation, the delicate layer under the epithelium (the basement membrane) becomes irreparably damaged, typically leading to chronic renal failure. Severe or pro-

longed lack of blood flow because of ischemia may lead to renal damage (ischemic parenchymal injury) and excess nitrogen in the blood (intrinsic renal azotemia).

Acute tubular necrosis, the precursor to intrarenal failure, can result from ischemic damage to renal parenchyma during unrecognized or poorly treated prerenal failure; or from obstetric complications, such as eclampsia, postpartum renal failure, septic abortion, or uterine hemorrhage.

The fluid loss causes hypotension, which leads to ischemia. The ischemic tissue generates toxic oxygen-free radicals, which cause swelling, injury, and necrosis.

Another cause of acute failure is the use of nephrotoxins, including analgesics, anesthetics, heavy metals, radiographic contrast media, organic solvents, and antimicrobials, particularly aminoglycoside antibiotics. These drugs can accumulate in the renal cortex, causing renal failure that manifests well after treatment or other toxin exposure. The necrosis caused by nephrotoxins tends to be uniform and limited to the proximal tubules, whereas ischemic necrosis tends to be patchy and distributed along various parts of the nephron.

Postrenal failure. Bilateral obstruction of urine outflow leads to postrenal failure. The cause may be in the bladder, ureters, or urethra.

Bladder obstruction can result from:

- anticholinergic drugs
- autonomic nerve dysfunction
- infection
- tumors.

Ureteral obstructions, which restrict urine flow from kidneys to bladder, can result from:

- blood clots
- calculi
- edema or inflammation
- necrotic renal papillae
- retroperitoneal fibrosis or hemorrhage
- surgery (accidental ligation and strictures)
- tumor or uric acid crystals.

Urethral obstruction can be the result of prostatic hyperplasia, tumor, or strictures.

The three types of acute renal failure (prerenal, intrarenal, or postrenal) usually pass through three distinct phases: oliguric, diuretic, and recovery.

Oliguric phase. Oliguria (excretion of a lessened amount of urine in relation to fluid intake) may be the result of one or several factors. Necrosis of the tubules can cause sloughing of cells, cast formations, and ischemic edema. The resulting tubular obstruction causes a retrograde increase in pressure and a decrease in GFR. Renal failure can occur within 24 hours from this effect. Glomerular filtration may remain normal in some cases of renal failure, but tubular reabsorption of filtrate may be accelerated. In this instance, ischemia may increase tubular permeability and cause back-leak. Another concept is that intrarenal release of angiotensin II or redistribution of blood flow from the cortex to the medulla may constrict the afferent arterioles, increasing glomerular permeability and decreasing GFR.

Urine output may remain at less than 30 ml/hour or 400 ml/day for a few days to weeks. Before damage occurs, the kidneys respond to decreased blood flow by conserving sodium and water.

Damage impairs the kidney's ability to conserve sodium. Fluid (water) volume excess, azotemia (elevated serum levels of urea, creatinine, and uric acid), and electrolyte imbalance occur. Ischemic or toxic injury leads to the release of mediators and intrarenal vasoconstriction. Medullary hypoxia results in the swelling of tubular and endothelial cells, adherence of neutrophils to capillaries and venules, and inappropriate platelet activation. Increasing ischemia and vasoconstriction further limit perfusion.

Injured cells lose polarity, and the ensuing disruption of tight junctions between the cells promotes back-leak of filtrate. Ischemia impairs the function of energy-dependent membrane pumps, and calcium accumulates in the cells. This excess calcium further stimulates vasoconstriction and activates proteases and other enzymes. Untreated prerenal oliguria may lead to acute tubular necrosis.

Diuretic phase. As the kidneys become unable to conserve sodium and water, the diuretic phase, marked by increased urine secretion of more than 400 ml/24 hours, ensues. GFR may be normal or increased, but tubular support mechanisms are abnormal. Excretion of dilute urine causes dehydration and electrolyte imbalances. High blood urea nitrogen (BUN) levels produce osmotic diuresis and consequent deficits of potassium, sodium, and water. The diuretic phase may last days or weeks.

Recovery phase. If the cause of the diuresis is corrected, azotemia gradually disappears and recovery occurs. The recovery phase is a gradual return to normal or near-normal renal function over 3 to 12 months.

▲ **AGE ALERT**
Even with treatment, the elderly patient is particularly susceptible to volume overload, precipitating acute pulmonary edema, hypertensive crisis, hyperkalemia, and infection.

SIGNS AND SYMPTOMS
Acute renal failure is a critical illness. Its early signs are oliguria, azotemia and, rarely, anuria. Electrolyte imbalance, metabolic acidosis, and other severe effects follow, as the patient becomes increasingly uremic and renal dysfunction disrupts other body systems.

■ anorexia, nausea, vomiting, diarrhea or constipation, stomatitis, bleeding, hematemesis, dry mucous membranes, uremic breath (GI)
■ headache, drowsiness, irritability, confusion, peripheral neuropathy, seizures, coma (central nervous system)
■ dryness, pruritus, pallor, purpura and, rarely, uremic frost (skin)
■ early in the disease, hypotension; later, hypertension, arrhythmias, fluid overload, heart failure, systemic edema, anemia, altered clotting mechanisms (cardiovascular)
■ pulmonary edema, Kussmaul's respirations (respiratory).

COMPLICATIONS
Renal failure affects many body processes. Complications may include:

- infection manifested by fever and chills (common),
- metabolic acidosis caused by decreased excretion of hydrogen ions
- anemia caused by erythropoietinemia, glomerular filtration of erythrocytes, or bleeding linked to platelet dysfunction; tissue hypoxia, stimulating increased ventilation and work of breathing
- sepsis because of decreased white blood cell–mediated immunity
- heart failure caused by fluid overload and anemia, which cause additional workload to the heart
- hypercoagulable state caused by abnormalities in quantities or function of anticoagulant proteins, coagulation factor, platelet, or endothelial mediators, resulting in bleeding or clotting difficulties
- altered mental status and peripheral sensation because of effects on the highly sensitive cells of nerves caused by retained toxins, hypoxia, electrolyte imbalance, and acidosis.

DIAGNOSIS

Diagnosis of acute renal failure is based on the following results:

- blood studies showing elevated BUN, serum creatinine, and potassium levels; decreased bicarbonate level, hematocrit, hemoglobin, and blood pH
- urine studies showing casts, cellular debris, and decreased specific gravity; in glomerular diseases, proteinuria and urine osmolality close to serum osmolality; urine sodium level less than 20 mEq/L (20 mmol/L) if oliguria results from decreased perfusion, and more than 40 mEq/L (40 mmol/L) if cause is intrarenal
- creatinine clearance test measuring GFR and reflecting the number of remaining functioning nephrons
- electrocardiogram (ECG) showing tall, peaked T waves, widening QRS complex, and disappearing P waves if hyperkalemia is present
- ultrasonography, plain films of the abdomen, kidney-ureter-bladder radiography, excretory urography, renal scan, retrograde pyelography, computed tomographic scans, and nephrotomography.

TREATMENT

Treatment of acute renal failure includes:

- high-calorie, low-protein, low-sodium, and low-potassium diet to meet metabolic needs
- careful monitoring of electrolytes; I.V. therapy to maintain and correct fluid and electrolyte balance
- fluid restriction to minimize edema
- diuretic therapy to treat oliguric phase
- sodium polystyrene sulfonate by mouth or enema to reverse hyperkalemia with mild hyperkalemic symptoms (malaise, loss of appetite, muscle weakness)
- hypertonic glucose, insulin, and sodium bicarbonate I.V.—for more severe hyperkalemic symptoms (numbness and tingling and ECG changes)

⬛ **CLINICAL ALERT**
Symptoms of hyperkalemia include malaise, anorexia, paresthesia, or muscle weakness and ECG changes, including tall, peaked T waves; widening QRS segment; and disappearing P waves. If the patient exhibits any of these symptoms, they must be reported immediately.

- hemodialysis or peritoneal dialysis to correct electrolyte and fluid imbalances.

Acute tubular necrosis

Acute tubular necrosis (ATN), also known as *acute tubulointerstitial nephritis*, accounts for about 75% of cases of acute renal failure and is the most common cause of acute renal failure in critically ill patients. ATN injures the nephron's tubular segment, causing renal failure and uremic syndrome. Mortality ranges from 40% to 70%, depending on complications from underlying diseases. Nonoliguric forms of ATN have a better prognosis.

CAUSES

ATN may result from:

- diseased tubular epithelium that allows leakage of glomerular filtrate across the membranes and reabsorption of filtrate into the blood
- obstruction of urine flow by the collection of damaged cells, casts, red blood cells (RBCs), and other cellular debris within the tubular walls

- ischemic injury to glomerular epithelial cells, resulting in cellular collapse and decreased glomerular capillary permeability
- ischemic injury to vascular endothelium, eventually resulting in cellular swelling and tubular obstruction.

PATHOPHYSIOLOGY
ATN results from ischemic or nephrotoxic injury, most commonly in debilitated patients, such as the critically ill or those who have undergone extensive surgery. In ischemic injury, disruption of blood flow to the kidneys may result from circulatory collapse, severe hypotension, trauma, hemorrhage, dehydration, cardiogenic or septic shock, surgery, anesthetics, or reactions to transfusions. Nephrotoxic injury may follow ingestion of certain chemical agents, such as contrasts administered during radiologic procedures or administration of antibiotics (aminoglycosides), or result from a hypersensitive reaction of the kidneys. Because nephrotoxic ATN doesn't damage the basement membrane of the nephron, it's potentially reversible, but ischemic ATN can damage the epithelial and basement membranes and can cause lesions in the renal interstitium.

SIGNS AND SYMPTOMS
ATN is usually difficult to recognize in its early stages because effects of the critically ill patient's primary disease may mask the symptoms of ATN. Signs and symptoms of ATN may include:
- decreased urine output, generally the first recognizable effect, because of reduced renal blood flow and glomerular filtration
- hyperkalemia because of disturbed renal tubular absorption
- uremic syndrome with oliguria (or, rarely, anuria) and confusion, which may progress to uremic coma, caused by renal failure
- dry mucous membranes and skin
- central nervous system symptoms, such as lethargy, twitching, or seizures.

COMPLICATIONS
Possible complications may include:
- heart failure
- uremic pericarditis

- pulmonary edema
- uremic lung
- anemia
- anorexia, intractable vomiting
- poor wound healing because of debilitation.

CLINICAL ALERT
Fever and chills may signal the onset of an infection, which is the leading cause of death in ATN.

DIAGNOSIS
Diagnosis is usually delayed until the condition has progressed to an advanced stage.
- The most significant laboratory clues are urinary sediment containing RBCs and casts, and dilute urine of a low specific gravity (1.010), low osmolality (less than 400 mOsm/kg [400 mmol/kg]), and high sodium level (40 to 60 mEq/L [40 to 60 mmol/L]).
- Blood studies reveal elevated blood urea nitrogen and serum creatinine levels, anemia, defects in platelet adherence, metabolic acidosis, and hyperkalemia.
- An electrocardiogram may show arrhythmias (caused by electrolyte imbalances) and, with hyperkalemia, widening QRS segment, disappearing P waves, and tall, peaked T waves.

TREATMENT
In the acute phase:
- vigorous supportive measures until normal kidney function resumes
- at first, possible administration of diuretics and infusion of a large volume of fluids to flush tubules of cellular casts and debris and to replace fluid loss (risk of fluid overload exists with this treatment).

Long-term fluid management:
- daily replacement of projected and calculated fluid losses (includes amounts for insensible loss)

Other appropriate measures to control complications include:
- transfusion of packed RBCs for anemia; epoetin alfa to stimulate RBC production as an alternative to blood transfusion
- administration of antibiotics for infection

■ emergency I.V. administration of 50% glucose, regular insulin, and sodium bicarbonate for hyperkalemia

■ sodium polystyrene sulfonate with sorbitol by mouth or by enema to reduce extracellular potassium levels

■ peritoneal dialysis or hemodialysis if the patient is catabolic or if hyperkalemia and fluid volume overload aren't controlled by other measures.

Chronic renal failure

Chronic renal failure is usually the end result of gradual tissue destruction and loss of renal function. It can also result from a rapidly progressing disease of sudden onset that destroys the nephrons and causes irreversible kidney damage.

Few symptoms develop until less than 25% of glomerular filtration remains. The normal parenchyma then deteriorates rapidly, and symptoms worsen as renal function decreases. This syndrome is fatal without treatment, but maintenance on dialysis or a kidney transplant can sustain life.

CAUSES
Chronic renal failure may be caused by:
■ chronic glomerular disease (glomerulonephritis)
■ chronic infection (such as chronic pyelonephritis and tuberculosis)
■ congenital anomalies (polycystic kidney disease)
■ vascular disease (hypertension, nephrosclerosis)
■ obstruction (renal calculi)
■ collagen disease (lupus erythematosus)
■ nephrotoxic agents (long-term aminoglycoside therapy)
■ endocrine disease (diabetic neuropathy).

PATHOPHYSIOLOGY
Chronic renal failure often progresses through four stages. Reduced renal reserve shows a glomerular filtration rate (GFR) of 35% to 50% of normal; renal insufficiency has a GFR of 20% to 35% of normal; renal failure has a GFR of 20% to 25% of normal; and end-stage renal disease has a GFR less than 20% of normal.

Nephron damage is progressive; damaged nephrons can't function and don't recover. The kidneys can maintain relatively normal function until about 75% of the nephrons are nonfunctional. Surviving nephrons hypertrophy and increase their rate of filtration, reabsorption, and secretion. Compensatory excretion continues as GFR lessens.

Urine may contain abnormal amounts of protein, red blood cells (RBCs), and white blood cells or casts. The major end products of excretion remain essentially normal, and nephron loss becomes significant. As GFR decreases, plasma creatinine levels increase proportionately without regulatory adjustment. As sodium delivery to the nephron increases, less is reabsorbed, and sodium deficits and volume depletion follow. The kidney becomes incapable of concentrating and diluting urine.

If tubular interstitial disease is the cause of chronic renal failure, primary damage to the tubules — the medullary portion of the nephron — precedes failure, as do such problems as renal tubular acidosis, salt wasting, and difficulty diluting and concentrating urine. If vascular or glomerular damage is the primary cause, proteinuria, hematuria, and nephrotic syndrome are more prominent.

Changes in acid-base balance affect phosphorus and calcium balance. Renal phosphate excretion and $1,25(OH)_2$ vitamin D_3 synthesis are decreased. Hypocalcemia results in secondary hypoparathyroidism, decreased GFR, and progressive hyperphosphatemia, hypocalcemia, and dissolution of bone. In early renal insufficiency, acid excretion and phosphate reabsorption increase to maintain normal pH. When GFR decreases by 30% to 40%, progressive metabolic acidosis develops and tubular secretion of potassium increases. Total-body potassium levels may increase to life-threatening levels requiring dialysis.

In glomerulosclerosis, distortion of filtration slits and erosion of the glomerular epithelial cells lead to increased fluid movement across the glomerular wall. Large proteins cross the slits but become trapped in glomerular basement membranes, obstructing the glomerular capillaries. Epithelial and endothelial injury cause proteinuria. Proliferation of mesangial cells (connective tissue cells in the glomerular capsule), increased production of extracellular matrix, and intraglomerular coagulation cause the sclerosis.

Tubulointerstitial injury occurs because of toxic or ischemic tubular damage, as with acute tubular necrosis. Debris and calcium deposits obstruct the tubules. The resulting defective tubular function is linked to interstitial edema, leukocyte infiltration, and tubular necrosis. Vascular injury causes diffuse or focal ischemia of the renal parenchyma, linked to thickening, fibrosis, or focal lesions of renal blood vessels. Decreased blood flow then leads to tubular atrophy, interstitial fibrosis, and functional disruption of glomerular filtration and concentration.

The structural changes trigger an inflammatory response. Fibrin deposits begin to form around the interstitium. Microaneurysms result from vascular wall damage and increased pressure caused by obstruction or hypertension. Eventual loss of the nephron triggers compensatory hyperfunction of uninjured nephrons, which begins a positive-feedback loop of growing vulnerability.

Eventually, the healthy glomeruli are so overburdened that they become sclerotic, stiff, and necrotic. Toxins accumulate and potentially fatal changes take place in all major organ systems.

Extrarenal consequences.
Physiologic changes affect more than one system, and the presence and severity of manifestations depend on the duration of renal failure and its response to treatment. In some fluid and electrolyte imbalances, the kidneys can't retain salt, and hyponatremia results. Dry mouth, fatigue, nausea, hypotension, loss of skin turgor, and listlessness can progress to somnolence and confusion. Later, as the number of functioning nephrons decreases, so does the capacity to excrete sodium and potassium. Sodium retention leads to fluid overload and edema; the potassium overload leads to muscle irritability and weakness, and life-threatening cardiac arrhythmias.

As the cardiovascular system becomes involved, hypertension occurs, and irregular distant heart sounds may be auscultated if pericardial effusion occurs. Crackles in the bases of both lungs and peripheral edema reflect heart failure.

Pulmonary changes include reduced macrophage activity and increasing susceptibility to infection. Decreased breath sounds in areas of consolidation reflect the presence of pneumonia. As the pleurae become more involved, the patient may experience pleuritic pain and friction rubs.

Kussmaul's respirations may be noted as a result of metabolic acidosis. The GI mucosa becomes inflamed and ulcerated, and gums may also be ulcerated and bleeding. Stomatitis, uremic fetor (an ammonia smell to the breath), hiccups, peptic ulcer, and pancreatitis in end-stage renal failure are believed to be caused by retention of metabolic acids and other metabolic waste products. Malnutrition may be caused by anorexia, malaise, and reduced dietary intake of protein. The reduced protein intake also affects capillary fragility, and results in decreased immune functioning and poor wound healing.

Normochromic normocytic anemia and platelet disorders with prolonged bleeding time follow as decreased erythropoietin secretion leads to reduced RBC production in the bone marrow. Uremic toxins linked to chronic renal failure shorten RBC survival time. The patient experiences lethargy and dizziness.

Demineralization of the bone (renal osteodystrophy) shown by bone pain and pathologic fractures is caused by several factors:
- decreased renal activation of vitamin D, decreasing absorption of dietary calcium
- retention of phosphate, increasing urinary loss of calcium
- increased circulation of parathyroid hormone because of decreased urinary excretion.

The skin turns grayish yellow as urine pigments (urochromes) accumulate. Inflammatory mediators released by retained toxins in the skin cause pruritus. Uric acid and other substances in the sweat crystallize and accumulate on the skin as uremic frost. High plasma calcium levels are also linked to pruritus.

Restless leg syndrome (abnormal sensation and spontaneous movement of the feet and lower legs), muscle weakness, and decreased deep tendon reflexes are believed to result from the effect of toxins on the nervous system.

CLINICAL ALERT
Restless leg syndrome is one of the first signs of peripheral neuropathy. This condition will eventually progress to paresthesia and motor nerve dysfunction (bilateral foot drop) unless dialysis is started.

Chronic renal failure increases the risk of death from infection. The increased risk is related to suppression of cell-mediated immunity and a reduction in the number and function of lymphocytes and phagocytes.

All hormone levels are impaired in excretion and activation. Women may be anovulatory, amenorrheic, or unable to carry pregnancy to full term. Men tend to have decreased sperm counts and impotence.

SIGNS AND SYMPTOMS
Signs and symptoms of chronic renal failure include:
- hypervolemia caused by sodium retention
- hypocalcemia and hyperkalemia because of electrolyte imbalance
- azotemia because of retention of nitrogenous wastes
- metabolic acidosis caused by loss of bicarbonate
- bone and muscle pain and fractures because of calcium-phosphorus imbalance and consequent parathyroid hormone imbalances
- peripheral neuropathy caused by accumulation of toxins
- dry mouth, fatigue, and nausea because of hyponatremia
- hypotension caused by sodium loss
- altered mental state caused by hyponatremia and toxin accumulation
- irregular heart rate because of hyperkalemia
- hypertension caused by fluid overload
- gum sores and bleeding because of coagulopathies

- yellow-bronze skin caused by altered metabolic processes
- dry, scaly skin and severe itching caused by uremic frost
- muscle cramps and twitching, including cardiac irritability, caused by hyperkalemia
- Kussmaul's respirations caused by metabolic acidosis

AGE ALERT
Growth retardation in children can occur because of endocrine abnormalities induced by renal failure. Impaired bone growth and bowlegs in children are also linked to rickets.

- infertility, decreased libido, amenorrhea, and impotence caused by endocrine disturbances
- GI bleeding, hemorrhage, and bruising because of thrombocytopenia and platelet defects
- pain, burning, and itching in legs and feet linked to peripheral neuropathy
- infection related to decreased macrophage activity.

COMPLICATIONS
Possible complications of chronic renal failure include:
- anemia
- peripheral neuropathy
- cardiopulmonary complications
- GI complications
- sexual dysfunction
- skeletal defects
- paresthesias
- motor nerve dysfunction, such as foot drop and flaccid paralysis
- pathologic fractures
- pericardial tamponade.

CLINICAL ALERT
Watch for the disappearance of friction rub, with a drop of 15 to 20 mm Hg during inspiration (paradoxical pulse) — an early sign of pericardial tamponade.

DIAGNOSIS
Blood study results that help diagnose chronic renal failure include:
- decreased arterial pH and bicarbonate, low hemoglobin levels and hematocrit
- decreased RBC survival time, mild thrombocytopenia, platelet defects

- elevated blood urea nitrogen, serum creatinine, sodium, and potassium levels
- increased aldosterone secretion related to increased renin production
- hyperglycemia (a sign of impaired carbohydrate metabolism)
- hypertriglyceridemia and low levels of high-density lipoprotein.

Urinalysis results aiding in diagnosis include:
- specific gravity fixed at 1.010
- proteinuria, glycosuria, presence of RBCs, leukocytes, casts, or crystals, depending on the cause.

Other study results used to diagnose chronic renal failure include:
- reduced kidney size on kidney-ureter-bladder radiography, excretory urography, nephrotomography, renal scan, or renal arteriography
- renal biopsy to identify underlying disease
- electroencephalography to identify metabolic encephalopathy.

TREATMENT
Treatment of chronic renal failure involves:
- low-protein diet, to limit accumulation of end products of protein metabolism that the kidneys can't excrete
- high-protein diet for patients receiving continuous peritoneal dialysis
- high-calorie diet, to prevent ketoacidosis and tissue atrophy
- sodium and potassium restrictions, to prevent elevated levels
- fluid restrictions, to maintain fluid balance
- loop diuretics, such as furosemide, to maintain fluid balance
- cardiac glycosides, such as digoxin, to mobilize fluids causing edema
- calcium carbonate or calcium acetate, to treat renal osteodystrophy by binding phosphate and supplementing calcium
- antihypertensives, to control blood pressure and edema
- antiemetics, to relieve nausea and vomiting
- famotidine or ranitidine, to decrease gastric irritation
- methylcellulose or docusate, to prevent constipation

- iron and folate supplements or RBC transfusion for anemia
- synthetic erythropoietin, to stimulate the bone marrow to produce RBCs; supplemental iron, conjugated estrogens, and desmopressin, to combat hematologic effects
- antipruritics, such as trimeprazine or diphenhydramine, to relieve itching
- aluminum hydroxide gel, to reduce serum phosphate levels
- supplementary vitamins, particularly B and D, and essential amino acids
- dialysis for hyperkalemia and fluid imbalances
- oral or rectal administration of cation exchange resins, such as sodium polystyrene sulfonate, and I.V. administration of calcium gluconate, sodium bicarbonate, 50% dextrose, and regular insulin, to reverse hyperkalemia
- emergency pericardiocentesis or surgery for cardiac tamponade
- intensive dialysis and thoracentesis, to relieve pulmonary edema and pleural effusion
- peritoneal or hemodialysis, to help control end-stage renal disease
- renal transplantation (usually the treatment of choice if a donor is available).

Congenital anomalies of the ureter, bladder, and urethra

Congenital anomalies of the ureter, bladder, and urethra are among the most common birth defects, occurring in about 5% of births. Some of these abnormalities are obvious at birth; others are recognized only after they produce symptoms.

CAUSES
Causes of these congenital anomalies are unknown.

PATHOPHYSIOLOGY
The most common malformations include duplicated ureter, retrocaval ureter, ectopic orifice of the ureter, stricture or stenosis of the ureter, ureterocele, exstrophy of the bladder, congenital bladder diverticulum, hypospadias, and epispadias. Their pathophysiology, signs and symptoms, diagnosis, and treatment vary. (See *Congenital urologic anomalies,* pages 506 to 508.)

(Text continues on page 508.)

Congenital urologic anomalies

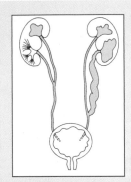

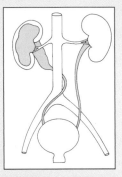

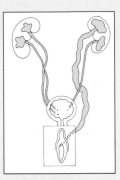

DUPLICATED URETER

Pathophysiology
◆ Most common ureteral anomaly
◆ Complete — a double collecting system with two separate renal pelves in a kidney, each with its own ureter and orifice
◆ Incomplete — two separate ureters from a kidney joining before entering bladder

Clinical features
◆ Persistent or recurrent infection
◆ Frequency, urgency, or burning on urination
◆ Diminished urine output
◆ Flank pain, fever, and chills

Diagnosis and treatment
◆ Excretory urography
◆ Voiding cystoscopy
◆ Cystoureterography
◆ Retrograde pyelography
◆ Surgery for obstruction, reflux, or severe renal damage

RETROCAVAL URETER (PREURETERAL VENA CAVA)

Pathophysiology
◆ Right ureter passing behind the inferior vena cava before entering the bladder (compression of the ureter between the vena cava and the spine causes dilation and elongation of the renal pelvis; hydroureter, hydronephrosis; fibrosis and stenosis of ureter in the compressed area)
◆ Relatively uncommon; higher incidence in males

Clinical features
◆ Right flank pain
◆ Recurrent urinary tract infection
◆ Renal calculi
◆ Hematuria

Diagnosis and treatment
◆ Excretory urography demonstrating superior ureteral enlargement with spiral appearance
◆ Surgical resection and anastomosis of ureter with renal pelvis, or reimplantation into bladder

ECTOPIC ORIFICE OF URETER

Pathophysiology
◆ Ureters single or duplicate; in females, ureteral orifice usually inserts in urethra or vaginal vestibule, beyond external urethral sphincter; in males, in prostatic urethra, or in seminal vesicles or vas deferens

Clinical features
◆ Symptoms rare when ureteral orifice opens between trigone and bladder neck
◆ Obstruction, reflux, and incontinence (dribbling) in 50% of females
◆ In males, flank pain, frequency, urgency

Diagnosis and treatment
◆ Excretory urography
◆ Urethroscopy, vaginoscopy
◆ Voiding cystourethrography
◆ Resection and ureteral reimplantation into bladder (for incontinence)

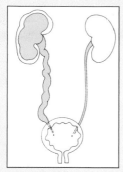 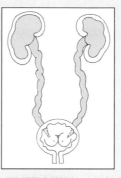 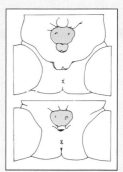

STRICTURES OR STENOSIS OF URETER

Pathophysiology
◆ Most common site, the distal ureter above ureterovesical junction; less common, ureteropelvic junction; rare, the midureter
◆ Discovered during infancy in 25% of patients; before puberty in most
◆ More common in males

Clinical features
◆ Megaloureter or hydroureter (enlarged ureter), with hydronephrosis when stenosis occurs in distal ureter
◆ Hydronephrosis alone when stenosis occurs at ureteropelvic junction

Diagnosis and treatment
◆ Ultrasound
◆ Excretory urography
◆ Voiding cystography
◆ Surgical repair of stricture; nephrectomy for severe renal damage

URETEROCELE

Pathophysiology
◆ Bulging of submucosal ureter into bladder can be 1 or 2 cm or can almost fill bladder
◆ Unilateral, bilateral, ectopic with resulting hydroureter and hydronephrosis

Clinical features
◆ Obstruction
◆ Persistent or recurrent infection

Diagnosis and treatment
◆ Voiding cystourethrography
◆ Excretory urography and cystoscopy showing thin, translucent mass
◆ Surgical excision or resection of ureterocele, with reimplantation of ureter

EXSTROPHY OF BLADDER

Pathophysiology
◆ Absence of anterior abdominal and bladder wall allowing the bladder to protrude onto abdomen
◆ In males, associated undescended testes and epispadias; in females, cleft clitoris, separated labia, or absent vagina
◆ Skeletal or intestinal anomalies possible

Clinical features
◆ Obvious at birth, with urine seeping onto abdominal wall from abnormal ureteral orifices
◆ Surrounding skin excoriated; exposed bladder mucosa ulcerated; infection; related abnormalities

Diagnosis and treatment
◆ Excretory urography
◆ Surgical closure of defect, and reconstruction of bladder and urethra during infancy to allow pubic bone fusion; alternative treatment: protective dressing and diapering; urinary diversion eventually necessary for most patients

(continued))

Congenital urologic anomalies (continued)

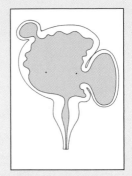

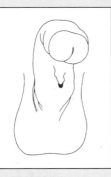

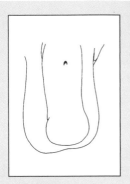

CONGENITAL BLADDER DIVERTICULUM

Pathophysiology
◆ Circumscribed pouch or sac (diverticulum) of bladder wall
◆ Occur anywhere in bladder, usually lateral to ureteral orifice (large diverticulum at orifice can cause reflux)

Clinical features
◆ Fever, frequency, and painful urination
◆ Urinary tract infection
◆ Cystitis, particularly in males

Diagnosis and treatment
◆ Excretory urography showing diverticulum
◆ Retrograde cystography showing vesicoureteral reflux in ureter
◆ Surgical correction for reflux

HYPOSPADIAS

Pathophysiology
◆ Urethral opening is on ventral surface of penis or, in females (rare), within the vagina
◆ Occurs in 1 in 300 live male births (genetic factor suspected in less severe cases)

Clinical features
◆ Usually linked to chordee (downward bowing of the penis), making normal urination with penis elevated impossible
◆ Absence of ventral prepuce
◆ Vaginal discharge in females

Diagnosis and treatment
◆ Mild disorder — no treatment
◆ Surgical repair of severe anomaly usually necessary before child reaches school age

EPISPADIAS

Pathophysiology
◆ Urethral opening on dorsal surface of penis; in females, a fissure of the upper wall of urethra
◆ A rare anomaly; usually developing in males; commonly accompanies bladder exstrophy

Clinical features
◆ In mild cases, orifice appearing along dorsum of glans; in severe cases, along dorsum of penis
◆ In females, bifid (in two parts or branches) clitoris and short, wide urethra

Diagnosis and treatment
◆ Surgical repair, in several stages, almost always necessary

Glomerulonephritis

Glomerulonephritis is a bilateral inflammation of the glomeruli, typically after a streptococcal infection. Acute glomerulonephritis is also called *acute poststreptococcal glomerulonephritis*.

Acute glomerulonephritis is most common in boys ages 3 to 7, but it can occur at any age. Of those affected, up to 95% of children and 70% of adults recover fully; the rest, especially elderly patients, may progress to chronic renal failure within months.

Rapidly progressive glomerulonephritis (RPGN) — also called *subacute, crescentic, or extracapillary glomerulonephritis* — most commonly occurs between ages 50 and 60. It may be idiopathic or linked to a proliferative glomerular disease such as poststreptococcal glomerulonephritis.

▲ **AGE ALERT**
Goodpasture's syndrome, a type of rapidly progressive glomerulonephritis, is rare but occurs most commonly in men ages 20 to 30.

Chronic glomerulonephritis is a slowly progressive disease characterized by inflammation, sclerosis, scarring and, eventually, renal failure. It usually remains undetected until the progressive phase, which is usually irreversible.

CAUSES

Causes of acute glomerulonephritis and RPGN include:
■ streptococcal infection of the respiratory tract
■ impetigo
■ immunoglobulin (Ig) A nephropathy (Berger's disease)
■ lipoid nephrosis.

Chronic glomerulonephritis is caused by:
■ membranoproliferative glomerulonephritis
■ membranous glomerulopathy
■ focal glomerulosclerosis
■ poststreptococcal glomerulonephritis
■ systemic lupus erythematosus
■ hemolytic uremic syndrome.

PATHOPHYSIOLOGY

In nearly all types of glomerulonephritis, the epithelial or podocyte layer of the glomerular membrane is disturbed. This results in a loss of negative charge. (See *Characteristics of glomerular lesions,*)

Acute poststreptococcal glomerulonephritis results from the entrapment and collection of antigen-antibody com-

---

Characteristics of glomerular lesions

The types of glomerular lesions and their characteristics include:
◆ diffuse lesions — relatively uniform, involve most or all glomeruli (for example, glomerulonephritis)
◆ focal lesions — involve only some glomeruli
◆ segmental-local — involve only one part of the glomerulus
◆ mesangial — deposits of immunoglobulins in mesangial matrix
◆ membranous — thickening of glomerular capillary wall
◆ proliferative lesions — increased number of glomerular cells
◆ sclerotic lesions — glomerular scarring from previous glomerular injury
◆ crescent lesions — accumulation of proliferating cells in Bowman's space.

---

plexes in the glomerular capillary membranes, after infection with a group A beta-hemolytic streptococcus. The antigens, which are endogenous or exogenous, stimulate the formation of antibodies. Circulating antigen-antibody complexes become lodged in the glomerular capillaries. (See *Glomerulonephritis,* page 510.)

Glomerular injury occurs when the complexes activate the complement system. Immunologic substances that lyse (cause the disintegration of) cells and increase membrane permeability are released. Antibody damage to basement membranes causes crescent (an intrusive crescent-shaped mass of cells) formation. The severity of glomerular damage and renal insufficiency is related to the size, number, location (focal or diffuse), duration of exposure, and type of antigen-antibody complexes.

Antibody or antigen-antibody complexes in the glomerular capillary wall activate biochemical mediators of inflammation — complement, leukocytes, and fibrin. Activated complement attracts neutrophils and monocytes, which release lysosomal

Glomerulonephritis

This illustration shows the immune complex deposits of glomerulonephritis.

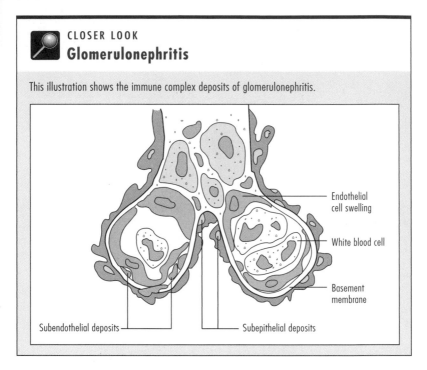

- Endothelial cell swelling
- White blood cell
- Basement membrane
- Subendothelial deposits
- Subepithelial deposits

enzymes that damage the glomerular cell walls and cause a proliferation of the extracellular matrix, affecting glomerular blood flow. Those events increase membrane permeability, which causes a loss of negative charge across the glomerular membrane as well as enhanced protein filtration.

Membrane damage leads to platelet aggregation, and platelet degranulation releases substances that increase glomerular permeability. Protein molecules and red blood cells (RBCs) can now pass into the urine, resulting in proteinuria and hematuria. Activation of the coagulation system leads to fibrin deposits in Bowman's space. The result is crescent formation and diminished renal blood flow and glomerular filtration rate (GFR). Glomerular bleeding causes acidic urine, which transforms hemoglobin to methemoglobin and results in brown urine without clots.

The inflammatory response decreases the GFR, which causes fluid retention and decreased urine output, extracellular fluid

volume expansion, and hypertension. Gross proteinuria is linked to nephrotic syndrome. After 10 to 20 years, renal insufficiency develops, followed by nephrotic syndrome and end-stage renal failure.

Goodpasture's syndrome is an RPGN in which antibodies are produced against the pulmonary capillaries and glomerular basement membrane. Diffuse intracellular antibody proliferation in Bowman's space leads to a crescent-shaped structure that obliterates the space. The crescent is composed of fibrin and endothelial, mesangial, and phagocytic cells, which compress the glomerular capillaries, diminish blood flow, and cause extensive scarring of the glomeruli. GFR is reduced, and renal failure occurs within weeks or months.

IgA nephropathy, or Berger's disease, is usually idiopathic. Plasma IgA level is elevated, and IgA and inflammatory cells are deposited into Bowman's space. The result is sclerosis and fibrosis of the glomerulus and a reduced GFR.

Lipid nephrosis causes disruption of the capillary filtration membrane and loss of its negative charge. This increased permeability with resultant loss of protein leads to nephrotic syndrome.

Systemic diseases, such as hepatitis B virus, systemic lupus erythematosus, or solid malignant tumors, cause a membranous nephropathy. An inflammatory process causes thickening of the glomerular capillary wall. Increased permeability and proteinuria lead to nephrotic syndrome.

Sometimes the immune complement further damages the glomerular membrane. The damaged and inflamed glomeruli lose the ability to be selectively permeable; as a result RBCs and proteins filter through as GFR decreases. Uremic poisoning may result. Renal function may deteriorate, especially in adults with sporadic acute poststreptococcal glomerulonephritis, commonly in the form of glomerulosclerosis accompanied by hypertension. The more severe the disorder, the more likely the occurrence of complications. Hypervolemia leads to hypertension, resulting from either sodium and water retention (caused by the decreased GFR) or inappropriate renin release. The patient develops pulmonary edema and heart failure. (See *Averting renal failure in glomerulonephritis,* page 512.)

SIGNS AND SYMPTOMS

Possible signs and symptoms of glomerulonephritis include:
- decreased urination or oliguria because of decreased GFR
- smoky or coffee-colored urine because of hematuria
- dyspnea and orthopnea because of pulmonary edema caused by hypervolemia
- periorbital edema caused by hypervolemia
- mild to severe hypertension caused by decreased GFR, sodium or water retention, or inappropriate release of renin
- bibasilar crackles caused by heart failure.

AGE ALERT
The presenting features of glomerulonephritis in children may be encephalopathy with seizures and local neurologic deficits. An elderly person with glomerulonephritis may report vague, nonspecific symptoms, such as nausea, malaise, and arthralgia.

COMPLICATIONS

Possible complications of glomerulonephritis include:
- pulmonary edema
- heart failure
- sepsis
- renal failure
- severe hypertension
- cardiac hypertrophy.

DIAGNOSIS

Blood study results that aid in diagnosis include:
- elevated electrolyte, blood urea nitrogen, and creatinine levels
- decreased serum protein level
- decreased hemoglobin levels in chronic glomerulonephritis
- elevated antistreptolysin-O titers (in 80% of patients), elevated streptozyme (a hemagglutination test that detects antibodies to several streptococcal antigens) and anti-DNase B (a test to determine a previous infection of group A beta-hemolytic streptococcus) titers, low serum complement levels indicating recent streptococcal infection.

Urinalysis results that help diagnose glomerulonephritis include:
- RBCs, white blood cells, mixed cell casts, and protein indicating renal failure
- fibrin-degradation products and C3 protein.

 AGE ALERT
Significant proteinuria isn't a common finding in an elderly patient.

Other results that help diagnose glomerulonephritis are:
- throat culture showing group A beta-hemolytic streptococcus
- bilateral kidney enlargement on kidney-ureter-bladder X-ray (acute glomerulonephritis)
- symmetric contraction of renal pelves with normal pelves and calyces (chronic glomerulonephritis) as seen on X-ray
- renal biopsy confirming the diagnosis or assessing renal tissue status.

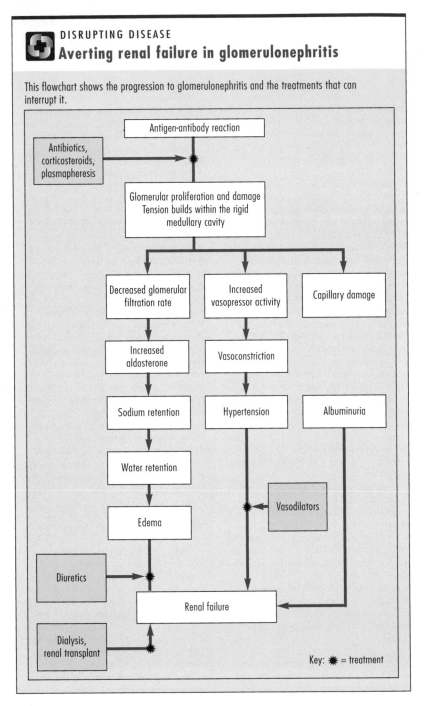

DISRUPTING DISEASE
Averting renal failure in glomerulonephritis

This flowchart shows the progression to glomerulonephritis and the treatments that can interrupt it.

Antigen-antibody reaction

Antibiotics, corticosteroids, plasmapheresis ✳

Glomerular proliferation and damage
Tension builds within the rigid medullary cavity

Decreased glomerular filtration rate

Increased vasopressor activity

Capillary damage

Increased aldosterone

Vasoconstriction

Sodium retention

Hypertension

Albuminuria

Water retention

Vasodilators ✳

Edema

Diuretics ✳

Renal failure

Dialysis, renal transplant ✳

Key: ✳ = treatment

TREATMENT

Treatment involves:
- treating the primary disease to alter immunologic cascade
- antibiotics for 7 to 10 days to treat infections contributing to ongoing antigen-antibody response
- anticoagulants, to control fibrin crescent formation in RPGN
- bed rest to reduce metabolic demands
- fluid restrictions to decrease edema
- dietary sodium restriction to prevent fluid retention
- correction of electrolyte imbalances
- loop diuretics, such as metolazone or furosemide, to reduce extracellular fluid overload
- vasodilators, such as hydralazine or nifedipine, to decrease hypertension
- dialysis or kidney transplantation for chronic glomerulonephritis
- corticosteroids to decrease antibody synthesis and suppress inflammatory response
- plasmapheresis in RPGN to suppress rebound antibody production, possibly combined with corticosteroids and cyclophosphamide.

Nephrotic syndrome

Marked proteinuria, hypoalbuminemia, hyperlipidemia, and edema characterize nephrotic syndrome. It results from a defect in the permeability of glomerular vessels. About 75% of cases result from primary (idiopathic) glomerulonephritis. The prognosis is highly variable, depending on the underlying cause.

AGE ALERT

Age has no part in the progression or prognosis of nephrotic syndrome. Primary nephrotic syndrome is found predominantly in the preschool child. It's more common in boys than in girls; incidence is 3 per 100,000 children per year. Incidence peaks between ages 2 and 3, and is rare after age 8.

Some forms of nephrotic syndrome may eventually progress to end-stage renal failure.

CAUSES

Causes of nephrotic syndrome include:
- lipid nephrosis (nil lesions)
- membranous glomerulonephritis

AGE ALERT

Lipid nephrosis is the main cause of nephrotic syndrome in children younger than age 8.

Membranous glomerulonephritis is the most common lesion in adult idiopathic nephrotic syndrome.
- focal glomerulosclerosis
- membranoproliferative glomerulonephritis
- metabolic diseases such as diabetes mellitus
- collagen-vascular disorders, such as systemic lupus erythematosus and periarteritis nodosa
- circulatory diseases, such as heart failure, sickle cell anemia, and renal vein thrombosis
- nephrotoxins, such as mercury, gold, and bismuth
- infections, such as tuberculosis and enteritis
- allergic reactions
- pregnancy
- hereditary nephritis
- neoplastic diseases such as multiple myeloma.

PATHOPHYSIOLOGY

In lipid nephrosis, the glomeruli appear normal by light microscopy, and some tubules may contain increased lipid deposits. Membranous glomerulonephritis is characterized by the appearance of immune complexes, seen as dense deposits in the glomerular basement membrane, and by the uniform thickening of the basement membrane. It eventually progresses to renal failure.

Focal glomerulosclerosis can develop spontaneously at any age, can occur after kidney transplantation, or may result from heroin injection. Ten percent of children with nephrotic syndrome, and up to 20% of adults, develop this condition. Lesions initially affect some of the deeper glomeruli, causing hyaline sclerosis. Involvement of the superficial glomeruli occurs later. These lesions usually cause slowly progressive deterioration in renal function, although remission may occur in children.

Membranoproliferative glomerulonephritis causes slowly progressive lesions in the subendothelial region of the basement membrane. This disorder may follow infection, particularly streptococcal infection, and occurs primarily in children and young adults.

Regardless of the cause, the injured glomerular filtration membrane allows the loss of plasma proteins, especially albumin and immunoglobulin. In addition, metabolic, biochemical, or physiochemical disturbances in the glomerular basement membrane result in the loss of negative charge as well as increased permeability to protein. Hypoalbuminemia results not only from urinary loss but also from decreased hepatic synthesis of replacement albumin. Hypoalbuminemia stimulates the liver to synthesize lipoprotein, resulting in hyperlipidemia, and clotting factors. Decreased dietary intake, as with anorexia, malnutrition, or concomitant disease, further contributes to decreased plasma albumin levels. Loss of immunoglobulin also increases susceptibility to infections.

Extensive proteinuria (more than 3.5 g/ day) and a low serum albumin level, caused by renal loss, lead to low serum colloid osmotic pressure and edema. The low serum albumin level also leads to hypovolemia and compensatory salt and water retention. Consequent hypertension may precipitate heart failure in compromised patients.

SIGNS AND SYMPTOMS
Possible signs and symptoms of nephrotic syndrome include:
- periorbital edema caused by fluid overload (generally occurs in the morning)
- mild to severe dependent edema of the ankles or sacrum resulting from fluid overload
- orthostatic hypotension caused by fluid imbalance
- ascites caused by fluid imbalance
- swollen external genitalia because of edema in dependent areas
- respiratory difficulty because of pleural effusion
- anorexia because of edema of intestinal mucosa
- pallor and shiny skin with prominent veins

- diarrhea caused by edema of intestinal mucosa
- frothy urine in children
- change in quality of hair related to protein deficiency
- pneumonia because of susceptibility to infections.

COMPLICATIONS
Possible complications include:
- malnutrition
- infection
- coagulation disorders
- thromboembolic vascular occlusion (especially in the lungs and legs)
- accelerated atherosclerosis
- hypochromic anemia caused by excessive urinary excretion of transferrin
- acute renal failure.

DIAGNOSIS
Diagnosis is based on:
- consistent heavy proteinuria (24-hour protein more than 3.5 mg/dl)
- urinalysis showing hyaline, granular and waxy fatty casts, and oval fat bodies
- increased serum cholesterol, phospholipid (especially low-density and very low-density lipoproteins), and triglyceride levels, and decreased albumin levels
- renal biopsy for histologic identification of the lesion.

TREATMENT
Treatment includes:
- correction of underlying cause, if possible
- nutritious diet, including 0.6 g of protein/kg of body weight
- restricted sodium intake to reduce edema
- diuretics to diminish edema
- antibiotics to treat infection
- 8-week course of a corticosteroid such as prednisone, followed by maintenance therapy or a combination of prednisone and azathioprine or cyclophosphamide
- treatment for hyperlipidemia (usually unsuccessful)
- paracentesis for ascites
- thoracentesis for pleural effusion.

Neurogenic bladder

All types of bladder dysfunction caused by an interruption of normal bladder innervation by the nervous system are referred to as neurogenic bladder. Other names for this disorder include neuromuscular dysfunction of the lower urinary tract, neurologic bladder dysfunction, and neuropathic bladder. Neurogenic bladder can be hyperreflexic (hypertonic, spastic, or automatic) or flaccid (hypotonic, atonic, or autonomous).

CAUSES

Many factors can interrupt bladder innervation. Cerebral disorders causing neurogenic bladder include:

- stroke
- brain tumor (meningioma and glioma)
- Parkinson's disease
- multiple sclerosis
- dementia
- incontinence linked to aging.

Spinal cord disease or trauma can also cause neurogenic bladder, including:

- spinal stenosis causing cord compression
- arachnoiditis (inflammation of the membrane between the dura and pia mater) causing adhesions between membranes covering the cord
- cervical spondylosis
- spina bifida
- poliomyelitis
- myelopathies from hereditary or nutritional deficiencies
- tabes dorsalis (degeneration of the dorsal columns of the spinal cord)
- disorders of peripheral innervation, including autonomic neuropathies, caused by endocrine disturbances such as diabetes mellitus (most common).

Other causes include:

- metabolic disturbances, such as hypothyroidism or uremia
- acute infectious diseases, such as Guillain-Barré syndrome or transverse myelitis (pathologic changes extending across the spinal cord)
- heavy metal toxicity
- chronic alcoholism
- collagen diseases such as systemic lupus erythematosus

- vascular diseases such as atherosclerosis
- distant effects of certain cancers such as primary oat cell carcinoma of the lung
- herpes zoster
- sacral agenesis (absence of a completely formed sacrum).

PATHOPHYSIOLOGY

An upper motor neuron lesion (at or above T12) causes spastic neurogenic bladder, with spontaneous contractions of detrusor muscles, increased intravesical voiding pressure, bladder wall hypertrophy with trabeculation (formation of strands of connective tissue, and urinary sphincter spasms. The patient may experience small urine volume, incomplete emptying, and loss of voluntary control of voiding. Urinary retention also sets the stage for infection.

A lower motor neuron lesion (at or below S2 to S4) affects the spinal reflex that controls micturition. The result is a flaccid neurogenic bladder with decreased intravesical pressure and increased bladder capacity, residual urine retention, and poor detrusor contraction. The bladder may not empty spontaneously. The patient experiences loss of voluntary and involuntary control of urination. Lower motor neuron lesions lead to overflow incontinence. When sensory neurons are interrupted, the patient can't perceive the need to void.

Interruption of the efferent nerves at the cortical, or upper motor neuron, level results in loss of voluntary control. Higher centers also control micturition, and voiding may be incomplete. Sensory neuron interruption leads to dribbling and overflow incontinence. (See *Types of neurogenic bladder,* page 516.) Altered bladder sensation often makes symptoms difficult to discern.

Retention of urine contributes to renal calculi as well as infection. Neurogenic bladder can lead to deterioration of renal function if not promptly diagnosed and treated.

SIGNS AND SYMPTOMS

Possible signs and symptoms of neurogenic bladder include:

Types of neurogenic bladder

NEURAL LESION	TYPE	CAUSE
Upper motor	Uninhibited	◆ Lack of voluntary control in infancy ◆ Multiple sclerosis
	Reflex or automatic	◆ Spinal cord transection ◆ Cord tumors ◆ Multiple sclerosis
Lower motor	Autonomous	◆ Sacral cord trauma ◆ Tumors ◆ Herniated disk ◆ Abdominal surgery with transection of pelvic parasympathetic nerves
	Motor paralysis	◆ Lesions at levels S2, S3, S4 ◆ Poliomyelitis ◆ Trauma ◆ Tumors
	Sensory paralysis	◆ Posterior lumbar nerve roots ◆ Diabetes mellitus ◆ Tabes dorsalis

■ some degree of incontinence, changes in initiation or interruption of micturition, or inability to completely empty the bladder caused by interrupted nerve impulse transmission

■ frequent urinary tract infections (UTIs) because of urine retention

■ hyperactive autonomic reflexes (autonomic dysreflexia) when the bladder is distended and the lesion is at upper thoracic or cervical level

■ severe hypertension, bradycardia, and vasodilation (blotchy skin) above the level of the lesion

■ piloerection and profuse sweating above the level of the lesion

■ involuntary or frequent, scant urination without a feeling of bladder fullness, caused by hyperreflexic neurogenic bladder

■ spontaneous spasms (caused by voiding) of the arms and legs because of hyperreflexic neurogenic bladder

■ increased anal sphincter tone caused by hyperreflexic neurogenic bladder

■ voiding and spontaneous contractions of the arms and legs caused by tactile stimulation of the abdomen, thighs, or genitalia

■ overflow incontinence and diminished anal sphincter tone because of flaccid neurogenic bladder

■ greatly distended bladder without feeling of bladder fullness because of sensory impairment.

COMPLICATIONS
Complications of neurogenic bladder may include:
■ incontinence
■ residual urine retention
■ UTI
■ calculus formation
■ renal failure.

DIAGNOSIS
The following studies may help diagnose neurogenic bladder:

- voiding cystourethrography to evaluate bladder neck function, vesicoureteral reflux, and continence
- urodynamic studies to evaluate how urine is stored in the bladder, how well the bladder empties urine, and the rate of movement of urine out of the bladder during voiding
- urine flow study (uroflow) to show diminished or impaired urine flow
- cystometry to evaluate bladder nerve supply, detrusor muscle tone, and intravesical pressures during bladder filling and contraction
- urethral pressure profile to determine urethral function with respect to the urethra's length and outlet pressure resistance
- sphincter electromyelography to correlate neuromuscular function of the external sphincter with bladder muscle function during bladder filling and contraction, and to evaluate how well the bladder and urinary sphincter muscles work together
- videourodynamic studies to correlate visual documentation of bladder function with pressure studies
- retrograde urethrography to show strictures and diverticula.

TREATMENT

Treatment includes:
- intermittent self-catheterization to empty the bladder
- anticholinergics and alpha-adrenergic stimulators for the patient with hyperreflexic neurogenic bladder, until intermittent self-catheterization is performed
- terazosin and doxazosin to facilitate bladder emptying in neurogenic bladder
- propantheline, methantheline, flavoxate, dicyclomine, imipramine, and pseudoephedrine to facilitate urine storage
- surgery to correct structural impairment through transurethral resection of the bladder neck, urethral dilation, external sphincterotomy, or urinary diversion procedures
- implantation of an artificial urinary sphincter may be necessary if permanent incontinence follows surgery.

Polycystic kidney disease

Polycystic kidney disease is an inherited disorder characterized by multiple, bilateral, grapelike clusters of fluid-filled cysts that enlarge the kidneys, compressing and eventually replacing functioning renal tissue. (See *Polycystic kidney.*)

The disease affects males and females equally and appears in two distinct forms. Autosomal dominant polycystic kidney disease (ADPKD) occurs in 1 in 1,000 to 1 in 3,000 people and accounts for about 10% of end-stage renal disease in the United States. The rare infantile form causes stillbirth or early neonatal death. The adult form has an insidious onset but usually becomes obvious between ages 30 and 50; rarely, it remains asymptomatic until the patient is in his 70s.

AGE ALERT
Renal deterioration is more gradual in adults than infants, but in both age groups, the disease progresses relentlessly to fatal uremia.

The prognosis in adults is extremely variable. Progression may be slow, even

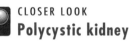

CLOSER LOOK
Polycystic kidney

This cross-sectional drawing shows multiple areas of cystic damage. Each indentation indicates a cyst.

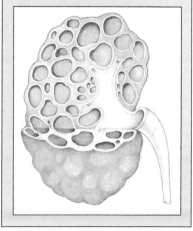

after symptoms of renal insufficiency appear. After uremia symptoms develop, polycystic disease usually is fatal within 4 years, unless the patient receives dialysis. Three genetic variants of the autosomal dominant form have been identified (see below).

CAUSES

Polycystic kidney disease is inherited as:
■ autosomal dominant trait (adult type)
■ autosomal recessive trait (infantile type).

PATHOPHYSIOLOGY

ADPKD occurs as ADPKD-1, mapped to the short arm of chromosome 16 and encoded for a 4,300–amino-acid protein; ADPKD-2, mapped to the short arm of chromosome 4 with later onset of symptoms; and a third variety not yet mapped. Autosomal recessive polycystic kidney disease occurs in 1 in 10,000 to 1 in 40,000 live births and has been localized to chromosome 6.

Grossly enlarged kidneys are caused by multiple spherical cysts, a few millimeters to centimeters in diameter, that contain straw-colored or hemorrhagic fluid. The cysts are distributed evenly throughout the cortex and medulla. Hyperplastic polyps and renal adenomas are common. Renal parenchyma may have varying degrees of tubular atrophy, interstitial fibrosis, and nephrosclerosis. The cysts cause elongation of the renal pelvis, flattening of the calyces, and indentations in the kidney.

Characteristically, an affected infant shows signs of respiratory distress, heart failure, and, eventually, uremia and renal failure. Accompanying hepatic fibrosis and intrahepatic bile duct abnormalities may cause portal hypertension and bleeding varices.

In most cases, about 10 years after symptoms appear, progressive compression of kidney structures by the enlarging mass causes renal failure.

Cysts also form elsewhere — such as on the liver, spleen, pancreas, and ovaries. Intracranial aneurysms, colonic diverticula, and mitral valve prolapse also occur.

In the autosomal recessive form, death in the neonatal period is most commonly caused by pulmonary hypoplasia.

SIGNS AND SYMPTOMS

Signs and symptoms in neonates include:
■ pronounced epicanthic folds (vertical fold of skin on either side of the nose); a pointed nose; small chin; and floppy, low-set ears (Potter facies), caused by genetic abnormalities
■ huge, bilateral, symmetrical masses on the flanks that are tense and can't be trans-illuminated caused by kidney enlargement
■ respiratory distress related to impaired renal function and fluid imbalance
■ uremia caused by renal failure.
Signs and symptoms in adults include:
■ hypertension caused by activation of the renin-angiotensin system
■ lumbar pain caused by enlarging kidney mass
■ widening abdominal girth caused by enlarged kidneys
■ swollen or tender abdomen caused by the enlarging kidney mass, worsened by exertion and relieved by lying down
■ grossly enlarged kidneys on palpation.

COMPLICATIONS

▲ **AGE ALERT**
A few infants with this disease survive for 2 years and then die of hepatic complications or renal, heart, or respiratory failure.

Possible complications in adults include:
■ pyelonephritis
■ recurrent hematuria
■ life-threatening retroperitoneal bleeding from cyst rupture
■ proteinuria
■ colicky abdominal pain from ureteral passage of clots or calculi
■ renal failure.

DIAGNOSIS

Diagnosis is based on the following test results:
■ excretory or retrograde urography showing enlarged kidneys with elongation of the renal pelvis, flattening of the caly-

ces, and indentations in the kidney caused by cysts
- excretory urography of the neonate showing poor excretion of contrast medium
- ultrasonography, tomography, and radioisotope scans showing kidney enlargement and cysts; tomography, computed tomography, and magnetic resonance imaging showing multiple areas of cystic damage
- urinalysis and creatinine clearance tests showing nonspecific results indicating abnormalities.

TREATMENT
Treatment includes:
- antibiotics for infections
- adequate hydration to maintain fluid balance
- surgical drainage of cystic abscess or retroperitoneal bleeding
- surgery for intractable pain (uncommon symptom) or analgesics for abdominal pain
- dialysis or kidney transplantation for progressive renal failure
- nephrectomy not recommended (polycystic kidney disease occurs bilaterally, and infection could recur in the remaining kidney).

Renal agenesis

Renal agenesis is the failure of a kidney to grow or develop. The kidney is usually polycystic and dysplastic. The disease may be unilateral or bilateral, random or hereditary, and occur in isolation or linked to other disorders. Unilateral renal agenesis occurs in 1 in 1,000 live births, and more commonly in boys than girls.

Bilateral renal agenesis is also called *Potter's syndrome.* It occurs in 1 of every 3,000 live births, and 75% of the cases are in boys. Bilateral renal agenesis isn't compatible with life, and most affected fetuses die in utero.

AGE ALERT
Neonates with Potter's syndrome rarely live longer than a few hours.

CAUSES
The causes of renal agenesis are unknown but suspected to be hereditary.

PATHOPHYSIOLOGY
In unilateral renal agenesis, the left kidney is usually absent. The remaining kidney may be completely normal. During the first years of life, this kidney hypertrophies to functionally compensate for the missing kidney. If the kidney has abnormalities of the collecting system, compensation is virtually impossible. Extrarenal congenital abnormalities are common with this type of agenesis.

SIGNS AND SYMPTOMS
There are no symptoms of unilateral renal agenesis if the remaining kidney is functioning appropriately. Signs and symptoms of Potter's syndrome are caused by a congenital anomaly and include:
- wide-set eyes
- parrot-beak nose
- low-set ears
- receding chin
- pulmonary pathophysiology.

COMPLICATIONS
A complication of renal agenesis is:
- renal failure.

DIAGNOSIS
Diagnosis is based on prenatal ultrasound.

TREATMENT
Treatment includes surgery for structural or functional defects in the remaining kidney.

Renal calculi

Renal calculi, or stones (nephrolithiasis), can form anywhere in the urinary tract, although they most commonly develop on the renal pelves or calyces. They may vary in size and may be solitary or multiple. (See *Renal calculi,* page 520.)

Renal calculi are more common in men than in women and rarely occur in children. Calcium calculi generally occur in middle-age men with a familial history of calculus formation.

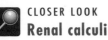

CLOSER LOOK
Renal calculi

Renal calculi vary in size and type. Small calculi may remain in the renal pelvis or pass down the ureter. A "staghorn" calculus (a cast of the calyceal and pelvic collecting system) may develop from a calculus that stays in the kidney.

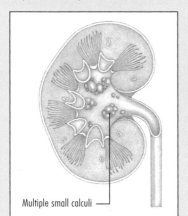

Multiple small calculi ⎯

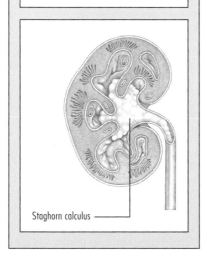

Staghorn calculus ⎯⎯

CULTURAL DIVERSITY
Renal calculi rarely occur in blacks. They're prevalent in certain geographic areas, such as the southeastern

United States (called the "stone belt"), possibly because a hot climate promotes dehydration and concentrates calculus-forming substances, or because of regional dietary habits.

CAUSES
Although the exact cause is unknown, predisposing factors of renal calculi include:
- dehydration
- infection
- changes in urine pH (calcium carbonate calculi, high pH; uric acid calculi, lower pH)
- obstruction to urine flow leading to stasis in the urinary tract
- immobilization causing calcium to be released into the blood, which is filtered by the kidneys
- metabolic factors
- dietary factors
- renal disease
- gout (a disease of increased uric acid production or decreased excretion).

PATHOPHYSIOLOGY
The major types of renal calculi are calcium oxalate and calcium phosphate, accounting for 75% to 80% of calculi; struvite (magnesium, ammonium, and phosphate), 15%; and uric acid, 7%. Cystine calculi are relatively rare, making up 1% of all renal calculi.

Calculi form when substances that are normally dissolved in the urine, such as calcium oxalate and calcium phosphate, precipitate. Dehydration may lead to renal calculi as calculus-forming substances concentrate in urine.

Calculi form around a nucleus or nidus in the appropriate environment. A crystal evolves in the presence of calculus-forming substances (calcium oxalate, calcium carbonate, magnesium, ammonium, phosphate, or uric acid) and becomes trapped in the urinary tract, where it attracts other crystals to form a calculus. A high urine saturation of these substances encourages crystal formation and results in calculus growth.

Calculi may be composed of different substances, and the pH of the urine affects the solubility of many calculus-forming substances. Formation of calcium oxalate and cystine calculi is independent of urine pH.

Calculi may occur on the papillae, renal tubules, calyces, renal pelves, ureter, or bladder. Many calculi are less than 5 mm in diameter and are usually passed in the urine. Staghorn calculi can continue to grow in the pelvis, extending to the calyces, forming a branching calculus, and ultimately resulting in renal failure if not surgically removed.

Calcium calculi are the smallest. Most are calcium oxalate or a combination of oxalate and phosphate. Although 80% are idiopathic, they commonly occur with hyperuricosuria (a high level of uric acid in the urine). Prolonged immobilization can lead to bone demineralization, hypercalciuria, and calculus formation. In addition, hyperparathyroidism, renal tubular acidosis, and excessive intake of vitamin D or dietary calcium may predispose to renal calculi.

Struvite calculi are typically precipitated by an infection, particularly with *Pseudomonas* or *Proteus* species. These urea-splitting organisms are more common in women. Struvite calculi can destroy renal parenchyma.

Uric acid calculi result from gout and high uric acid concentrations in the urine. Diets high in purine (such as meat, fish, and poultry) elevate levels of uric acid in the body. Regional enteritis and ulcerative colitis can lead to the formation of uric acid calculi. These diseases commonly result in fluid loss and loss of bicarbonate, leading to metabolic acidosis. Acidic urine enhances the formation of uric acid calculi.

Cystinuria is a rare hereditary disorder in which a metabolic error causes decreased tubular reabsorption of cystine. This causes an increased amount of cystine in the urine. Because cystine is a relatively insoluble substance, its presence contributes to calculus formation.

Infected, scarred tissue may be an ideal site for calculus development. In addition, infected calculi (usually magnesium ammonium phosphate or staghorn calculi) may develop if bacteria serve as the nucleus in calculus formation.

Urinary stasis allows calculus constituents to collect and adhere and encourages infection, which compounds the obstruction.

Calculi may either enter the ureter or remain in the renal pelvis, where they damage or destroy renal parenchyma and may cause pressure necrosis.

In ureters, calculi cause obstruction with resulting hydronephrosis and tend to recur. Intractable pain and serious bleeding also can result from calculi and the damage they cause. Large, rough calculi occlude the opening to the ureteropelvic junction and increase the frequency and force of peristaltic contractions, causing hematuria from trauma. The patient usually reports pain traveling from the costovertebral angle to the flank and then to the suprapubic region and external genitalia (classic renal colic pain). Pain intensity fluctuates and may be excruciating at its peak. The patient with calculi in the renal pelvis and calyces may report a constant dull pain. He may also report back pain if calculi are causing obstruction within a kidney and severe abdominal pain from calculi traveling down a ureter. Infection can develop in static urine or after trauma as the calculus abrades surfaces. If the calculus lodges and blocks urine, hydronephrosis can occur.

SIGNS AND SYMPTOMS
Possible signs and symptoms of renal calculi include:

- severe pain resulting from obstruction
- nausea and vomiting
- fever and chills from infection
- hematuria when calculi abrade a ureter
- abdominal distention caused by obstruction and bladder filling
- anuria from bilateral obstruction or obstruction linked to a person's only kidney.

COMPLICATIONS
Complications include:

- damage or destruction of renal parenchyma
- pressure necrosis
- obstruction by the calculus
- hydronephrosis
- bleeding

- pain
- infection.

DIAGNOSIS
The following tests may be used to diagnose renal calculi:
- kidney-ureter-bladder (KUB) radiography to show most renal calculi
- excretory urography to help confirm the diagnosis and determine the size and location of calculi
- kidney ultrasonography to detect obstructive changes, such as unilateral or bilateral hydronephrosis and radiolucent calculi not seen on KUB radiography
- urine culture showing pyuria, a sign of urinary tract infection
- 24-hour urine collection test for calcium oxalate, phosphorus, and uric acid excretion levels
- calculus analysis for mineral content
- serial blood calcium and phosphorus levels to diagnose hyperparathyroidism and increased calcium relative to normal serum protein
- blood protein levels to determine the level of free calcium unbound to protein.

TREATMENT
Treatment may include:
- increasing fluid intake to more than 3 qt/day (3 L/day) to promote hydration
- antimicrobial agents to treat infection, varying with the cultured organism
- analgesics, such as meperidine or morphine, for pain
- diuretics to prevent urinary stasis and further calculus formation; thiazides to decrease calcium excretion into the urine
- low-calcium diet to prevent recurrence
- oxalate-binding cholestyramine for absorptive hypercalciuria
- parathyroidectomy for hyperparathyroidism
- allopurinol for uric acid calculi
- daily small doses of ascorbic acid to acidify urine
- cystoscopy with manipulation of the calculus to remove renal calculi too large for natural passage
- percutaneous ultrasonic lithotripsy, extracorporeal shock wave lithotripsy, or laser therapy to shatter the calculus into

fragments for removal by suction or natural passage
- surgical removal of cystine calculi or large calculi or placement of urinary diversion around the calculus to relieve obstruction.

Vesicoureteral reflux
In vesicoureteral reflux, urine flows from the bladder back into the ureters and eventually into the renal pelvis or the parenchyma. When the bladder empties only part of the stored urine, urinary tract infection (UTI) may result.

 AGE ALERT
This disorder is most common during infancy in boys and during early childhood (ages 3 to 7) in girls. Up to 25% of asymptomatic siblings of children with diagnosed primary vesicoureteral reflux also have the disorder.

Primary vesicoureteral reflux that results from congenital anomalies is more common in females. Secondary vesicoureteral reflux occurs in adults.

CULTURAL DIVERSITY
Vesicoureteral reflux is extremely rare in blacks.

CAUSES
Primary vesicoureteral reflux is caused by congenital anomalies of the ureters or bladder, including:
- short or absent intravesical ureters
- ureteral ectopia lateralis (ureter that is located more laterally in the bladder wall)
- ureteral duplication
- ureterocele
- gaping or "golf-hole" ureteral orifice.
  Secondary vesicoureteral reflux is caused by damage by:
- bladder outlet obstruction
- iatrogenic injury
- trauma
- inadequate detrusor muscle buttress in the bladder
- cystitis, repeated infections
- neurogenic bladder.

PATHOPHYSIOLOGY
Incompetence of the ureterovesical junction and shortening of intravesical ureteral musculature allow backflow of urine into the ureters when the bladder contracts

during voiding. Congenital paraurethral bladder diverticulum, acquired diverticulum (from outlet obstruction), flaccid neurogenic bladder, and high intravesical pressure may cause inadequate detrusor muscle contraction in the bladder from outlet obstruction or an unknown cause.

Vesicoureteral reflux may also result from cystitis; inflammation of the intravesical ureter causes edema and intramural ureter fixation. This usually leads to reflux in people with congenital ureteral or bladder anomalies or other predisposing conditions. Recurrent UTIs can lead to acute or chronic pyelonephritis and renal damage caused by renal scarring, hypertension, or calculi.

SIGNS AND SYMPTOMS

Signs and symptoms of vesicoureteral reflux most commonly reflect an infection of the urinary tract and include:

- urinary frequency and urgency caused by UTI
- burning and pain upon urination caused by UTI
- hematuria resulting from irritation of the urinary tract
- foul-smelling urine because of infection
- high fever and chills caused by UTI
- flank pain
- vomiting
- malaise
- palpation showing a hard, thickened bladder if posterior urethral valves are causing an obstruction in males.

 AGE ALERT
Infants with vesicoureteral reflux may have dark, concentrated urine because of retention. In children, fever, nonspecific abdominal pain, and diarrhea may be the only clinical effects. In children younger than age 5, repeated UTIs are suggestive of reflux.

COMPLICATIONS

Possible complications include:
- recurrent UTIs
- pyelonephritis
- anemia
- hypertension
- renal obstruction
- renal failure.

DIAGNOSIS

The following test results help diagnose vesicoureteral reflux:

- clean-catch urinalysis showing bacterial count more than 100,000/ml, sometimes without pyuria; microscopic examination showing red and white blood cells and increased urine pH (active infection); specific gravity less than 1.010 caused by inability to concentrate urine
- elevated serum creatinine (more than 1.2 mg/dl [115 mmol/L]) and blood urea nitrogen (more than 20 mg/dl [7.5 mmol/L] levels caused by advanced renal dysfunction

The following tests are also useful in diagnosis:

- voiding cystourethrography to identify and determine the degree of reflux, show when reflux occurs, and define the anomaly causing the reflux
- catheterization of the bladder after the patient voids to determine the amount of residual urine (post-void residual or PVR)
- excretory urography to visualize vesicoureteral reflux and to show a dilated lower ureter, a ureter visible for its entire length, hydronephrosis, calyceal distortion, and renal scarring
- cystoscopy (may confirm diagnosis)
- radioisotope scanning and renal ultrasonography to detect reflux and screen the upper urinary tract for damage caused by infection and other renal abnormalities.

TREATMENT

Treatment of vesicoureteral reflux includes:

- antibiotics to treat reflux caused by infection or related to neurogenic bladder and, in children, a short intravesical ureter (disappears spontaneously with growth)
- long-term prophylactic antibiotic therapy for recurrent infection
- vesicoureteral reimplantation to treat recurrent infection despite prophylactic antibiotic therapy
- transurethral sphincterotomy to relieve obstructed outlet
- bladder augmentation to decrease intravesical pressure.

Sensory system

Through the sensory system, a person receives stimuli that help him interact with the surrounding world. Afferent pathways connect specialized sensory receptors in the eyes, ears, nose, and mouth to the brain—the final station for continuous processing of sensory stimuli. Alterations in sensory function can lead to dysfunctions of sight and hearing as well as smell, taste, balance, and coordination.

PATHOPHYSIOLOGIC CHANGES

Alterations can occur in all the senses.

Vision

Vision disorders include alterations in ocular movement, visual acuity (clarity), accommodation, refraction, and color vision.

OCULAR MOVEMENT

When the eyes view an object, they constantly move to keep the image of the object on the *fovea*, a small area of the retina that is responsible for the best peripheral visual acuity. The six extraocular muscles that move each eye are innervated by three cranial nerves: oculomotor (III), trochlear (IV), and abducens (VI). (See *Extraocular control of eye movement.*) Alterations in ocular movement include strabismus, diplopia, and nystagmus.

Strabismus. Strabismus occurs when one eye deviates from its normal position because of the absence of normal, parallel, or coordinated movement. The eyes may have an uncoordinated appearance, and the person may experience diplopia (the perception of two images of a single object, "double vision").

In children, types of strabismus include:
- *concomitant,* in which the degree of deviation doesn't vary with the direction of gaze
- *nonconcomitant,* in which the degree of deviation varies with the direction of gaze
- *congenital* (present at birth or during the first 6 months)
- *acquired* (present during the first 2½ years)
- *latent* (phoria; apparent only when the child is tired or sick)
- constant.

Tropia, or constant strabismus, is divided into four categories: esotropia (inward deviation), exotropia (outward deviation), hypertropia (upward deviation), and hypotropia (downward deviation).

Strabismic amblyopia, "lazy" eye, is characterized by the loss of central vision in one eye; it typically results in esotropia (caused by fixation in the dominant eye and suppression of images in the deviating eye). Strabismic amblyopia may result from hyperopia (farsightedness) or anisometropia (unequal refractive power).

Esotropia may result from muscle imbalance and can be congenital or ac-

524

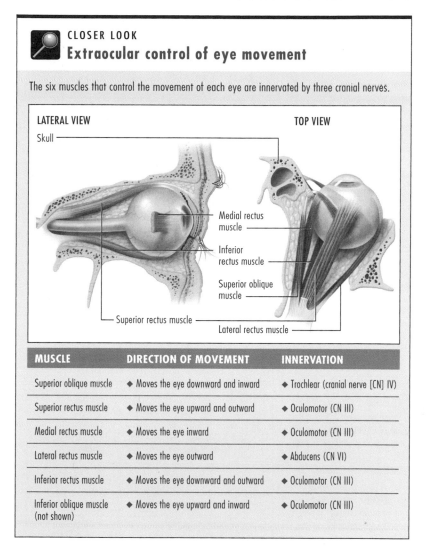

CLOSER LOOK
Extraocular control of eye movement

The six muscles that control the movement of each eye are innervated by three cranial nerves.

LATERAL VIEW

Skull

Medial rectus muscle
Inferior rectus muscle
Superior oblique muscle
Superior rectus muscle
Lateral rectus muscle

TOP VIEW

MUSCLE	DIRECTION OF MOVEMENT	INNERVATION
Superior oblique muscle	◆ Moves the eye downward and inward	◆ Trochlear (cranial nerve [CN] IV)
Superior rectus muscle	◆ Moves the eye upward and outward	◆ Oculomotor (CN III)
Medial rectus muscle	◆ Moves the eye inward	◆ Oculomotor (CN III)
Lateral rectus muscle	◆ Moves the eye outward	◆ Abducens (CN VI)
Inferior rectus muscle	◆ Moves the eye downward and outward	◆ Oculomotor (CN III)
Inferior oblique muscle (not shown)	◆ Moves the eye upward and inward	◆ Oculomotor (CN III)

quired. In accommodative esotropia, the child's attempt to compensate for the far-sightedness affects the convergent reflex, and the eyes "cross."

Strabismus is usually an inherited characteristic, but its cause is unknown. In adults, strabismus may result from trauma. The incidence of strabismus is higher in persons with central nervous system disorders, such as cerebral palsy, mental retardation, and Down syndrome.

Muscle imbalances may be corrected by glasses, patching, or surgery, depending on the cause, but residual defects in vision and extraocular muscle alignment may persist even after treatment.

AGE ALERT
In the absence of early intervention, children with strabismus may develop amblyopia as a result of cerebral suppression of visual stimuli. Deviation of an eye is the second most common

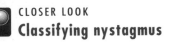

CLOSER LOOK
Classifying nystagmus

Nystagmus is classified as pendular or jerk. Each type has further classifications.

PENDULAR NYSTAGMUS
Oscillating: slow, steady oscillations of equal velocity around a center point; caused by congenital loss of visual acuity or multiple sclerosis.

Vertical or seesaw: rapid, seesaw movement in which one eye appears to rise while the other appears to fall; suggests an optic chiasm lesion.

JERK NYSTAGMUS
Convergence-retraction: irregular jerking of the eyes back into the orbit during upward gaze; can reflect midbrain tegmental (roof of the midbrain) damage.

Downbeat: irregular downward jerking of the eyes during downward gaze; can signal lower medullary damage.

Vestibular: horizontal or rotary movements of the eyes; suggests vestibular disease or cochlear dysfunction.

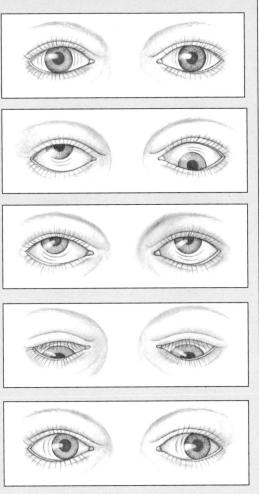

symptom in a child with retinoblastoma. Therefore, acquired strabismus should always be checked.

Diplopia. Diplopia, or double vision, results when the extraocular muscles fail to work together and images fall on noncorresponding parts of the retinas. Diplopia usually begins intermittently or affects near or far vision exclusively. It can be classified as monocular (persisting when one eye is covered) or, more commonly, binocular (clearing when one eye is covered). Monocular diplopia may result from an early cataract, retinal edema or scarring, subluxated lens (partial dislocation of the lens of the eye), poorly fitting contact lens, or uncorrected refractive error. Binocular diplopia may result from ocular deviation or displacement, extraocular muscle palsies, psychological disorders, or after retinal surgery. Other causes of binocular diplopia include infection, neoplastic disease, metabolic disorders, degenerative disease, inflammatory disorders, and vascular disease.

Nystagmus. Nystagmus refers to involuntary oscillations or alternating movements of one or both eyes. These oscillations are usually rhythmic and may be horizontal, vertical, rotary, or mixed. They may be transient or sustained and may occur spontaneously or on deviation or fixation. Nystagmus may be classified as pendular (oscillations are equal in rate in both directions) or jerk (faster movements in one direction than in the opposite direction). Nystagmoid movements usually have a fast and a slow component. The direction of the nystagmus is given by the fast component. (See *Classifying nystagmus.*)

Nystagmus is a supranuclear ocular palsy resulting from pathology in the visual perceptual area, vestibular system, or cerebellum. Causes of nystagmus include brain stem or cerebellar lesions, labyrinthine disease, stroke, encephalitis, Ménière's disease, multiple sclerosis, and alcohol and drug toxicity, including barbiturate, phenytoin, or carbamazepine toxicity.

▲ **AGE ALERT**
In children, pendular nystagmus may be idiopathic or may result from early impairment of vision linked to such disorders as optic atrophy, albinism, congenital cataracts, and severe astigmatism.

Visual acuity

Visual acuity refers to the ability to see clearly. A lack of visual acuity is commonly linked to refractive errors. In nearsightedness, or myopia, the eye focuses the visual image in front of the retina, causing objects in close view to be seen clearly and those at a distance to be blurry. In farsightedness, or hyperopia, the eye focuses the visual image behind the retina, causing objects in close view to be blurry and those at a distance to be clear. Both problems are caused by an alteration in the normal shape of the eyeball. Other causes of reduced visual acuity include aging, amblyopia, cataracts, glaucoma, papilledema, dark adaptation, and scotoma (an area of diminished visual acuity surrounded by an area of normal vision within the visual field).

Amblyopia is severely decreased visual acuity or virtual blindness in a structurally intact eye. It may be caused by toxins (including alcohol and tobacco) or may accompany such systemic diseases as diabetes mellitus or renal failure.

▲ **AGE ALERT**
With age, the pupil becomes smaller, which decreases the amount of light that reaches the retina. Older adults need about three times as much light as a younger person to see objects clearly.

ACCOMMODATION

Accommodation occurs as the thickness of the eye's lens changes to maintain visual acuity. For near vision, the ciliary body contracts and relaxes the zonules, the lens becomes spherical, the pupil constricts, and the eyes converge. For far vision, the ciliary body relaxes, the zonules tighten, the lens becomes flatter, the eyes straighten, and the pupils dilate. The oculomotor nerve and coordinated brain stem pathways account for accommodation. Alterations in accommodation may be caused by pressure, inflammation, the aging process, or disorders affecting the oculomotor nerve. The result of impaired accommodation may be diplopia, blurred vision, or headache.

REFRACTION

Refraction is the process of bending light rays so that they fall on the retina. As rays of light reach the surface of the cornea from all directions, the cornea directs them toward the lens. The lens further bends the light and directs the light rays

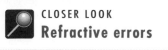

CLOSER LOOK
Refractive errors

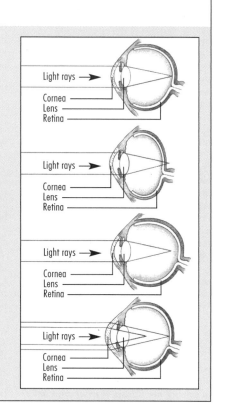

NORMAL REFRACTION
In the normal eye, light rays are focused exactly on the retina.

Light rays →
Cornea
Lens
Retina

HYPEROPIA
In hyperopia, the light rays focus behind the retina.

Light rays →
Cornea
Lens
Retina

MYOPIA
In myopia, light rays focus in front of the retina.

Light rays →
Cornea
Lens
Retina

ASTIGMATISM
In astigmatism, light rays don't come to a single focus on the retina.

Light rays →
Cornea
Lens
Retina

to one spot on the retina. The greater the refractive power, the more the light rays are bent. Emmetropia is a condition in which light rays fall exactly on the retina—that is, are focused. Refractive errors are present when light isn't properly focused on the retina. Causes include abnormalities in curvature of the cornea, focusing of the lens, and eye length. Results include myopia, hyperopia, and astigmatism. (See *Refractive errors.*)

Hyperopia. Hyperopia, or farsightedness, occurs when light rays are focused behind the retina. Distant objects appear clear, and nearby objects are blurred. This condition occurs when the eye is too short or the refractive power of the cornea or lens is

too low, and may be corrected with a convex lens that bends light rays inward.

▲ **AGE ALERT**
Presbyopia is a form of hyperopia that begins in middle-age as the eye's lens becomes firm and loses its elasticity. As a result, the refractive power of the lens is reduced, the eye loses its ability to accommodate, and near objects appear blurred. This condition is treated with a convex lens that bends light rays in different directions so they focus in a single point.

Myopia. Myopia, or nearsightedness, occurs when light rays are focused in front of the retina. Near objects can be seen clearly, and distant objects appear blurry. This condition may occur if the eye is too long or the refractive power of the cornea or lens is too great.

Myopia may also occur if hyperglycemia in uncontrolled diabetes causes lens swelling. A concave lens that bends light rays outward is used to correct myopia.

Astigmatism. Astigmatism occurs when unequal curvature of the cornea or eyeball causes light rays to focus on different points on the retina, resulting in distorted images. Astigmatism may occur along with other refractive disorders.

COLOR VISION

The retina's cones (or cone cells) are responsible for color vision. Each cone contains one of three different visual pigments (red, green, or blue) that absorb light waves of different wavelengths.

Color blindness is inherited on the X chromosome and therefore usually affects males. Acquired color blindness may also be caused by diabetes, bilateral strokes affecting the ventral portion of the occipital lobe, or disease of the macula or optic nerve.

▲ **AGE ALERT**
Older adults typically experience impaired color vision, especially in the blue and green ranges, because cones in the retina deteriorate. Yellowing of the aging lens also impairs color vision.

Hearing

Sound waves normally enter the external auditory canal, then travel to the tympanic membrane in the middle ear, causing it to vibrate. This vibration causes the malleus to move, setting in motion the incus and, in turn, the stapes. The malleus, incus, and stapes are collectively referred to as the ossicles. The stapes presses on the oval window of the inner ear, setting in motion the fluid of the cochlea and stimulating hair cells. The hair cells carry impulses through the cochlear division of the auditory cranial nerve (VIII) to the brain. This type of sound transmission to the inner ear, called air conduction, is usually better than transmission through bone (bone conduction).

Alterations in hearing are classified as conductive or sensorineural. Mixed hearing loss combines aspects of conductive and sensorineural hearing loss.

Taste and smell

The senses of taste and smell are also subject to alterations.

TASTE

The sensory receptors for taste are the taste buds, concentrated over the surface of the tongue and scattered over the palate, pharynx, and larynx. These buds can differentiate among sweet, salty, sour, and bitter stimuli. Taste and olfactory receptors together perceive more complex flavors. Much of what's considered taste is actually smell; food odors typically stimulate the olfactory system more strongly than related food tastes stimulate the taste buds.

A factor interrupting the transmission of taste stimuli to the brain may cause taste abnormalities. (See *Taste pathways to the brain,* page 530.) Taste abnormalities may result from trauma, infection, vitamin or mineral deficiencies, neurologic or oral disorders, and the effects of drugs. Moreover, because tastes are most accurately perceived in a fluid medium, dryness of the mouth may interfere with taste. Two major causes of impaired taste are aging, which normally reduces the number of taste buds, and heavy smoking (especially pipe smoking), which dries the tongue.

Alterations in taste may include:
■ *ageusia*—a complete loss of taste
■ *hypogeusia*—a partial loss of taste
■ *dysgeusia*—a distorted sense of taste
■ *cacogeusia*—an unpleasant or revolting taste of food.

▲ **AGE ALERT**
Young children typically can't differentiate between an abnormal taste sensation and a simple taste dislike.

SMELL

As air travels between the septum and the turbinates of the nose, it touches sensory hairs (cilia) and olfactory nerve endings in the mucosal surface. The resulting stimulation of cranial nerve I sends im-

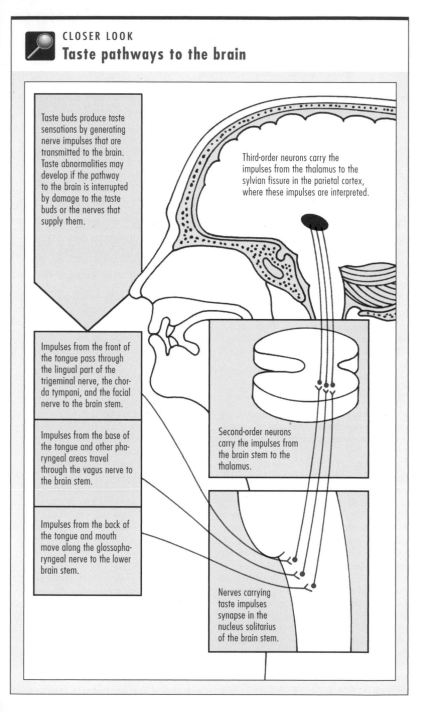

CLOSER LOOK
Taste pathways to the brain

Taste buds produce taste sensations by generating nerve impulses that are transmitted to the brain. Taste abnormalities may develop if the pathway to the brain is interrupted by damage to the taste buds or the nerves that supply them.

Third-order neurons carry the impulses from the thalamus to the sylvian fissure in the parietal cortex, where these impulses are interpreted.

Impulses from the front of the tongue pass through the lingual part of the trigeminal nerve, the chorda tympani, and the facial nerve to the brain stem.

Impulses from the base of the tongue and other pharyngeal areas travel through the vagus nerve to the brain stem.

Impulses from the back of the tongue and mouth move along the glossopharyngeal nerve to the lower brain stem.

Second-order neurons carry the impulses from the brain stem to the thalamus.

Nerves carrying taste impulses synapse in the nucleus solitarius of the brain stem.

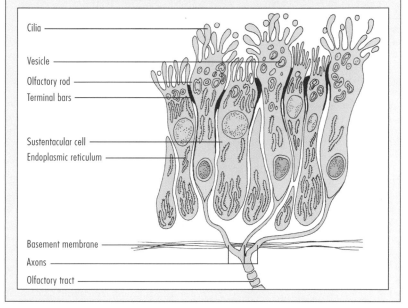

CLOSER LOOK
Olfactory perception

The exact mechanism of olfactory perception remains unknown. The most likely theory suggests that the sticky mucus covering the olfactory cells traps airborne odorous molecules. As the molecules fit into appropriate receptors on the cell surface, the opposite end of the cell transmits an electrical impulse to the brain by way of the olfactory nerve (cranial nerve I).

Cilia

Vesicle

Olfactory rod

Terminal bars

Sustentacular cell

Endoplasmic reticulum

Basement membrane

Axons

Olfactory tract

pulses to the brain's olfactory-receiving area, primarily in the frontal cortex. (See *Olfactory perception.*)

Temporary impairment in the sense of smell can result from a condition that irritates and causes swelling of the nasal mucosa and obstructs the olfactory area in the nose, such as heavy smoking, rhinitis, or sinusitis. Permanent alterations in the sense of smell usually result when the olfactory neuroepithelium or a part of the olfactory nerve is destroyed. Permanent or temporary loss can also result from inhaling irritants, such as cocaine or acid fumes, that paralyze nasal cilia. Conditions, such as aging, Parkinson's disease, Alzheimer's disease, or Kallmann's syndrome (a congenital disorder), may also alter the sense of smell. Because combined stimulation of taste buds and olfactory cells produces the sense of taste, the loss of the sense of smell is usually accompanied by the loss of the sense of taste.

Alterations in smell include:
■ *anosmia*—a total loss of the sense of smell
■ *hyposmia*—an impaired sense of smell
■ *pyarosmia*—an abnormal sense of smell.

DISORDERS

The most common disorders of vision are age-related macular degeneration, cataract, and glaucoma. Other common sensory disorders include hearing loss, Ménière's disease, and otosclerosis.

Age-related macular degeneration

Macular degeneration—atrophy or degeneration of the macular disk—is the most common cause of legal blindness in adults. Commonly affecting both eyes, it accounts for about 12% of blindness in the United States and for about 17% of new blindness. It's also one of the causes of severe irreversible and unpreventable loss of central vision in elderly persons.

Two types of age-related macular degeneration occur. The dry, or atrophic, form is characterized by atrophic pigment epithelial changes and typically causes mild, gradual visual loss. The wet, exudative form rapidly causes severe vision loss. It's characterized by the subretinal formation of new blood vessels (neovascularization) that cause leakage, hemorrhage, and fibrovascular scar formation.

CAUSES
The causes of macular degeneration are unknown but may include:
- aging
- inflammation
- injury
- infection
- nutritional factors.

PATHOPHYSIOLOGY
Age-related macular degeneration results from hardening and obstruction of retinal arteries, which probably reflect normal degenerative changes. The formation of new blood vessels in the macular area obscures central vision. Underlying pathologic changes occur primarily in the retinal pigment epithelium, Bruch's membrane, and choriocapillaris in the macular region.

The dry form develops as yellow extracellular deposits, or drusen, accumulate beneath the pigment epithelium of the retina; they may be prominent in the macula. Drusen are common in elderly persons. Over time, drusen grow and become more numerous. Vision loss occurs as the retinal pigment epithelium detaches and becomes atrophic.

Exudative macular degeneration develops as new blood vessels in the choroid project through abnormalities in Bruch's membrane and invade the potential space underneath the retinal pigment epithelium. As these vessels leak, fluid in the retinal pigment epithelium is increased, resulting in blurry vision.

SIGNS AND SYMPTOMS
Signs and symptoms of macular degeneration include:
- changes in central vision caused by neovascularization such as a blank spot (scotoma) in the center of a page when reading
- distorted appearance of straight lines caused by relocation of retinal receptors
- worsening intermittent blurred vision.

COMPLICATIONS
Possible complications include:
- visual impairment progressing to blindness
- nystagmus (if the macular degeneration is bilateral).

DIAGNOSIS
Diagnosis is based on the following test results:
- indirect ophthalmoscopy, to show gross macular changes, opacities, hemorrhage, neovascularization, retinal pallor, or retinal detachment
- I.V. fluorescein angiography sequential photographs, to show leaking vessels as fluorescein dye flows into the tissues from the subretinal neovascular net
- Amsler's grid test, to show central visual field loss.

TREATMENT
Treatment includes:
- argon laser photocoagulation, to reduce the incidence of severe visual loss in persons with subretinal neovascularization (exudative form)
- currently no cure for the atrophic form.

Cataract
A cataract is a gradually developing opacity of the lens or lens capsule of the eye. Light shining through the cornea is blocked by this opacity, and a blurred im-

age is cast onto the retina. As a result, the brain interprets a hazy image. Cataracts commonly occur bilaterally, and each progresses independently. Exceptions are traumatic cataracts, which are usually unilateral, and congenital cataracts, which may remain stationary. Cataracts are most prevalent in people older than age 70, as part of the aging process. The prognosis is generally good; surgery improves vision in 95% of affected persons.

CAUSES

Causes of cataracts include:
- aging (senile cataracts)
- congenital disorders
- genetic abnormalities
- maternal rubella during the first trimester of pregnancy
- trauma such as a lens rupture
- foreign-body injury
- disease process
- uveitis
- glaucoma
- retinitis pigmentosa
- retinal detachment
- diabetes mellitus
- hypoparathyroidism
- myotonic dystrophy
- atopic dermatitis
- exposure to ionizing radiation or infrared rays
- drugs that are toxic to the lens, including
  - prednisone
  - ergot alkaloids
  - dinitrophenol
  - naphthalene
  - phenothiazines
  - pilocarpine
- exposure to ultraviolet rays.

PATHOPHYSIOLOGY

Pathophysiology can vary with each form of cataract. Congenital cataracts are particularly challenging. (See *Congenital cataracts*.) Senile cataracts show evidence of protein aggregation, oxidative injury, and increased pigmentation in the center of the lens. In traumatic cataracts, phagocytosis of the lens or inflammation may occur when a lens ruptures. The mechanism of a complicated cataract varies with the disease process; for example, in dia-

---

Congenital cataracts

Congenital cataracts may be caused by:
- chromosomal abnormalities
- metabolic disease (such as galactosemia)
- intrauterine nutritional deficiencies
- infection of the mother during pregnancy (such as rubella).

Congenital cataracts may not be apparent at birth unless the eye is examined by funduscope.

If the cataract is removed within a few months of birth, the infant will be able to develop proper retinal fixation and cortical visual responses. After surgery, the child is likely to favor the normal eye; the brain suppresses the poor image from the affected eye, leading to underdeveloped vision (amblyopia) in that eye. Postoperatively, in the child with bilateral cataracts, vision develops equally in both eyes.

---

betes, increased glucose in the lens causes it to absorb water.

Typically, cataracts develop through four stages:
- *immature* — the lens isn't totally opaque
- *mature* — the lens is completely opaque and vision loss is significant
- *tumescent* — the lens is filled with water; this stage may lead to glaucoma
- *hypermature* — the lens proteins deteriorate, causing peptides to leak through the lens capsule; glaucoma may develop if intraocular fluid outflow is obstructed.

SIGNS AND SYMPTOMS

Possible signs and symptoms of cataracts include:
- gradual painless blurring and loss of vision because of lens opacity
- milky white pupil because of lens opacity
- blinding glare from headlights at night caused by the inefficient reflection of light rays by the opacities
- poor reading vision caused by reduced clarity of images

Comparing methods of cataract removal

Cataracts can be removed by extracapsular or intracapsular techniques.

EXTRACAPSULAR CATARACT EXTRACTION

The surgeon may use irrigation and aspiration or phacoemulsification.

To irrigate and aspirate, he makes an incision at the limbus, opens the anterior lens capsule with a cystotome, and exerts pressure from below to express the lens. He then irrigates and suctions the remaining lens cortex.

In phacoemulsification, he uses an ultrasonic probe to break the lens into minute particles and aspirates the particles.

INTRACAPSULAR CATARACT EXTRACTION

The surgeon makes a partial incision at the superior limbus arc. He then removes the lens using specially designed forceps or a cryoprobe, which adheres to the lens to facilitate its removal.

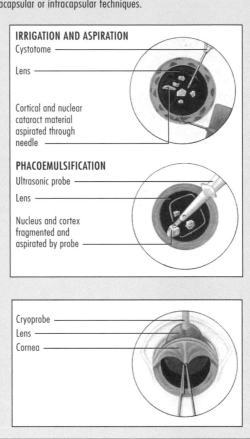

IRRIGATION AND ASPIRATION
Cystotome
Lens
Cortical and nuclear cataract material aspirated through needle

PHACOEMULSIFICATION
Ultrasonic probe
Lens
Nucleus and cortex fragmented and aspirated by probe

Cryoprobe
Lens
Cornea

■ better vision in dim light than in bright light in patients with central opacity; as pupils dilate, patients can see around the opacity.

AGE ALERT
Elderly people with reduced vision may become depressed and withdraw from social activities rather than complain about reduced vision.

COMPLICATIONS
Complications of cataracts include:
■ blindness

■ glaucoma.
Surgical complications may include:
■ loss of vitreous humor
■ wound dehiscence (separation of the layers of a wound) from loosening of sutures, with prolapse of flat anterior chamber or iris into the wound
■ hyphema, which is a hemorrhage into the eye's anterior chamber
■ vitreous-block glaucoma
■ retinal detachment
■ infection.

DIAGNOSIS

Diagnosis is based on the following tests:

- physical examination (shining a pen-light on the pupil to show the white area behind the pupil, which remains unnoticeable until the cataract is advanced)
- indirect ophthalmoscopy and slit-lamp examination to show a dark area in the normally homogeneous red reflex
- visual acuity test to confirm vision loss.

TREATMENT

Cataract treatment may include:

- extracapsular cataract extraction to remove the anterior lens capsule, and cortex and intraocular lens (IOL) implant in the posterior chamber, typically performed by using phacoemulsification to fragment the lens with ultrasonic vibrations, then aspirating the pieces (see *Comparing methods of cataract removal*)
- intracapsular cataract extraction to remove the entire lens within the intact capsule by cryoextraction (the moist lens sticks to an extremely cold metal probe for easy and safe extraction; rarely performed today). An IOL may be placed in the anterior or posterior chamber after lens removal; or, a contact lens or aphakic glasses may be used to enhance vision.
- laser surgery after an extracapsular cataract extraction to restore visual acuity when a secondary membrane forms in the posterior lens capsule that has been left intact
- discission (an incision) and aspiration may still be used in children with soft cataracts
- contact lenses or lens implantation after surgery to improve visual acuity, binocular vision, and depth perception.

Glaucoma

Glaucoma is a group of disorders characterized by an abnormally high intraocular pressure (IOP) that damages the optic nerve and other structures inside the eye. Untreated, it leads to a gradual loss of vision and, ultimately, blindness. Glaucoma occurs in several forms: chronic open-angle (primary), acute angle-closure, congenital (inherited as an autosomal recessive trait), and glaucoma resulting from other causes. Chronic open-angle glaucoma is usually bilateral, with insidious onset and a slowly progressive course. Acute angle-closure glaucoma typically has a rapid onset and is an ophthalmic emergency. Unless treated promptly, this acute form of glaucoma causes blindness in 3 to 5 days.

In the United States, about 2.5 million people have diagnosed glaucoma; another 1 million people have the disease but it is undiagnosed. Glaucoma accounts for 12% of new cases of blindness in the United States. The prognosis is good with early treatment.

CULTURAL DIVERSITY

Blacks have the highest incidence of glaucoma, and it's the single most common cause of blindness in this group.

CAUSES

Risk factors for chronic open-angle glaucoma include:

- genetics
- hypertension
- diabetes mellitus
- aging
- black ethnicity
- severe myopia.

Precipitating factors for acute angle-closure glaucoma include:

- drug-induced mydriasis (extreme dilation of the pupil)
- emotional excitement, which can lead to hypertension.

Secondary glaucoma may result from:

- uveitis
- trauma
- steroids
- diabetes
- infections
- surgery.

PATHOPHYSIOLOGY

Chronic open-angle glaucoma results from overproduction or obstruction of the outflow of aqueous humor through the trabecular meshwork or Schlemm's canal, causing increased IOP and damage to the optic nerve. (See *Normal flow of aqueous humor,* page 536.) In secondary glaucoma, such conditions as trauma and surgery increase the risk of obstruction of intraocular fluid outflow caused by edema or other abnormal processes.

CLOSER LOOK
Normal flow of aqueous humor

Aqueous humor, a transparent fluid produced by the ciliary epithelium of the ciliary body, flows from the posterior chamber through the pupil to the anterior chamber. It then flows peripherally and filters through the trabecular meshwork to Schlemm's canal, through which the fluid ultimately enters venous circulation.

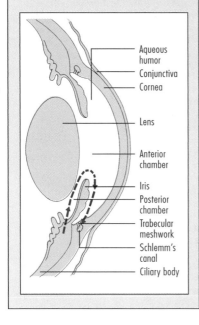

- Aqueous humor
- Conjunctiva
- Cornea
- Lens
- Anterior chamber
- Iris
- Posterior chamber
- Trabecular meshwork
- Schlemm's canal
- Ciliary body

AGE ALERT
In older persons, partial closure of the angle may also occur, so that two forms of glaucoma may coexist.

SIGNS AND SYMPTOMS
Clinical manifestations of chronic open-angle glaucoma typically are bilateral and include:
- mild aching in the eyes caused by increased IOP
- loss of peripheral vision caused by compression of retinal rods and nerve fibers
- halos around lights as a result of corneal edema
- reduced visual acuity, especially at night, not correctable with glasses.

Clinical manifestations of acute angle-closure glaucoma have a rapid onset, are usually unilateral, and include:
- inflammation and red, painful eye caused by an abrupt elevation of IOP
- sensation of pressure over the eye caused by increased IOP
- moderate pupillary dilation nonreactive to light
- cloudy cornea caused by compression of intraocular components
- blurring and decreased visual acuity caused by aberrant neural conduction
- photophobia caused by abnormal intraocular pressures
- halos around lights caused by corneal edema
- nausea and vomiting caused by increased IOP.

COMPLICATIONS
A complication of glaucoma is:
- blindness.

DIAGNOSIS
Glaucoma may be diagnosed using the following tests:
- pressure measurement tonometry using an applanation, Schiøtz, or pneumatic tonometer; fingertip tension to estimate IOP (on gentle palpation of closed eyelids, one eye feels harder than the other in acute angle-closure glaucoma)
- slit-lamp examination of the eye's anterior structures, including the cornea, iris, and lens

Acute angle-closure glaucoma results from obstruction to the outflow of aqueous humor.

Obstruction may be caused by anatomically narrow angles between the anterior iris and the posterior corneal surface, shallow anterior chambers, a thickened iris that causes angle closure on pupil dilation, or a bulging iris that presses on the trabeculae, closing the angle (peripheral anterior synechiae). Any of these may cause IOP to increase suddenly. (See *Congenital glaucoma*.)

■ gonioscopy, to determine the angle of the eye's anterior chamber, enabling differentiation between chronic open-angle glaucoma and acute angle-closure glaucoma (normal angle in chronic open-angle glaucoma and abnormal angle in acute angle-closure glaucoma (see *Optic disk changes in chronic glaucoma,* page 538)

■ ophthalmoscopy, to show cupping of the optic disk in chronic open-angle glaucoma; pale disk suggesting acute angle-closure glaucoma

■ perimetry or visual field tests to detect loss of peripheral vision caused by chronic open-angle glaucoma

■ fundus photography, to monitor the disk for changes.

TREATMENT

Treatment of chronic open-angle glaucoma may include:

■ beta-adrenergic blockers, such as timolol or betaxolol (a beta$_1$-receptor antagonist), to decrease aqueous humor production

■ alpha adrenergic agonists, such as brimonidine or apraclonidine, to reduce intraocular pressure

■ carbonic anhydrase inhibitors, such as dorzolamide or acetazolamide, to decrease the formation and secretion of aqueous humor

■ epinephrine to reduce IOP by improving aqueous outflow

■ prostaglandins such as latanoprost to reduce IOP

■ miotic eye drops such as pilocarpine to reduce IOP by aiding the outflow of aqueous humor.

When medical therapy fails to reduce IOP, the following surgical procedures may be performed:

■ argon laser trabeculoplasty of the trabecular meshwork of an open angle to produce a thermal burn that changes the surface of the meshwork and increases the outflow of aqueous humor

■ trabeculectomy to remove scleral tissue, followed by a peripheral iridectomy to produce an opening for aqueous outflow under the conjunctiva, creating a filtering bleb.

Congenital glaucoma

Congenital glaucoma, a rare disease, occurs when a congenital defect in the angle of the anterior chamber obstructs the outflow of aqueous humor. Congenital glaucoma is usually bilateral, with an enlarged cornea that may be cloudy and bulging. Symptoms in a neonate, although difficult to assess, may include tearing, pain, and photophobia.

Untreated, congenital glaucoma causes damage to the optic nerve and blindness. Surgical intervention (such as goniotomy, goniopuncture, trabeculotomy, or trabeculectomy) is necessary to reduce intraocular pressure and prevent vision loss.

 CLINICAL ALERT

Acute angle-closure glaucoma is an ocular emergency requiring immediate intervention to reduce high IOP.

Treatment of acute angle-closure glaucoma includes:

■ I.V. mannitol (20%) or oral glycerin (50%) to reduce IOP by creating an osmotic pressure gradient between the blood and intraocular fluid

■ steroid drops to reduce inflammation

■ acetazolamide, a carbonic anhydrase inhibitor, to reduce IOP by decreasing the formation and secretion of aqueous humor

■ pilocarpine, to constrict the pupil, forcing the iris away from the trabeculae and allowing fluid to escape

■ timolol, a beta-adrenergic blocker, to decrease IOP

■ opioid analgesics to reduce pain if necessary

■ laser iridotomy or surgical peripheral iridectomy, if drug therapy doesn't reduce IOP, to relieve pressure and preserve vision by promoting outflow of aqueous humor

■ cycloplegic drops, such as apraclonidine, in the affected eye (only after laser peripheral iridectomy), to relax the ciliary muscle and reduce inflammation to prevent adhesions.

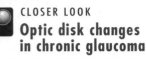

CLOSER LOOK
Optic disk changes in chronic glaucoma

Ophthalmoscopy and slit-lamp examination show cupping of the optic disk, which is characteristic of chronic glaucoma.

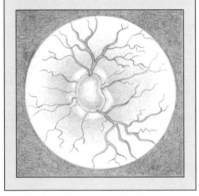

CLINICAL ALERT
Cycloplegics must be used only in the affected eye after a peripheral iridectomy. The use of these drops in the normal eye may bring on an attack of acute angle-closure glaucoma in this eye, threatening the patient's residual vision.

Hearing loss

Hearing loss, or deafness, results from a mechanical or nervous impediment to the transmission of sound waves and is the most common pathologic process linked to hearing alteration. Hearing loss is further defined as an inability to perceive the range of sounds audible to an individual with normal hearing. Types of hearing loss include congenital hearing loss, sudden deafness, noise-induced hearing loss, and presbycusis.

CAUSES
Congenital hearing loss may be transmitted as a dominant, autosomal dominant, autosomal recessive, or sex-linked recessive trait. Hearing loss in neonates may also result from trauma, toxicity, or infection during pregnancy or delivery. Predisposing factors include:
- maternal exposure to rubella or syphilis during pregnancy
- maternal use of ototoxic drugs during pregnancy
- trauma or prolonged fetal anoxia during delivery
- congenital abnormalities of the ears, nose, or throat
- prematurity or low birth weight
- serum bilirubin levels above 20 mg/dl.

Sudden deafness refers to rapid hearing loss in a person with no prior hearing impairment. This condition is considered a medical emergency because prompt treatment may restore full hearing. Its causes and predisposing factors may include:
- acute infections, especially mumps (most common cause of unilateral sensorineural hearing loss in children); other bacterial and viral infections, such as rubella, rubeola, influenza, herpes zoster, and infectious mononucleosis; and *Mycoplasma* infections
- metabolic disorders (diabetes mellitus, hypothyroidism, hyperlipoproteinemia)
- vascular disorders (hypertension, arteriosclerosis)
- head trauma or brain tumors
- ototoxic drugs (tobramycin, streptomycin, quinine, gentamicin, furosemide, ethacrynic acid)
- neurologic disorders (multiple sclerosis, neurosyphilis)
- blood dyscrasias (leukemia, hypercoagulation).

Noise-induced hearing loss, which may be transient or permanent, may occur after:
- prolonged exposure to loud noise (85 to 90 decibels [dB])
- brief exposure to extremely loud noise (greater than 90 dB).

Such hearing loss is common in workers subjected to constant industrial noise and in military personnel, hunters, and rock musicians.

Presbycusis, an otologic effect of aging, results from a loss of hair cells in the organ of Corti. This disorder causes progressive, symmetrical, bilateral sensorineural hearing loss, usually of high-frequency tones.

PATHOPHYSIOLOGY

The major forms of hearing loss are classified as:

■ *conductive loss*—interrupted passage of sound from the external ear to the junction of the stapes and oval window caused by wax, or otitis media or externa

■ *sensorineural loss*—impaired cochlea or acoustic (eighth cranial) nerve dysfunction causing failure of transmission of sound impulses within the inner ear or brain

■ *mixed loss*—combined dysfunction of conduction and sensorineural transmission.

Hearing loss also may be classified as partial or total.

SIGNS AND SYMPTOMS

Although congenital hearing loss may produce no obvious signs of hearing impairment at birth, a deficient response to auditory stimuli generally becomes apparent within 2 to 3 days.

Other clinical features of hearing loss include:

■ impaired speech development caused by inability to discriminate sounds

■ loss of perception of certain frequencies (around 4,000 hertz [Hz]) depending on severity of hearing loss

■ tinnitus (a "ringing" in the ear)

■ inability to understand the spoken word.

▲ AGE ALERT
A deaf infant's behavior can appear normal and mislead the parents as well as the professional, especially if the infant has autosomal recessive deafness and is the first child of carrier parents.

COMPLICATIONS

Complications may include:

■ increased hearing loss

■ total deafness

■ chronic ear problems

■ chronic tinnitus.

DIAGNOSIS

■ Patient, family, and occupational histories and a complete audiologic examination usually provide ample evidence of hearing loss and suggest possible causes or predisposing factors.

■ Weber, Rinne, and specialized audiologic tests differentiate between conductive and sensorineural hearing loss.

TREATMENT

After the underlying cause is identified, therapy for congenital hearing loss not treatable with surgery consists of:

■ developing the patient's ability to communicate through sign language, speech reading, or other effective means

■ phototherapy and exchange transfusions for hyperbilirubinemia

■ aggressively immunizing children against rubella to reduce the risk of maternal exposure during pregnancy; educating pregnant women about the dangers of exposure to drugs, chemicals, or infection; and careful monitoring during labor and delivery to prevent fetal anoxia.

Treatment of sudden deafness requires prompt identification of the underlying cause. Prevention necessitates educating patients and health care professionals about the many causes of sudden deafness and the ways to recognize and treat it.

For patients with noise-induced hearing loss:

■ Overnight rest usually restores normal hearing in those who have been exposed to noise levels greater than 90 dB for several hours.

■ Reduction of exposure to loud noises generally prevents high-frequency hearing loss.

■ Repeated exposure to such noise may require speech and hearing rehabilitation, because hearing aids are seldom helpful.

For patients with presbycusis:

■ Amplifying sound, such as with a hearing aid, helps some patients.

■ Many patients are intolerant of loud noise and aren't helped by a hearing aid.

Ménière's disease

Ménière's disease, an inner ear disease that results from a labyrinthine dysfunction (also known as *endolymphatic hydrops*), causes severe vertigo, sensorineural hearing loss, and tinnitus.

▲ AGE ALERT

Ménière's disease usually affects adults between ages 30 and 60, is slightly more common in men than in

Normal vestibular function

The semicircular canals and vestibule of the inner ear are responsible for equilibrium and balance. Each of the three semicircular canals lies at a 90-degree angle to the others. When the head is moved, endolymph inside each semicircular canal moves in an opposite direction. The movement stimulates hair cells, which send electrical impulses to the brain through the vestibular portion of cranial nerve VIII. Head movement also causes movement of the vestibular otoliths (crystals of calcium salts) in their gel medium, which tugs on hair cells, initiating the transmission of electrical impulses to the brain through the vestibular nerve. Together, these two organs help detect the body's present position as well as a change in direction or motion.

women, and rarely occurs in children. Usually, only one ear is involved. After multiple attacks over several years, residual tinnitus and hearing loss can be incapacitating.

CAUSES

The cause of Ménière's disease is unknown. It may be linked to:
- family history
- immune disorder
- migraine headaches
- middle ear infection
- head trauma
- autonomic nervous system dysfunction
- premenstrual edema.

PATHOPHYSIOLOGY

Ménière's disease may result from overproduction or decreased absorption of endolymph—the fluid contained in the labyrinth of the ear. Accumulated endolymph dilates the semicircular canals, utricle, and saccule and causes degeneration of the vestibular and cochlear hair cells. Overstimulation of the vestibular branch of cranial nerve VIII impairs pos-

tural reflexes and stimulates the vomiting reflex. (See *Normal vestibular function*.) Perception of sound is impaired as a result of this excessive cranial nerve stimulation, and injury to sensory receptors for hearing may affect auditory acuity.

This condition may also stem from autonomic nervous system dysfunction that produces a temporary constriction of blood vessels supplying the inner ear.

CLINICAL ALERT
In some women, premenstrual edema may bring on outbreaks of Ménière's disease.

SIGNS AND SYMPTOMS

Signs and symptoms of Ménière's disease include:
- sudden severe spinning, whirling vertigo, lasting from 10 minutes to several hours, caused by increased endolymph (attacks may occur several times per year, or remissions may last as long as several years)
- tinnitus caused by altered firing of sensory auditory neurons (may have residual tinnitus between attacks)
- hearing impairment caused by sensorineural loss (hearing may be normal between attacks, but repeated attacks may progressively cause permanent hearing loss)
- feeling of fullness or blockage in the affected ear preceding an attack, a result of changing sensitivity of pressure receptors
- severe nausea, vomiting, sweating, and pallor during an acute attack caused by autonomic dysfunction
- nystagmus caused by asymmetry and intensity of impulses reaching the brain stem
- loss of balance and falling to the affected side because of vertigo.

COMPLICATIONS

Complications include:
- continued tinnitus
- hearing loss.

DIAGNOSIS

Diagnosis of Ménière's disease is based on:
- patient history of signs and symptoms
- audiometric testing showing a sensorineural hearing loss and loss of discrimination and recruitment (an increase in

perceived sound intensity out of proportion to the actual sound increase)
■ electronystagmography showing normal or reduced vestibular response on the affected side
■ cold caloric testing showing impairment of oculovestibular reflex
■ electrocochleography showing increased ratio of summating potential to action potential
■ brain stem evoked response audiometry test to rule out acoustic neuroma, brain tumor, and vascular lesions in the brain stem
■ computed tomography scan and magnetic resonance imaging to rule out acoustic neuroma as a cause of symptoms.

TREATMENT
During an acute attack, treatment may include:
■ lying down to minimize head movement, and avoiding sudden movements and glaring lights to reduce dizziness
■ promethazine or prochlorperazine to relieve nausea and vomiting
■ atropine to control an attack by reducing autonomic nervous system function
■ dimenhydrinate to control vertigo and nausea
■ central nervous system depressants, such as lorazepam or diazepam during an acute attack to reduce excitability of vestibular nuclei
■ antihistamines, such as meclizine or diphenhydramine, to reduce dizziness and vomiting.
Long-term management may include:
■ diuretics, such as triamterene or acetazolamide, to reduce endolymph pressure
■ betahistine dihydrochloride to alleviate vertigo, hearing loss, and tinnitus
■ vasodilators to dilate blood vessels supplying the inner ear
■ sodium restriction to reduce endolymphatic hydrops
■ antihistamines or mild sedatives to prevent attacks
■ systemic streptomycin to produce chemical ablation of the sensory neuroepithelium of the inner ear and thereby control vertigo in patients with bilateral disease for whom no other treatment can be considered.

In Ménière's disease that persists despite medical treatment or produces incapacitating vertigo, the following surgical procedures may be performed:
■ endolymphatic drainage and shunt procedures to reduce pressure on the hair cells of the cochlea and prevent further sensorineural hearing loss
■ vestibular nerve resection in patients with intact hearing to reduce vertigo and prevent further hearing loss
■ labyrinthectomy for relief of vertigo in patients with incapacitating symptoms and poor or no hearing, because destruction of the cochlea results in a total loss of hearing in the affected ear
■ cochlear implantation to improve hearing in patients with profound deafness caused by Ménière's disease.

Otosclerosis

The most common cause of chronic, progressive, conductive hearing loss, otosclerosis is the slow formation of spongy bone in the otic capsule, particularly at the oval window.

CULTURAL DIVERSITY
Otosclerosis occurs in at least 10% of people of European descent and is three times as prevalent in females as in males.

The onset is usually between ages 15 and 30. Occurring unilaterally at first, the disorder may progress to bilateral conductive hearing loss. With surgery, the prognosis is good.

CAUSES
Causes include:
■ autosomal dominant trait
■ pregnancy.

AGE ALERT
Children with osteogenesis imperfecta, an inherited condition characterized by brittle bones, may also have otosclerosis.

PATHOPHYSIOLOGY
In otosclerosis, the normal bone of the otic capsule is gradually replaced with a highly vascular spongy bone. This spongy bone immobilizes the footplate of the normally mobile stapes, disrupting the conduction of vibrations from the tympanic

membrane to the cochlea. Because the sound pressure vibrations aren't transmitted to the fluid of the inner ear, the result is conductive hearing loss. If the inner ear becomes involved, sensorineural hearing loss may develop.

SIGNS AND SYMPTOMS

Signs and symptoms of otosclerosis include:

- progressive hearing loss—which starts unilaterally and may become bilateral without evidence of a middle ear infection—caused by interference with vibration transmission
- bilateral conductive hearing loss caused by the disruption of the conduction of vibrations from the tympanic membrane to the cochlea
- tinnitus caused by overstimulation of cranial nerve VIII afferents
- ability to hear a conversation better in a noisy environment than in a quiet one (paracusis of Willis) as a result of masking effects.

COMPLICATIONS

A complication of otosclerosis is:
- deafness.

DIAGNOSIS

Diagnosis is based on:

- otoscopic examination showing a normal-appearing tympanic membrane; occasionally, the tympanic membrane may appear pinkish-orange (Schwartze's sign) as a result of vascular and bony changes in the middle ear
- Rinne test showing bone conduction lasting longer than air conduction (normally, the reverse is true); as otosclerosis progresses, bone conduction also deteriorates
- audiometric testing showing hearing loss ranging from 60 dB in early stages to total loss
- Weber's test to detect sounds lateralizing to the more affected ear.

AGE ALERT
Audiometric testing should be performed in late adolescence when otosclerosis and noise-induced hearing may start to occur.

TREATMENT

Treatment of otosclerosis may include:
- prevention of infection with prophylactic antibiotics
- stapedectomy (removal of the stapes) and insertion of a prosthesis to restore partial or total hearing
- stapedotomy (creation of a small hole in the footplate of the stapes) and insertion of a wire and piston as a prosthesis to help restore hearing
- hearing aid (air conduction aid with molded ear insertion receiver) if surgery isn't possible, to permit hearing of conversation in normal surroundings.

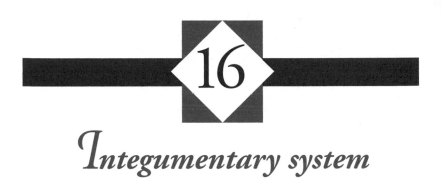

Integumentary system

The integumentary system, the largest and heaviest body system, includes the skin — the integument, or external covering of the body — and the epidermal appendages, including the hair and nails as well as sebaceous, eccrine, and apocrine glands. It protects the body against injury and invasion by microorganisms, harmful substances, and radiation; regulates body temperature; serves as a reservoir for food and water; and synthesizes vitamin D. Emotional well-being, including one's responses to the daily stresses of life, is reflected in the skin.

SKIN

The skin is composed of three layers: the epidermis, the dermis, and subcutaneous tissue. The epidermis is the outermost layer. It's thin and contains sensory receptors for pain, temperature, touch, and vibration. The epidermal layer has no blood vessels and relies on the dermal layer for nutrition. The dermis contains connective tissue, the sebaceous glands, and some hair follicles. The subcutaneous tissue lies beneath the dermis; it contains fat and sweat glands and the rest of the hair follicles. The subcutaneous layer can store calories for future use in the body. (See *Close-up view of the skin,* page 544.)

HAIR AND NAILS

The hair and nails are considered appendages of the skin. Both have protective functions in addition to their cosmetic appeal. The cuticle of the nail, for example, functions as a seal, protecting the area below it from external hazards. (See *Nail structure,* page 545.)

GLANDS

The sebaceous glands, found on all areas of the skin except the palms and soles, produce sebum, a semifluid material composed of fat and epithelial cells. Sebum is secreted into the hair follicle and exits to the skin surface. It helps waterproof the hair and skin and promotes the absorption of fat-soluble substances into the dermis.

The eccrine glands produce sweat, an odorless, watery fluid. Glands in the palms and soles secrete sweat primarily in response to emotional stress. The other remaining eccrine glands respond mainly to thermal stress, effectively regulating temperature.

Located mainly in the axillary and anogenital areas, apocrine glands have a coiled secretory portion that lies deeper in the dermis than the eccrine glands. These

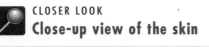

CLOSER LOOK
Close-up view of the skin

The skin is composed of two major layers — the epidermis and dermis. The epidermis consists of five strata, shown below. Subcutaneous tissue lying beneath the dermis consists of loose connective tissue that attaches the skin to underlying structures.

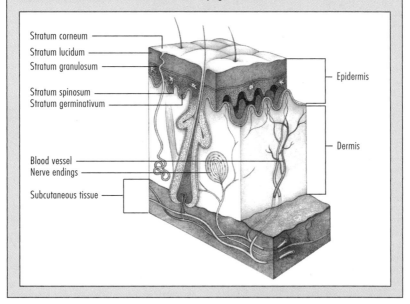

Stratum corneum
Stratum lucidum
Stratum granulosum

Stratum spinosum
Stratum germinativum

Blood vessel
Nerve endings

Subcutaneous tissue

Epidermis

Dermis

glands begin to function at puberty and have no known biological function. Bacterial decomposition of the apocrine fluid produced by these glands causes body odor.

Skin color depends on four pigments: melanin, carotene, oxyhemoglobin, and deoxyhemoglobin. Each pigment is unique in its function and effect on the skin. For example, the amount of melanin, the brownish pigment of the skin, is genetically determined, though it can be altered by sunlight exposure. Excessive dietary carotene (from carrots, sweet potatoes, and leafy vegetables) causes a yellowing of the skin. Excessive oxyhemoglobin in the blood causes a reddening of the skin, and excessive deoxyhemoglobin (not bound to oxygen) causes a bluish discoloration.

$\mathcal{P}$ATHOPHYSIOLOGIC CHANGES

Clinical manifestations of skin dysfunction include the inflammatory reaction of the skin and the formation of lesions.

Inflammatory reaction of the skin

An inflammatory reaction occurs with injury to the skin. The reaction can occur only in living organisms. Although it's a beneficial response, it's usually accompanied by some degree of discomfort at the site. Irritation changes the epidermal structure, with a resulting increase of immunoglobulin E activity. Other classic signs of inflammatory skin responses are

Nail structure

This illustration shows the anatomic components of a fingernail.

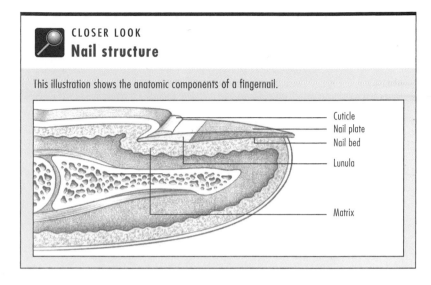

Cuticle
Nail plate
Nail bed
Lunula
Matrix

erythema, edema, and warmth, caused by bioamines released from the granules of tissue mast cells and basophils.

Formation of lesions

Primary skin lesions appear on previously healthy skin in response to disease or external irritation. They're classified by their appearance as macules, papules, plaques, patches, nodules, tumors, wheals, comedones, cysts, vesicles, pustules, or bullae. (See *Recognizing primary skin lesions,* pages 546 and 547.)

Modified lesions are described as secondary skin lesions. These lesions occur as a result of rupture, mechanical irritation, extension, invasion, or normal or abnormal healing of primary lesions. These include atrophy, erosions, ulcers, scales, crusts, excoriation, fissures, lichenification, and scars. (See *Recognizing secondary skin lesions,* pages 548 and 549.)

*D*ISORDERS

Trauma, abnormal cellular function, infection, and systemic disease may cause disruptions in skin integrity.

Acne

Acne is a chronic inflammatory disease of the sebaceous glands. It's usually linked to a high rate of sebum secretion and occurs on areas of the body that have sebaceous glands, such as the face, neck, chest, back, and shoulders. There are two types of acne: *inflammatory,* in which the hair follicle is blocked by sebum, causing bacteria to grow and eventually rupture the follicle; and *noninflammatory,* in which the follicle doesn't rupture but remains dilated.

AGE ALERT
Acne occurs in both males and females. Acne vulgaris develops in 80% to 90% of adolescents or young adults, primarily between ages 15 and 18. Although the lesions can appear as early as age 8, acne primarily affects adolescents.

Although the severity and overall incidence of acne is usually greater in males, it tends to start at an earlier age and lasts longer in females.

The prognosis varies and depends on the severity and underlying causes; with treatment, the prognosis is usually good.

CAUSES
The cause of acne is multifactorial. Diet isn't believed to be an activating factor. Possible causes of acne include increased
(Text continues on page 549.)

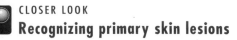

CLOSER LOOK
Recognizing primary skin lesions

BULLA
Fluid-filled lesion more than 2 cm in diameter (also called a *blister*) (severe poison oak or ivy dermatitis, bullous pemphigoid, second-degree burn)

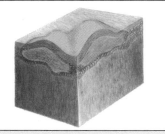

MACULE
Flat, pigmented, circumscribed area less than 1 cm in diameter (freckle, rubella)

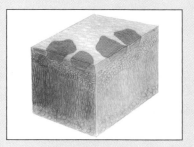

COMEDO
Plugged pilosebaceous duct, exfoliative, formed from sebum and keratin (blackhead [open comedo], whitehead [closed comedo])

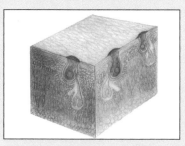

NODULE
Firm, raised lesion; deeper than a papule, extending into dermal layer; 0.5 to 2 cm in diameter (intradermal nevus)

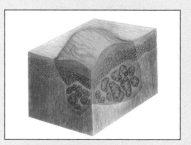

CYST
Semisolid or fluid-filled encapsulated mass extending deep into the dermis (sebaceous cyst, cystic acne)

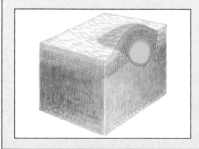

PAPULE
Firm, inflammatory, raised lesion up to 0.5 cm in diameter, may be same color as skin or pigmented (acne papule, lichen planus)

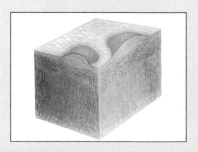

PATCH
Flat, pigmented, circumscribed area more than 1 cm in diameter (herald patch [pityriasis rosea])

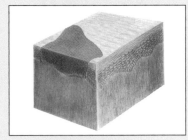

PLAQUE
Circumscribed, solid, elevated lesion more than 1 cm in diameter; elevation above skin surface occupies larger surface area compared with height (psoriasis)

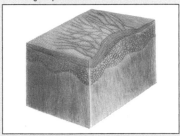

PUSTULE
Raised, circumscribed lesion usually less than 1 cm in diameter; containing purulent material, making it a yellow-white color (acne pustule, impetigo, furuncle)

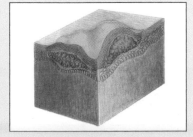

TUMOR
Elevated solid lesion more than 2 cm in diameter, extending into dermal and subcutaneous layers (dermatofibroma)

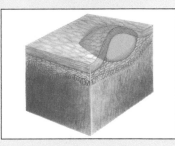

VESICLE
Raised, circumscribed, fluid-filled lesion less than 0.5 cm in diameter (chickenpox, herpes simplex)

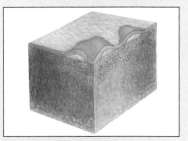

WHEAL
Raised, firm lesion with intense localized skin edema, varying in size and shape; color ranging from pale pink to red, disappears in hours (hive [urticaria], insect bite)

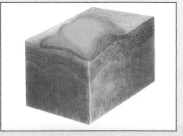

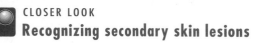

CLOSER LOOK
Recognizing secondary skin lesions

ATROPHY
Thinning of skin surface at site of disorder (striae, aging skin)

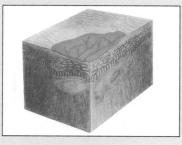

CRUST
Dried sebum, serous, sanguineous, or purulent exudate overlying an erosion or weeping vesicle, bulla, or pustule (impetigo)

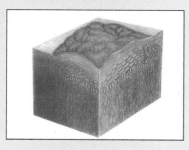

EROSION
Circumscribed lesion involving loss of superficial epidermis (rug burn, abrasion)

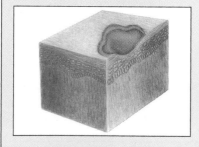

EXCORIATION
Linear scratched or abraded areas, usually self-induced (abraded acne, eczema)

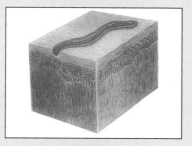

FISSURE
Linear cracking of the skin extending into the dermal layer (hand dermatitis [chapped skin])

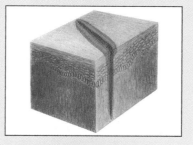

LICHENIFICATION
Thickened, prominent skin markings by constant rubbing (chronic atopic dermatitis)

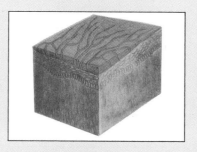

SCALE
Thin, dry flakes of shedding skin (psoriasis, dry skin, newborn desquamation)

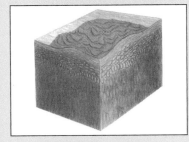

SCAR
Fibrous tissue caused by trauma, deep inflammation, or surgical incision; red and raised (recent), pink and flat (6 weeks), and depressed (old [on a healed surgical incision])

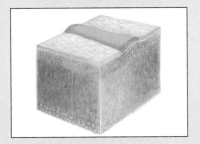

ULCER
Epidermal and dermal destruction may extend into subcutaneous tissue; usually heals with scarring (pressure ulcer)

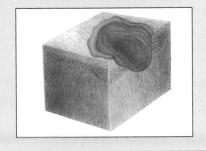

activity of sebaceous glands and blockage of the pilosebaceous ducts (hair follicles).

Factors that may predispose to acne include:
- heredity
- androgen stimulation
- certain drugs, including corticosteroids, corticotropin, androgens, iodides, bromides, trimethadione, phenytoin, isoniazid, lithium, and halothane
- cobalt irradiation
- hyperalimentation
- exposure to heavy oils, greases, or tars
- trauma or rubbing from tight clothing
- cosmetics
- emotional stress
- tropical climate
- hormonal contraceptive use. (Many women experience acne flare-up during their first few menses after starting or stopping hormonal contraceptives.)

PATHOPHYSIOLOGY
Androgens stimulate sebaceous gland growth and the production of sebum, which is secreted into hair follicles that contain bacteria. The bacteria, usually *Propionibacterium acne* and *Staphylococcus epidermis,* are normal skin flora that secrete lipase. This enzyme interacts with sebum to produce free fatty acids, which provoke inflammation. Hair follicles also produce more of the substance keratin, which joins with the sebum to form a plug in the dilated follicle.

SIGNS AND SYMPTOMS
The acne plug may appear as:
- a closed comedo, or whitehead (not protruding from the follicle and covered by the epidermis)
- an open comedo, or blackhead (protruding from the follicle and not covered by the epidermis; melanin or pigment of the follicle causes the black color).

Rupture or leakage from an infected follicle into the epidermis produces inflammation, characteristic acne pustules, papules or, in severe forms, acne cysts or abscesses (chronic, recurring lesions producing acne scars).

In women, signs and symptoms may include increased severity just before or during menstruation when estrogen levels are at the lowest.

COMPLICATIONS

Complications of acne may include:
- acne conglobata
- scarring (when acne is severe)
- impaired self-esteem
- abscesses or secondary bacterial infections.

DIAGNOSIS

Diagnosis of acne vulgaris is confirmed by characteristic acne lesions, especially in adolescents.

TREATMENT

Topical treatments of acne include the application of antibacterial agents, such as benzoyl peroxide, clindamycin, or benzoyl peroxide plus erythromycin. These may be applied alone or with tretinoin, which is a keratolytic. Keratolytic agents, such as benzoyl peroxide and tretinoin, dry and peel the skin to help open blocked follicles, moving the sebum up to the skin level.

Systemic therapy consists primarily of:
- antibiotics, usually tetracycline, to decrease bacterial growth (Dosage is reduced for long-term maintenance when the condition is in remission.)
- culture to identify a possible secondary bacterial infection (Look for exacerbation of pustules or abscesses in a person receiving tetracycline or erythromycin drug therapy.)
- oral isotretinoin to inhibit sebaceous gland function and keratinization (A 16- to 20-week course of isotretinoin is limited to patients with severe papulopustular or cystic acne not responding to conventional therapy, because of its severe adverse effects. Because this drug is known to cause birth defects, the manufacturer, with Food and Drug Administration approval, recommends the following precautions: pregnancy testing before dispensing; dispensing only a 30-day supply; repeat pregnancy testing throughout treatment period; effective contraception during treatment; and informed consent. Because of its effects on the liver, a serum triglyc-

eride level should be drawn before and periodically during treatment.)
- for women only, antiandrogens: birth control pills, such as norgestimate/ethinyl estradiol or spironolactone
- cleaning with an abrasive sponge to dislodge superficial comedones
- surgery to remove comedones and to open and drain pustules (usually performed on an outpatient basis)
- dermabrasion (for severe acne scarring) with a high-speed metal brush to smooth the skin (performed only by a well-trained dermatologist or plastic surgeon)
- bovine collagen injections into the dermis beneath the scarred area to fill in affected areas and even out the skin surface (not recommended by all dermatologists).

Burns

Burns are classified as first-degree, second-degree superficial, second-degree full thickness, third-degree full thickness, and fourth-degree. A first-degree burn is limited to the epidermis. The most common example of a first-degree burn is sunburn, which results from exposure to the sun. In a second-degree burn, the epidermis and part of the dermis are damaged. A third-degree burn damages the epidermis and dermis, and vessels and tissue are visible. In fourth-degree burns, the damage extends through deeply charred subcutaneous tissue to muscle and bone. A major burn is a horrifying injury that requires painful treatment and a long period of rehabilitation.

Each year about 2 million people in the United States receive burn injuries. Of these, 300,000 are burned seriously, and more than 6,000 die, making burns the third leading cause of accidental death in the United States. About 60,000 people are hospitalized each year for burns. Most significant burns occur in the home; home fires account for the highest burn fatality rate.

People younger than age 4 and older than age 60 have a higher incidence of complications with burns and thus a higher mortality rate. Immediate, aggressive burn treatment increases the patient's chance for survival. Later, supportive measures and strict sterile technique can mini-

CLOSER LOOK
Classifications of burns

The depth of skin and tissue damage determines burn classification. This illustration shows the four degrees of burn classification.

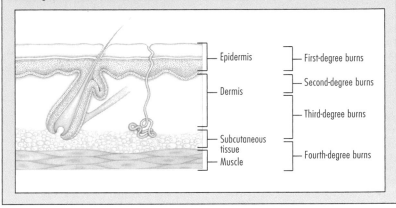

mize infection. Meticulous, comprehensive burn care can make the difference between life and death. Survival and recovery from a major burn are more likely after the burn wound is reduced to less than 20% of the total body surface area (BSA).

CAUSES

Thermal burns, the most common type, typically result from:

■ residential fires
■ automobile crashes
■ playing with matches
■ improper handling of firecrackers
■ improper handling of gasoline
■ scalding injuries and kitchen injuries (such as a child climbing on top of a stove, grasping a hot iron, spilling a container of hot liquid)
■ parental abuse (in children), or abuse of elderly people
■ clothes that have caught on fire.

Chemical burns result from contact, ingestion, inhalation, or injection of acids, alkalis, or vesicants.

Electrical burns usually result from contact with faulty electrical wiring or high-voltage power lines. Sometimes young children chew electrical cords.

Friction or abrasion burns occur when the skin rubs harshly against a coarse surface.

Sunburn results from excessive exposure to sunlight.

PATHOPHYSIOLOGY

The injuring agent denatures cellular proteins. Some cells die because of traumatic or ischemic necrosis. Loss of collagen cross-linking also occurs with denaturation, creating abnormal osmotic and hydrostatic pressure gradients, which cause the movement of intravascular fluid into interstitial spaces. Cellular injury triggers the release of mediators of inflammation, contributing to local and, in the case of major burns, systemic increases in capillary permeability. Specific pathophysiologic events depend on the cause and classification of the burn. (See *Classifications of burns.*)

First-degree burns

A first-degree burn causes localized injury or destruction to the skin (epidermis only) by direct (such as chemical splash) or indirect (such as sunlight) contact. The barrier function of the skin remains intact, and these burns aren't life-threatening.

Second-degree superficial partial-thickness burns. These burns involve destruction to the epidermis and some dermis. Thin-walled, fluid-filled blisters develop within a few minutes of the injury. As these blisters break, nerve endings become exposed to the air. Because pain and tactile responses remain intact, subsequent treatments are painful. The barrier function of the skin is lost.

Second-degree full thickness burns. These burns involve destruction of the epidermis and dermis, producing blisters and mild to moderate edema and pain. The hair follicles are still intact, so hair will grow again. Compared with second-degree superficial partial-thickness burns, less pain sensation is present with this burn because the sensory neurons have undergone extensive destruction. The areas around the burn injury are still sensitive to pain. The barrier function of the skin is lost.

Third- and fourth-degree burns. A major burn affects every body system and organ. A third-degree burn extends through the epidermis and dermis and into the subcutaneous tissue layer. A fourth-degree burn involves muscle, bone, and interstitial tissues. Within only hours, fluids and protein shift from capillary to interstitial spaces, causing edema. There's an immediate immunologic response to a burn injury, making burn wound sepsis a potential threat. Finally, an increase in calorie demand after a burn injury increases the metabolic rate.

SIGNS AND SYMPTOMS
Signs and symptoms depend on the type of burn and may include:
■ localized pain and erythema caused by injury from direct or indirect contact with a burn source, usually without blisters in the first 24 hours (first-degree burn)
■ chills, headache, localized edema, and nausea and vomiting (more severe first-degree burn)

■ thin-walled, fluid-filled blisters appearing within minutes of the injury, with mild to moderate edema and pain (second-degree superficial partial-thickness burn)
■ white, waxy appearance to damaged area (second-degree full-thickness burn)
■ white, brown, or black leathery tissue and visible thrombosed vessels caused by destruction of skin elasticity (dorsum of hand most common site of thrombosed veins), without blisters (third-degree burn)
■ silver-colored, raised area, usually at the site of electrical contact (electrical burn)
■ evidence of smoke inhalation, such as singed nasal hairs, mucosal burns, voice changes, coughing, wheezing, soot in mouth or nose, and darkened sputum.

COMPLICATIONS
Possible complications of burns include:
■ loss of function (burns to face, hands, feet, and genitalia)
■ total occlusion of circulation in extremity (caused by edema from circumferential burns)
■ airway obstruction (neck burns) or restricted respiratory expansion (chest burns)
■ pulmonary injury (from smoke inhalation or pulmonary embolism)
■ adult respiratory distress syndrome (caused by left-sided heart failure or myocardial infarction)
■ greater damage than indicated by the surface burn (electrical and chemical burns) or internal tissue damage along the conduction pathway (electrical burns)
■ cardiac arrhythmias (caused by electrical shock and fluid shifts)
■ hypotension, caused by shock or hypovolemia
■ infected burn wound
■ stroke, heart attack, or pulmonary embolism (caused by formation of blood clots resulting from slower blood flow)
■ burn shock (caused by fluid shifts out of the vascular compartments, possibly leading to kidney damage and renal failure)
■ peptic ulcer disease or ileus (caused by decreased blood supply in the abdominal area)

- disseminated intravascular coagulation (more severe burn states)
- added pain, depression, and financial burden (caused by psychological component of burn or disfigurement).

DIAGNOSIS

Diagnosis involves determining the size and classification of the wound. The following methods are used to determine size:

- percentage of BSA covered by the burn using the Rule of Nines chart
- Lund-Browder chart (more accurate because it allows BSA changes with age); correlation of the burn's depth and size to estimate its severity. (See *Using the Rule of Nines and the Lund-Browder chart,* pages 554 and 555.)

Major burns are classified as:

- third-degree burns over more than 10% of BSA
- second-degree burns over more than 25% of adult BSA (over 20% in children)
- burns of hands, face, feet, or genitalia
- burns complicated by fractures or respiratory damage
- electrical burns
- all burns in poor-risk patients.

Moderate burns are classified as:

- third-degree burns over 2% to 10% of BSA
- second-degree burns over 15% to 25% of adult BSA (10% to 20% in children).

Minor burns are classified as:

- third-degree burns over less than 2% of BSA
- second-degree burns over less than 15% of adult BSA (10% in children).

TREATMENT

Initial burn treatments are based on the type of burn and may include:

- immersing the burned area in cool water (55° F [12.8° C]) or applying cool compresses (minor burns)
- administering pain medication as needed or anti-inflammatory medications
- covering the area with an antimicrobial agent and a nonstick bulky dressing (after debridement); prophylactic tetanus injection as needed

- preventing hypoxia by maintaining an open airway; assessing airway, breathing, and circulation; checking for smoke inhalation immediately on receipt of the patient; assisting with endotracheal intubation; and giving 100% oxygen (first immediate treatment for moderate and major burns)
- controlling active bleeding
- covering partial-thickness burns over 30% of BSA or full-thickness burns over 5% of BSA with a clean, dry, sterile bed sheet; *don't* cover large burns with saline-soaked dressings because these dressings can cause a drastic reduction in body temperature
- removing smoldering clothing (first soaking with saline solution if clothing is stuck to the patient's skin), rings, and other constricting items
- providing immediate I.V. therapy to prevent hypovolemic shock and maintain cardiac output (commonly, lactated Ringer's solution in amounts determined by a fluid replacement formula)
- monitoring results of tests including complete blood count, electrolytes, glucose, blood urea nitrogen, and serum creatinine levels; arterial blood gas analysis; blood typing and cross-matching; urinalysis for myoglobinuria and hemoglobinuria
- closely monitoring fluid intake and output, frequently checking vital signs (every 15 minutes), possibly inserting indwelling urinary catheter
- using nasogastric tube to decompress the stomach and avoid aspiration of stomach contents
- irrigating the wound with copious amounts of normal saline solution (chemical burns).
- providing surgical intervention, including skin grafts and more thorough surgical cleaning (major burns).

Cellulitis

Cellulitis is an infection of the dermis or subcutaneous layer of the skin. It may follow damage to the skin, such as a bite or wound. As the cellulitis spreads, fever, erythema, and lymphangitis may occur.

(Text continues on page 556.)

Using the Rule of Nines and the Lund-Browder chart

You can quickly estimate the extent of an adult patient's burn by using the Rule of Nines. This method divides an adult's body surface area into percentages. To use this method, mentally transfer your patient's burns to the body chart shown below, then add up the corresponding percentages for each burned body section. The total, an estimate of the extent of your patient's burn, enters into the formula to determine his initial fluid replacement needs.

You can't use the Rule of Nines for infants and children because their body section percentages differ from those of adults. For example, the head accounts for about 17% of the total body surface area in an infant compared with 7% in an adult. Instead, use the Lund-Browder chart.

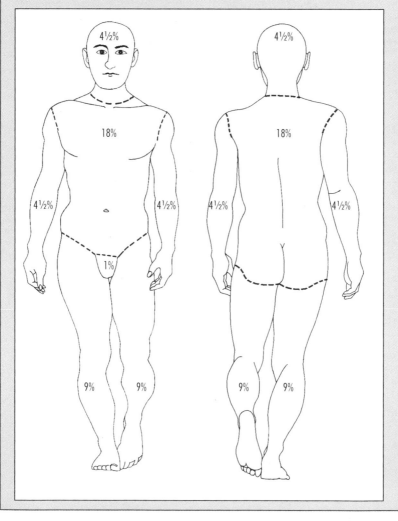

LUND-BROWDER CHART

To determine the extent of an infant's or child's burns, use the Lund-Browder chart shown here.

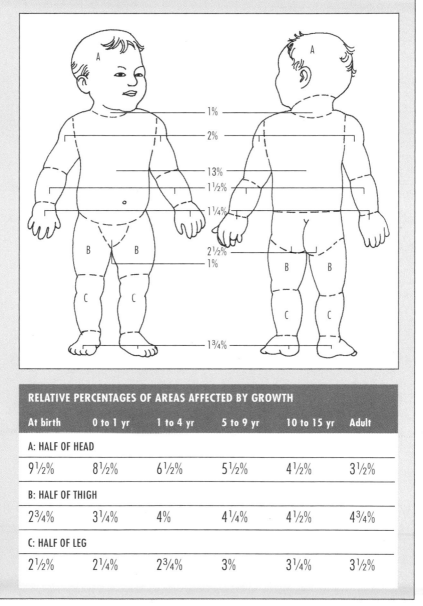

RELATIVE PERCENTAGES OF AREAS AFFECTED BY GROWTH					
At birth	0 to 1 yr	1 to 4 yr	5 to 9 yr	10 to 15 yr	Adult
A: HALF OF HEAD					
$9\frac{1}{2}$%	$8\frac{1}{2}$%	$6\frac{1}{2}$%	$5\frac{1}{2}$%	$4\frac{1}{2}$%	$3\frac{1}{2}$%
B: HALF OF THIGH					
$2\frac{3}{4}$%	$3\frac{1}{4}$%	4%	$4\frac{1}{4}$%	$4\frac{1}{2}$%	$4\frac{3}{4}$%
C: HALF OF LEG					
$2\frac{1}{2}$%	$2\frac{1}{4}$%	$2\frac{3}{4}$%	3%	$3\frac{1}{4}$%	$3\frac{1}{2}$%

If treated in a timely manner, the prognosis is usually good. People with other contributing health factors, such as diabetes, immunodeficiency, impaired circulation, and neuropathy, have an increased risk of developing or spreading cellulitis.

CAUSES
Possible causes of cellulitis are bacterial and fungal infections, typically group A streptococcus and *Staphylococcus aureus.*

PATHOPHYSIOLOGY
As the offending organism invades the compromised area, it overwhelms the defensive cells (neutrophils, eosinophils, basophils, and mast cells) that break down the cellular components, and which normally contain and localize the inflammation. As cellulitis progresses, the organism invades tissue around the initial wound site.

SIGNS AND SYMPTOMS
Signs and symptoms of cellulitis include:
- erythema and edema caused by inflammatory responses to the injury (classic signs)
- pain at the site and possibly surrounding area due edema and subsequent increased pressure
- fever and warmth because of temperature increase caused by infection.

COMPLICATIONS
Possible complications of cellulitis include:
- sepsis (untreated cellulitis)
- progression of cellulitis to involve more tissue area
- local abscesses
- thrombophlebitis
- lymphangitis in recurrent cellulitis.

DIAGNOSIS
Diagnosis is based on:
- visual examination and inspection of the affected area
- white blood cell count showing mild leukocytosis with a left shift
- mildly elevated erythrocyte sedimentation rate
- culture and Gram stain results of fluid from abscesses and bulla positive for the offending organism.

TREATMENT
Treatment of cellulitis may include:
- oral or I.V. penicillin (drug of choice for initial treatment) unless the patient has a known penicillin allergy
- warm soaks to the site to help relieve pain and decrease edema by increasing vasodilation
- pain medication as needed to promote comfort
- elevation of infected extremity to promote comfort and decrease edema
- modified bed rest
- protective footwear for ambulation.

AGE ALERT
Cellulitis of the lower extremity is more likely to develop into thrombophlebitis in an elderly patient.

Dermatitis
Dermatitis is an inflammation of the skin that occurs in several forms: atopic (see "Atopic dermatitis" in chapter 12), seborrheic, nummular, contact, chronic, localized neurodermatitis (lichen simplex chronicus), exfoliative, and stasis. (See *Types of dermatitis.*)

Folliculitis, furuncles, and carbuncles
Folliculitis is a bacterial infection of a hair follicle that causes a pustule to form. The infection can be superficial (follicular impetigo or Bockhart's impetigo) or deep (sycosis barbae).

Furuncles, also known as *boils*, are another form of deep folliculitis. Carbuncles are a group of interconnected furuncles. (See *Follicular skin infection,* page 560.)

The incidence of folliculitis in the general population is difficult to determine because many affected people never seek treatment.

With appropriate treatment, the prognosis for patients with folliculitis is good. The disorder usually resolves in 2 to 3 weeks. The prognosis for patients with carbuncles depends on the severity of the infection and the patient's physical condition and ability to resist infection.

(Text continues on page 560.)

Types of dermatitis

TYPE AND CHARACTERISTICS	CAUSE	SIGNS AND SYMPTOMS	TREATMENT AND INTERVENTION
Seborrheic dermatitis A subacute skin disease affecting the scalp, face, and occasionally other areas that's characterized by lesions covered with yellow or brownish-gray scales.	◆ Unknown; stress, immunodeficiency, and neurologic conditions may be predisposing factors; related to the yeast *Pityrosporum ovale* (normal flora)	◆ Eruptions in areas with many sebaceous glands (usually scalp, face, chest, axillae, and groin) and in skin folds ◆ Itching, redness, and inflammation of affected areas; lesions may appear greasy; fissures may occur ◆ Indistinct, occasionally yellowish scaly patches from excess stratum corneum (dandruff may be a mild seborrheic dermatitis)	◆ Removal of scales with frequent washing and shampooing with selenium sulfide suspension (most effective), zinc pyrithione, ketoconazole 2%, or tar and salicylic acid shampoo ◆ Application of topical corticosteroids and antifungals to involved area
Nummular dermatitis A chronic form of dermatitis characterized by inflammation in coin shaped, scaling, or vesicular patches, usually pruritic.	◆ Possibly brought on by stress, dry skin, irritants, or scratching	◆ Round, nummular (coin-shaped), red lesions, usually on arms and legs, with distinct borders of crusts and scales ◆ Possible oozing and severe itching ◆ Summertime remissions common, with wintertime recurrence	◆ Elimination of known irritants ◆ Measures to relieve dry skin: increased humidification, limited frequency of baths, use of bland soap and bath oils, and application of emollients ◆ Application of wet dressings in acute phase ◆ Topical corticosteroids (occlusive dressings or intralesional injections) for persistent lesions ◆ Tar preparations and antihistamines to control itching ◆ Antibiotics for secondary infection

(continued)

Types of dermatitis *(continued)*

TYPE AND CHARACTERISTICS	CAUSE	SIGNS AND SYMPTOMS	TREATMENT AND INTERVENTION
Contact dermatitis Commonly sharply demarcated inflammation of the skin resulting from contact with an irritating chemical or atopic allergen (a substance producing an allergic reaction in the skin) and irritation of the skin resulting from contact with concentrated substances to which the skin is sensitive, such as perfumes, soaps, or chemicals.	◆ Mild irritants: chronic exposure to detergents or solvents ◆ Strong irritants: damage on contact with acids or alkalis ◆ Allergens: sensitization after repeated exposure	◆ Erythema and small vesicles that ooze, scale, and itch — with mild irritants and allergens ◆ Blisters and ulcerations — with strong irritants ◆ Classic allergic response: clearly defined lesions, with straight lines following points of contact ◆ Severe allergic reaction: marked erythema, blistering, and edema of affected areas	◆ Elimination of known allergens and decreased exposure to irritants, wearing protective clothing such as gloves, and washing immediately after contact with irritants or allergens ◆ Topical anti-inflammatory agents (including corticosteroids), systemic corticosteroids for edema and bullae, antihistamines, and local applications of Burow's solution (for blisters)
Hand or foot dermatitis Skin disease characterized by inflammatory eruptions of the hands or feet.	◆ In many cases unknown but may result from irritant or allergic contact ◆ Excessively dry skin often a contributing factor ◆ 50% of patients atopic	◆ Redness and scaling of the palms or soles ◆ Possible production of painful fissures ◆ Blisters as presenting symptom sometimes (dyshidrotic eczema)	◆ Same as for nummular dermatitis ◆ Systemic steroids possibly required for severe cases
Localized neurodermatitis (lichen simplex chronicus, essential pruritus) Superficial inflammation of the skin characterized by itching and papular eruptions that appear on thickened, hyperpigmented skin.	◆ Chronic scratching or rubbing of a primary lesion or insect bite or other skin irritation ◆ May be psychogenic	◆ Intense, sometimes continual scratching ◆ Thick, sharp-bordered, possibly dry, scaly lesions with raised papules and accentuated skin lines (lichenification) ◆ Usually affecting easily reached areas, such as ankles, lower legs, anogenital area, back of neck, and ears ◆ One or several lesions present; asymmetric distribution	◆ Cessation of scratching; then lesions disappear in about 2 weeks ◆ Fixed dressings or Unna's boot to cover affected areas ◆ Topical corticosteroids under occlusion or by intralesional injection ◆ Antihistamines and open wet dressings ◆ Emollients ◆ Patient informed about underlying cause

Types of dermatitis (continued)

TYPE AND CHARACTERISTICS	CAUSE	SIGNS AND SYMPTOMS	TREATMENT AND INTERVENTION
Exfoliative dermatitis Severe skin inflammation characterized by redness and widespread erythema and scaling, covering virtually the entire skin surface.	◆ Preexisting skin lesions progressing to exfoliative stage, such as in contact dermatitis, drug reaction, lymphoma, leukemia, or atopic dermatitis ◆ May be idiopathic	◆ Generalized dermatitis, with acute loss of stratum corneum, erythema, and scaling ◆ Sensation of tight skin ◆ Hair loss ◆ Possible fever, sensitivity to cold, shivering, gynecomastia, and lymphadenopathy	◆ Hospitalization, with protective isolation and hygienic measures to prevent secondary bacterial infection ◆ Open wet dressings, with colloidal baths ◆ Bland lotions over topical corticosteroids ◆ Maintenance of constant environmental temperature to prevent chilling or overheating ◆ Careful monitoring of renal and cardiac status ◆ Systemic antibiotics and steroids
Stasis dermatitis A condition usually caused by impaired circulation and characterized by eczema of the legs with edema, hyperpigmentation, and persistent inflammation.	◆ Resulting from peripheral vascular diseases affecting the legs, such as recurrent thrombophlebitis and resultant chronic venous insufficiency	◆ Varicosities and edema common, but obvious vascular insufficiency not always present ◆ Usual site: the lower leg just above internal malleolus or sites of trauma or irritation ◆ Early signs: dusky-red deposits of hemosiderin in skin, with itching and dimpling of subcutaneous tissue ◆ Later signs: edema, redness, and scaling of large areas of legs ◆ Possible fissures, crusts, and ulcers	◆ Measures to prevent venous stasis: avoidance of prolonged sitting or standing, use of support stockings, weight reduction in obesity, and leg elevation ◆ Corrective surgery for underlying cause ◆ After ulcer develops, rest periods with legs elevated, open wet dressings, Unna's boot (zinc gelatin dressing provides continuous pressure to affected areas), and antibiotics for secondary infection after wound culture

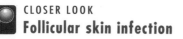

CLOSER LOOK
Follicular skin infection

The degree of hair follicle involvement in bacterial skin infection ranges from superficial erythema and pustule of a single follicle to deep abscesses (carbuncles) involving several follicles.

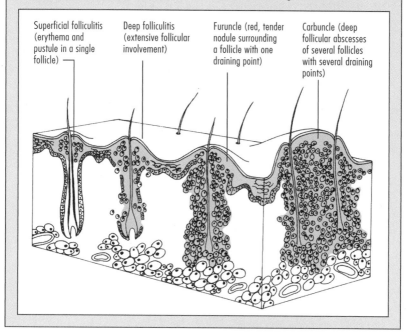

Superficial folliculitis (erythema and pustule in a single follicle)

Deep folliculitis (extensive follicular involvement)

Furuncle (red, tender nodule surrounding a follicle with one draining point)

Carbuncle (deep follicular abscesses of several follicles with several draining points)

CAUSES

The most common cause of folliculitis, furuncles, and carbuncles is coagulase-positive *Staphylococcus aureus.*

Other causes may include:

- *Klebsiella, Enterobacter*, or *Proteus* organisms (These organisms cause gram-negative folliculitis in patients receiving long-term antibiotic therapy such as for acne.)

- *Pseudomonas aeruginosa* (This organism thrives in a warm environment with a high pH and low chlorine content—"hot tub folliculitis.")

Predisposing risk factors include:
- infected wound
- poor hygiene
- debilitation
- tight clothes
- friction
- immunosuppressive therapy
- exposure to certain solvents
- diabetes.

PATHOPHYSIOLOGY

The affecting organism enters the body, usually at a break in the skin barrier (such as a wound site). The organism then causes an inflammatory reaction within the hair follicle.

SIGNS AND SYMPTOMS

Folliculitis, furuncles, and carbuncles have different signs and symptoms depending on the degree of the inflammatory reaction involving the hair follicle.

- Folliculitis shows as pustules on the scalp, arms, and legs in children and the trunk, buttocks, and legs in adults.
- Furuncles show as hard, painful nodules, commonly on the neck, face, axillae, and buttocks. The nodules enlarge for several days, then rupture, discharging pus and necrotic material; after the nodules rupture, pain subsides but erythema and edema persist for days or weeks.
- Carbuncles show as painful, deep abscesses draining through multiple openings onto the skin surface, usually around several hair follicles; with accompanying fever and malaise. Carbuncles are now rare.

COMPLICATIONS

Possible complications include:

- scarring
- bacteremia or cellulitis
- metastatic seeding of a cardiac valve defect or arthritic joint.

DIAGNOSIS

Diagnosis is based on:

- patient history showing preexistent furuncles (carbuncles)
- physical examination showing the presence of the skin lesion to diagnose either folliculitis or carbuncle
- wound cultures of the infected site (usually showing *S. aureus*)
- possibly elevated white blood cell count (leukocytosis).

TREATMENT

Appropriate treatments include:

- cleaning the infected area thoroughly with antibacterial soap and water
- applying warm, wet compresses to promote vasodilation and drainage from the lesions
- applying topical antibiotics, such as mupirocin ointment or clindamycin or erythromycin solution.

Specific treatments include:

- folliculitis (extensive infection) — use of systemic antibiotics, such as a cephalosporin or dicloxacillin
- furuncles — incision and drainage of ripe lesions after applying warm, wet compresses, then giving systemic antibiotics

- carbuncles — systemic antibiotic therapy and incision and drainage.

Fungal infections

Fungal infections of the skin are commonly regarded as superficial infections affecting the hair, nails, and dermatophytes (the dead top layer of the skin). They are unique in that they infect and survive on the keratin within these structures. The most common fungal infections are tinea and candidiasis.

Tinea infections are classified by the body location in which they occur. Tinea commonly infects children and adolescents. Obese patients are also at greater risk for these infections, especially in skin folds that are constantly moist. Some forms, such as tinea cruris (a fungal infection of the groin), infect one gender more than the other. Tinea cruris occurs more commonly in males.

Candidiasis can infect the skin or mucous membranes. These infections are also classified according to the infected site or area. *Candida* organisms are the normal flora found in some people (on the skin, in the mouth, GI tract, and genitalia).

Candidiasis usually occurs in children and immunosuppressed individuals. There are also higher rates of candidiasis in pregnant women and in patients with diabetes mellitus as well as those with indwelling catheters and I.V. lines.

The prognosis for tinea and candidiasis is very good. These infections usually respond well to appropriate drug therapy and resolve completely. Reducing risk factors is important to obtain a good outcome from the infection. Antifungal therapy usually resolves candidiasis, but if risk factors aren't avoided, a chronic condition can develop.

CAUSES

Tinea infections are caused by:

- *Microsporum, Trichophyton,* or *Epidermophyton* organisms
- contact with contaminated objects or surfaces.

Risk factors for tinea include:

- obesity
- exposure to the causative organisms

- antibiotic therapy with suppression of normal flora
- softened skin from prolonged water contact, such as with water sports or diaphoresis.

Causes of candidiasis include:
- overgrowth of *Candida* organisms and infection because of depletion of the normal flora (such as with antibiotic therapy)
- neutropenia and bone marrow suppression in immunocompromised patients (at greater risk for the disseminating form)
- *Candida albicans,* normal GI flora (causes candidiasis in susceptible patients)
- *Candida* overgrowth in the mouth (thrush).

PATHOPHYSIOLOGY
In tinea infections, the tinea fungi attack the outer, dead skin layers. These fungi prefer a dark, warm, moist environment. Tinea infections can be spread from human to human, animal to human, or soil to human. Tinea corpus, for example, can be contracted from animals infected with *Microsporum canis or Trichophyton mentagrophytes,* and also from humans infected with *Trichophyton rubrum.*

In candidiasis, the *Candida* organism penetrates the epidermis after it binds to integrin receptors and adhesion molecules. The secretion of proteolytic enzymes by the organism facilitates tissue invasion. An inflammatory response results from the attraction of neutrophils to the area and from activation of the complement cascade.

SIGNS AND SYMPTOMS
Signs and symptoms of tinea include:
- erythema and pustules in a ring-like formation
- itching, commonly severe
Signs and symptoms of candidiasis include:
- superficial papules and pustules caused by proteolytic enzyme destruction of keratin
- erythematous and edematous areas of the infected epidermis or mucous membrane (with progression of inflammation, a white-yellow, curdlike crust covering the infected area) caused by release of possible toxins by the fungus

- severe pruritus and pain at the lesion sites (common) caused by inflammation
- white coating of the tongue and possibly lesions in the mouth (thrush).

COMPLICATIONS
Possible complications include:
- secondary bacterial infections of wounds opened by scratching
- ulcers with chronic forms (candidiasis lesions)
- candidal meningitis, endocarditis, or septicemia caused by systemic disseminating candidiasis.

DIAGNOSIS
Diagnosis is based on:
- culture to determine the causative organism and suggest the mode of infection transmission (tinea infection)
- microscopic examination of a potassium hydroxide-treated skin scraping and culture (tinea and candidal infections).

TREATMENT
Treatment includes:
- topical antifungal agents such as ketoconazole, believed to inhibit yeast growth by altering cell membrane permeability (tinea pedis, tinea cruris, and tinea corporis)
- oral therapy with griseofulvin if no response to topical treatment, to arrest fungal cell activity by disrupting its miotic spindle structure (tinea)
- oral ketoconazole for infections resistant to griseofulvin therapy, to make the fungus more susceptible to osmotic pressure; other oral medications include fluconazole and terbinafine
- eliminating risk factors (tinea and candidiasis)
- oral nystatin and topical antifungals such as miconazole (candidiasis)
- I.V. amphotericin B or oral ketoconazole (systemic infections).

Pressure ulcers

Pressure ulcers, commonly called *pressure sores* or *bedsores,* are localized areas of cellular necrosis that occur most commonly in the skin and subcutaneous tissue over bony prominences. These ulcers may be superficial, caused by local skin irritation with subsequent surface maceration, or deep, originating in underlying tissue. Deep lesions commonly go undetected until they penetrate the skin, but by then, they have usually caused subcutaneous damage. (See *Staging pressure ulcers,* pages 564 and 565.)

Most pressure ulcers develop over five body locations: sacral area, greater trochanter, ischial tuberosity, heel, and lateral malleolus. Collectively, these areas account for 95% of all pressure ulcer sites. Patients who have contractures are at an increased risk for developing pressure ulcers because of the added pressure on the tissue and the alignment of the bones.

▲ **AGE ALERT**
Age also plays a role in the incidence of pressure ulcers. Muscle is lost with aging, and skin elasticity decreases. Both of these factors increase the risk of developing pressure ulcers.

Partial-thickness ulcers usually involve the dermis and epidermis; with treatment, these wounds heal within a few weeks. Full-thickness ulcers also involve the dermis and epidermis, but in these wounds, the damage is more severe and complete. There may also be damage to the deeper tissue layers. Ulcers of the subcutaneous tissue and muscle may require several months to heal. If the damage has affected the bone in addition to the skin layers, osteomyelitis may occur, which will prolong healing time.

CAUSES
Possible causes of pressure ulcers include:
- immobility and decreased level of activity
- friction or shearing forces causing damage to the epidermal and upper dermal skin layers
- constant moisture on the skin causing tissue maceration
- impaired hygiene status, such as with urinary or fecal incontinence, leading to skin breakdown
- malnutrition (linked to pressure ulcer development)
- medical conditions, such as diabetes and orthopedic injuries (These conditions may predispose the patient to pressure ulcer development.)

- psychological factors, such as depression and chronic emotional stresses. (Certain factors may play a role in pressure ulcer development.)

PATHOPHYSIOLOGY
A pressure ulcer is caused by an injury to the skin and its underlying tissues. The pressure exerted on the area causes ischemia and hypoxemia to the affected tissues because of decreased blood flow to the site. As the capillaries collapse, thrombosis occurs, which subsequently leads to tissue edema and progression to tissue necrosis. Ischemia also adds to an accumulation of waste products at the site, which in turn leads to the production of toxins. The toxins further break down the tissue and eventually lead to the death of the cells.

SIGNS AND SYMPTOMS
Signs and symptoms of pressure ulcers may include:
- blanching erythema, varying from pink to bright red depending on the patient's skin color; when the examiner's finger presses on the reddened area, the pressed-on area whitens and color returns in 1 to 3 seconds if capillary refill is good.

 CULTURAL DIVERSITY
In dark-skinned people, purple discoloration or a darkening of normal skin color is typically the first clinical sign.

- pain at the site and surrounding area caused by increased pressure from edema
- localized edema caused by the inflammatory response
- increased body temperature caused by initial inflammatory response (in more severe cases, cool skin caused by more severe damage or necrosis)
- nonblanching erythema (more severe cases) ranging from dark red to purple or cyanotic; indicates deeper dermal involvement
- blisters, crusts, or scaling as the skin deteriorates and the ulcer progresses
- skin usually a dusky red, not bleeding easily, warm to the touch, and possibly mottled (deep ulcer originating at the bony prominence below the skin surface)

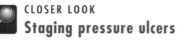

CLOSER LOOK
Staging pressure ulcers

The staging system described here is based on the recommendations of the National Pressure Ulcer Advisory Panel (NPUAP) (Consensus Conference, 1991) and the Agency for Health Care Policy and Research (Clinical Practice Guidelines for Treatment of Pressure Ulcers, 1992). The stage 1 definition was updated by the NPUAP in 1997.

STAGE I
A stage I pressure ulcer is an observable pressure-related alteration of intact skin. The indicators, compared with the adjacent or opposite area on the body, may include changes in one or more of the following factors: skin temperature (warmth or coolness), tissue consistency (firm or boggy feel), or sensation (pain or itching). The ulcer appears as a defined area of persistent redness in lightly pigmented skin; in darker skin, the ulcer may appear with persistent red, blue, or purple hues.

STAGE II
A stage II pressure ulcer is characterized by partial-thickness skin loss involving the epidermis or dermis. The ulcer is superficial and appears as an abrasion, blister, or shallow crater.

STAGE III
A stage III pressure ulcer is characterized by full-thickness skin loss involving damage or necrosis of subcutaneous tissue, which may extend down to, but not through, the underlying fascia. The ulcer appears as a deep crater with or without undermining of adjacent tissue.

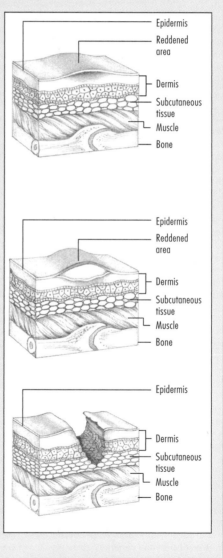

Staging pressure ulcers *(continued)*

STAGE IV
Full-thickness skin loss with extensive destruction, tissue necrosis, or damage to muscle, bone, or support structures (for example, tendon or joint capsule) characterize a stage IV pressure ulcer. Tunneling and sinus tracts may also occur in stage IV pressure ulcers.

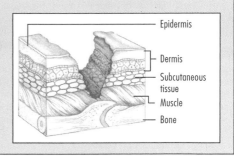

- possible foul-smelling, purulent drainage from the ulcerated lesion
- eschar (sloughing or shredded) tissue on and around the lesion because of the necrotic tissue that prevents healthy tissue growth.

COMPLICATIONS
Possible complications of pressure ulcers include:
- progression of the pressure ulcer to a more severe state
- secondary infections such as sepsis
- loss of limb from bone involvement
- osteomyelitis.

DIAGNOSIS
Diagnosis is based on:
- physical examination showing presence of the ulcer
- wound culture with exudate or evidence of infection
- elevated white blood cell count with infection
- possibly elevated erythrocyte sedimentation rate
- total serum protein and serum albumin levels showing severe hypoproteinemia
- elevated temperature with infection.

TREATMENT
Treatment for pressure ulcers includes:
- repositioning by the caregiver every 2 hours or more often if indicated, with support of pillows for immobile patients; a pillow and encouragement to change position for those able to move
- movement and range-of-motion (ROM) exercises to promote circulation
- foam, gel, or air mattress to aid in healing by reducing pressure on the ulcer site and reducing the risk of more ulcers
- foam, gel, or air mattress on chairs and wheelchairs as indicated
- nutritional assessment and dietary consult as indicated; nutritional supplements, such as vitamin C and zinc, for the malnourished patient; monitoring serum albumin and protein markers and body weight
- adequate fluid intake (I.V. if indicated) and increased fluids for a dehydrated patient
- good skin care and hygiene practices (for example, meticulous hygiene and skin care for the incontinent patient to prevent breakdown of the affected tissue and skin.)
- cover ulcer with transparent film, polyurethane foam, or hydrocolloid dressing (stage II ulcer)
- loosely fill wound with saline- or gel-moistened gauze, manage exudate with absorbent dressing (moist gauze or foam) and cover with secondary dressing (stage II or IV ulcer)
- clean, bulky dressing for certain types of ulcers
- surgical debridement for deeper wounds (stage III or IV ulcer) as indicated.

Psoriasis
Psoriasis is a chronic, recurrent disease marked by epidermal proliferation and

characterized by recurring partial remissions and exacerbations. Flare-ups are commonly related to specific systemic and environmental factors, but may be unpredictable. Widespread involvement is called *exfoliative* or *erythrodermic psoriasis*.

Psoriasis affects about 21% of the population in the United States. Although this disorder usually affects young adults, it may strike at any age, including infancy. Genetic factors predetermine the incidence of psoriasis; researchers have discovered a significantly greater incidence of certain human leukocyte antigens (HLAs) in families with psoriasis.

Flare-ups can usually be controlled with therapy. Appropriate treatment depends on the type of psoriasis, extent of the disease, the patient's response, and the effect of the disease on the patient's life style. No permanent cure exists, and all methods of treatment are palliative.

CAUSES
Causes of psoriasis include:
- genetically determined tendency to develop psoriasis
- possible immune disorder, as shown in the HLA type in families
- environmental factors
- isomorphic effect or Koebner's phenomenon, in which lesions develop at sites of injury caused by trauma
- flare-up of guttate (drop-shaped) lesions caused by infections, especially beta-hemolytic streptococci.

Other contributing factors include:
- pregnancy
- endocrine changes
- climate (cold weather tends to exacerbate psoriasis)
- emotional stress.

PATHOPHYSIOLOGY
A skin cell normally takes 14 days to move from the basal layer to the stratum corneum, where it's sloughed off after 14 days of normal wear and tear. Thus, the life cycle of a normal skin cell is 28 days compared with only 4 days for a psoriatic skin cell. This markedly shortened cycle doesn't allow time for the cell to mature. Consequently, the stratum corneum becomes

thick and flaky, producing the cardinal manifestations of psoriasis.

SIGNS AND SYMPTOMS
Possible signs and symptoms include:
- itching and occasional pain from dry, cracked, encrusted lesions (most common)
- erythematous and usually well-defined plaques, sometimes covering large areas of the body (psoriatic lesions)
- lesions most commonly on the scalp, chest, elbows, knees, back, and buttocks
- plaques with characteristic silver scales that either flake off easily or thicken, covering the lesion; scale removal can produce fine bleeding
- occasional small guttate lesions (usually thin and erythematous, with few scales), either alone or with plaques.

COMPLICATIONS
Possible complications of psoriasis include:
- spread to fingernails, producing small indentations or pits and yellow or brown discoloration (about 60% of patients)
- accumulation of thick, crumbly debris under the nail, causing it to separate from the nail bed (onycholysis)
- infection, from scratching.

Rarely, psoriasis becomes pustular, taking one of two forms:
- localized pustular psoriasis, with pustules on the palms and soles that remain sterile until opened
- generalized pustular (Von Zumbusch) psoriasis, typically occurring with fever, leukocytosis, and malaise, with groups of pustules coalescing to form lakes of pus on red skin (also remain sterile until opened), commonly involving the tongue and oral mucosa
- erythrodermic psoriasis (least common form), which is an inflammatory form of the disorder characterized by periodic fiery erythema and exfoliation of the skin with severe itching and pain
- arthritic symptoms, usually in one or more joints of the fingers or toes, the larger joints, or sometimes the sacroiliac joints, which may progress to spondylitis, and morning stiffness (some patients).

DIAGNOSIS

Diagnosis is based on the following factors:

- patient history, appearance of the lesions and, if needed, the results of skin biopsy
- serum uric acid level (usually elevated in severe cases because of accelerated nucleic acid degradation), but without indications of gout
- Serum HLA-Cw6, -B13, and -Bw57 (may be present in early-onset familial psoriasis).

TREATMENT

Treatment may include:

- ultraviolet B (UVB) or natural sunlight exposure to retard rapid cell production to the point of minimal erythema
- tar preparations or crude coal tar applications to the affected areas about 15 minutes before exposure to UVB, or left on overnight and wiped off the next morning
- gradually increasing exposure to UVB (outpatient treatment or day treatment avoids long hospitalizations and prolongs remission)
- steroid creams and ointments applied twice daily, preferably after bathing to facilitate absorption, and overnight use of occlusive dressings to control symptoms of psoriasis
- intralesional steroid injection for small, stubborn plaques
- anthralin ointment or paste mixture for well-defined plaques (not applied to unaffected areas because of injury and staining of normal skin); petroleum jelly around affected skin before applying anthralin
- anthralin and steroids (anthralin application at night and steroid use during the day)
- calcipotriene ointment, a vitamin D analogue (best when alternated with a topical steroid)
- combination of tar baths or anthralin and UVB treatments to help achieve remission and clear the skin (severe chronic psoriasis)
- administration of psoralens (plant extracts that accelerate exfoliation) with exposure to high-intensity ultraviolet A (UVA) (psoralen plus UVA [PUVA] therapy)
- cytotoxin, usually methotrexate (last-resort treatment for refractory psoriasis)
- acitretin, a retinoid compound (extensive psoriasis)
- cyclosporine, an immunosuppressant (in resistive cases)
- low-dose antihistamines, oatmeal baths, emollients, and open wet dressings to help relieve pruritus
- aspirin and local heat to help alleviate the pain of psoriatic arthritis; nonsteroidal anti-inflammatory drugs in severe cases
- tar shampoo followed by a steroid lotion (psoriasis of the scalp)
- no effective topical treatment for psoriasis of the nails.

Scleroderma

Scleroderma (also known as *systemic sclerosis*) is an uncommon disease of diffuse connective tissue disease characterized by inflammatory and then degenerative and fibrotic changes in the skin, blood vessels, synovial membranes, skeletal muscles, and internal organs (especially the esophagus, intestinal tract, thyroid, heart, lungs, and kidneys). There are several forms of scleroderma, including diffuse systemic sclerosis, localized, linear, chemically induced localized, eosinophilia-myalgia syndrome, toxic oil syndrome, and graft-versus-host disease.

Scleroderma is an uncommon disease. It affects women three to four times more commonly than men, especially between ages 30 and 50. The peak incidence of occurrence is between ages 50 and 60.

Scleroderma usually progresses slowly. When the condition is limited to the skin, the prognosis is usually favorable, but about 30% of patients with scleroderma die within 5 years of onset. Death is usually caused by infection or renal or heart failure.

CAUSES

The cause of scleroderma is unknown, but some possible causes include:

- systemic exposure to silica dust or polyvinyl chloride
- anticancer agents, such as bleomycin, or nonnarcotic analgesics such as pentazocine
- fibrosis caused by an abnormal immune system response

- underlying vascular problems causing tissue changes.

PATHOPHYSIOLOGY

Scleroderma usually begins in the fingers and extends proximally to the upper arms, shoulders, neck, and face. The skin atrophies, edema and infiltrates containing CD4+ T cells surround the blood vessels, and inflamed collagen fibers become edematous, losing strength and elasticity, and degenerate. The dermis becomes tightly bound to the underlying structures, resulting in atrophy of the affected appendages and destruction of the fingers by osteoporosis. As the disease progresses, this atrophy can affect other areas. For example, in some patients, muscles and joints become fibrotic.

SIGNS AND SYMPTOMS

Possible signs and symptoms of scleroderma include:
- skin thickening, commonly limited to the distal extremities and face, but which can also involve internal organs (limited systemic sclerosis)
- CREST syndrome (a benign subtype of limited systemic sclerosis): *C*alcinosis, *Ray*naud's phenomenon, *E*sophageal dysfunction, *S*clerodactyly, and *T*elangiectasia
- generalized skin thickening and involvement of internal organs (diffuse systemic sclerosis)
- patchy skin changes with a teardrop-like appearance known as *morphea* (localized scleroderma)
- band of thickened skin on the face or extremities that severely damages underlying tissues, causing atrophy and deformity (linear scleroderma)

▲ **AGE ALERT**
Atrophy and deformity with scleroderma are most common in children.

- Raynaud's phenomenon (blanching, cyanosis, and erythema of the fingers and toes when exposed to cold or stress); progressive phalangeal resorption may shorten the fingers (early symptoms)
- pain, stiffness, and swelling of fingers and joints (later symptoms)
- taut, shiny skin over the entire hand and forearm because of skin thickening
- tight and inelastic facial skin, causing a mask-like appearance and "pinching" of the mouth; contractures with progressive tightening
- thickened skin over proximal limbs and trunk (diffuse systemic sclerosis)
- frequent reflux, heartburn, dysphagia, and bloating after meals because of GI dysfunction
- abdominal distention, diarrhea, constipation, and malodorous floating stool.

COMPLICATIONS

Complications of scleroderma include:
- compromised circulation caused by abnormal thickening of the arterial intima, possibly causing slowly healing ulcerations on fingertips or toes leading to gangrene
- decreased food intake and weight loss because of GI symptoms
- arrhythmias and dyspnea caused by cardiac and pulmonary fibrosis; malignant hypertension caused by renal involvement (called *renal crisis* [may be fatal if untreated; advanced disease]).

DIAGNOSIS

Diagnosis of scleroderma may include:
- typical skin changes (the first clue to diagnosis.)
- slightly elevated erythrocyte sedimentation rate, positive rheumatoid factor in 25% to 35% of patients, and positive antinuclear antibody test results
- urinalysis showing proteinuria, microscopic hematuria, and casts (with renal involvement)
- hand X-rays showing terminal phalangeal tuft resorption, subcutaneous calcification, and joint space narrowing and erosion
- chest X-rays showing bilateral basilar pulmonary fibrosis
- GI X-rays showing distal esophageal hypomotility and stricture, duodenal loop dilation, small-bowel malabsorption pattern, and large diverticula
- pulmonary function studies showing decreased diffusion and vital capacity
- electrocardiogram showing nonspecific abnormalities related to myocardial fibrosis
- skin biopsy showing changes consistent with disease progression, such as marked

thickening of the dermis and occlusive vessel changes.

TREATMENT

There's no cure for scleroderma. Treatment aims to preserve normal body func tions and minimize complications and may include:

■ biologic therapy, such as alefacept for moderate to severe plaque psoriasis and etanercept for psoriatic arthritis

■ immunosuppressants, such as cyclosporine or chlorambucil (common palliative medications)

■ vasodilators and antihypertensives; such as nifedipine, prazosin, or topical nitroglycerin; digital sympathectomy; or rarely, cervical sympathetic blockade to treat Raynaud's phenomenon

■ plaster casting of fingers to immobilize the area, minimize trauma, and maintain cleanliness; possible surgical debridement for chronic digital ulceration

■ antacids (to reduce total acid level in GI tract), omeprazole (proton pump inhibitor to block the formation of gastric acid), periodic dilation, and a soft, bland diet for esophagitis with stricture

■ broad-spectrum antibiotics to treat small-bowel involvement with erythromycin or tetracycline (preferred drugs) to counteract the bacterial overgrowth in the duodenum and jejunum related to hypomotility

■ short-term benefit from vasodilators, such as nifedipine or hydralazine, to decrease contractility and oxygen demand, and cause vasodilation (for pulmonary hypertension)

■ angiotensin-converting enzyme inhibitor to preserve renal function (early intervention in renal crisis)

■ physical therapy to maintain function and promote muscle strength, heat therapy to relieve joint stiffness, and patient teaching to make performance of daily activities easier (for hand debilitation).

Warts

Warts, also known as *verrucae*, are common, benign, viral infections of the skin and adjacent mucous membranes. Although their incidence is greatest in children and young adults, warts can

occur at any age. The prognosis varies; many types of warts resolve spontaneously, whereas others need more vigorous and prolonged treatment. Most people eventually develop an immune response to the virus, which causes the warts to disappear spontaneously. An immune response may develop to some types of warts, but this immune response can be delayed for many years.

CAUSES

Warts are caused by:

■ human papillomavirus (HPV)

■ transmission by touch and skin-to-skin contact

■ autoinoculation causing spreading on the affected person

PATHOPHYSIOLOGY

HPV replicates in the epidermal cells, causing irregular thickening of the stratum corneum in the infected areas. People who lack the virus-specific immunity are susceptible to the virus.

SIGNS AND SYMPTOMS

Signs and symptoms depend on the type of wart and its location and may include:

■ rough, elevated, rounded surface, most frequently occurring on extremities, particularly hands and fingers; most prevalent in children and young adults (common warts [verruca vulgaris])

■ single, thin, threadlike projection; commonly occurring around the face and neck (filiform)

■ rough, irregularly shaped, elevated surface, occurring around edges of fingernails and toenails (when severe, extending under the nail and lifting it off the nail bed, causing pain [periungual wart])

■ multiple groupings of up to several hundred slightly raised lesions with smooth, flat, or slightly rounded tops, common on the face, neck, chest, knees, dorsa of hands, wrists, and flexor surfaces of the forearms (usually occur in children but can affect adults); typically a linear distribution from being spread by scratching or shaving (flat or juvenile)

■ slightly elevated or flat; occurring singly or in large clusters (mosaic warts), primarily at pressure points of the feet (plantar)

- fingerlike, horny projection arising from a pea-shaped base, occurring on scalp or near hairline (digitate)
- usually small, pink to red, moist, and soft, occurring singly or in large cauliflower-like clusters on the penis, scrotum, vulva, and anus; although transmitted through sexual contact, it isn't always venereal in origin (condyloma acuminatum [moist wart]).

COMPLICATIONS
Possible complications include:
- autoinoculation
- scar formation
- chronic pain after plantar wart removal and scar formation
- nail deformity after injury to nail matrix
- cervical cancer, with increased risk if a woman smokes (certain strains of HPV)
- esophageal warts (in neonates exposed to genital warts during delivery).

 AGE ALERT
The presence of perianal warts in children may be a sign of sexual abuse.

DIAGNOSIS
Diagnosis is based on:
- physical examination of the patient
- sigmoidoscopy with recurrent anal warts to rule out internal involvement necessitating surgery.

TREATMENT
If immunity develops, warts resolve by themselves. Treatments may include:
- skin irritants, such as salicylic acid or formaldehyde, applied to the wart to try to stimulate an immune response
- curettage or cryosurgery
- podophyllin 25% in compound benzoin tincture for venereal warts
- carbon dioxide laser treatment for recalcitrant warts on the feet, groin, or nail bed
- sexual abstinence or condom use until warts are eradicated; partners should also be examined and treated as needed (genital warts).

Reproductive system

The reproductive system must function properly to ensure survival of the species. The male reproductive system produces sperm and delivers them to the female reproductive tract. The female reproductive system produces the ovum. If a sperm fertilizes an ovum, this female system also nurtures and protects the embryo and developing fetus and delivers it at birth. The functioning of the reproductive system is determined not only by anatomic structure but also by complex hormonal, neurologic, vascular, and psychogenic factors.

Anatomically, the main distinction between the male and female is the presence of conspicuous external genitalia in the male. In contrast, the major reproductive organs of the female lie within the pelvic cavity.

MALE REPRODUCTIVE SYSTEM

The male reproductive system consists of the organs that produce and maintain sperm, transfer mature sperm from the testes, and introduce them into the female reproductive tract, where fertilization occurs.

Besides supplying male sex cells (in a process called *spermatogenesis*), the male

reproductive system plays a part in the secretion of male sex hormones. The penis also functions in urine elimination.

In males, the reproductive and urinary systems are structurally integrated; most disorders of either system, therefore, affect both systems. Congenital abnormalities or prostate enlargement may impair both sexual and urinary function. Abnormal findings in the pelvic area may result from pathologic changes in other organ systems, such as the upper urinary and GI tracts, endocrine glands, and neuromusculoskeletal system.

Reproductive organs

The male reproductive organs include the penis, scrotum, testes, duct system, and accessory reproductive glands.

PENIS

The penis consists of three cylinders of erectile tissue: two corpora cavernosa, and the corpus spongiosum, which contains the urethra. The glans, or tip, of the penis contains the urethral meatus, through which urine and semen pass to the exterior, and many nerve endings for sexual sensation.

SCROTUM

The scrotum, which contains the testes, epididymis, and lower spermatic cords, maintains the proper testicular temperature for spermatogenesis (creating sperm) through relaxation and contraction. This control of temperature is important because excessive heat reduces the sperm count.

TESTES

The testes (also called *gonads* or *testicles*) produce sperm in the seminiferous tubules. Complete spermatogenesis develops in most males by age 15 or 16.

The testes form in the abdominal cavity of the male fetus and descend into the scrotum during the seventh month of gestation.

The testes produce and secrete hormones, especially testosterone, in their interstitial cells (Leydig's cells). Testosterone affects the development and maintenance of secondary sex characteristics and sex drive. It also regulates metabolism, stimulates protein anabolism (encouraging skeletal growth and muscular development), inhibits pituitary secretion of the gonadotropins (follicle-stimulating hormone and interstitial cell-stimulating hormone), promotes potassium excretion, and mildly influences renal sodium reabsorption.

DUCT SYSTEM

The vas deferens connects the epididymis, in which sperm mature and ripen for up to 6 weeks, and the ejaculatory ducts. The seminal vesicles—two convoluted membranous pouches—secrete a viscous liquid of fructose-rich semen, which provides energy for sperm, and prostaglandins that probably facilitate fertilization.

ACCESSORY REPRODUCTIVE GLANDS

The prostate gland secretes the thin alkaline substance that comprises most of the seminal fluid; this fluid also protects sperm from acidity in the male urethra and in the vagina, thus increasing sperm motility.

The bulbourethral (Cowper's) glands secrete an alkaline ejaculatory fluid, probably similar in function to that produced by the prostate gland. The spermatic cords are cylindrical fibrous coverings in the inguinal canal containing the vas deferens, blood vessels, and nerves.

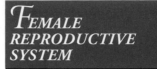

FEMALE REPRODUCTIVE SYSTEM

Female reproductive structures include the mammary glands, external genitalia, and internal genitalia. Hormonal influences determine the development and function of these structures and affect fertility, childbearing, and the ability to experience sexual pleasure.

In no other part of the body do so many interrelated physiologic functions occur so near each other as in the region of the female reproductive tract. Besides the internal genitalia, the female pelvis contains the organs of the urinary and GI systems (bladder, ureters, urethra, sigmoid colon, and rectum). The reproductive tract and its surrounding area are thus the site of urination, defecation, menstruation, ovulation, copulation, impregnation, and parturition.

Mammary glands

Located in the breasts, the mammary glands are specialized accessory glands that secrete milk. Although present in both sexes, they normally function only in females.

External structures

Female genitalia include the following external structures, collectively known as the *vulva*: mons pubis (or mons veneris), labia majora, labia minora, clitoris, and the vestibule. The perineum is the external region between the vulva and the anus. The size, shape, and color of these structures—as well as pubic hair distribution and skin texture and pigmentation—vary greatly among individuals. Furthermore, these external structures undergo distinct changes during the life cycle.

MONS PUBIS

The mons pubis is the pad of fat over the symphysis pubis (pubic bone), which is usually covered by the base of the inverted triangular patch of pubic hair that grows over the vulva after puberty.

LABIA MAJORA

The labia majora are the two thick, longitudinal folds of fatty tissue that extend from the mons pubis to the posterior aspect of the perineum. The labia majora protect the perineum and contain large sebaceous glands that help maintain lubrication. Virtually absent in the young child, their development is a characteristic sign of onset of puberty. The skin of the more prominent parts of the labia majora is pigmented and darkens after puberty.

LABIA MINORA

The labia minora are the two thin, longitudinal folds of skin that border the vestibule. Firmer than the labia majora, they extend from the clitoris to the posterior fourchette.

CLITORIS

The clitoris is the small, protuberant organ located just beneath the arch of the mons pubis. The clitoris contains erectile tissue, venous cavernous spaces, and specialized sensory corpuscles that are stimulated during coitus. It's a counterpart to the male penis.

VESTIBULE

The vestibule is the oval space bordered by the clitoris, labia minora, and fourchette. The urethral meatus is located in the anterior portion of the vestibule, and the vaginal meatus is in the posterior portion. The hymen is the elastic membrane that partially obstructs the vaginal meatus in virgins. Its absence doesn't necessarily imply a history of coitus, nor does its presence obstruct menstrual blood flow.

Several glands lubricate the vestibule. Skene's glands (also known as the *paraurethral glands*) open on both sides of the urethral meatus; Bartholin's glands, on both sides of the vaginal meatus.

The fourchette is the posterior junction of the labia majora and labia minora. The perineum, which includes the underlying muscles and fascia, is the external surface of the floor of the pelvis, extending from the fourchette to the anus.

Internal structures

The internal structures of the female genitalia include the vagina, cervix, uterus, fallopian tubes (or oviducts), and ovaries.

VAGINA

The vagina occupies the space between the bladder and the rectum. A muscular, membranous tube about 2″ to 3″ (5 to 7.5 cm) long, the vagina connects the uterus with the vestibule of the external genitalia. It serves as a passageway for sperm to the fallopian tubes, a conduit for the discharge of menstrual fluid, and the birth canal during parturition (childbirth).

CERVIX

The cervix, the narrow neck of the uterus, protrudes into the upper vaginal canal, providing a passageway between the vagina and the uterine cavity.

UTERUS

The uterus is the hollow, pear-shaped organ in which the conceptus (products of fertilization—fertilized ovum, embryo, fetus, and associated membranes) grows during pregnancy. The thick uterine wall consists of mucosal, muscular, and serous layers. The inner mucosal lining (the endometrium) undergoes cyclic changes based on hormonal activity to facilitate and maintain pregnancy.

The smooth muscular middle layer (the myometrium) interlaces the uterine and ovarian arteries and veins that circulate blood through the uterus. During pregnancy, this vascular system expands dramatically. After abortion or childbirth, the myometrium contracts to constrict the vasculature and control loss of blood.

The outer serous layer (the parietal peritoneum) covers all of the fundus, part of the corpus, but none of the cervix. This incompleteness allows surgical entry into the uterus without incision of the peritoneum (reducing the risk of peritonitis in the days before effective antibiotic therapy).

FALLOPIAN TUBES

The two fallopian tubes extend from the sides of the fundus and terminate near the ovaries. Each tube has a fimbriated (fringe-

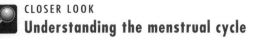

CLOSER LOOK
Understanding the menstrual cycle

The menstrual cycle is divided into three distinct phases.
◆ During the menstrual phase, which starts on the first day of menstruation, the top layer of the endometrium breaks down and flows out of the body. This flow consists of blood and unneeded mucous tissue.
◆ During the proliferative (follicular) phase, the endometrium begins to thicken, and the

level of estrogen in the blood increases, surging at midcycle. Estrogen production decreases, the follicle matures, and ovulation occurs.
◆ During the secretory (luteal) phase, the endometrium begins to thicken to nourish an embryo should fertilization occur. Without fertilization, the top layer of the endometrium breaks down and the menstrual phase of the cycle begins again.

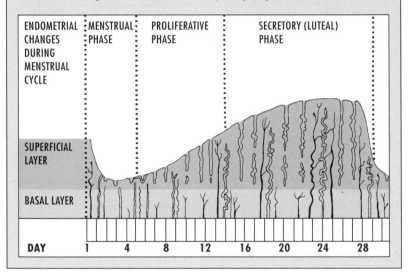

like) end adjacent to the ovary that serves to capture an oocyte after ovulation. Through ciliary and muscular action, these small tubes carry ova from the ovaries to the uterus and facilitate the movement of sperm from the uterus toward the ovaries. The same ciliary and muscular action helps move a zygote (fertilized ovum) down to the uterus, where it may implant in the blood-rich inner uterine lining, the endometrium.

OVARIES

The ovaries are two almond-shaped organs, one on each side of the pelvis, situated behind and below the fallopian tubes.

The ovaries produce ova and two primary hormones — estrogen and progesterone — in addition to small amounts of androgen. These hormones in turn produce and maintain secondary sex characteristics, prepare the uterus for pregnancy, and stimulate mammary gland development. The ovaries are connected to the uterus by the utero-ovarian ligament.

In the 30th week of gestation, the female fetus has about 7 million follicles (ova precursors), which degenerate, leaving about 2 million present at birth. By puberty, only 400,000 follicles remain, and these become graafian follicles in response to the effects of pituitary gonadotropic hormones (follicle-stimulating hormone [FSH] and luteinizing hormone [LH]). Fewer than 500 of each woman's ova mature and become potentially fertile.

The menstrual cycle

Maturation of the hypothalamus and the resulting increase in hormone levels initiate puberty. In the young girl, the appearance of pubic and axillary hair (pubarche) and the characteristic adolescent growth spurt follow breast development (thelarche) — the first sign of puberty. The reproductive system begins to undergo a series of hormone-induced changes that result in menarche, or the onset of menstruation (or menses).

The menstrual cycle consists of three different phases: menstrual, proliferative (estrogen-dominated), and secretory (progesterone-dominated). (See *Understanding the menstrual cycle*.)

At the end of the secretory phase, the uterine lining is ready to receive and nourish a zygote. If fertilization doesn't occur, increasing estrogen and progesterone levels decrease LH and FSH production. Because LH is needed to maintain the corpus luteum, a decrease in LH production causes the corpus luteum to atrophy and halt the secretion of estrogen and progesterone. The thickened uterine lining then begins to slough off, and menstruation begins.

In the nonpregnant female, LH controls the secretions of the corpus luteum, thereby increasing progesterone levels in the bloodstream. In the pregnant woman, human chorionic gonadotropin (hCG), produced by the nascent (coming into existence) placenta, controls these secretions.

If fertilization and pregnancy occur, the endometrium grows even thicker and vascular ingrowth occurs. After implantation of the zygote (about 5 or 6 days after fertilization), the endometrium becomes the decidua. Trophoblastic cells produce hCG soon after implantation, stimulating the corpus luteum to continue secreting estrogen and progesterone, thus preventing further ovulation and menstruation.

hCG continues to stimulate the corpus luteum until the placenta (the vascular organ that develops to carry materials to and from the fetus) forms and starts producing its own estrogen and progesterone. After the placenta takes over hormonal production, secretions of the corpus luteum are no longer needed to maintain the pregnancy, and the corpus luteum gradually decreases its function and begins to degenerate. This change, called the *luteoplacental shift*, commonly occurs by the end of the first trimester.

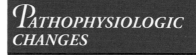

PATHOPHYSIOLOGIC CHANGES

Alterations may occur in the structure, process, or function of both the male and female reproductive systems.

Sexual maturation alteration

Sexual maturation, or puberty, can be affected by various congenital and endocrine disorders. The timing of puberty may be too early (precocious puberty) or too late (delayed puberty). Precocious puberty is the onset of sexual maturation before age 9 in boys and before age 8 in girls. It occurs more often in girls than boys. In girls, the cause is most commonly idiopathic, whereas in boys it's more likely to be organic. (See "Precocious puberty," page 593.)

In delayed puberty, there's no evidence of the development of secondary sex characteristics in boys by age 14 or girls by age 13. There's usually no evidence of hormonal abnormalities. The hypothalamic-pituitary-gonadal axis, a system that stimulates and regulates the production of hormones necessary for normal sexual development and function, is intact, but maturation is slow. The cause is unknown.

Hormonal alterations

Complex hormonal interactions determine the normal function of the female reproductive tract and require an intact hypothalamic-pituitary-ovarian axis. A defect or malfunction of this system can cause infertility because of insufficient gonadotropin secretions (both LH and FSH).

The ovary controls, and is controlled by, the hypothalamus through a system of negative and positive feedback mediated by estrogen production. Insufficient gonadotropin levels may result from infections, tumors, or neurologic disease of the hypothalamus or pituitary gland. A mild hormonal imbalance in gonadotropin production and regulation, possibly caused by polycystic disease of the ovary or abnormalities in the adrenal or thyroid gland that adversely affect hypothalamic-pituitary functioning, may sporadically inhibit ovulation. Because gonadotropins are released in a pulsatile (rhythmic) fashion, a significant disturbance in this rhythm will adversely affect ovulatory function. (See also *Gonadotropin deficiency* in chapter 13, page 467.)

Male hypogonadism, or an abnormal decrease in gonad size and function, results from decreased androgen production in males, which may impair spermatogenesis (causing infertility) and inhibit the development of normal secondary sex characteristics. The clinical effects of androgen deficiency depend on age at onset. Primary hypogonadism results directly from interstitial (Leydig's cell) cellular or seminiferous tubular damage of the testes from faulty development or mechanical damage. Androgen deficiency causes increased secretion of gonadotropins by the pituitary in an attempt to increase the testicular functional state and is therefore termed hypergonadotropic hypogonadism. This form of hypogonadism includes Klinefelter's syndrome (typically linked to chromosome 47 XXY), Reifenstein's syndrome, male Turner's syndrome, Sertoli-cell–only syndrome, anorchism (absence of the testis), orchitis, and sequelae of irradiation. (See also *Gonadotropin deficiency* in chapter 13, page 467.)

Secondary hypogonadism is caused by faulty interaction within the hypothalamic-pituitary axis, resulting in failure to secrete normal levels of gonadotropins, and is therefore termed hypogonadotropic hypogonadism. This form of hypogonadism includes hypopituitarism, isolated FSH deficiency, isolated LH deficiency, Kallmann's syndrome, and Prader-Willi syndrome. Depending on the patient's age at onset, hypogonadism may cause eunuchism (complete gonadal failure) or eunuchoidism (partial failure).

Symptoms vary depending on the specific cause of hypogonadism. Some characteristic findings may include delayed bone maturation; delayed puberty; infantile penis and small, soft testes; less than average muscle development and strength; fine, sparse facial hair; scant or absent axillary, pubic, and body hair; and a high-pitched, effeminate voice. In an adult, hypogonadism diminishes sex drive and potency and causes regression of secondary sex characteristics. (See also *Gonadotropin deficiency* in chapter 13, page 467.)

Menstrual alterations

Alterations in menstruation include the absence of menses, abnormal bleeding patterns, or painful menstruation. Menopause is the cessation of menstruation. It results from a complex continuum of physiologic changes — the climacteric — caused by declining ovarian function. The climacteric produces various changes in the body, the most dramatic being the cessation of menses.

▲ **AGE ALERT**
The climacteric, a normal gradual reduction in ovarian function because of aging, begins in most women between ages 40 and 50 and results in infrequent ovulation, decreased menstrual function, and, eventually, cessation of menstruation (usually between ages 45 and 55).

Premature menopause, the gradual or abrupt cessation of menstruation before age 35, occurs without apparent cause in about 5% of women in the United States. Certain diseases, especially autoimmune diseases such as premature ovarian failure, may be a cause. Other factors that may bring on premature menopause include malnutrition, debilitation, extreme emotional stress, pelvic irradiation, and surgical procedures that impair ovarian blood supply. Radiation therapy or surgical procedures such as removal of both ovaries (bilateral oophorectomy) may lead to artificial menopause. Hysterectomy decreases the interval before menopause even when the ovaries aren't removed, and it may also decrease ovarian blood flow in some way.

Ovarian failure, in which no ova are produced, may result from a functional ovarian disorder caused by premature menopause. Amenorrhea is a natural consequence of ovarian failure.

Pain is commonly linked to the menstrual cycle; in many common diseases of the female reproductive tract, such pain may follow a cyclic pattern. A patient with endometriosis, for example, may report increasing premenstrual pain that decreases at the end of menstruation. For a description of the types of abnormal menstrual bleeding, see *Abnormal premenopausal bleeding*.

Sexual dysfunction in women

Sexual dysfunction in women includes arousal problems, orgasmic problems, and sexual pain (dyspareunia, vaginismus). Dysfunction may be caused by a general medical condition, psychological condition, substance use or abuse, or a combination of these factors.

Arousal disorder is an inability to experience sexual pleasure. According to the *Diagnostic and Statistical Manual of Mental Disorders,* Fourth Edition, *Text Revision* (*DSM-IV-TR*), the essential feature is a persistent or recurrent inability to attain or to maintain an adequate lubrication-swelling response of sexual excitement until completion of the sexual act. Orgasmic disorder, according to the *DSM-IV-TR*, is a persistent or recurrent delay in or absence of orgasm after a normal sexual excitement phase.

Arousal and orgasmic disorders are considered primary if they exist in a female who has never experienced sexual arousal or orgasm; they are secondary when a physical, mental, or situational condition has inhibited or obliterated a previously normal sexual function. The prognosis is good for temporary or mild disorders resulting from misinformation or situational stress but is guarded for disorders that result from intense anxiety, chronically discordant relationships, psychological disturbances, or drug or alcohol abuse in either partner.

Abnormal premenopausal bleeding

Causes of abnormal premenopausal bleeding vary with the type of bleeding:

◆ Oligomenorrhea (infrequent menses) and polymenorrhea (menses occurring too frequently) usually result from anovulation caused by an endocrine or systemic disorder.

◆ Hypomenorrhea (decreased amount of menstrual fluid) results from local, endocrine, or systemic disorders or blockage caused by partial obstruction by the hymen or cervical obstruction.

◆ Hypermenorrhea (excessive bleeding occurring at regular intervals) usually results from local lesions, such as uterine leiomyomas, endometrial polyps, and endometrial hyperplasia. It may also result from endometritis, salpingitis, and anovulation.

◆ Cryptomenorrhea (no external bleeding, although menstrual symptoms are present) may result from an imperforate hymen or cervical stenosis.

◆ Metrorrhagia (bleeding occurring at irregular intervals) usually results from slight physiologic bleeding from the endometrium during ovulation but may also result from local disorders, such as uterine malignancy, cervical erosions, polyps (which tend to bleed after intercourse), or inappropriate estrogen therapy.

Complications of pregnancy can also cause premenopausal bleeding, which may be as mild as spotting or as severe as hypermenorrhea.

The following factors, alone or in combination, may cause arousal or orgasmic disorder:

■ certain drugs, including central nervous system depressants, alcohol, street drugs, and, rarely, oral contraceptives

■ general systemic illnesses, diseases of the endocrine or nervous system, or diseases that impair muscle tone or contractility

- gynecologic factors, such as chronic vaginal or pelvic infection or pain, congenital anomalies, and genital cancers
- stress and fatigue
- inadequate or ineffective stimulation
- psychological factors, such as performance anxiety, guilt, depression, or unconscious conflicts about sexuality
- relationship problems, such as poor communication, hostility, or ambivalence toward the partner, fear of abandonment or independence, or boredom with sex.

All these factors may contribute to involuntary inhibition of the orgasmic reflex. Another crucial factor is the fear of losing control of feelings or behavior. Whether these factors produce sexual dysfunction and the type of dysfunction depend on how well the woman copes with the resulting pressures. Physical factors may also cause arousal or orgasmic disorder.

Female sexual function and responses decline, along with estrogen levels, in the perimenopausal period. The decrease in estradiol levels during menopause affects nerve transmission and response in the peripheral vascular system. As a result, the timing and degree of vasoconstriction during the sexual response is affected, vasocongestion decreases, muscle tension decreases, lubrication decreases, and contractions are fewer and less intense during orgasm.

A woman with arousal disorder has limited or absent sexual desire and experiences little or no pleasure from sexual stimulation. Physical signs of this disorder include lack of vaginal lubrication or absence of signs of genital vasocongestion.

Dyspareunia is genital pain linked to intercourse. Insufficient lubrication is the most common cause. Other physical causes of dyspareunia include:
- endometriosis (See "Endometriosis," page 586.)
- genital, rectal, or pelvic scar tissue
- acute or chronic infections of the genitourinary tract
- disorders of the surrounding viscera (including residual effects of pelvic inflammatory disease or disease of the adnexal and broad ligaments).

Other possible physical causes include:

- deformities or lesions of the introitus or vagina
- benign and malignant growths and tumors
- intact hymen
- radiation to the pelvis
- allergic reactions to diaphragms, condoms, or other contraceptives.

Psychological causes include:
- fear of pain or injury during intercourse
- previous painful experience, including sexual abuse
- guilty feelings about sex
- fear of pregnancy or injury to the fetus during pregnancy
- anxiety caused by a new sexual partner or technique
- mental or physical fatigue.

Vaginismus is an involuntary spastic constriction of the lower vaginal muscles, usually from fear of vaginal penetration. This disorder may coexist with dyspareunia and, if severe, may prevent intercourse (a common cause of unconsummated marriages). Vaginismus may be physical or psychological in origin. It may occur spontaneously as a protective reflex to pain or result from organic causes, such as hymenal abnormalities, genital herpes, obstetric trauma, and atrophic vaginitis.

Psychological causes may include:
- childhood and adolescent exposure to rigid, punitive, and guilt-ridden attitudes toward sex
- fear resulting from painful or traumatic sexual experiences, such as incest or rape
- early traumatic experience with pelvic examinations
- fear of pregnancy, sexually transmitted disease, or cancer.

Sexual dysfunction in men

In men, the normal sexual response involves penile erection, emission (passage of semen and accessory gland secretions in the urethra), and ejaculation (expulsion of seminal fluid from the urethra). Sexual dysfunction is the impairment of one or all of these processes. Erectile dysfunction, or impotence, refers to inability to attain or maintain penile erection sufficient to complete intercourse. Transient periods of impotence aren't considered dysfunction and probably occur among half of adult males. Erectile dysfunction affects all age groups but increases in frequency with age.

Psychogenic factors (guilt, fear, depression) are responsible for about 50% to 60% of the cases of erectile dysfunction, organic factors for the rest. In some patients, psychogenic and organic factors (chronic disease, paralysis, consequence of a surgical procedure) coexist, making isolation of the primary cause difficult. (See "Erectile dysfunction," page 588.)

Problems with emission and ejaculation usually have structural causes.

Male structural alterations

Structural defects of the male reproductive system may be congenital or acquired. Testicular disorders, such as cryptorchidism or torsion, may result in infertility.

In cryptorchidism, a congenital disorder, one or both testes fail to descend into the scrotum, remaining in the abdomen or inguinal canal or at the external ring. If untreated, cryptorchidism can lead to significant problems. (See "Cryptorchidism," page 584 and "Testicular torsion," page 599.)

AGE ALERT
The testes of an older man may be slightly smaller than those of a younger man, but the testes should be equal in size, smooth, freely moveable, and soft, without nodules. The left testis is commonly lower than the right.

Benign prostatic hyperplasia is a disorder of prostate enlargement caused by androgen-induced growth of prostate cells. It's more prevalent with aging and may result in urinary obstructive symptoms. (See "Benign prostatic hyperplasia," page 582.)

Hypospadias is the most common penile structural abnormality. The midline fusion of the urethral folds is incomplete, so the urethral meatus opens on the ventral (anterior, or "belly") surface of the penis. In epispadias, the urethral meatus is located on the dorsal (posterior, or "back") surface of the penis.

Priapism is prolonged, painful erection in the absence of sexual stimulation. It results from arteriovenous shunting within the corpus cavernosum that leads to obstructed venous outflow from the penis. In adults it's usually idiopathic. In children it may be linked to sickle cell disease. Without prompt treatment it can lead to ischemic fibrosis and infertility.

A urethral stricture is a narrowing of the urethra caused by scarring. It may result from trauma, surgery (adhesions), or infection. Common complications include prostatitis and secondary infection.

During the first 3 years of life, congenital adhesions between the foreskin and the glans penis separate naturally with penile erections. Phimosis is a condition in which the foreskin can't be retracted over the glans penis; poor hygiene and chronic infection can cause it. Paraphimosis is a condition in which the foreskin is retracted and can't be reduced to cover the glans; the penis becomes constricted, causing edema of the glans. Severe paraphimosis is a surgical emergency.

To prevent threatened spontaneous abortion, millions of women took diethylstilbestrol (DES) between 1946 and 1971. Men whose mothers took DES during their 8th to 16th weeks of pregnancy have experienced structural abnormalities, such as urethral meatal stenosis, hypospadias, epididymal cysts, varicoceles, cryptorchidism, and decreased fertility.

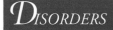

*D*ISORDERS

Disorders of the reproductive system may affect sexual, reproductive, or urinary function.

Abnormal uterine bleeding

Abnormal uterine bleeding refers to abnormal endometrial bleeding without recognizable organic lesions. Abnormal uterine bleeding is the indication for almost 25% of gynecologic surgical procedures. The prognosis varies with the cause. Correction of hormonal imbalance or structural abnormality yields a good prognosis.

CAUSES
Abnormal uterine bleeding usually results from an imbalance in the hormonal-endometrial relationship in which persistent and unopposed stimulation of the en-

dometrium by estrogen occurs. Disorders that cause sustained high estrogen levels include:

- polycystic ovary syndrome
- obesity (because enzymes present in peripheral adipose tissue convert the androgen androstenedione to estrogen precursors)
- immaturity of the hypothalamic-pituitary-ovarian mechanism (postpubertal teenagers)
- anovulation (women in their late 30s or early 40s).

Other causes of abnormal uterine bleeding include:

- trauma (foreign object insertion or direct trauma)
- endometriosis
- coagulopathy such as thrombocytopenia or leukemia (rare)
- drug-induced coagulopathy.

PATHOPHYSIOLOGY

Irregular bleeding is linked to hormonal imbalance and anovulation (failure of ovulation to occur). When progesterone secretion is absent but estrogen secretion continues, the endometrium proliferates and become hypervascular. When ovulation doesn't occur, the endometrium is randomly broken down, and exposed vascular channels cause prolonged and excessive bleeding. In most cases of abnormal uterine bleeding, the endometrium shows no pathologic changes, but in chronic unopposed estrogen stimulation (as from a hormone-producing ovarian tumor), the endometrium may show hyperplastic or malignant changes.

SIGNS AND SYMPTOMS

Abnormal uterine bleeding usually occurs as:

- metrorrhagia (episodes of vaginal bleeding between menses)
- hypermenorrhea (heavy or prolonged menses, longer than 8 days, also incorrectly termed menorrhagia)
- chronic polymenorrhea (menstrual cycle less than 18 days) or oligomenorrhea (infrequent menses)
- fatigue caused by anemia
- oligomenorrhea and infertility because of anovulation.

(For a review of the types of abnormal menstrual bleeding, see *Abnormal premenopausal bleeding*, page 577.)

COMPLICATIONS

Possible complications include:

- iron deficiency anemia (blood loss of more than 1.6 L over a short period) and hemorrhagic shock or right-sided heart failure (rare)
- endometrial adenocarcinoma caused by chronic estrogen stimulation.

DIAGNOSIS

Abnormal uterine bleeding may be caused by anovulation. Diagnosis of anovulation is based on:

- history of abnormal bleeding, bleeding in response to a brief course of progesterone, absence of ovulatory cycle body temperature changes, and low serum progesterone levels
- diagnostic studies ruling out other causes of excessive vaginal bleeding, such as organic, systemic, psychogenic, and endocrine causes, including certain cancers, polyps, pregnancy, and infection
- dilatation and curettage (D&C) or office endometrial biopsy to rule out endometrial hyperplasia and cancer in women over age 35
- endometrial biopsy to rule out endometrial adenocarcinoma (the patient age 35 and older)
- hemoglobin levels and hematocrit to determine the need for blood transfusion or iron supplementation.

TREATMENT

Possible treatment of abnormal uterine bleeding includes:

- high-dose estrogen-progestogen combination therapy (hormonal contraceptives) to control endometrial growth and reestablish a normal cyclic pattern of menstruation (usually given four times daily for 5 to 7 days even though bleeding usually stops in 12 to 24 hours; drug choice and dosage determined by patient's age and cause of bleeding); maintenance therapy with lower dose combination hormonal contraceptives
- progestogen therapy (alternative in many women, such as those susceptible

to such adverse effects of estrogen as thrombophlebitis)
- I.V. estrogen followed by progesterone or combination hormonal contraceptives if the patient is young (more likely to be anovulatory) and severely anemic (if oral drug therapy is ineffective)
- D&C (short-lived treatment and not clinically useful, but an important diagnostic tool) with hysteroscopy as a useful adjunct
- iron supplementation or transfusions of packed cells or whole blood, as indicated, because of anemia caused by recurrent or excessive bleeding
- explanation to patient about the importance of following the prescribed hormonal therapy; D&C or endometrial biopsy procedure and purpose (if ordered)
- continued regular checkups to assess the effectiveness of treatment.

Amenorrhea

Amenorrhea is the abnormal absence or suppression of menstruation. Absence of menstruation is normal before puberty, after menopause, or during pregnancy and lactation; it's abnormal, and therefore pathologic, at any other time. Primary amenorrhea is the absence of menarche in an adolescent (age 16 and older). Secondary amenorrhea is the absence of menstruation for 3 months in a previously established menstrual pattern (secondary amenorrhea). Primary amenorrhea occurs in 0.3% of women; secondary amenorrhea is seen in 1% to 3% of women. Prognosis is variable, depending on the specific cause. Surgical correction of outflow tract obstruction is usually curative.

CAUSES
Amenorrhea usually results from:
- anovulation caused by hormonal abnormalities, such as decreased secretion of estrogen, gonadotropins, luteinizing hormone, and follicle-stimulating hormone (FSH)
- lack of ovarian response to gonadotropins
- constant presence of progesterone or other endocrine abnormalities.
Amenorrhea may also result from:
- absence of a uterus

- damage to the endometrium
- ovarian, adrenal, or pituitary tumors
- emotional disorders (common in the patient with severe disorders such as depression and anorexia nervosa); mild emotional disturbances, tending to distort the ovulatory cycle; severe psychic trauma abruptly changing the bleeding pattern or completely suppressing one or more full ovulatory cycles
- malnutrition and intense exercise, causing an inadequate hypothalamic response.

PATHOPHYSIOLOGY
The mechanism varies depending on the cause and whether the defect is structural, hormonal, or both. Women who have adequate estrogen levels but a progesterone deficiency don't ovulate and are thus infertile. In primary amenorrhea, the hypothalamic-pituitary-ovarian axis is dysfunctional. Because of anatomic defects of the central nervous system, the ovary doesn't receive the hormonal signals that normally initiate the development of secondary sex characteristics and the beginning of menstruation.

Secondary amenorrhea can result from several central factors (hypogonadotropic hypoestrogenic anovulation), uterine factors (as with Asherman syndrome, in which the endometrium is sufficiently scarred that no functional endometrium exists), cervical stenosis, premature ovarian failure, and others.

SIGNS AND SYMPTOMS
Amenorrhea may result from many disorders; signs and symptoms depend on the specific cause and include:
- absence of menstruation
- vasomotor flushes, vaginal atrophy, hirsutism (abnormal hairiness), and acne (secondary amenorrhea).

COMPLICATIONS
Complications of amenorrhea include:
- infertility
- endometrial adenocarcinoma (amenorrhea linked to anovulation that gives rise to unopposed estrogen stimulation of the endometrium).

DIAGNOSIS

Diagnosis of amenorrhea is based on:

■ history of failure to menstruate in females age 16 and older, if consistent with bone age (confirms primary amenorrhea)

■ absence of menstruation for 3 months in a previously established menstrual pattern (secondary amenorrhea)

■ physical and pelvic examination and sensitive pregnancy test ruling out pregnancy, as well as anatomic abnormalities (such as cervical stenosis) that may cause false amenorrhea (cryptomenorrhea), in which menstruation occurs without external bleeding

■ onset of menstruation (spotting) within 1 week after giving pure progestational agents such as medroxyprogesterone (Provera), indicating enough estrogen to stimulate the lining of the uterus (if menstruation doesn't occur, special diagnostic studies, such as gonadotropin levels, are indicated)

■ blood and urine studies showing hormonal imbalances, such as lack of ovarian response to gonadotropins (elevated pituitary gonadotropin levels), failure of gonadotropin secretion (low pituitary gonadotropin levels), and abnormal thyroid levels (without suspicion of premature ovarian failure or central hypogonadotropism, gonadotropin levels aren't clinically meaningful because they're released in a pulsatile fashion; at a given time of day, levels may be elevated, low, or average)

■ complete medical workup, including appropriate X-rays, laparoscopy, and biopsy, to identify ovarian, adrenal, and pituitary tumors.

Tests to identify dominant or missing hormones include:

■ "ferning" of cervical mucus on microscopic examination (an estrogen effect)

■ vaginal cytologic examination

■ endometrial biopsy

■ serum progesterone level

■ serum androgen level

■ elevated urinary 17-ketosteroid levels with excessive androgen secretions

■ plasma FSH level more than 50 IU/L, depending on the laboratory (suggests primary ovarian failure); or normal or low FSH level (possible hypothalamic or pituitary abnormality, depending on the clinical situation).

TREATMENT

Treatment of amenorrhea may include:

■ appropriate hormone replacement to reestablish menstruation

■ treatment of the cause of amenorrhea not related to hormone deficiency (for example, surgery for amenorrhea because of a tumor or obstruction)

■ ovulation induction; with intact pituitary gland, clomiphene citrate may induce ovulation in women with secondary amenorrhea caused by gonadotropin deficiency, polycystic ovarian disease, or excessive weight loss or gain if it's reversed

■ FSH and human menopausal gonadotropins for women with pituitary disease

■ improvement of nutritional status

■ modification of exercise routine.

Benign prostatic hyperplasia

Although most men age 50 and older have some prostatic enlargement, in benign prostatic hyperplasia (BPH) — also known as *benign prostatic hypertrophy* — the prostate gland enlarges enough to compress the urethra and cause overt urinary obstruction. Depending on the size of the enlarged prostate, the age and health of the patient, and the extent of obstruction, BPH is treated symptomatically or surgically. BPH is common, affecting up to 50% of men age 50 and older, and 75% of men age 80 and older.

CAUSES

The main cause of BPH may be age-associated changes in hormone activity. Androgenic hormone production decreases with age, causing imbalance in androgen and estrogen levels and high levels of dihydrotestosterone, the main prostatic intracellular androgen.

Other causes include:

■ arteriosclerosis

■ inflammation

■ metabolic or nutritional disturbances.

PATHOPHYSIOLOGY

Regardless of the cause, BPH begins with nonmalignant changes in periurethral prostatic glandular tissue. The growth of the fibroadenomatous nodules (masses of fibrous glandular tissue) progresses to compress the remaining normal gland (nodular hyperplasia). The hyperplastic tissue is mostly glandular, with some fibrous stroma and smooth muscle. As the prostate enlarges, it may extend into the bladder and obstruct urinary outflow by compressing or distorting the prostatic urethra. Periodic increases occur in sympathetic stimulation of the smooth muscle of the prostatic urethra and bladder neck. Progressive bladder distention may also cause a pouch to form in the bladder that retains urine when the rest of the bladder empties. This retained urine may lead to calculus formation or cystitis.

SIGNS AND SYMPTOMS

Clinical features of BPH depend on the extent of prostatic enlargement and the lobes affected. Characteristically, the condition starts with a group of symptoms known as prostatism, which are caused by enlargement and include:

- reduced urinary stream caliber and force
- urinary hesitancy
- difficulty starting micturition (resulting in straining, feeling of incomplete voiding, and an interrupted stream).

As the obstruction increases, it causes:

- frequent urination with nocturia
- sense of urgency
- dribbling
- urine retention
- incontinence
- possible hematuria.

COMPLICATIONS

As BPH worsens, a common complication is complete urinary obstruction after infection or while using decongestants, tranquilizers, alcohol, antidepressants, or anticholinergics.

Other complications include:

- infection
- hydronephrosis, renal insufficiency, and, if untreated, renal failure
- urinary calculi
- hemorrhage
- shock.

DIAGNOSIS

Diagnosis includes physical examination showing:

- visible midline mass above the symphysis pubis (This is a sign of an incompletely emptied bladder.)
- enlarged prostate on rectal palpation.

Clinical features and a rectal examination are usually sufficient for diagnosis. Other findings that help confirm BPH may include:

- excretory urography or cystoscopy (if patient is unable to cooperate) to rule out urinary tract obstruction, hydronephrosis (distention of the renal pelvis and calices caused by obstruction of the ureter and consequent retention of urine), calculi or tumors, and filling and emptying defects in the bladder
- elevated blood urea nitrogen and serum creatinine levels (suggest renal dysfunction)
- elevated prostate-specific antigen (PSA) (Prostatic carcinoma must be ruled out.)
- urinalysis and urine cultures showing hematuria, pyuria and, with bacterial count more than 100,000/µl, urinary tract infection (UTI)
- cystourethroscopy for severe symptoms (definitive diagnosis) showing prostate enlargement, bladder wall changes, and a raised bladder. (Cystourethroscopy is only done immediately before surgery to help determine the best procedure.)

TREATMENT

Conservative therapy includes:

- prostate massages
- sitz baths
- fluid restriction to prevent bladder distention
- antimicrobial agents to treat infection
- regular ejaculation to help relieve prostatic congestion
- alpha blockers, such as terazosin and prazosin, to improve urine flow rates to relieve bladder outlet obstruction by preventing contractions of the prostatic capsule and bladder neck
- finasteride to possibly reduce the size of the prostate in some patients
- continuous drainage with an indwelling urinary catheter to alleviate urine retention (high-risk patients).

Surgery is the only effective therapy to relieve acute urine retention, hydronephrosis, severe hematuria, recurrent UTIs, and other intolerable symptoms. The following procedures involve open surgical removal:

- transurethral resection (if the prostate weighs less than 2 oz [56.7 g]); tissue removed with a wire loop and electric current using a resectoscope
- suprapubic (transvesical) resection (Incision made into the bladder through which prostate gland is removed.)
- retropubic (extravesical) resection allowing direct visualization (Potency and continence are usually maintained.)
- balloon dilation of the urethra and use of prostatic stents to maintain urethral patency (occasionally)
- laser excision to relieve prostatic enlargement
- nerve-sparing surgical techniques to reduce common complications such as erectile dysfunction.

Cryptorchidism

Cryptorchidism is a congenital disorder in which one or both testes fail to descend into the scrotum, remaining in the abdomen or inguinal canal or at the external ring. Although this condition may be bilateral, it more commonly affects the right testis. True undescended testes remain along the path of normal descent, while ectopic testes deviate from that path.

Cryptorchidism occurs in 30% of premature male neonates, but in only 3% of those born at term. In about 80% of affected infants, the testes descend spontaneously during the first year; in the rest, the testes may descend later. If indicated, surgical therapy is successful in up to 95% of the cases if the infant is treated early enough.

CAUSES

The mechanism by which the testes descend into the scrotum is still unexplained. Possible causes of cryptorchidism include:

- hormonal factors, most likely androgenic hormones from the placenta, maternal or fetal adrenals, or the immature fetal testis and possibly maternal progesterone

or gonadotropic hormones from the maternal pituitary

- testosterone deficiency resulting in a defect in the hypothalamic-pituitary-gonadal axis, causing failure of gonadal differentiation and gonadal descent
- structural factors impeding gonadal descent, such as ectopic location of the testis or short spermatic cord
- genetic predisposition in a small number of cases (greater incidence of cryptorchidism in infants with neural tube defects)
- premature neonates most commonly affected, because descent of testes into the scrotum usually occurs between gestational weeks 34 and 38.

PATHOPHYSIOLOGY

A prevalent but still unsubstantiated theory links undescended testes to the development of the gubernaculum, a fibromuscular band that connects the testes to the scrotal floor. Normally in the male fetus, testosterone stimulates the formation of the gubernaculum. This band probably helps pull the testes into the scrotum by shortening as the fetus grows. Thus, cryptorchidism may result from inadequate testosterone levels or a defect in the testes or the gubernaculum. Because the undescended testis is maintained at a higher temperature, spermatogenesis is impaired, leading to reduced fertility.

SIGNS AND SYMPTOMS

Possible signs and symptoms of cryptorchidism include:

- testis on the affected side not palpable in the scrotum; underdeveloped scrotum (unilateral cryptorchidism)
- scrotum enlarged on the unaffected side because of compensatory hypertrophy (occasionally)
- infertility after puberty because of prevention of spermatogenesis (uncorrected bilateral cryptorchidism) despite normal testosterone levels.

COMPLICATIONS

Bilateral cryptorchidism that is untreated into adolescence may result in:

- irreversible sterility because of testicular temperature higher than optimal for spermatogenesis
- significantly increased risk for testicular cancer because the higher temperatures can cause abnormal division of germ cells
- increased vulnerability of the testes to trauma

DIAGNOSIS

Physical examination confirms cryptorchidism after sex is determined by the following laboratory tests:
- buccal smear (cells from oral mucosa) to determine genetic sex (a male sex chromatin pattern)
- serum gonadotropin to confirm the presence of testes by showing presence of circulating hormone.

TREATMENT

If the testes don't descend spontaneously by age 1, surgical correction is generally indicated. Treatment includes:
- orchiopexy to secure the testes in the scrotum and to prevent sterility, excessive trauma from abnormal positioning, and harmful psychological effects (usually before age 4; optimum age, 1 to 2 years)
- human chorionic gonadotropin I.M. to stimulate descent (rarely); ineffective for testes located in the abdomen.

Dysmenorrhea

Dysmenorrhea is painful menstruation linked to ovulation that isn't related to pelvic disease. It's the most common gynecologic complaint and a leading cause of absenteeism from school (affecting 10% of high school girls each month) and work (estimated 140 million work hours lost annually) in the United States. The incidence peaks in women in their early 20s and then slowly decreases.

Dysmenorrhea can occur as a primary disorder or be the result of an underlying disease. Because primary dysmenorrhea is self-limiting, the prognosis is generally good. The prognosis for secondary dysmenorrhea depends on the underlying disorder.

CAUSES

Although primary dysmenorrhea is unrelated to proven, identifiable cause, possible contributing factors include:
- hormonal imbalance
- psychogenic factors.

Dysmenorrhea may also be caused by such gynecologic disorders as:
- endometriosis
- cervical stenosis
- uterine leiomyomas (benign fibroid tumors)
- pelvic inflammatory disease
- pelvic tumors.

PATHOPHYSIOLOGY

The pain of dysmenorrhea probably results from increased prostaglandin secretion in menstrual blood, which intensifies normal uterine contractions. Prostaglandins intensify myometrial smooth muscle contraction and uterine blood vessel constriction, thereby worsening the uterine hypoxia normally linked to menstruation. This combination of intense muscle contractions and hypoxia causes the intense pain of dysmenorrhea. Prostaglandins and their metabolites can also cause GI disturbances, headache, and syncope.

Because dysmenorrhea almost always follows an ovulatory cycle, both the primary and secondary forms are rare during the anovulatory cycle of menses. After age 20, dysmenorrhea is usually secondary.

SIGNS AND SYMPTOMS

Possible signs and symptoms of dysmenorrhea include sharp, intermittent, cramping, lower abdominal pain, usually radiating to the back, thighs, groin, and vulva, and typically starting with or immediately before menstrual flow and peaking within 24 hours.

Dysmenorrhea may also be linked to signs and symptoms suggestive of premenstrual syndrome, including:
- urinary frequency
- nausea
- vomiting
- diarrhea
- headache
- backache
- chills

- abdominal bloating
- painful breasts
- depression
- irritability.

COMPLICATIONS
A possible but rare complication is dehydration caused by nausea, vomiting, and diarrhea.

DIAGNOSIS
Diagnosis of dysmenorrhea may include:
- pelvic examination and a detailed patient history to help suggest the cause
- ruling out secondary causes for menses painful since menarche (primary dysmenorrhea)
- tests, such as laparoscopy, hysteroscopy, and pelvic ultrasound, to diagnose underlying disorders in secondary dysmenorrhea.

TREATMENT
Initial treatment aims to relieve pain and may include:
- analgesics such as nonsteroidal anti-inflammatory drugs for mild to moderate pain (most effective when taken 24 to 48 hours before onset of menses), especially effective because of inhibiting prostaglandin synthesis through inhibition of the enzyme cyclooxygenase
- opioids for severe pain (infrequently used)
- prostaglandin inhibitors (such as mefenamic acid and ibuprofen) to relieve pain by decreasing the severity of uterine contractions
- heat applied locally to the lower abdomen (may relieve discomfort in mature women), used cautiously in young adolescents because appendicitis may mimic dysmenorrhea.

For primary dysmenorrhea:
- sex steroids (effective alternative to treatment with antiprostaglandins or analgesics), such as hormonal contraceptives, to relieve pain by suppressing ovulation and inhibiting endometrial prostaglandin synthesis (the patient attempting pregnancy should rely on antiprostaglandin therapy)
- psychological evaluation and appropriate counseling because of possible psychogenic cause of persistently severe dysmenorrhea.

Treatment of secondary dysmenorrhea is designed to identify and correct the underlying cause and may include surgical treatment of underlying disorders, such as endometriosis or uterine leiomyomas (after conservative therapy fails).

Endometriosis
Endometriosis is the presence of endometrial tissue outside the lining of the uterine cavity. Ectopic (outside its normal location) tissue is usually confined to the pelvic area — usually around the ovaries, uterovesical peritoneum, uterosacral ligaments, and cul-de-sac — but it can appear anywhere in the body.

Active endometriosis may occur at any age, including adolescence. As many as 50% of infertile women may have endometriosis, although the true incidence in both fertile and infertile women remains unknown.

Severe symptoms of endometriosis may have an abrupt onset or may develop over many years. Infertility occurs in 30% to 40% of women with endometriosis. Endometriosis usually appears during the menstrual years; after menopause, it tends to subside. Hormonal treatment of endometriosis (continuous use of oral contraceptives, danazol, and gonadotropin-releasing hormone [Gn-RH] antagonists) is potentially effective in relieving discomfort, although treatment for advanced stages of endometriosis usually isn't as successful because of impaired follicular development. Surgery appears to be the more effective way to enhance fertility, although definitive evidence doesn't currently exist. Pharmacologic and surgical treatment of endometriosis may be beneficial for managing chronic pelvic pain.

CAUSES
The cause of endometriosis remains unknown. The main theories to explain this disorder (one or more are perhaps true for certain populations of women) include:
- retrograde menstruation with implantation at ectopic sites (retrograde menstruation alone may not be sufficient for endometriosis to occur because it occurs

in women with no clinical evidence of endometriosis)
- genetic predisposition and depressed immune system (may predispose to endometriosis)
- coelomic metaplasia (repeated inflammation inducing metaplasia of mesothelial cells to the endometrial epithelium)
- lymphatic or hematogenous spread of endometrial tissue (extraperitoneal disease).

PATHOPHYSIOLOGY
The ectopic endometrial tissue responds to normal stimulation in the same way as the endometrium, but more unpredictably. The endometrial cells respond to estrogen and progesterone with proliferation and secretion. During menstruation, the ectopic tissue bleeds, which causes inflammation of the surrounding tissues. This inflammation causes fibrosis, leading to adhesions that can produce pain and infertility.

SIGNS AND SYMPTOMS
Signs and symptoms of endometriosis include:
- dysmenorrhea, abnormal uterine bleeding, and infertility (classic symptoms) caused by inflammation from bleeding ectopic tissue
- pain that begins 5 to 7 days before menses peaks and lasts for 2 to 3 days (varies among patients); severity of pain not indicative of extent of disease.

Other signs and symptoms depend on the location of the ectopic tissue and may include:
- infertility and profuse menses (ovaries and oviducts)
- deep-thrust dyspareunia (ovaries or cul-de-sac)
- suprapubic pain, dysuria, and hematuria (bladder)
- abdominal cramps, pain on defecation, constipation; bloody stools caused by bleeding of ectopic endometrium in the rectosigmoid musculature (large bowel and appendix)
- bleeding from endometrial deposits in the cervix, vagina, and perineum during menses; pain on intercourse.

COMPLICATIONS
Complications of endometriosis include:
- infertility caused by fibrosis, scarring, and adhesions (major complication)
- chronic pelvic pain
- ovarian carcinoma (rare).

DIAGNOSIS
The only definitive way to diagnose endometriosis is through laparoscopy or laparotomy. Pelvic examination may suggest endometriosis or be unremarkable. Findings suggestive of endometriosis include:
- multiple tender nodules on uterosacral ligaments or in the rectovaginal septum (in one-third of the patients)
- ovarian enlargement in the presence of endometrial cysts on the ovaries.

Although laparoscopy is recommended to diagnose and determine the extent of disease, some clinicians recommend:
- empiric trial of Gn-RH agonist therapy to confirm or refute the impression of endometriosis before resorting to laparoscopy (controversial, but may be cost-effective)
- biopsy at the time of laparoscopy (helpful to confirm the diagnosis), although in some instances, diagnosis is confirmed by visual inspection.

TREATMENT
Treatment of endometriosis varies according to the stage of the disease and the patient's age and desire to have children. Conservative therapy for young women who want to have children includes:
- androgens such as danazol
- progestins and continuous combined hormonal contraceptives (pseudopregnancy regimen) to relieve symptoms by causing a regression of endometrial tissue
- Gn-RH agonists to induce pseudomenopause (medical oophorectomy), causing remission of the disease (commonly used).

No pharmacologic treatment has been shown to cure the disease or be effective in all women. Some disadvantages of nonsurgical therapy include:
- adverse reaction to drug-induced menopause (including osteoporosis if used for more than 6 months), high expense of use for an extended duration, and possible

recurrence of endometriosis after discontinuation of Gn-RH agonists
- high expense and weight gain when using danazol
- lowest fertility rates of any medical treatment for endometriosis when using continuous oral contraceptive pills
- weight gain and depressive symptoms when using progestin (but as effective as Gn-RH antagonists).

When ovarian masses are present, surgery must rule out cancer. Conservative surgery includes:
- laparoscopic removal of endometrial implants with conventional or laser techniques (no benefit shown for laser laparoscopy over electrocautery or suture methods)
- presacral neurectomy for central pelvic pain; effective in about 50% or fewer appropriate candidates
- laparoscopic uterosacral nerve ablation (LUNA) also for central pelvic pain, although definitive studies supporting the efficacy of LUNA are lacking
- total abdominal hysterectomy with or without bilateral salpingo-oophorectomy, although success rates vary; it's unclear whether ovarian conservation is appropriate (treatment of last resort for women who don't want to have children or for extensive disease).

Erectile dysfunction

Erectile dysfunction, or impotence, refers to a male's inability to attain or maintain penile erection sufficient to complete intercourse. The patient with primary impotence has never achieved a sufficient erection. Secondary impotence is more common, but no less disturbing than the primary form, and implies that the patient has succeeded in completing intercourse in the past.

Transient periods of impotence aren't considered dysfunction and probably occur in half of adult males. Erectile disorder affects all age groups but increases in frequency with age. The prognosis for erectile in the dysfunction patient depends on the severity and duration of their impotence and the underlying causes.

CAUSES

Causes of erectile dysfunction include psychogenic factors (50% to 60% of cases), organic causes, or both psychogenic and organic factors in some patients. This complexity makes the isolation of the primary cause difficult.

Psychogenic causes of erectile dysfunction include:
- intrapersonal psychogenic causes reflecting personal sexual anxieties and generally involving guilt, fear, depression, or feelings of inadequacy resulting from previous traumatic sexual experience, rejection by parents or peers, exaggerated religious orthodoxy, abnormal mother-son intimacy, or homosexual experiences
- psychogenic factors reflecting a disturbed sexual relationship, possibly stemming from differences in sexual preferences between partners, lack of communication, insufficient knowledge of sexual function, or nonsexual personal conflicts
- situational impotence, a temporary condition in response to stress.

Organic causes include:
- chronic diseases that cause neurologic and vascular impairment, such as cardiopulmonary disease, diabetes, multiple sclerosis, or renal failure
- liver cirrhosis causing increased circulating estrogen because of reduced hepatic inactivation of the hormone
- spinal cord trauma
- complications of surgery, particularly radical prostatectomy
- drug- or alcohol-induced dysfunction
- genital anomalies or central nervous system defects (rare).

PATHOPHYSIOLOGY

Neurologic dysfunction results in lack of the autonomic signal and, in combination with vascular disease, interferes with arteriolar dilation. The blood is shunted around the sacs of the corpus cavernosum into medium-sized veins, a process that prevents the sacs from filling completely. Also, perfusion of the corpus cavernosum is hindered from the start by partial obstruction of small arteries, leading to loss of erection before ejaculation.

Psychogenic causes may exacerbate emotional problems in a circular pattern;

anxiety causes fear of erectile dysfunction, which causes further emotional problems.

SIGNS AND SYMPTOMS

Secondary erectile disorder is classified as:
- *partial*—inability to achieve or sustain a full erection
- *intermittent*—sometimes potent with the same partner
- *selective*—potent only with certain partners.

Some men lose erectile function suddenly, and others lose it gradually. If the cause isn't organic, erection may still be achieved through masturbation.

Immediately before a sexual encounter, the patient with psychogenic impotence may:
- feel anxious
- perspire
- have palpitations
- lose interest in sexual activity.

COMPLICATIONS

A complication of erectile dysfunction is severe depression (the patient with psychogenic or organic drug-induced erectile dysfunction), causing the impotence or resulting from it. Erectile dysfunction may also place a strain on sexual relationships.

DIAGNOSIS

A detailed sexual history helps differentiate between organic and psychogenic factors and primary and secondary impotence. (See *Questions to include in a sexual history*.)

Diagnosis also includes:
- ruling out such chronic diseases as diabetes and other vascular, neurologic, or urogenital problems
- fulfilling the diagnostic criteria of the *Diagnostic and Statistical Manual of Mental Disorders*, Fourth Edition, *Text Revision* (*DSM-IV-TR*) for the disorder (when the disorder causes marked distress or interpersonal difficulty).

TREATMENT

Treatment for psychogenic impotence includes:
- sex therapy including both partners (course and content of therapy depend

---

Questions to include in a sexual history

When gathering information about a patient's erectile dysfunction, be sure to include these important questions in the sexual history:
- ◆ Does the patient have intermittent or selective nocturnal or early morning erections?
- ◆ Can he achieve erections through other sexual activity?
- ◆ When did his dysfunction begin, and what was his life situation at that time?
- ◆ Did erectile problems occur suddenly or gradually?
- ◆ What prescription or nonprescription drugs is he taking?
- ◆ How often and how much alcohol does he drink?

---

on the specific cause of dysfunction and nature of the partner relationship)
- teaching or helping the patient to improve verbal communication skills, eliminate unreasonable guilt, or reevaluate attitudes toward sex and sexual roles.

Treatment for organic impotence includes:
- reversing the cause, if possible
- psychological counseling to help the couple deal realistically with their situation and explore alternatives for sexual expression if reversing the cause isn't possible
- sildenafil or other similar medications, such as vardenafil, to cause vasodilation within the penis (This may effectively manage erectile dysfunction in appropriate patients.)
- adrenergic antagonist, yohimbine, to enhance parasympathetic neurotransmission
- testosterone supplementation for hypogonadal men

CLINICAL ALERT
Testosterone supplementation isn't given to men with prostate cancer because often prostatic tumors are hormone dependent.

- prostaglandin E injected directly into the corpus cavernosum (This may induce an erection for 30 to 60 minutes in some men.)
- surgically inserted inflatable or noninflatable penile implants. (Used in some patients with organic impotence.)

Gynecomastia

Gynecomastia is the enlargement of breast tissue in males. Gynecomastia is typically bilateral, but in men over age 50, it's usually unilateral. Usually the cause is physiologic. Gynecomastia often resolves spontaneously in 6 to 12 months.

CAUSES

Gynecomastia may be caused by excessive estrogen production from conditions including:
- testicular tumors
- obesity
- pituitary tumors
- some hypogonadism syndromes.

Systemic disorders linked to gynecomastia that may alter the estrogen-testosterone ratio include:
- liver disease causing inability to break down normal male estrogen secretions
- chronic renal failure
- chronic obstructive lung disease.

Pharmacologic agents that may cause gynecomastia include marijuana and exogenous estrogen, as given for prostatic malignancy.

PATHOPHYSIOLOGY

A disturbance in the normal ratio of active androgen to estrogen results in proliferation of the fibroblastic stroma and the duct system of the breast.

SIGNS AND SYMPTOMS

Signs and symptoms of gynecomastia are caused by the imbalance in hormone levels and include:
- enlarged breast tissue (at least ¾" [2 cm] in diameter), either unilateral or bilateral, beneath the areola
- bilateral enlargement (hormone-induced gynecomastia).

COMPLICATIONS

A possible complication of gynecomastia is malignant changes in the breast tissue.

DIAGNOSIS

Diagnosis depends on:
- biopsy to rule out malignancy
- excessively high estrogen levels and normal testosterone levels (in drug- and tumor-induced hyperestrogenism)
- very low testosterone levels and normal estrogen levels (hypergonadism).

TREATMENT

Gynecomastia usually resolves spontaneously without treatment. If indicated, treatments include:
- treatment of the cause to reduce excess breast tissue
- resection of extra breast tissue for cosmetic reasons.

HYDROCELE

A hydrocele is a collection of fluid between the visceral and parietal layers of the tunica vaginalis of the testicle or along the spermatic cord. It's the most common cause of scrotal swelling.

CAUSES

Possible causes of hydrocele include:
- congenital malformation (infants)
- trauma to the testes or epididymis
- infection of the testes or epididymis
- testicular tumor.

PATHOPHYSIOLOGY

Congenital hydrocele occurs because of a patency (open area or passage) between the scrotal sac and the peritoneal cavity, allowing peritoneal fluids to collect in the scrotum. The exact mechanism of congenital hydrocele is unknown.

In adults, the fluid accumulation may be caused by infection, trauma, tumor, an imbalance between the secreting and absorptive capacities of scrotal tissue, or an obstruction of lymphatic or venous drainage in the spermatic cord. Fluid accumulation leads to a displacement of fluid in the scrotum, outside the testes. Subsequent swelling results, leading to reduced blood flow to the testes.

SIGNS AND SYMPTOMS
Possible signs and symptoms of hydrocele include:
- scrotal swelling and feeling of heaviness caused by fluid accumulation
- inguinal hernia (often present in congenital hydrocele)
- size of hydrocele ranges from slightly larger than the testes to the size of a grapefruit or larger
- fluid collection with either flaccid or tense mass
- pain with acute epididymal infection or testicular torsion
- scrotal tenderness because of severe swelling.

COMPLICATIONS
Complications may include:
- epididymitis
- testicular atrophy.

DIAGNOSIS
Diagnosis of hydrocele may include:
- transillumination to distinguish fluid-filled from solid mass (a tumor doesn't transilluminate)
- ultrasound to visualize the testes and determine the presence of a tumor
- fluid biopsy to determine the cause and differentiate between normal cells and malignancy.

TREATMENT
Usually, no treatment of congenital hydrocele is indicated, because this condition frequently resolves spontaneously by age 1. Otherwise, possible treatments for hydrocele include:
- surgical repair to avoid strangulation of the bowel (inguinal hernia with bowel present in the sac)
- aspiration of fluid and injection of sclerosing drug into the scrotal sac for a tense hydrocele that impedes blood circulation or causes pain
- excision of the tunica vaginalis for recurrent hydroceles
- suprainguinal excision for testicular tumor detected by ultrasound.

Ovarian cysts

Ovarian cysts are usually nonneoplastic sacs on an ovary that contain fluid or semisolid material. Although these cysts are usually small and produce no symptoms, they may require thorough investigation as possible sites of malignant change. Cysts may be single or multiple (polycystic ovarian disease). Common physiologic ovarian cysts include follicular cysts, theca-lutein cysts, and corpus luteum cysts. Ovarian cysts can develop any time between puberty and menopause, including during pregnancy. The prognosis for nonneoplastic ovarian cysts is excellent. The risk for ovarian malignancy isn't increased with a functional (physiologic) ovarian cyst.

CAUSES
Possible causes of ovarian cyst include:
- granulosa-lutein cysts, which occur within the corpus luteum, are functional (arising during some variation of the ovulatory process), nonneoplastic enlargements of the ovaries caused by excessive accumulation of blood during the hemorrhagic phase of the menstrual cycle
- theca-lutein cysts are commonly bilateral and filled with clear, straw-colored liquid; they are often linked to hydatidiform mole, choriocarcinoma, or hormone therapy (with human chorionic gonadotropin [hCG] or clomiphene citrate).

PATHOPHYSIOLOGY
Follicular cysts are generally very small and arise from follicles that overdistend, either because they haven't ruptured or have ruptured and resealed before their fluid was reabsorbed. (See *Follicular cyst*, page 592.)

Luteal cysts develop if a mature corpus luteum persists abnormally and continues to secrete progesterone. They consist of blood or fluid that accumulates in the cavity of the corpus luteum and are typically more symptomatic than follicular cysts. When such cysts persist into menopause, they secrete excessive amounts of estrogen in response to the hypersecretion of follicle-stimulating hormone and luteinizing hormone that normally occurs during menopause.

CLOSER LOOK
Follicular cyst

A common type of ovarian cyst, a follicular cyst is usually semitransparent and overdistended, with watery fluid visible through its thin walls

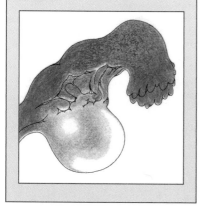

SIGNS AND SYMPTOMS
Possible signs and symptoms of ovarian cysts include:
- no symptoms (small ovarian cysts such as follicular cysts)
- mild pelvic discomfort, lower back pain, dyspareunia, or abnormal uterine bleeding, caused by a disturbed ovulatory pattern (large or multiple cysts)
- acute abdominal pain similar to that of appendicitis (ovarian cysts with torsion)
- unilateral pelvic discomfort (from granulosa-lutein cysts appearing early in pregnancy and growing as large as 5 to 6 cm in diameter), delayed menses, followed by prolonged or irregular bleeding (granulosa-lutein cysts in nonpregnant women).

COMPLICATIONS
Complications of ovarian cysts may include torsion or rupture, causing signs of an acute abdomen (abdominal tenderness, distention, and rigidity) because of massive intraperitoneal hemorrhage or peritonitis. Other complications include infertility and amenorrhea.

DIAGNOSIS
Generally, characteristic clinical features suggest ovarian cysts. They're confirmed by visualization of the ovary through ultrasound, laparoscopy, or surgery (usually for another condition).

TREATMENT
Treatment depends on the type of cyst and symptoms and may include:
- no treatment because of tendency of cyst to disappear spontaneously within one to two menstrual cycles; persisting cyst indicates excision to rule out malignancy (follicular cysts)
- hormonal treatment (commonly used, but no proven benefit in ovarian cyst management)
- analgesics to relieve symptoms (functional cysts that occur during pregnancy); cysts usually shrink during the third trimester (rarely needing surgery)
- elimination of the hydatidiform mole, destruction of choriocarcinoma, or discontinuation of hCG or clomiphene citrate therapy (theca-lutein cysts)
- laparoscopy or exploratory laparotomy with possible ovarian cystectomy or oophorectomy for persistent or suspicious ovarian cyst (These may be performed during pregnancy, if necessary. Optimal timing for surgery is the second trimester; laparoscopic management during pregnancy is promising.)
- surgery for ongoing hemorrhage from ruptured corpus luteum cyst. (Otherwise, ruptured ovarian cysts may be treated by draining intraperitoneal fluid through culdocentesis in the emergency department or office setting.)

Polycystic ovary syndrome
Polycystic ovary syndrome is a metabolic disorder characterized by multiple ovarian cysts. About 22% of the women in the United States have the disorder, and obesity is present in 50% to 80% of these women. More than 75% of women who seek treatment for infertility have some degree of polycystic ovary syndrome, usually appearing as anovulation alone. The outlook is good for ovulation and fertility with appropriate treatment.

CAUSES

The precise cause of polycystic ovary syndrome is unknown. Theories include:
- abnormal enzyme activity triggering excess androgen secretion from the ovaries and adrenal glands
- endocrine abnormalities causing all of the signs and symptoms of polycystic ovarian disease; amenorrhea, polycystic ovaries on ultrasound, hyperandrogenism (part of the Stein-Leventhal syndrome).

PATHOPHYSIOLOGY

A general feature of all anovulation syndromes is a lack of pulsatile release of gonadotropin-releasing hormone. Initial ovarian follicle development is normal. Many small follicles begin to accumulate because there's no selection of a dominant follicle. These follicles may respond abnormally to the hormonal stimulation, causing an abnormal pattern of estrogen secretion during the menstrual cycle. Endocrine abnormalities may be the cause of polycystic ovary syndrome or cystic abnormalities; muscle and adipose tissue are resistant to the effects of insulin, and lipid metabolism is abnormal.

SIGNS AND SYMPTOMS

Signs and symptoms are related to abnormal hormonal secretions that occur during the cycle. Those of classic polycystic ovary syndrome (Stein-Leventhal syndrome) include:
- mild pelvic discomfort
- lower back pain
- dyspareunia
- abnormal uterine bleeding because of disturbed ovulatory pattern
- hirsutism
- acne
- male-pattern hair loss.

COMPLICATIONS

Possible complications of polycystic ovary syndrome include:
- malignancy caused by sustained estrogenic stimulation of the endometrium
- increased risk of cardiovascular disease and type 2 diabetes mellitus because of insulin resistance.

Polycystic ovary syndrome may produce:

- secondary amenorrhea
- oligomenorrhea
- infertility.

DIAGNOSIS

Diagnosis of polycystic ovary syndrome includes:
- history and physical examination showing bilaterally enlarged polycystic ovaries and menstrual disturbance, usually dating back to menarche
- visualization of the ovary through ultrasound, laparoscopy, or surgery, often for another condition (may confirm ovarian cysts)
- slightly elevated urinary 17-ketosteroid levels
- anovulation (shown by basal body temperature graphs and endometrial biopsy)
- elevated ratio of luteinizing hormone to follicle-stimulating hormone (usually 3:1 or greater), and elevated levels of testosterone and androstenedione
- unopposed estrogen action during the menstrual cycle because of anovulation
- direct visualization by laparoscopy to rule out paraovarian cysts of the broad ligament, salpingitis, endometriosis, and neoplastic cysts.

TREATMENT

Treatment of polycystic ovary syndrome includes monitoring patient's weight to maintain a normal body mass index in order to reduce risks linked to insulin resistance. (This treatment alone may cause spontaneous ovulation in some women.)

Treatment of polycystic ovary syndrome may include the administration of drugs, such as:
- clomiphene to induce ovulation
- medroxyprogesterone for 10 consecutive days each month for a patient wanting to become pregnant
- low-dose hormonal contraceptives to treat abnormal bleeding for the patient needing reliable contraception.

Precocious puberty

Precocious puberty may occur in boys or girls. With this disorder, boys begin to mature sexually before age 9. This disorder occurs most commonly as true precocious puberty — early maturation of the hypothalamic-pituitary-gonadal axis, development of secondary sex characteristics, gonadal development, and spermatogenesis — or as pseudoprecocious puberty, marked by development of secondary sex characteristics without gonadal development. Males with true precocious puberty are reported to have fathered children as early as age 7.

In most males with precocious puberty, sexual characteristics develop in essentially normal sequence; these children function normally when they reach adulthood.

Precocious puberty is five times more common in females than males. In females, precocious puberty is the early onset of pubertal changes, such as breast development, pubic and axillary hair development, and menarche, before age 8. Normally, the mean age for menarche is 13. In true precocious puberty, the ovaries mature and pubertal changes progress in an orderly manner.

In pseudoprecocious puberty, pubertal changes occur without corresponding ovarian maturation. (See *Precocious puberty*.) In many cases, precocious puberty can be reversed.

Prostatitis

Prostatitis, or inflammation of the prostate gland, may be acute or chronic. Acute prostatitis most commonly results from gram-negative bacteria and is easy to recognize and treat. Chronic prostatitis, the most common cause of recurrent urinary tract infections (UTIs) in men, is less easy to recognize. As many as 35% of men age 50 and older have chronic prostatitis. Granulomatous prostatitis (tuberculous prostatitis), nonbacterial prostatitis, and prostatodynia (painful prostate) are other classifications of the disease.

CAUSES

Bacterial prostatitis is caused by:
- *Escherichia coli* (80% of cases)
- Klebsiella, Enterobacter, Proteus, Pseudomonas, Streptococcus, or Staphylococcus organisms (20% of cases).

These organisms probably spread to the prostate by:
- an ascending urethral infection or through the blood stream

- invasion of rectal bacteria through lymphatics
- reflux of infected bladder urine into prostate ducts
- infrequent or excessive sexual intercourse
- procedures, such as cystoscopy or catheterization (less commonly)
- bacterial invasion from the urethra (chronic prostatitis).

Granulomatous prostatitis is caused by *Mycobacterium tuberculosis,* a gram-positive acid-fast bacillus. The cause of nonbacterial prostatitis is unknown but possible causes include infection by a protozoa or virus. The cause of prostatodynia is also unknown.

 AGE ALERT
Acute prostatitis is linked to benign prostatic hyperplasia in older men.

PATHOPHYSIOLOGY

Spasms in the genitourinary tract or tension in the pelvic floor muscles may cause inflammation and nonbacterial prostatitis.

Bacterial prostatic infections can be the result of a previous or concurrent infection. The bacteria ascend from the infected urethra, bladder, lymphatics, or blood through the prostatic ducts and into the prostate. Infection stimulates an inflammatory response in which the prostate becomes larger, tender, and firm. Inflammation is usually limited to a few of the gland's excretory ducts.

SIGNS AND SYMPTOMS

Acute prostatitis begins with:
- chills
- lower back pain, especially when standing, because of compression of the prostate gland
- perineal fullness and suprapubic tenderness caused by inflammation and prostatic enlargement
- frequent and urgent urination caused by pressure from enlarged prostate
- dysuria, nocturia, and urinary obstruction caused by blocked urethra from enlarged prostate
- cloudy urine because of infection
  Signs of systemic infection include:
- fever

(Text continues on page 598.)

Precocious puberty

Although precocious puberty occurs in boys and girls, the origins of the disorder are different, so treatment varies.

	GIRLS	BOYS
Causes	True precocious puberty is idiopathic in 85% of cases. Pathologic causes may include: ◆ central nervous system (CNS) disorders resulting from tumors, trauma, infection, or other lesions. Pseudoprecocious puberty may result from: ◆ increased levels of sex hormones from ovarian and adrenocortical tumors ◆ adrenal cortical virilizing hyperplasia ◆ estrogen or androgen ingestion ◆ increased end-organ sensitivity to low levels of circulating sex hormones (estrogens promoting premature breast development, androgens promoting premature pubic and axillary hair growth).	True precocious puberty may be: ◆ idiopathic and genetically transmitted as a dominant trait ◆ cerebral (neurogenic). Pseudoprecocious puberty may result from: ◆ testicular tumors (hyperplasia, adenoma, or carcinoma) that produce excessive testosterone levels ◆ congenital adrenogenital syndrome, producing high levels of adrenocortical steroids.
Pathophysiology	Idiopathic precocious puberty results from early development and activation of the endocrine glands without corresponding abnormality.	Idiopathic precocious puberty results from pituitary or hypothalamic intracranial lesions that cause excessive secretion of gonadotropin.
Signs and symptoms	Changes that may occur independently or simultaneously, before age 8 include: ◆ rapid growth spurt ◆ thelarche (breast development) ◆ pubarche (pubic hair development) ◆ menarche.	Signs and symptoms may include: ◆ early bone development, causing an initial growth spurt ◆ early muscle development ◆ premature closure of the epiphyses, and thus stunted adult stature ◆ adult hair pattern, penile growth, and bilateral enlarged testes. Symptoms of precocity from cerebral lesions include: ◆ nausea, vomiting ◆ headache, vision disturbances ◆ internal hydrocephalus. Symptoms of pseudoprecocity from testicular tumors include: ◆ adult hair patterns, acne

(continued)

Precocious puberty *(continued)*

	GIRLS	BOYS
Signs and symptoms (continued)		◆ discrepancy in testis size (enlarged testis feels hard or contains a palpable, isolated nodule). Adrenogenital syndrome produces: ◆ adult skin tone, excessive hair and beard, deepened voice ◆ stocky, muscular appearance ◆ penile, scrotal sac, and prostate (but not the testes) enlargement.
Complications	Development of ovarian or adrenal malignancy.	Testicular tumors or, in precocious puberty caused by a brain tumor, possibly death.
Diagnosis	Diagnosis requires: ◆ complete patient history ◆ thorough physical examination ◆ special tests to differentiate between true and pseudoprecocious puberty and to indicate the necessary treatment ◆ X-rays of the hands, wrists, knees, and hips to determine bone age and possible premature epiphyseal closure ◆ ultrasound, laparoscopy, or exploratory laparotomy to verify a suspected abdominal lesion ◆ EEG, ventriculography, pneumoencephalography, computed axial tomography scan, or angiography to detect CNS disorders. Other tests detect abnormally high hormonal levels for the patient's age and may include: ◆ vaginal smear for estrogen secretion ◆ urinary tests for gonadotropic activity and excretion of 17-ketosteroids ◆ radioimmunoassay for both luteinizing and follicle-stimulating hormones.	Diagnosis requires: ◆ complete physical examination ◆ detailed patient history to evaluate the patient's recent growth pattern, behavior changes, family history of precocious puberty, or ingestion of hormones. In true precocity, laboratory results include: ◆ elevated serum levels of luteinizing and follicle-stimulating hormones and corticotropin ◆ elevated plasma testosterone levels (equal to that of a man) ◆ ejaculate showing the presence of live spermatozoa ◆ possible CNS tumors on brain scan, skull X-rays, and EEG ◆ skull and hand X-rays showing advanced bone age. In pseudoprecocity, diagnosis includes: ◆ chromosomal karyotype analysis showing abnormal pattern of autosomes and sex chromosomes ◆ elevated levels of 24-hour urinary 17-ketosteroids and other steroids.
Treatments	Constitutional true precocious puberty may require medroxyprogesterone (Provera) to reduce gonadotropin secretion and prevent menstruation. Depending on the cause of precocious puberty and its stage of development, other therapy may include:	No medical treatment is usually needed for idiopathic precocious puberty. No physical complications occur in adulthood. Supportive psychological counseling is the most important therapy.

Precocious puberty *(continued)*

	GIRLS	BOYS
Treatments (continued)	◆ cortical or adrenocortical steroid replacement for adrenogenital syndrome ◆ surgery to remove ovarian and adrenal tumors, resulting in regression of secondary sex characteristics, especially in young children ◆ surgery and chemotherapy for choriocarcinomas ◆ thyroid extract or levothyroxine to decrease gonadotropic secretions in hypothyroidism ◆ stop ingestion of estrogens or androgens ◆ no treatment in precocious thelarche and pubarche. Interventions to help the child undergoing these changes and her family include: ◆ encouraging the patient and family to express their feelings about these changes ◆ explaining diagnostic procedures and telling patient and family that surgery may be necessary ◆ explaining the condition to the child in terms she can understand to prevent feelings of shame and loss of self-esteem ◆ providing appropriate sex education, including information on menstruation and related hygiene ◆ emphasizing to parents that the child's social and emotional development should remain consistent with her chronological age, not with physical development; advising parents not to place unrealistic demands on the child ◆ suggesting that parents continue to dress their daughter in age-appropriate clothes that don't call attention to her physical development ◆ reassuring parents that precocious puberty doesn't usually precipitate precocious sexual behavior.	Interventions for specific conditions Include: ◆ reassessing regularly for possible tumors in a child with an initial diagnosis of idiopathic precocious puberty ◆ neurosurgery for brain tumors (they commonly resist treatment) ◆ removing the affected testis (orchiectomy) for testicular tumors; chemotherapy and lymphatic radiation therapy for malignant tumors (poor prognosis) ◆ lifelong therapy with maintenance doses of glucocorticoids (cortisol) to inhibit corticotropin production in adrenogenital syndrome causing precocious puberty. Interventions to help the child undergoing these changes and his family include: ◆ emphasizing to parents that the child's social and emotional development should remain consistent with his chronological age, not with his physical development; advising parents not to place unrealistic demands on the child ◆ reassuring the child that although his body is changing more rapidly than those of other boys, they too will eventually experience the same changes ◆ helping him feel less self-conscious about his changing body; suggesting clothing that de-emphasizes sexual development ◆ providing sex education for the child with true precocity ◆ explaining adverse effects of medication (cushingoid symptoms) to family if a child must take glucocorticoids for the rest of his life.

- myalgia
- fatigue
- arthralgia.

Signs and symptoms of chronic bacterial prostatitis may include:
- the same urinary symptoms as the acute form but to a lesser degree
- recurrent symptomatic cystitis.

Other possible signs include:
- evidence of UTI, such as urinary frequency, burning, cloudy urine
- painful ejaculation
- bloody semen
- persistent urethral discharge
- sexual dysfunction.

COMPLICATIONS

Possible complications of prostatitis include:
- UTI (common)
- infected and abscessed testis (removed surgically).

DIAGNOSIS

Diagnosis of prostatitis may include:
- rectal examination finding evidence of acute prostatitis, such as very tender, warm, and enlarged prostate (characteristic)
- rectal examination finding firm, irregularly shaped, and slightly enlarged prostate caused by fibrosis (chronic bacterial prostatitis)
- palpation showing normal prostate gland by exclusion (nonbacterial prostatitis)
- pelvic X-ray showing prostatic calculi
- urine culture identifying the causative infectious organism
- urine culture identifying no UTI or causative organism (nonbacterial prostatitis).

Firm diagnosis depends on a comparison of urine cultures of four specimens:
- first specimen when the patient starts voiding (voided bladder one)
- second specimen midstream
- third specimen after the patient stops voiding and the physician massages the prostate to produce secretions (expressed prostate secretions)
- final voided specimen

A significant increase in colony count in the prostatic specimens confirms prostatitis.

TREATMENT

Systemic antibiotic therapy is the treatment of choice for acute prostatitis, and may include:
- co-trimoxazole orally for 30 days (for culture showing sensitivity)
- I.V. co-trimoxazole or I.V. gentamicin plus ampicillin until sensitivity test results are known (sepsis)
- parenteral therapy for 48 hours to 1 week; then oral agent for 30 more days (with favorable test results and clinical response)
- co-trimoxazole for at least 6 weeks (chronic prostatitis caused by *E. coli*).

Supportive therapy includes:
- bed rest
- adequate hydration
- analgesics
- antipyretics
- sitz baths
- stool softeners as necessary.

In symptomatic chronic prostatitis, treatment may include:
- increased fluid intake of at least eight glasses of water daily
- regular careful massage of the prostate to relieve discomfort (vigorous massage may cause secondary epididymitis or septicemia)
- regular ejaculation to help promote drainage of prostatic secretions
- anticholinergic drugs and analgesics to help relieve nonbacterial prostatitis symptoms
- alpha-adrenergic blockers and muscle relaxants to relieve pain
- continuous low-dose anabolic steroid therapy (effective in some men).

If drug therapy is unsuccessful, surgical treatment may include:
- transurethral resection of the prostate removing all infected tissue (not usually performed on young adults; may cause retrograde ejaculation and sterility)
- total prostatectomy (curative but may cause impotence and incontinence).

Testicular torsion

Testicular torsion is an abnormal twisting of the spermatic cord caused by rotation of a testis or the mesorchium (a fold in the area between the testis and epididymis), which causes strangulation and, if left untreated, eventual infarction of the testis. Onset may be spontaneous or may follow physical exertion or trauma

AGE ALERT
This condition is almost always (90%) unilateral. The greatest risk is during the neonatal period and again between ages 12 and 18 (puberty), but the disorder may occur at any age. Infants with torsion of one testis have a greater incidence of torsion of the other testis later in life than do males in the general population.

The prognosis is good with early detection and prompt treatment.

CAUSES

In intravaginal torsion (the most common type of testicular torsion in adolescents), testicular twisting may result from:
- abnormality of the coverings of the testis and abnormally positioned testis
- incomplete attachment of the testis and spermatic fascia to the scrotal wall, leaving the testis free to rotate around its vascular pedicle.

In extravaginal torsion (most common in neonates):
- loose attachment of the tunica vaginalis to the scrotal lining causing spermatic cord rotation above the testis
- sudden forceful contraction of the cremaster muscle (may precipitate this condition).

PATHOPHYSIOLOGY

Normally, the tunica vaginalis envelops the testis and attaches to the epididymis and spermatic cord. Normal contraction of the cremaster muscle causes the left testis to rotate counterclockwise and the right testis to rotate clockwise. In testicular torsion, the testis rotates on its vascular pedicle and twists the arteries and vein in the spermatic cord, causing an interruption of circulation to the testis. Vascular engorgement and ischemia develop, causing scrotal swelling unrelieved by rest or

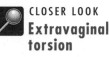

CLOSER LOOK
Extravaginal torsion

In extravaginal torsion, rotation of the spermatic cord above the testis causes strangulation and, eventually, infarction of the testis.

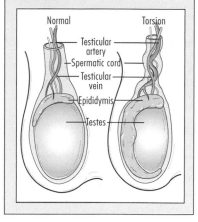

elevation of the scrotum. If manual reduction is unsuccessful, surgical correction must take place within 6 hours after the onset of symptoms to preserve testicular function (70% salvage rate). After 12 hours, the testis becomes dysfunctional and necrotic. (See *Extravaginal torsion.*)

SIGNS AND SYMPTOMS

Signs and symptoms of testicular torsion include:
- excruciating pain in the affected testis or iliac fossa of the pelvis because of ischemia
- edematous, elevated, and ecchymotic (showing a small hemorrhagic spot in the skin forming a bluish or purplish patch) scrotum with loss of the cremasteric reflex (in which stimulation of the skin on the inner thigh retracts the testis on the same side) on the affected side.

Associated symptoms include:
- abdominal pain
- nausea and vomiting.

COMPLICATIONS
Possible complications of testicular torsion include:
- testicular infarction and necrosis
- infertility.

DIAGNOSIS
Diagnosis of testicular torsion is based on:
- physical examination showing tense, tender swelling in the scrotum or inguinal canal; persistent reddening of the overlying skin; possibly palpable twisting of the spermatic cord (when examined before severe edema develops)
- Doppler ultrasonography to help distinguish testicular torsion from strangulated hernia, undescended testes, or epididymitis (absent blood flow and avascular testis in torsion)

TREATMENT
Treatment consists of immediate surgical repair by:
- orchiopexy (fixation of a viable testis to the scrotum and prophylactic fixation of the contralateral testis)
- orchiectomy (excision of a nonviable testis) to decrease the risk for autoimmune response to necrotic testis and its contents, damage to unaffected testis, and subsequent infertility
- manual manipulation of the testis counterclockwise in order to improve blood flow before surgery (not always possible).

Uterine leiomyomas

Uterine leiomyomas, the most common benign tumors in women, are also known as myomas, fibromyomas, or fibroids. They're tumors composed of smooth muscle that usually occur in the uterine corpus, although they may appear on the cervix or on the round or broad ligament (supporting structure of the pelvic cavity). Uterine leiomyomas occur in 20% to 25% of women of reproductive age and may affect three times as many Blacks as Whites, although the true incidence in either population is unknown.

The tumors become malignant (leiomyosarcoma) in less than 0.1% of the patient, a figure that should comfort women concerned with the possibility of a uterine malignancy in association with a fibroid.

CAUSES
The cause of uterine leiomyomas is unknown, but some factors implicated as regulators of leiomyoma growth include:
- several growth factors, including epidermal growth factor
- steroid hormones, including estrogen and progesterone (leiomyomas typically arise after menarche and regress after menopause, implicating estrogen as a promoter of leiomyoma growth).

PATHOPHYSIOLOGY
Leiomyomas are classified according to location. They may be located within the uterine wall (intramural) or protrude into the endometrial cavity (submucous) or from the serosal surface of the uterus (subserous). Their size varies. They're usually firm and surrounded by a pseudocapsule composed of compressed but otherwise normal uterine myometrium. When leiomyomas are present, the uterine cavity may become larger, increasing the endometrial surface area. This enlarged surface can cause increased uterine bleeding.

SIGNS AND SYMPTOMS
Most leiomyomas are asymptomatic. Signs and symptoms of leiomyoma include:
- abnormal bleeding, typically menorrhagia with disrupted submucosal vessels (most common symptom)
- isolated pain, linked to torsion of a pedunculated (stemmed) subserous tumor or leiomyomas undergoing degeneration (The fibroid outgrows its blood supply and shrinks in size. This process can be artificially induced through myolysis, a laparoscopic procedure to shrink fibroids, or uterine artery embolization.)
- pelvic pressure and impingement on adjacent viscera (indications for treatment, depending on severity) resulting in mild hydronephrosis. (This isn't believed to be an indication for treatment because renal failure rarely, if ever, results.)

COMPLICATIONS

Various disorders have been attributed to uterine leiomyomas, including:
- recurrent spontaneous abortion
- preterm labor
- malposition of the fetus
- anemia from excessive bleeding
- bladder compression
- infection (if tumor protrudes out of the vaginal opening)
- secondary infertility (rare)
- bowel obstruction.

DIAGNOSIS

Diagnosis of leiomyoma may be based on:
- clinical findings (enlarged uterus) and patient history suggesting uterine leiomyomas
- blood studies showing anemia from abnormal bleeding (may support the diagnosis)
- bimanual examination showing enlarged, firm, nontender, and irregularly contoured uterus (also seen in adenomyosis and other pelvic abnormalities)
- ultrasound for accurate assessment of the dimension, number, and location of tumors
- magnetic resonance imaging (especially sensitive with regard to fibroid imaging).

Other diagnostic procedures include:
- hysterosalpingography
- hysteroscopy
- endometrial biopsy (to rule out endometrial cancer in the patient older than age 35 with abnormal uterine bleeding)
- laparoscopy.

TREATMENT

Treatment depends on the severity of symptoms; size and location of the tumors; and the patient's age, parity, pregnancy status, desire to have children, and general health.

Treatment options include nonsurgical as well as surgical procedures. Pharmacologic treatment isn't usually effective in the long term for fibroids. Progestational agents are ineffective as primary treatment for fibroids.

Besides observation, nonsurgical methods include:

- gonadotropin-releasing hormone agonists to rapidly suppress pituitary gonadotropin release, which leads to profound hypoestrogenemia, a 50% reduction in uterine volume (peak effects occurring in the 12th week of therapy), consequent benefit of reductions in tumor size before surgery and blood loss during surgery, and an increase in preoperative hematocrit (This treatment isn't a cure, because tumors increase in size after cessation of therapy. [Increases in tumor size *during* therapy can indicate uterine sarcoma.] The treatment is best used preoperatively or for up to 6 months in a perimenopausal woman who might soon experience a natural menopause and thus avoid surgery.)
- nonsteroidal anti-inflammatory drugs for dysmenorrhea or pelvic discomfort.

Surgical procedures include:
- open abdominal, laparoscopic, or hysteroscopic myomectomy (removal of tumors in the uterine muscle) for a patient of any age who wants to preserve her uterus
- myolysis (a laparoscopic procedure to treat fibroids without hysterectomy or major surgery, performed on an outpatient basis) to coagulate the fibroids and preserve the uterus and childbearing potential
- uterine artery embolization (radiologically assisted procedure) to block uterine arteries using small pieces of polyvinyl chloride (This is a promising alternative to surgery in many women, but no long-term studies exist to establish long-term success or side effects or to confirm if this procedure is appropriate in women who want to become pregnant later. Recent data suggest decreased time to menopause after embolization.)
- hysterectomy (Although this is the definitive treatment for symptomatic women who have completed childbearing, it's critical to inform women of all their choices because hysterectomy usually isn't the only available option.)
- blood transfusions (with severe anemia caused by excessive bleeding).

Varicocele

A mass of dilated and tortuous varicose veins in the spermatic cord is called a *varicocele*. It's classically described as a "bag of worms." Thirty percent of all men diagnosed with infertility have a varicocele. In 95% of cases, varicocele occurs in the left spermatic cord. It occurs in 10% to 15% of all males, usually between ages 13 and 18.

CAUSES

Causes of varicocele include:
- incompetent or congenitally absent valves in the spermatic veins
- tumor or thrombus obstructing the inferior vena cava (unilateral left-sided varicocele).

PATHOPHYSIOLOGY

Because of a valvular disorder in the spermatic vein, blood pools in the pampiniform plexus of veins that drain each testis rather than flowing into the venous system. One function of the pampiniform plexus is to keep the testes slightly cooler than body temperature—the optimal temperature for sperm production. Incomplete blood flow through the testis thus interferes with spermatogenesis. Testicular atrophy also may occur because of the reduced blood flow.

SIGNS AND SYMPTOMS

Usually, no symptoms are linked to a varicocele. Occasionally, symptoms may include:
- feeling of heaviness on the affected side because of blood pooling
- testicular pain and tenderness on palpation.

COMPLICATIONS

Possible complications of a varicocele include:
- infertility because of the elevated temperature caused by increased blood flow to the testes.

DIAGNOSIS

Physical examination shows:
- palpation of "bag of worms" when the patient is in an upright position
- nonpalpable varicocele when the patient is in a recumbent position.

TREATMENT

Possible treatment includes:
- conservative treatment with a scrotal support to relieve discomfort (in mild varicocele and infertility not an issue)
- surgical repair or removal involving ligation of the spermatic cord at the internal inguinal ring (if infertility is an issue).

APPENDICES

SELECTED REFERENCES

INDEX

LESS COMMON DISORDERS

DISEASE AND CAUSES	PATHOPHYSIOLOGY	SIGNS AND SYMPTOMS
Adenoid hyperplasia ◆ Cause unknown; may be hereditary or caused by chronic infections or irritations	Increased mitosis leads to an increase in cell numbers in adenoid tissue resulting in enlarged adenoid glands.	◆ Respiratory obstruction, especially mouth breathing, snoring at night, and frequent, prolonged nasal congestion ◆ Persistent mouth breathing during the formative years ◆ Sinusitis, frequent otitis media
Adrenogenital syndrome ◆ Autosomal recessive disorder that causes a 21-hydroxylase deficiency or 11-b hydroxylase deficiency ◆ Tumor of the adrenal glands	Lack of an enzyme needed to synthesize cortisol causes an excessive ACTH response through the negative feedback loop to the pituitary. The continual ACTH message to the adrenal glands results in hyperplasia of adrenal tissue. Excessive androgen production is stimulated because the adrenal pathway to androgen production is not blocked. Hypersecretion of androgens results in somatic masculinization.	◆ Enlarged external genitalia in neonate from excessive androgen production. Girls may have slightly enlarged clitoris or clitoris with a penile shape and labia fused to appear as a scrotum, whereas boys have enlarged genitals. ◆ Severe electrolyte imbalance, dehydration, vomiting, wasting, and shock from adrenal crisis at 5 to10 days
Albinism ◆ Autosomal recessive inheritance	Absence of the enzyme tyrosine results in a defect in melanin formation. There can be a partial or total lack of melanin pigment.	◆ Extremely fair skin color ◆ Fine, white hair ◆ Gray or blue irises of the eye ◆ Strabismus, nystagmus, photophobia ◆ Persistent loss of visual acuity
Alpha$_1$-antitrypsin deficiency ◆ Autosomal recessive inheritance	Reduced or absent levels of alpha$_1$-antitrypsin, which is needed to inhibit proteolytic enzymes, leads to the unopposed action of protease on the liver and lungs.	*In children:* ◆ Cholestasis ◆ Hepatitis ◆ Portal hypertension *In young adults:* ◆ Emphysema ◆ Cirrhosis
Amblyopia ◆ Strabismus in children ◆ Excessive alcohol or tobacco use in adults	Acuity is reduced because of a toxic reaction in the orbital portion of the optic nerve or by cerebral blockage of the visual stimuli.	◆ Visual dimness, photophobia, and ocular discomfort ◆ Small central or pericentral scotoma enlarges slowly ◆ Temporal disk pallor ◆ Possible blindness

DISEASE AND CAUSES	PATHOPHYSIOLOGY	SIGNS AND SYMPTOMS
Amyloidosis ◆ Pressure due to accumulation and infiltration of amyloid causes atrophy of nearby cells. Abnormal immunoglobulin synthesis and reticuloendothelial cell dysfunction may occur ◆ Familial inheritance in persons with Portuguese ancestry ◆ May occur with tuberculosis, chronic infection, rheumatoid arthritis, multiple myeloma, Hodgkin's disease, paraplegia, brucellosis, and Alzheimer's disease	A rare, chronic disease of abnormal fibrillar scleroprotein (a waxy, starchlike glycoprotein) accumulation that infiltrates body organs and soft tissues. Perireticular type affects the inner coats of blood vessels whereas pericollagen type affects the outer coats. Amyloidosis can result in permanent, even life-threatening, organ damage.	◆ Proteinuria, leading to nephrotic syndrome, eventually to renal failure ◆ Heart failure from cardiomegaly, arrhythmias, and amyloid deposits in subendocardium, endocardium, and myocardium ◆ Stiffness and enlargement of tongue, decreased intestinal motility, malabsorption, bleeding, abdominal pain, constipation, and diarrhea ◆ Appearance of peripheral neuropathy ◆ Liver enlargement, often with azotemia, anemia, albuminuria and, rarely, jaundice
Ankylosing spondylitis ◆ Cause unknown; strongly associated with presence of human leukocyte antigen (HLA)-B27 ◆ Familial inheritance	Fibrous tissue of the joint capsule is infiltrated by inflammatory cells that erode the bone and fibrocartilage. Repair of the cartilaginous structures begins with the proliferation of fibroblasts, which synthesize and secrete collagen. The collagen forms fibrous scar tissue that eventually undergoes calcification and ossification, causing the joint to fuse or lose flexibility.	◆ Intermittent lower back pain that's most severe after inactivity or in the morning ◆ Stiffness, limited lumbar spine motion ◆ Pain and limited expansion of chest ◆ Peripheral arthritis in shoulders, hips, and knees ◆ Kyphosis in advanced stages ◆ Hip deformity and limited range of motion ◆ Mild fatigue, fever, and anorexia or weight loss ◆ Dyspnea if the costovertebral joints are involved
Aspergillosis ◆ Fungal infection due to *Aspergillus* species; transmitted by inhalation of fungal spores or invasion of spores through wounds or injured tissue	*Aspergillus* species produce extracellular enzymes such as proteases and peptidases that contribute to tissue invasion, leading to hemorrhage and necrosis.	◆ Incubation is a few days to weeks; may be asymptomatic or mimic tuberculosis, causing a productive cough and purulent or blood-tinged sputum, dyspnea, empyema, and lung abscesses ◆ Allergic aspergillosis causes wheezing, dyspnea, pleural pain, and fever ◆ Aspergillosis endophthalmitis appears 2 to 3 weeks after eye surgery ◆ Cloudy vision, eye pain, reddened conjunctiva, purulent exudate

DISEASE AND CAUSES	PATHOPHYSIOLOGY	SIGNS AND SYMPTOMS
Behçet's syndrome ◆ Cause unknown; environmental factor or unknown virus can initiate process if genetic predisposition exists ◆ Family members may exhibit similar symptoms.	Overactive immune system produces sudden inflammation of small blood vessels; symptoms based on location of inflammation. Behçet's syndrome is more apparent in persons with Mediterranean, Middle East, and Far East ancestry. Onset is usually ages 10 to 20; five times more common in males.	◆ Recurrent genital ulcerations ◆ Recurrent oral ulcerations ◆ Eye inflammation and skin lesions ◆ Subcutaneous thrombophlebitis ◆ Epididymitis and deep vein thrombosis ◆ Arterial occlusion and aneurysm ◆ Severe headache and fatigue ◆ Bloating, diarrhea, cramping, and bloody stools ◆ Movement and speech difficulties
Blastomycosis ◆ Fungal infection from *Blastomyces dermatitidis;* usually infects the lungs and produces bronchopneumonia. ◆ May disseminate through blood causing osteomyelitis and central nervous system (CNS), skin, and genital disorders	Inhalation of the conidia leads to clearing of the organism by alveolar macrophages that kill conidia. Conidia that aren't killed convert to yeast forms that trigger an inflammatory response resulting in the formation of noncaseating granulomas.	◆ Dry, hacking, or productive cough ◆ Pleuritic chest pain, dyspnea ◆ Fever, shaking, chills, night sweats, malaise, and anorexia ◆ Small, painless, nonpruritic, and nondistinctive macules or papules on exposed body parts ◆ Painful swelling of testes, epididymis, or prostate; deep perineal pain, pyuria, and hematuria
Bronchiectasis ◆ Conditions associated with continued damage to bronchial walls and abnormal mucociliary clearance cause tissue breakdown to adjacent airways; such conditions include cystic fibrosis, immunologic disorders, and recurrent bacterial respiratory tract infections	Inflammation and destruction of the structural components of the bronchial wall lead to chronic abnormal dilatation.	*In early stages:* ◆ Asymptomatic with complaints of frequent pneumonia or hemoptysis ◆ Chronic cough producing copious, foul-smelling, mucopurulent secretions, hemoptysis ◆ Coarse crackles during inspiration ◆ Wheezing, dyspnea, sinusitis, fever, chills *In advanced stage:* ◆ Chronic malnutrition and right-sided heart failure from hypoxic pulmonary vasoconstriction

DISEASE AND CAUSES	PATHOPHYSIOLOGY	SIGNS AND SYMPTOMS
Bronchiolitis ◆ Acute viral infection of the lower respiratory tract; most commonly Infection from respiratory syncytial virus or parainfluenza virus; may be associated with specific diseases or conditions, such as bone marrow, heart or lung transplants, rheumatoid arthritis, lupus erythematosus, and Crohn's disease	Infection or other unknown factors cause necrosis of the bronchial epithelium and destruction of ciliated epithelial cells. As the submucosa becomes edematous, cellular debris and fibrin form plugs in the bronchioles.	*Subacute symptoms:* ◆ Fever, persistent nonproductive cough, dyspnea, malaise, and anorexla ◆ Physical assessment reveals dry crackles *Less common symptoms:* ◆ Tachypnea, tachycardia, intercostal and subcostal retractions ◆ Productive cough, hemoptysis, chest pain, general aches, and night sweat
Brucellosis ◆ Caused by gram-negative, aerobic *Brucella bacterium* that's transmitted by consumption of unpasteurized dairy products and meat or contact with infected animals or their secretions or excretions	Nonmotile, nonspore-forming, gram-negative coccobacilli of *Brucella* species cause an acute febrile illness.	◆ Usually insidious *In acute phase:* ◆ Fever, chills, profuse sweating, fatigue, headache, backache, enlarged lymph nodes ◆ Anorexia, joint pain, enlarged spleen *In chronic phase:* ◆ Depression, sleep disturbances, and sexual impotence
Cancer of the vulva ◆ Cause unknown; affects external female reproductive organs ◆ Usually occurs after menopause ◆ Accounts for 3% to 4% of all cancers of the female reproductive system	Squamous and basal cell carcinomas (90% squamous, 4% basal, 6% rare carcinomas) that usually begin on skin surface and are mostly slow-growing. Untreated, cancer spreads to vagina, urethra, anus, or lymph nodes.	◆ Unusual lumps or sores ◆ Vulvar pruritus ◆ Bleeding ◆ Small painful, infected ulcer ◆ Groin pain ◆ Abnormal urination and defecation
Celiac disease ◆ Results from a complex interaction involving dietary, genetic, and immunologic factors	The body can't hydrolyze peptides contained in fluten. Ingestion of gluten causes injury to the villi in the upper small intestine, leading to a decreased surface area and malabsorption of most nutrients. Inflammatory enteritis also results, leading to osmotic diarrhea and secretory diarrhea.	◆ Recurrent diarrhea, abdominal distention, stomach cramps, weakness, muscle wasting, or increased appetite without weight gain ◆ Normochromic, hypochromic, or macrocytic anemia ◆ Osteomalacia, osteoporosis, tetany, and bone pain in lower back, rib cage, pelvis ◆ Peripheral neuropathy, paresthesia, or seizures ◆ Dry skin, eczema, psoriasis, dermatitis herpetiformis, and acne rosacea ◆ Amenorrhea, hypometabolism, and adrenocortical insufficiency ◆ Extreme lethargy, mood changes and irritability

DISEASE AND CAUSES	PATHOPHYSIOLOGY	SIGNS AND SYMPTOMS
Cervical cancer ◆ Cause unknown; predisposing factors include intercourse under age 16, multiple sex partners, multiple pregnancies, and venereal infections ◆ Two types of cervical cancer: preinvasive and invasive	Preinvasive cancer is curable with early detection causing minimal cervical dysplasia in the lower third of the epithelium. Invasive cancer penetrates basement membrane to disseminate throughout the body via lymphatic routes. Histologic type is 95% squamous cell carcinoma.	*Preinvasive cancer:* ◆ Early invasive cancer shows no clinical changes or symptoms ◆ Abnormal vaginal bleeding ◆ Persistent vaginal discharge ◆ Postcoital pain and bleeding *Advanced stages:* ◆ Pelvic pain ◆ Vaginal leakage of urine or feces from fistula ◆ Anorexia, weight loss, and anemia
Cervical spondylosis ◆ Caused by narrowing of cervical canal or neural foramina due to degenerative changes in the intervertebral disk and annulus and to bony osteophytes	Progressive myelopathy leads to cord compression, causing a spastic gait.	◆ Pain or loss of feeling in the affected arm and shoulder, stiffness of the cervical spine ◆ Arm weakness and atrophy with reflex loss ◆ Hyperreflexia and increased tone ◆ Plantar extensor response in legs
Chalazion ◆ Caused by obstruction of the meibomian (sebaceous) gland duct	Blockage of the meibomian gland leads to the formation of granulation tissue.	◆ Local swelling, mild irritation ◆ Blurred vision ◆ Red-yellow elevation on conjunctival surface under eyelid
Chédiak-Higashi syndrome ◆ Linked to consanguinity and transmitted as an autosomal recessive trait	A genetic defect that manifests in morphologic changes in the granulocytes and causes delayed chemotaxis and impaired intracellular digestion of organisms; diminished inflammatory response results.	◆ Recurrent bacterial infections, primarily in the skin, lungs, and subcutaneous tissue ◆ Fever, significant photophobia ◆ Thrombocytopenia, neutropenia, and hepatosplenomegaly ◆ Motor and sensory neuropathies ◆ Cellular proliferation of liver, spleen, and bone marrow is fatal
Cholera ◆ Acute enterotoxin-mediated GI infection caused by gramnegative bacillus (*Vibrio cholerae*), which is transmitted through water and food contaminated with fecal material from carriers or people with active infections	After ingestion of a significant inoculum, colonization of the small intestine occurs. The secretion of a potent enterotoxin results in a massive outpouring of isotonic fluid from the mucosal surface of the small intestine. Profuse diarrhea, vomiting, and fluid and electrolyte loss occurs and may lead to hypovolemic shock, metabolic acidosis, and death.	◆ Incubation period is several hours to 5 days ◆ Acute, painless, profuse watery diarrhea, and vomiting ◆ Intense thirst, weakness, loss of skin tone; dehydration; electrolyte imbalances; oliguria ◆ Muscle cramps ◆ Cyanosis ◆ Tachycardia ◆ Falling blood pressure, fever, and hypoactive bowel sounds

DISEASE AND CAUSES	PATHOPHYSIOLOGY	SIGNS AND SYMPTOMS
Chronic fatigue and immune dysfunction syndrome ◆ Cause unknown; may be found in human herpesvirus-6 or other herpesviruses, enteroviruses, or retroviruses	Infectious agents or environmental factors trigger an abnormal immune response and hormonal alterations.	◆ Constellation of symptoms including myalgia, arthralgia with arthritis, low grade fever, pain, cervical adenopathy, sore throat, headache, memory deficits, and sleep disturbances ◆ Prolonged, overwhelming fatigue
Coccidioidomycosis ◆ Fungal infection from possible inhalation of *Coccidioides limmitis* spores from the soil or in plaster casts or dressing of infected people	*C. immitis* induces a granulomatous reaction that results in caseous necrosis.	◆ Dry cough, pleuritic chest pain, dyspnea, pleural effusion ◆ Fever, sore throat, chills, malaise, headache, and itchy macular rash ◆ Tender red nodules on legs with joint pain in knees and ankles in white women ◆ Chronic pulmonary cavitation ◆ Anorexia, weight loss
Colorado tick fever ◆ Virus is transmitted to human by a hard-shelled wood tick, *Dermacentor andersoni.* Tick acquires the virus when it bites an infected rodent and remains a permanently infected vector	Virus circulates inside of erythropoietic cells, producing typical febrile symptoms.	◆ Incubation is 3 to 6 days; symptoms begin abruptly ◆ Chills, high temperature, severe back, arm and leg aches, and lethargy ◆ Headache with ocular movement ◆ Photophobia, abdominal pain, nausea, and vomiting
Common variable immunodeficiency ◆ Characterized by progressive deterioration of B-cell (humoral) immunity, resulting in increased susceptibility to infection ◆ Cause unknown; may be associated with autoimmune diseases, such as systemic lupus erythematosus, rheumatoid arthritis, hemolytic anemia, and pernicious anemia, and with cancers, such as leukemia and lymphoma	Most patients have a normal circulating B-cell count but defective synthesis or release of immunoglobulins. Many also exhibit progressive deterioration of T-cell (cell-mediated) immunity revealed by delayed hypersensitivity skin testing.	◆ Chronic, rather than acute, pyogenic bacterial infections ◆ Recurrent sinopulmonary infections, chronic bacterial conjunctivitis, and malabsorption — usually the first clues

DISEASE AND CAUSES	PATHOPHYSIOLOGY	SIGNS AND SYMPTOMS
Complement deficiencies ◆ Primary complement deficiencies inherited as autosomal recessive traits; however, C1 esterase inhibitor is autosomal dominant ◆ Secondary deficiencies may follow complement-fixing reactions ◆ May be associated with such illnesses as acute post-streptococcal glomerulonephritis or acute systemic lupus erythematosus	Series of circulating enzymatic serum proteins with nine functional components labeled C1–C9. Deficiencies may increase susceptibility to infections and certain auto-immune disorders.	Clinical effects vary with deficiency. *C5 deficiency (familial defect in infants):* ◆ Diarrhea and seborrheic dermatitis *C1 esterase inhibitor deficiency:* ◆ Swelling in face, hands, abdomen, or throat; possibly fatal laryngeal edema *C2 and C3 deficiencies and C5 familial dysfunction:* ◆ Increase susceptibility to bacterial infection *C2 and C4 deficiencies:* ◆ Collagen vascular disease (lupus and chronic renal failure)
Costochondritis ◆ Cause unknown	An inflammatory process of the costochondral or costosternal joints is initiated, causing localized pain and tenderness.	◆ Sharp pain in chest wall ◆ Area is sensitive to touch ◆ Pain may radiate into arm ◆ Pain worsens with movement ◆ Reproducible pain
Creutzfeldt-Jakob disease ◆ Rare, degenerative invariably fatal brain disorder	Prior infects the CNS, leading to myelin destruction and neuronal loss.	◆ Myoclonic jerking, ataxia, aphasia, visual disturbances, paralysis, and early abnormal EEG ◆ May progress to dementia
Croup ◆ Childhood disease involving severe inflammation and obstruction of the upper airway, occurring as acute laryngotracheobronchitis, laryngitis, and acute spasmodic laryngitis ◆ Usually results from a viral infection (parainfluenza viruses, adenoviruses, respiratory syncytial virus, and influenza and measles viruses) or bacterial infection (pertussis, diphtheria, and mycoplasma)	Inflammatory swelling and spasms constrict the larynx, thereby reducing airflow. Inflammatory changes almost completely obstruct the larynx (which includes the epiglottis) and significantly narrow the trachea.	◆ Inspiratory stridor, hoarse or muffled vocal sounds, and varying degrees of laryngeal obstruction and respiratory distress ◆ Characteristic sharp, barking, seallike cough ◆ With progression, inflammatory edema and, possibly, spasm, which can obstruct the upper airway and severely compromise ventilation

DISEASE AND CAUSES	PATHOPHYSIOLOGY	SIGNS AND SYMPTOMS
Cryptococcosis ◆ Fungal infection caused by *Cryptococcus neoformans*, which is transmitted in particles of dust contamination by pigeon feces ◆ Transmission by inhalation of cryptococci	An asymptomatic pulmonary infection disseminates to extrapulmonary sites, usually CNS, but also skin, bones, prostate gland, liver, or kidneys. Untreated, infection progresses from coma to death from cerebral edema or hydrocephalus.	◆ Fever, cough with pleuritic pain, and weight loss ◆ Severe frontal and temporal headache, diplopia, blurred vision, dizziness, aphasia, and vomiting ◆ Skin abscesses and painful lesions of the long bones, skull, spine, and joints
Cystic echinococcosis ◆ Infection caused by tapeworm larvae, *Echinococcus gramulosus, E. multilocularis,* or *E. vogeli* ◆ Mainly transmitted by dogs that ingested the viscera of infected sheep ◆ Also found in coyotes, wolves, dingoes, and jackals	*E. granulosus* forms cysts in the liver, lungs, kidneys, and spleen; infection can be treated with surgery. *E. multilocularis* (alveolar hydatid disease) forms parasite tumors in the liver, lungs, brain, and other organs; infection can be fatal.	◆ Slow-growing cysts may be asymptomatic for years. Symptoms reflect location and size of cysts
Cystinuria ◆ Inherited autosomal recessive defect; more prevalent in persons of short stature (cause unknown)	Impaired function of membrane carrier proteins essential for transport of cystine and other dibasic amino acids results in excessive amino acid concentration in urine and excessive urinary excretion of cystine.	◆ Dull flank pain and capsular distention from acute renal colic; hematuria ◆ Tenderness in the costovertebral angle or over the kidneys ◆ Urinary obstruction with secondary infection (fever, chills, frequency, and foul-smelling urine)
DiGeorge syndrome ◆ Partial or total absence of cell-mediated immunity that results from a deficiency of T-lymphocytes	Abnormal fetal development of the third and fourth pharyngeal pouches interferes with thymus formation. The thymus is absent or partially present in an abnormal site, causing deficient cell-mediated immunity. Without a fetal thymus transplant, patients die by age 2.	*At birth:* ◆ Low-set ears, notches in ear pinna, fish-shaped mouth, an undersized jaw and abnormally wide-set eyes ◆ Great vessel anomalies and tetralogy of Fallot ◆ Hypocalcemia ◆ CNS and early heart failure

DISEASE AND CAUSES	PATHOPHYSIOLOGY	SIGNS AND SYMPTOMS
Encephalitis ◆ Severe inflammation of the brain, usually caused by a mosquito- or tick-borne virus; also by ingestion of infected goat's milk and accidental injection or inhalation of the virus ◆ Results from infection with arboviruses, enteroviruses, herpesvirus, mumps virus, HIV, adenoviruses, and demyelinating diseases after measles, varicella, rubella, or vaccination	Intense lymphocytic infiltration of brain tissues and the leptomeninges causes cerebral edema, degeneration of the brain's ganglion cells, and diffuse nerve cell destruction.	◆ Acute illness begins with sudden onset of fever, headache, and vomiting ◆ Progresses to signs and symptoms of meningeal irritation (stiff neck and back) and neuronal damage (drowsiness, coma, paralysis, seizures, ataxia, tremors, nausea, vomiting, and organic psychoses) ◆ After acute illness, coma may persist for days or weeks
Epicondylitis ◆ Inflammation of the extensor tendons of the forearm or inflammation at the origin of the flexor muscles of the wrist ◆ Common among tennis players or persons whose activities require a forceful grasp, wrist extension against resistance, or frequent forearm rotation	This disorder probably begins as a partial tear of the tendon or muscle. Untreated epicondylitis may become disabling as adherent fibers form between the tendons and the elbow capsule.	◆ Elbow pain that gradually worsens and usually radiates to the forearm and back of the hand whenever grasping an object or twisting the elbow ◆ Tenderness over the involved lateral or medial epicondyle or over the head of the radius and a weak grasp
Epidermolysis bullosa ◆ Cause unknown ◆ Nonscarring forms result from an autosomal dominant inheritance, except for junctional epidermolysis bullosa (recessively inherited) and dystrophic epidermolysis bullosa (results from X-linked recessive inheritance)	Vesicles and bullae occur from frictional trauma or heat; prognosis depends on severity. Disease is fatal in infant and child but becomes less severe as patient matures.	◆ Vesicles and bullae appear on hands, feet, knees, or elbows, and occur in GI, respiratory, or genitourinary tracts ◆ Eyelid blisters, conjunctivitis, adhesions, and corneal opacities ◆ Sloughing of large areas of neonatal skin ◆ Scars and contractures may result upon healing
Epiglottiditis ◆ Acute inflammation of the epiglottis that tends to cause airway obstruction; typically strikes children between ages 2 and 8 ◆ Usually results from infection with *Haemophilus influenzae* type B and, occasionally, pneumococci and group A streptococci	Sometimes preceded by an upper respiratory infection, epiglottiditis may rapidly progress to complete upper airway obstruction within 2 to 5 hours. Laryngeal obstruction results from inflammation and edema of the epiglottis.	◆ High fever, stridor, sore throat, dysphagia, irritability, restlessness, and drooling ◆ To relieve severe respiratory distress, child may hyperextend his neck, sit up, and lean forward with his mouth open, tongue protruding, and nostrils flaring ◆ Inspiratory retractions and rhonchi

DISEASE AND CAUSES	PATHOPHYSIOLOGY	SIGNS AND SYMPTOMS
Esophageal varices ◆ Portal hypertension	Shunting of blood to the venae cavae because portal hypertension leads to a complex of enlarged, swollen, and tortuous veins at the lower end of the esophagus.	◆ Hemorrhage and subsequent hypotension ◆ Compromised oxygen supply ◆ Altered level of consciousness ◆ Hematemesis
Fanconi's syndrome ◆ Inherited renal tubular transport disorder	Changes in the proximal renal tubules from atrophy of epithelial cells and loss of proximal tube volume results in a shortened connection to glomeruli by an unusually narrow segment. Malfunction of the proximal renal tubules leads to hyperkalemia, hypernatremia, glycosuria, phosphaturia, aminoaciduria, uricosuria, acidosis, retarded growth, and rickets.	◆ Mostly normal appearance at birth with slightly lower birth weights ◆ After 6 months, weakness, failure to thrive, dehydration, cystine crystals in the corners of the eye, and retinal pigment degeneration ◆ Yellow skin with little pigmentation ◆ Slow linear growth
Galactosemia ◆ Inherited autosomal recessive defects ◆ Inability to metabolize galactose (a sugar formed mainly by digestion of the disaccharaide lactose that's present in milk)	Galactose-1-phosphate and galactose accumulate in the tissues leading to decreased hepatic output of glucose and hypoglycemia.	◆ Nausea, vomiting, and diarrhea ◆ Jaundice and hepatomegaly ◆ Mental retardation, malnourishment, progressive hepatic failure, and death
Gallbladder and bile duct carcinoma ◆ Rare cancer in patients with cholecystitis ◆ Rapidly progressive and fatal ◆ Cause of extrahepatic bile duct carcinoma unknown	Direct extension to liver, cystic and common bile ducts, stomach and colon causes obstructions and consequent progressive, profound jaundice and epigastric and right upper quadrant pain.	◆ Ulcerative colitis; difficult to distinguish from cholecystitis ◆ Pain in epigastrium or upper right quadrant ◆ Weight loss, anorexia, chills, fever ◆ Nausea, vomiting, jaundice ◆ Pruritus, skin excoriations
Gas gangrene ◆ Local infection in devitalized tissue from *Clostridium perfringens*	Bacteria produce hydrolytic enzymes and toxins that destroy connective tissue and cellular membranes and cause gas bubbles to form in muscle cells. Enzymes also lyse red blood cell (RBC) membranes, destroying their oxygen-carrying capacity.	◆ Myositis, soft-tissue anaerobic cellulitis ◆ Crepitus ◆ Severe localized pain, swelling, and distortion ◆ Bullae and necrosis form after 36 hours ◆ Skin over wound may rupture, exposing dark red or black necrotic muscle and a foul-smelling watery or frothy discharge ◆ Intravascular hemolysis, thrombosis of blood vessels, toxemia, hypovolemia ◆ Toxic delirium

DISEASE AND CAUSES	PATHOPHYSIOLOGY	SIGNS AND SYMPTOMS
Gastric cancer ◆ Cause unknown; often associated with gastritis resulting from gastric cancer ◆ May be genetic in people with type A blood	An increase in nitrosoamines damages the DNA of mucosal cells, promoting metaplasia and neoplasia.	*In early stage:* ◆ Chronic dyspepsia and epigastric discomfort *In later stage:* ◆ Weight loss, anorexia, fullness after eating, anemia, fatigue ◆ Dysphagia, vomiting, blood in stool
Gastritis ◆ Chronic ingestion of irritating foods, aspirin, other nonsteroidal anti-inflammatory drug caffeine, corticosteroids, and poisons and endotoxins released by infecting bacteria ◆ Chronic gastritis associated with peptic ulcer disease or gastrostomy, causing chronic reflux of pancreatic secretions	An acute or chronic inflammation of gastric mucosa produces mucosal bleeding, edema, hemorrhage, and erosion.	◆ Onset is rapid after eating ◆ Epigastric discomfort, indigestion, cramping, anorexia, nausea, vomiting, and hematemesis
Giant cell arteritis ◆ Immune-mediated process ◆ Possible infectious etiology ◆ Genetic factors apparent with HLA-DR4 genotype; twice as common in women; incidence increases sharply with age	Lymphocytes, plasma cells, and multinucleated giant cells infiltrate affected vessels. Patchy or segmental changes overcome the medium and large arteries of the head and neck and may extend into the carotids and aorta. A cell-mediated immune response directed toward antigens in or near the elastic tissue component of the arterial wall may account for this disorder.	◆ Continuous, throbbing, intractable temporal headache ◆ Ischemia of masseter muscles, tongue, and pharynx ◆ Necrosis and ulceration of scalp ◆ Ocular or orbital pain ◆ Transient loss of vision, visual field defects, blurring, and hallucinations ◆ Tender, red, swollen, and nodular temporal arteries with diminished pulses ◆ Sudden blindness ◆ Pale, swollen optic disk surrounded by pericapillary hemorrhage ◆ Depression, difficulty in chewing, weight loss, fever
Gilbert's disease ◆ Genetic defect resulting in reduced bilirubin UDP-glucuronosyltransferase-1	Impaired hepatic bilirubin clearance results in hyperbilirubinemia.	◆ Mild jaundice without dark urine ◆ Nausea and vomiting ◆ Portal hypertension, ascites, and skin or endocrine changes ◆ Abdominal pain, anorexia, malaise

DISEASE AND CAUSES	PATHOPHYSIOLOGY	SIGNS AND SYMPTOMS
Globoid cell leukodystrophy ◆ Galactosylceramidase deficiency	Deficiency leads to rapid cerebral demyelination with large globoid bodies in the white matter and CNS.	◆ Irritability, rigidity, blindness, tonic-clonic seizures, deafness, mental deterioration
Goodpasture's syndrome ◆ Cause unknown; associated with exposure to hydrocarbons or type 2 influenza	Abnormal production of autoantibodies directed against alveolar and glomerular basement membranes leads to immune-mediated inflammation of lung and kidney tissues.	◆ Cough, bloody sputum, dyspnea ◆ Anemia ◆ Peripheral edema ◆ Hematuria, elevated serum creatinine and protein levels, progressive renal failure
Hand, foot, and mouth disease ◆ Highly contagious, common disease in infants and children due to Coxsackie A 16	RNA virus produces fever and vesicles in the oropharynx and on the hands and feet.	◆ Painful vesicular lesions on the mouth, tongue, hands, and feet
Hemothorax ◆ Blood in the chest that usually results from blunt or penetrating chest trauma	Blood from damaged intercostal, pleural, mediastinal, and (infrequently) lung parenchymal vessels enters the pleural cavity. Depending on the amount of bleeding and the underlying cause, hemothorax may be associated with varying degrees of lung collapse and mediastinal shift. Pneumothorax commonly accompanies hemothorax.	◆ Chest pain, tachypnea, and mild to severe dyspnea ◆ Marked blood loss producing hypotension and shock ◆ Affected side of the chest expands and stiffens, whereas the unaffected side rises and falls with the patient's breaths
Hereditary hemorrhagic telangiectasia ◆ An inherited vascular disorder transmitted by autosomal dominant inheritance ◆ May be lethal in its homozygous state ◆ Signs present in childhood but increase in severity with age	Venules and capillaries dilate to form fragile masses of thin convoluted vessels (telangiectases), resulting in an abnormal tendency to hemorrhage.	◆ Localized clusters of dilated capillaries appearing on the face, ears, scalp, hands, arms, and feet; under the nails; and on the mucous membranes of the nose, mouth, and stomach, causing frequent epistaxis, hemoptysis, and GI bleeding ◆ Characteristic telangiectases are violet, bleed spontaneously, may be flat or raised, blanch on pressure, and are nonpulsatile ◆ Generalized capillary fragility, as evidenced by spontaneous bleeding, petechiae, ecchymoses, and spider hemangiomas of varying sizes; may exist without overt telangiectasia

DISEASE AND CAUSES	PATHOPHYSIOLOGY	SIGNS AND SYMPTOMS
Herpangina ◆ Acute infection caused by group A Coxsackievirus transmitted by fecal-oral route	RNA virus produces fever and vesicles in the posterior portion of the oropharynx.	◆ Sore throat, pain with swallowing ◆ Fever (100° to 104° F [37.8° to 40° C]) lasting 1 to 4 days, febrile seizures ◆ Anorexia, malaise, vomiting, diarrhea ◆ Gray-white papulovesicles on soft palate ◆ Headache ◆ Pain in abdomen, neck, and extremities
Hiatal hernia ◆ Diaphragmatic malformation or weakening	Weakening of anchors from the gastroesophageal junction to the diaphragm or increased abdominal pressure allow herniation of part of the stomach through the esophageal hiatus in the diaphragm.	◆ Reflux of gastric contents with associated indigestion (heart burn) ◆ Dysphagia ◆ Chest pain
Hirsutism ◆ Androgen excess caused by heredity, endocrine (such as Cushing's or acromegaly) causes, or pharmacologic adverse effects	Minoxidil, androgenic steroids, or testosterone ingestion can cause signs of masculinization, pituitary dysfunction (precocious puberty), and adrenal dysfunction (Cushing's syndrome).	◆ Excessive hair growth in women or children, typically in an adult male distribution pattern
Hydronephrosis ◆ An abnormal dilation of the renal pelvis and the calyces of one or both kidneys, caused by an obstruction of urine flow in the genitourinary tract (such as from benign prostatic hyperplasia, urethral strictures, and calculi)	Partial obstruction and hydronephrosis may not produce initial symptoms, but pressure built up behind the area of obstruction results in symptomatic renal dysfunction. Total obstruction of urine flow with dilation of the collecting system ultimately causes complete cortical atrophy and cessation of glomerular filtration.	◆ No symptoms or only mild pain and slightly decreased urinary flow ◆ Severe, colicky renal pain or dull flank pain that may radiate to the groin and gross urinary abnormalities, such as hematuria, pyuria, dysuria, alternating oliguria and polyuria, or complete anuria ◆ Nausea, vomiting, abdominal fullness ◆ Pain on urination, dribbling, or hesitancy, infection caused by urinary stasis

DISEASES AND CAUSES	PATHOPHYSIOLOGY	SIGNS AND SYMPTOMS
Hypersplenism ◆ Increased activity of the spleen, where all types of blood cells are removed from circulation because of chronic myelogenous leukemia, lymphomas, Gaucher's disease, hairy cell leukemia, and sarcoidosis ◆ May also be associated with portal hypertension, malaria, tuberculosis, and various connective tissue and inflammatory diseases	Spleen growth may be stimulated by an increase in its workload, such as the trapping and destroying of abnormal RBCs.	◆ Enlarged spleen ◆ Cytopenia ◆ Abdominal pain on left side ◆ Fullness after eating small amounts of food
Idiopathic pulmonary fibrosis ◆ Chronic progressive lung disease associated with inflammation and fibrosis ◆ Cause unknown, but may follow an earlier infection of tuberculosis or pneumoconiosis	Interstitial inflammation consists of an alveolar septal infiltrate of lymphocytes, plasma cells, and histiocytes. Fibrotic areas are composed of dense acellular collagen. Areas of honeycombing that form are composed of cystic fibrotic air spaces, frequently lined with bronchiolar epithelium and filled with mucus. Smooth muscle hyperplasia may occur in areas of fibrosis and honeycombing.	◆ Dyspnea ◆ Nonproductive cough ◆ Chest heaviness ◆ Wheezing ◆ Anorexia ◆ Weight loss
Intussusception ◆ A telescoping (invagination) of a portion of the bowel into an adjacent distal portion ◆ Cause usually unknown; may be linked to viral infection, alterations in intestinal motility, hemangioma, lymphosarcoma, lymphoid hyperplasia, or Meckel's diverticulum in children and benign or malignant tumors in adults	When a bowel segment invaginates, peristalsis propels it along the bowel, pulling more bowel along with it. This invagination produces edema, hemorrhage from venous engorgement, incarceration, and obstruction. If treatment is delayed for longer than 24 hours, strangulation of the intestine usually occurs, causing gangrene, shock, and perforation.	◆ Intermittent attacks of colicky pain ◆ Vomiting ◆ "Currant jelly" stools, containing a mixture of blood and mucus ◆ Tender, distended abdomen, with a palpable, sausage-shaped abdominal mass
Kaposi's sarcoma ◆ Malignant, acquired immunodeficiency syndrome–related cancer	Arising from vascular endothelial cells, Kaposi's sarcoma affects endothelial tissue, which compromises all blood vessels.	◆ Red-purple or brown circular lesions, slightly raised on the face, arms, neck, and legs ◆ Internal lesions, especially in GI tract, identified by biopsy
Keratitis ◆ Inflammation of cornea from microorganisms, trauma, or autoimmune disorders	Bacterial infection leads to ulceration of the cornea.	◆ Decreased visual acuity ◆ Pain ◆ Photophobia

DISEASE AND CAUSES	PATHOPHYSIOLOGY	SIGNS AND SYMPTOMS
Kidney cancer ◆ Renal cell carcinoma associated with obesity and cigarette smoking	Tumors of various cell types and patterns that are usually aggressive in growth and affect younger patients	◆ Hematuria, flank pain, increased erythrocyte sedimentation rate ◆ Palpable mass ◆ Weight loss, anemia, fever, hypertension
Kyphosis ◆ An excessive curvature of the spine with convexity backward resulting from a congenital anomaly, tuberculosis, syphilis, malignant or compression fracture, arthritis, or rickets	Related to causative factor	◆ Abnormally rounded thoracic curve ◆ Possible back pain
Lassa fever ◆ High contagious viral infection from *Lassa* species	An epidemic hemorrhagic fever transmitted to humans by contact with infected rodent urine, feces, or saliva	◆ Fever lasting 2 to 3 weeks ◆ Exudative pharyngitis, oral ulcers, dysphagia, swelling of face and neck ◆ Lymphadenopathy ◆ Purpura, ecchymoses ◆ Conjunctivitis ◆ Bradycardia, shock, peripheral collapse ◆ Pleural effusion and renal involvement
Legionnaires' disease ◆ Infection from gram-negative bacillus, *Legionella pneumophila*	Transmission occurs with inhalation of organism carried in aerosols produced by air-conditioning units, water faucets, shower heads, humidifiers, and contaminated respiratory equipment.	◆ Dry cough ◆ Myalgia ◆ GI distress, diarrhea ◆ Pneumonia ◆ Cardiovascular collapse
Leprosy ◆ Infection from *Mycobacterium leprae*	Chronic, systemic infection with progressive cutaneous lesions, attacking the peripheral nervous system.	◆ Skin lesions ◆ Anesthesia ◆ Muscle weakness ◆ Paralysis
Mastocytosis ◆ Cause unknown	Proliferation of mast cells systemically and within skin.	◆ Urticaria pigmentosa, flushing ◆ Diarrhea, abdominal pain, ascites ◆ Headache, vascular collapse
Mastoiditis ◆ Bacterial infection of the mastoid antrum	An inflammation and infection of the air cells of the mastoid antrum.	◆ Dull ache and tenderness around the mastoid process, facial paralysis, labyrinthitis ◆ Headache, low-grade fever ◆ Thick purulent drainage ◆ Brain abscess, meningitis

DISEASE AND CAUSES	PATHOPHYSIOLOGY	SIGNS AND SYMPTOMS
Medullary sponge kidney ◆ Genetic disorder	Collecting ducts in the renal pyramids dilate, forming cavities, clefts, and cysts that produce complications of calcium oxylate stones and infections.	◆ Renal calculi ◆ Hematuria ◆ Infection (fever, chills, and malaise)
Melasma ◆ Hypermelanotic skin disorder associated with increased hormonal levels with pregnancy, hormonal contraceptive use, and ovarian cancer	Thought to be caused by the effects of estrogen and progesterone on melanin production.	◆ Patchy, nonraised, hypermelanotic rash
Multiple endocrine neoplasia ◆ Hereditary disorder in which two or more endocrine glands develop hyperplasia, adenoma, or carcinoma, concurrently or consecutively ◆ Caused by autosomal dominant inheritance	Two of the types are well documented: multiple endocrine neoplasia (MEN) I (Werner's syndrome) (most common) involves hyperplasia and adenomatosis of the pituitary and parathyroid glands, islet cells of the pancreas, and, rarely, the thyroid and adrenal glands; MEN II (Sipple's syndrome) involves medullary carcinoma of the thyroid, with hyperplasia and adenomatosis of the adrenal medulla (pheochromocytoma) and parathyroid glands.	MEN I signs and symptoms include: ◆ Signs of hyperparathyroidism, including hypercalcemia ◆ Ulcer caused by Zollinger-Ellison syndrome ◆ Hypoglycemia MEN II signs and symptoms include: ◆ Enlarged thyroid mass, with resultant increased calcitonin and, occasionally, ectopic corticotropin, causing Cushing's syndrome ◆ With adrenal medulla tumors, headache, tachyarrhythmias, and hypertension; with adenomatosis or hyperplasia of the parathyroids, symptoms result from renal calculi
Myelitis and acute transverse myelitis ◆ Caused by acute infections (measles or pneumonia) or primary lesions of the spinal cord (syphilis or acute disseminated encephalomyc-litis); can accompany demyelinating diseases (acute multiple sclerosis) and inflammatory and necrotizing disorders of the spinal cord (hematomyelia) ◆ May result from certain toxic agents (such as carbon monoxide, lead, arsenic); other infections, such as poliovirus, herpes zoster, herpesvirus B; disorders that cause meningeal inflammation; or smallpox or polio vaccination	Myelitis is an inflammation of the spinal cord that can result from several diseases. Only the cord's gray matter may be affected, producing motor dysfunction, or the white matter may be affected, producing sensory dysfunction. These types of myelitis can attack any level of the spinal cord, causing partial destruction or scattered lesions. Acute transverse myelitis, which affects the entire thickness of the spinal cord, produces motor and sensory dysfunctions. It has a rapid onset and is the most devastating form of myelitis.	*Myelitis:* ◆ Sensory or motor dysfunction, depending on the site of damage to the spinal cord *Acute transverse myelitis:* ◆ Rapid motor and sensory dysfunctions below the level of spinal cord damage appear in 1 to 2 days ◆ Flaccid paralysis of the legs with loss of sensory and sphincter functions ◆ Reflexes disappear, but may reappear later ◆ Extent of damage depends on the level of the spinal cord affected ◆ If spinal cord damage is severe, shock may occur (hypotension and hypothermia)

DISEASE AND CAUSES	PATHOPHYSIOLOGY	SIGNS AND SYMPTOMS
Myelodysplastic syndromes ◆ Caused by genetic factors and exposure to chemicals or radiation	Preleukemic disorders that progress to leukemia	◆ Pancytopenia, anemia ◆ Weakness, fatigue, palpitations ◆ Dizziness, irritability
Narcolepsy ◆ Familial disorder	Chronic, recurrent attacks of drowsiness and sleep during the daytime.	◆ Drowsiness, daytime sleepiness ◆ Sudden loss of muscle tone ◆ Extreme strong emotions
Necrotizing enterocolitis ◆ Diffuse or patchy intestinal necrosis, accompanied by sepsis in about one-third of cases ◆ Exact cause unknown; suggested predisposing factors include birth asphyxia, postnatal hypotension, umbilical vessel catheterization, exchange transfusion, or patent ductus arteriosus; may also be a response to significant prenatal stress, such as premature rupture of membranes, placenta previa, preeclampsia, or maternal sepsis	According to current theory, necrotizing enterocolitis develops when the infant suffers perinatal hypoxemia caused by shunting of blood from the gut to more vital organs. Subsequent mucosal ischemia provides an ideal medium for bacterial growth. As the bowel swells and breaks down, gas-forming bacteria invade damaged areas, producing free air in the intestinal wall. This may result in fatal perforation and peritonitis.	◆ Distended (especially tense or rigid) abdomen with gastric retention ◆ Increasing residual gastric contents, which may contain bile ◆ Bile-stained vomitus ◆ Occult blood in the stool ◆ Thermal instability, lethargy, metabolic acidosis, jaundice, and disseminated intravascular coagulation
Neurofibromatosis ◆ Inherited autosomal dominant disorder	Group of developmental disorders of the nervous system, muscles, bones, and skin that affects the cell growth of neural tissue.	◆ Café-au-lait spots ◆ Multiple, pediculated, soft tumors (neurofibromas) ◆ Hearing loss ◆ Bone changes, skeletal deformities
Neurogenic arthropathy ◆ Progressive degenerative disease of peripheral and axial joints, resulting from impaired sensory innervation ◆ Caused by diabetes mellitus, tabes dorsalis, syringomyelia, myelopathy of pernicious anemia, spinal cord trauma, paraplegia, hereditary sensory neuropathy, and Charcot-Marie-Tooth disease	The loss of sensation in the joints causes progressive deterioration, resulting from trauma or primary disease, which leads to laxity of supporting ligaments and eventual disintegration of the affected joints.	◆ Swelling, warmth, decreased mobility, and instability in a single joint or in many joints ◆ Progression to deformity ◆ Pain is minimal despite deformity
Orbital cellulitis ◆ Bacterial infection typically caused by streptococcal, staphylococcal, and pneumococcal organisms	Inflammation and infection of the fatty orbital tissues and eyelids.	◆ Unilateral eyelid edema ◆ Hyperemia ◆ Redden eyelids, matted lashes

DISEASE AND CAUSES	PATHOPHYSIOLOGY	SIGNS AND SYMPTOMS
Osgood-Schlatter disease ◆ Probably results from trauma before complete fusion of the epiphysis to the main bone has occurred (between ages 10 and 15); such trauma may be a single violent action or repeated knee flexion against a tight quadriceps muscle	This painful, incomplete separation of the epiphysis of the tibial tubercle from the tibial shaft is most common in active adolescent boys. Severe disease may cause permanent tubercle enlargement.	◆ Constant aching and pain and tenderness below the kneecap ◆ Obvious soft-tissue swelling and localized heat and tenderness
Paraphilia ◆ Psychosexual disorder	Dependence on unusual behaviors or fantasies to achieve sexual excitement.	◆ Exhibitionism, voyeurism ◆ Fetishism, transvestic fetishism ◆ Frottage ◆ Pedophilia ◆ Sexual masochism, sexual sadism
Pediculosis ◆ Infestation by lice	Louse attaches itself to the hair shaft with claws and feeds on blood several times daily; resides close to the scalp to maintain its body temperature. Itching may be from an allergic reaction to louse saliva or irritability.	◆ Itching, inflammation ◆ Eczematous dermatitis ◆ Tiredness, irritability, weakness ◆ Lice present in hair (head, axilla, and pubic)
Penile cancer ◆ Preceded by chronic irritation, condylomata acuminata, or phimosis in uncircumcised men	Neoplasms may be benign or malignant; latter are usually squamous cell carcinomas.	◆ Painless ulcerations on the glans or foreskin; small, warty plaque ◆ Dysuria, purulent discharge, and obstruction
Phenylketonuria ◆ Inborn error in phenylalanine metabolism resulting in the accumulation of high serum phenylalanine levels ◆ Transmitted by an autosomal recessive gene	Because of insufficient hepatic phenylalanine hydroxylase, an enzyme that acts as a catalyst in the conversion of phenylalanine to tyrosine, phenylalanine and its metabolites accumulate in the blood, causing mental retardation if left untreated. The exact mechanism that causes this retardation is unclear.	◆ By age 4 months, infant shows signs of arrested brain development, including mental retardation and, later, personality disturbances (schizoid and antisocial personality patterns and uncontrollable temper) ◆ Lighter complexion, blue eyes ◆ Microcephaly; eczematous skin lesions or dry, rough skin; musty (mousy) odor ◆ Abnormal EEG patterns and, possibly, seizures
Pheochromocytoma ◆ Polyglandular multiple endocrine neoplasia	Tumor of the chromaffin cells of the adrenal medulla that causes an increased production of catecholamines.	◆ Hypertension, high blood sugar and lipid levels ◆ Headache, palpitations, sweating, dizziness, syncope, anxiety, constipation

DISEASES AND CAUSES	PATHOPHYSIOLOGY	SIGNS AND SYMPTOMS
Pilonidal disease ◆ May develop congenitally from a tendency to hirsutism, or it may be acquired from stretching or irritation of the sacrococcygeal area from prolonged rough exercise, heat, excessive perspiration, or constricting clothing	A coccygeal cyst forms in the intergluteal cleft on the posterior surface of the lower sacrum. It usually contains hair and becomes infected, producing an abscess, a draining sinus, or a fistula.	◆ Generally, no symptoms until the cyst becomes infected ◆ Local pain, tenderness, swelling, or heat ◆ Continuous or intermittent purulent drainage ◆ Abscess development, chills, fever, headache, and malaise
Pituitary tumor ◆ Cause unknown	Tumors are usually macroadenomas with self-secreting thyroid-stimulating hormone.	◆ Signs of hyperthyroidism without skin and eye manifestations ◆ Goiters ◆ High free thyroxine levels
Pleurisy ◆ Several causes including lupus, rheumatoid arthritis, and tuberculosis	Inflammation of the visceral and parietal pleurae that line the inside of the thoracic cage and envelop the lungs	◆ Sharp, stabbing chest pain ◆ Dyspnea ◆ Pleural friction rub
Pneumoconioses ◆ Inhalation of dust particles, usually in an occupational setting	Chronic and permanent disposition of particles in the lungs causes a tissue reaction, which may be harmless or destructive.	◆ Critical exposure ◆ Emphysema ◆ Shortness of breath, cough ◆ Fatigue, weakness ◆ Weight loss
Polymyositis ◆ Cause unknown; may be from viral or autoimmune reaction	Damage of skeletal muscle by an inflammatory process dominated by lymphocytic infiltration leads to progressive muscle weakness.	◆ Proximal muscle weakness, dysphonia, dysphagia, and regurgitation ◆ Polyarthralgias, joint effusions, and Raynaud's phenomenon ◆ Rash associated with muscular pain, tenderness, and induration
Postherpetic neuralgia ◆ Complication of the chronic phase of herpes zoster	Varicella virus in ganglia of the posterior nerve roots reactivates, multiplies, and spreads down the sensory nerves to the skin.	◆ Intractable neurologic pain lasting over 6 weeks after disappearance of herpes zoster rash
Proctitis ◆ Contributing factors that allow the normal mucosa to break down include trauma, infection, allergies, drugs, radiation, stress, and sexually transmitted diseases	Acute or chronic inflammation of the rectal mucosa.	◆ Mild rectal pain, mucous discharge, bleeding, feeling of rectal fullness, and tenesmus ◆ Urge to pass stool with inability to do so ◆ Pus, blood, or mucous in stools
Pseudogout ◆ Cause unknown; associated with conditions that cause degenerative or metabolic changes in cartilage	Calcium pyrophosphate crystals deposit in periarticular joint structures. It commonly invades knee joint.	◆ Sudden joint pain and swelling in larger peripheral joints; mimics other form of arthritis

DISEASE AND CAUSES	PATHOPHYSIOLOGY	SIGNS AND SYMPTOMS
Pseudomembranous enterocolitis ◆ Acute inflammation and necrosis of the small and large intestines, usually affecting the mucosa but may extend into submucosa and, rarely, other layers ◆ Exact cause unknown; *Clostridium difficile* may produce a toxin that could play a role in development	Necrotic mucosa is replaced by a pseudomembrane filled with staphylococci, leukocytes, mucus, fibrin, and inflammatory cells.	◆ Copious watery or bloody diarrhea, abdominal pain, and fever ◆ Severe dehydration, electrolyte imbalance, hypotension, shock, and colonic perforation
Ptosis ◆ Due to congenital (autosomal dominant trait or anomaly) or acquired (age, mechanical, myogenic, neurogenic, or nutritional) factors	Stretching of eyelid skin or aponeurotic tendon causes upper eyelid to droop. Lesion affects innervation of either of two muscles that open the eyelid.	◆ Drooping of upper eyelid
Pyloric stenosis ◆ Congenital; cause unknown	Pyloric sphincter muscle fibers thicken and become inelastic, leading to a narrowed opening. The extra peristaltic effort needed leads to hypertrophied muscle layers of the stomach.	◆ Progressive nonbilious vomiting, leading to projectile vomiting at ages 2 to 4 weeks
Rectal prolapse ◆ Protrusion of one or more layers of mucous membrane through the anus due to conditions that affect the pelvic floor or rectum	Increased intra-abdominal pressure triggers the circumferential protrusion of one or more layers of the mucous membrane.	◆ Lower abdominal pain caused by ulceration, bloody diarrhea, or tissue protruding from rectum during defecation or walking
Reiter's syndrome ◆ Cause unknown; mostly follows a venereal or enteric infection ◆ Genetic factor (HLA-B27) increases risk of acquiring disorder	An infection (caused by *Mycoplasma, Shigella, Salmonella, Yersinia,* or *Chlamydia* organisms) is thought to initiate an aberrant and hyperactive immune response that produces inflammation in involved target organs.	*General:* ◆ Low-grade fever, unexplained diarrhea ◆ Superficial lesions on palms or soles *Urogenital tract:* ◆ Burning sensation with urination, penile discharge, and prostatitis in men ◆ Cervicitis, urethritis, and vulvovaginitis in women *Joint symptoms or arthritis:* ◆ Affects knees, ankles, feet ◆ Inflammation where tendon attaches to bone *Eye involvement:* ◆ Conjunctivitis, uveitis

DISEASE AND CAUSES	PATHOPHYSIOLOGY	SIGNS AND SYMPTOMS
Renal infarction ◆ Formation of a coagulated, necrotic area in one or both kidneys ◆ Caused by renal artery embolism in 75% of patients; less common causes include atherosclerosis, with or without thrombus formation; and thrombus from flank trauma, sickle cell anemia, scleroderma, polyarteritis nodosa, and arterionephrosclerosis	Results from renal blood vessel occlusion that reduces blood flow to renal tissue and leads to ischemia. The location and size of the infarction depend on the site of vascular occlusion; usually, infarction affects the renal cortex, but it can extend into the medulla. Residual renal function after infarction depends on the extent of the damage from the infarction.	◆ May be asymptomatic ◆ Typically, severe abdominal or gnawing flank pain and tenderness, costovertebral tenderness ◆ Fever, anorexia, nausea, and vomiting ◆ Gross hematuria
Renal tubular acidosis ◆ *Distal (type I):* familial with another genetic disease or an isolated autosomal dominant disease ◆ *Proximal (type II):* accompanies several inherited diseases, multiple myeloma, vitamin D deficiency, chronic hypocalcemia, after renal transplantation, and after treatment with certain drugs	In type I, the distal tubule is unable to secrete hydrogen ions across the tubular membrane, causing decreased excretion of titratable acids and ammonium and increased loss of potassium and bicarbonate. Prolonged acidosis leads to hypercalciuria and renal calculi. In type II, defective reabsorption of bicarbonate in proximal tubule causes bicarbonate to flood the distal tubule, leading to impaired formation of titratable acids and ammonium for excretion.	*In infants:* ◆ Vomiting, fever, constipation, anorexia, weakness, polyuria, growth retardation, nephrocalcinosis, and rickets *In children and adults:* ◆ Growth problems, urinary tract infections, and rickets
Renal vein thrombosis ◆ Clotting in the renal vein ◆ Caused by a tumor that obstructs the renal vein, thrombophlebitis of the inferior vena cava or blood vessels of the legs, heart failure, and periarteritis ◆ In infants, caused by diarrhea, leading to severe dehydration	Results in renal congestion, engorgement, possible infarction. Acute or chronic, may affect both kidneys. Chronic thrombosis usually impairs renal function, causing nephrotic syndrome. Abrupt onset with extensive damage may precipitate rapidly fatal renal infarction. Less severe thrombosis affecting only one kidney, or gradual progression allowing circulation to develop, may preserve partial renal function.	*With rapid onset:* ◆ Severe lumbar pain and tenderness in epigastric region and costovertebral angle ◆ Fever, leukocytosis, pallor, hematuria, proteinuria, peripheral edema ◆ Enlarged kidneys, easily palpable *With gradual onset:* ◆ Symptoms of nephrotic syndrome ◆ Pain generally absent ◆ Proteinuria, hypoalbuminemia, and hyperlipidemia *In infants:* ◆ Enlarged kidneys, oliguria ◆ Renal insufficiency that may progress to acute or chronic renal failure

DISEASE AND CAUSES	PATHOPHYSIOLOGY	SIGNS AND SYMPTOMS
Renovascular hypertension ◆ A rise in systemic blood pressure resulting from stenosis of the major renal arteries or their branches or from intrarenal atherosclerosis ◆ Caused by atherosclerosis and fibromuscular diseases of the renal artery wall layers; other causes include arteritis, anomalies of the renal arteries, embolism, trauma, tumor, and dissecting aneurysm	Stenosis or occlusion of the renal artery stimulates the affected kidney to release the enzyme renin, which converts angiotensinogen (a plasma protein) to angiotensin I. As angiotensin I circulates through the lungs and liver, it converts to angiotensin II, which causes peripheral vasoconstriction, increased arterial pressure and aldosterone secretion and, eventually, hypertension.	◆ Elevated systemic blood pressure ◆ Headache, palpitations, tachycardia, anxiety, light-headedness, decreased tolerance of temperature extremes, retinopathy, and mental sluggishness
Retinal detachment ◆ Caused by trauma, after cataract surgery, severe uveitis, and primary or metastatic choroidal tumors; may also occur as a result of internal changes in the vitreous chamber associated with aging	The neural retina separates from the underlying retinal pigment epithelium.	◆ Floaters, flashing lights, scotoma in peripheral visual field (painless) and, eventually, a curtain or veil occurs in the field of vision
Retinitis pigmentosa ◆ Autosomal recessive disorder in 80% of affected children ◆ Less commonly transmitted as an X-linked trait	Slow, degenerative changes in rods cause the retina and pigment epithelium to atrophy. Irregular black deposits of clumped pigment are in equatorial region of retina and eventually in the macular and peripheral areas.	◆ Progressive night blindness, visual field constriction with ring scotoma, and loss of acuity progressing to blindness
Rocky Mountain spotted fever ◆ Infection from *Rickettsia rickettsii* carried by several tick species	*R. rickettsii* multiplies within endothelial cells and spreads via the bloodstream. Focal areas of infiltration lead to thrombosis and leakage of RBCs into surrounding tissue.	◆ Fever, headache, mental confusion, and myalgia ◆ Rash develops as small macules that progress to maculopapules and petechiae (Starts on wrists and ankles, spreads to trunk. Diagnostic rash on palms and soles.) ◆ Constipation and abdominal distension
Rosacea ◆ Cause unknown	Small facial blood vessels, usually the nose and cheeks, become flushed and dilated.	◆ Pronounced flushing of nose, cheeks, and forehead ◆ Papules, pustules, telangiectases can be superimposed

DISEASE AND CAUSES	PATHOPHYSIOLOGY	SIGNS AND SYMPTOMS
Sarcoidosis ◆ Cause unknown ◆ Evidence suggests that disease is result of exaggerated cellular immune response to limited class of antigens	Organ dysfunction results from an accumulation of T lymphocytes, mononuclear phagocytes, and nonsecreting epithelial granulomas, which distort normal tissue architecture.	◆ Mainly generalized, most commonly involving the lung with resulting respiratory symptoms ◆ Fever, fatigue, and malaise
Scabies ◆ Human itch mite (*Sarcoptes scabiei* var. *hominis*)	Mite burrows superficially beneath stratum corneum depositing eggs that hatch, mature, and reinvade the skin. Sensitization reaction against mite excreta results.	◆ Intense itching that worsens at night ◆ Threadlike lesions on wrists, between fingers, and on elbows, axillae, belt line, buttocks, and male genitalia ◆ Secondary bacterial infection may occur
Schistosomiasis ◆ Blood flukes of the class Trematoda; *Schistosoma mansoni* and *S. japonicum* infect intestinal tract, whereas *S. haematobium* infects the urinary tract	Infection follows contact by bathing with free swimming cercariae of the parasite, which penetrate the skin, migrate to intrahepatic portal circulation, and mature. Adult worms lodge in venules of bladder or intestines.	Depends on infection site and stage. *In initial stage:* ◆ Pruritic papular dermatitis at penetration site; fever; cough *In later stage:* ◆ Hepatosplenomegaly and lymphadenopathy ◆ May cause seizures and skin abscesses
Septic arthritis ◆ Infectious arthritis ◆ Common infecting organisms include gram-positive cocci and *Staphylococcus aureus, Streptococcus pyogenes,* and *S. pneumoniae* in children; in adults, *Neisseria gonorrhoeae, S. aureus,* and streptococci ◆ Predisposing factors include concurrent bacterial infection or serious chronic illness, diseases that depress the immune system and immunosuppressive therapy, recent articular trauma, joint surgery, intra-articular injections, and local joint abnormalities	This disorder occurs when bacterial invasion of a joint causes inflammation of the synovial lining, effusion and pyogenesis, and destruction of bone and cartilage. Septic arthritis can lead to ankylosis and even fatal septicemia without prompt treatment.	◆ Intense pain, inflammation, and swelling of the affected joint ◆ Low-grade fever ◆ Migratory polyarthritis

DISEASES AND CAUSES	PATHOPHYSIOLOGY	SIGNS AND SYMPTOMS
Severe combined immunodeficiency syndrome ◆ Both cell-mediated (T-cell) and humoral (B-cell) immunity are deficient or absent, resulting in susceptibility to infection from all classes of microorganisms during infancy ◆ Usually transmitted as an autosomal recessive trait, although it may be X-linked	In most cases, genetic defect seems associated with failure of the stem cell to differentiate into T and B lymphocytes. Many molecular defects, such as mutation of the kinase ZAP-70, can cause this disorder. X-linked severe combined immunodeficiency syndrome is due to a mutation of a subunit of the interleukin (IL)-2, IL-4, and IL-7 receptors. Less commonly, it results from an enzyme deficiency.	◆ Extreme susceptibility to infection ◆ Failure to thrive and chronic otitis, sepsis, watery diarrhea (from *Salmonella* or *Escherichia coli*), recurrent pulmonary infections, persistent oral candidiasis and, possibly, fatal viral infections (such as chickenpox) ◆ *Pneumocystis carinii* pneumonia
Shigellosis ◆ Acute infectious inflammatory colitis from *Shigella* organisms	*Shigella* is transmitted by oral or fecal-oral route. Invasion of colonic epithelial cells and cell-to-cell spread of infection results in characteristic mucosal ulcerations.	*In children:* ◆ Fever, watery diarrhea, nausea, vomiting, irritability, abdominal pain and distention *In adults:* ◆ Intermittent severe abdominal pain, tenesmus and, in severe cases, headache and prostration; fever is rare ◆ Pus, blood, or mucous in stools
Silicosis ◆ Exposure to high concentrations of respirable silica dust	Alveolar macrophages engulf respirable particles of free silica, causing release of cytotoxic enzymes. This attracts other macrophages and produces fibrous tissue in the lung parenchyma. *Note:* Silicosis is associated with a high incidence of active tuberculosis.	*In simple nodular silicosis:* ◆ Cough that raises sputum; usually no other symptoms *In conglomerate silicosis:* ◆ Severe shortness of breath, cough, and sputum; may lead to pulmonary hypertension and cor pulmonale
Sjögren's syndrome ◆ Autoimmune rheumatic disorder with unknown cause; genetic and environmental factors may be involved	Lymphocytic infiltration of exocrine glands causes tissue damage that results in xerostomia and dry eyes.	*In xerostomia:* ◆ Dry mouth; difficulty swallowing and speaking; ulcers of tongue, buccal mucosa and lips; severe dental caries *In ocular involvement:* ◆ Dry eyes; gritty, sandy feeling; decreased tearing; burning, itching, redness, photosensitivity *Extraglandular:* ◆ Arthralgias, Raynaud's phenomenon, lymphadenopathy, and lung involvement

DISEASE AND CAUSES	PATHOPHYSIOLOGY	SIGNS AND SYMPTOMS
Sleep apnea ◆ Caused by occlusion of airway (obstructive), absence of respiratory effort (central), or both	Airflow ceases because of upper airway narrowing and glottal obstruction as a result of obesity or congenital abnormalities of the upper airway. When primary brain stem medullary failure occurs, sleeping patient may breathe insufficiently or not at all.	*In obstructive sleep apnea:* ◆ Snoring, excessive daytime sleepiness, intellectual impairment, memory loss, and cardiorespiratory symptoms *In central sleep apnea:* ◆ Sleeping poorly, morning headache, and daytime fatigue
Spinal ischemia or infarction ◆ Caused by direct vascular compression (tumors and acute disc compression) or by remote occlusion (aortic surgery and dissecting aneurysm)	Major arterial branches that supply the spinal cord become compressed or occluded, decreasing blood flow to the spinal cord, causing cord ischemia and motor and sensory deficiencies.	◆ Sudden back pain and pain in distribution of affected segment followed by bilateral flaccid weakness and dissociated sensory loss below level of infarct

Sporotrichosis
◆ Fungal infection caused by *Sporothrix schenckii*, which occurs in soil, wood, sphagnum moss, and decaying vegetation
	Inflammatory response includes both the clustering of neutrophils and a marked granulomatous response, with epithelioid cells and giant cells producing nodular erythematous primary lesions and secondary lesions along lymphatic channels in cutaneous lymphatic type.
	    In pulmonary sporotrichosis, inflammatory response produces pulmonary lesions and nodules.
	    In disseminated sporotrichosis, multifocal lesions spread from skin or lungs.
		In cutaneous or lymphatic sporotrichosis:
		◆ Subcutaneous, movable, painless nodule on hands or fingers that grows progressively larger, discolors, and eventually ulcerates; additional lesions form on the adjacent lymph node chain
		In pulmonary sporotrichosis:
		◆ Productive cough, lung cavities and nodules, pleural effusion, fibrosis, and formation of fungus ball
		In disseminated sporotrichosis:
		◆ Weight loss, anorexia, synovial or bony lesions and, possibly, arthritis or osteomyelitis

Stickler syndrome ◆ Autosomal dominant chondrodysplasia caused by structural defects in collagen, an essential component of connective tissue ◆ Characterized by ocular, skeletal, auditory, and craniofacial abnormalities	Collagen defect is typically caused by a mutation in the type II collagen gene (COL2A I) located on chromosome 12q13.11to 12q13.2. Others show linkage to the COLIIA2 gene located on chromosome 6p21.3 and others to COLIIAI gene located on chromosome lp2l. COL11A2 and COLIIAI are expressed in the hyaline cartilage, vitreous, intervertebral disc, and inner ear.	◆ Ocular symptoms: myopia, vitreal abnormalities, and retinal detachment resulting in blindness ◆ Auditory symptoms: conductive hearing loss or sensorineural hearing loss ◆ Craniofacial features: micrognathia and a flattened midface and nasal bridge ◆ Skeletal symptoms: joint hypermobility, spondyloepiphyseal dysplasia, and degenerative arthropathy

DISEASE AND CAUSES	PATHOPHYSIOLOGY	SIGNS AND SYMPTOMS
Stomatitis ♦ Results from the herpes simplex virus ♦ Aphthous cause unknown; predisposing factors include stress, fatigue, fever, trauma, and overexposure to sun	Inflammation of the cells of the oral mucosa, buccal mucosa, lips and palate with resulting ulcers.	♦ Papulovesicular ulcers in mouth and throat, mouth pain, malaise, anorexia, and swelling of mucous membranes
Strabismus ♦ Eye malalignment that is frequently inherited; controversy exists whether amblyopia is caused by or results from strabismus	In paralytic (nonconcomitant) strabismus, paralysis of one or more ocular muscles may be from an oculomotor nerve lesion. In nonparalytic (concomitant) strabismus, unequal ocular muscle tone is caused by supranuclear abnormality within the CNS.	♦ Noticeable eye malalignment by external eye examination, ophthalmoscopic observation of the corneal light reflex in center of pupils, diplopia, and other vision disturbances ♦ Visual acuity diminishes with decreased use of an eye
Thrombocythemia ♦ Primary: cause unknown ♦ Secondary: from chronic inflammatory disorders, iron deficiency, acute infection, neoplasm, hemorrhage, or postsplenectomy	A clonal abnormality of a multipotent hematopoietic stem cell results in increased platelet production, although platelet survival is usually normal. If combined with degenerative vascular disease, may lead to serious bleeding or thrombosis.	♦ Weakness, hemorrhage, nonspecific headache, paresthesia, dizziness, and easy bruising
Thrombophlebitis ♦ Caused by endothelial damage, accelerated blood clotting, and reduced blood flow	Alteration in epithelial lining causes platelet aggregation and fibrin entrapment of RBCs, white blood cells, and additional platelets; the thrombus initiates a chemical inflammatory process in the vessel epithelium that leads to fibrosis, which may occlude the vessel lumen or may embolize.	♦ Varies with site and length of affected vein ♦ Affected area usually extremely tender, swollen, and red
Tinea versicolor ♦ Caused by *Pityrosporum orbiculare* (*Melassezia furfur*), which occurs normally in human skin ♦ Unclear whether caused by infection or by proliferation of normal skin fungi	Nondermatophyte dimorphic fungus converts to the hyphal form and causes characteristic lesions. Invasion of the stratum corneum by the yeast produces C9 and C11 dicarboxylic acids that inhibit tyrosinase in vitro.	♦ Asymptomatic, well-delineated, hyperpigmented or hypopigmented macules occur on upper trunk and arms

DISEASE AND CAUSES	PATHOPHYSIOLOGY	SIGNS AND SYMPTOMS
Torticollis ◆ *Congenital:* from malposition of head in utero, prenatal injury, fibroma, and interruption of blood supply ◆ *Acquired* or *acute*: inflammatory diseases and cervical spinal lesions that produce scar tissue ◆ *Hysterical:* psychogenic inability to control neck muscles ◆ *Spasmodic:* organic CNS disorder	Contraction of the sternocleido-mastoid neck muscles produces twisting of the neck and unnatural position of the head.	*Congenital:* ◆ Firm, nontender, palpable enlargement of the sternocleidomastoid muscle visible at birth *Acquired:* ◆ Recurring unilateral stiffness of neck muscles ◆ Drawing sensation that pulls head to affected side ◆ Severe neuralgic pain of head and neck
Tourette syndrome ◆ Autosomal dominant multiple-tic disorder	Obscure pathology; dopaminergic excess suggested because tics may respond to treatment with dopamine-blocking drugs.	◆ Single or multiple motor tics that commonly affect the face and phonic tics ◆ Involuntary arm and shoulder movements
Trachoma ◆ Infection from *Chlamydia trachomatis*	Chronic conjunctivitis from *C. trachomatis* that leads to inflammatory leukocytic infiltration and superficial vascularization of the cornea, conjunctival scarring, and eyelid distortion. This causes lashes to abrade the cornea, which progresses to corneal ulceration, scarring, and blindness.	◆ Mild infection resembling bacterial conjunctivitis; red and edematous eyelids, pain, photophobia, tearing, and exudation
Trichomoniasis ◆ Infection of the genitourinary tract from *Trichomonas vaginalis*	In women, *T. vaginalis* infects the vagina, urethra and, possibly, the endocervix, bladder, or Bartholin's or Skene's glands. In men, it infects the lower urethra and possibly the prostate gland, seminal vesicles, and epididymis.	*In women:* ◆ Malodorous, greenish yellow vaginal discharge; irritation of vulva, perineum, and thighs; dyspareunia; and dysuria *In men:* ◆ Generally asymptomatic; some transient frothy or purulent urethral discharge with dysuria and frequency; recurrent urethritis
Trigeminal neuralgia ◆ Cause unknown, possibly a compression neuropathy ◆ At surgery or autopsy, the intracranial arterial and venous loops are found to compress the trigeminal nerve root at the brain stem	Painful disorder along the distribution of one or more of the trigeminal nerve's sensory divisions, most often the maxillary	◆ Searing or burning pain lasting seconds to 2 minutes at the trigeminal nerve distribution ◆ Touching a trigger point usually elicits pain

DISEASES AND CAUSES	PATHOPHYSIOLOGY	SIGNS AND SYMPTOMS
Uveitis ◆ Cause unknown but associated with many autoimmune diseases or from allergy, bacteria, viruses, fungi, chemicals, trauma, or surgery	An inflammation of any part of the uveal tract. Inflammatory cells floating in aqueous humor or deposited on corneal endothelium affect the uveal tract.	*Anterior:* ◆ Pain, redness, photophobia, and decreased vision *Intermediate:* ◆ Floaters, decreased vision *Posterior:* ◆ Diverse symptoms, most commonly floaters and decreased vision
Vaginal cancer ◆ Cause unknown; tumor development has been linked to intrauterine exposure to diethylstilbestrol and to human papilloma virus	Usually squamous cell carcinoma (sometimes melanoma, sarcoma, or adenocarcinoma), progresses from intraepithelial tumor to invasive cancer.	◆ Abnormal bleeding and discharge ◆ Firm, ulcerated lesion in the vagina
Vaginismus ◆ Cause related to physical (hymenal abnormalities, genital herpes, obstetric trauma, or atrophic vaginitis) or psychological (conditioned response to traumatic sexual experience) factors	An involuntary spastic constriction of the lower vaginal muscles, tightly closing the vaginal introitus	◆ Muscle spasm with pain when an object is inserted into the vagina ◆ Lack of sexual interest or desire
Variola ◆ Infection from *Poxvirus variola*	Virus is transmitted by respiratory droplets or direct contact. Replicates in the body and causes viremia.	◆ Fever, vomiting, sore throat, CNS symptoms (such as headache, malaise, stupor, and coma), macular rash progressing to vesicular, and pustular lesions
Velocardiofacial syndrome ◆ A chromosomal microdeletion syndrome caused by a submicroscopic deletion of chromosome 22ql 1.2	The chromosome deletion is too small to be detected by routine chromosome analysis. The deleted region, containing 1.5 to 3 megabases, is thought to contain a number of genes. Because infants with DiGeorge syndrome often test positive for a 22ql 1.2 deletion, DiGeorge syndrome represents the severe end of the syndrome's clinical spectrum.	◆ Severe form: complex heart malformations, dysmorphic features, hypocalcemia, missing thymus, and renal abnormalities ◆ Cardiac anomalies: conotruncal defects (tetrology of Fallot, interrupted aortic arch, and truncus arteriosus) ◆ Craniofacial features: palatal abnormalities, dysmorphic facial features, and dysphagia ◆ Neuropsychological symptoms: hypotonia, cognitive symptoms, and psychiatric disorders

DISEASES AND CAUSES	PATHOPHYSIOLOGY	SIGNS AND SYMPTOMS
Vitiligo ◆ Cause unknown; usually acquired but may be familial (autosomal dominant) ◆ Possible immunologic and neurochemical basis	Destruction of melanocytes (humoral or cellular) and circulating antibodies against melanocytes results in hypopigmented areas.	◆ Progressive, symmetric areas of complete pigment loss with sharp borders, generally appearing in periorifical areas, flexor wrists, and extensor distal extremities
Volvulus ◆ Cause may be unknown or may result from an anomaly of rotation, an ingested foreign body, or an adhesion	Twisting of the intestinal tract at least 180 degrees on its mesentery causes blood vessel compression and ischemia. In adults, most common site is the sigmoid bowel; in children, the small bowel. Other common sites are the stomach and cecum.	◆ Vomiting and rapid, marked abdominal distension ◆ Sudden onset of severe abdominal pain
Vulvovaginitis ◆ Caused by bacterial or viral infection, vaginal atrophy, or various traumas or irritations	Infectious diseases and other conditions cause an inflammatory reaction of the vaginal mucosa and vulva.	◆ Vaginal discharge; consistency, odor, and color vary with causative agent ◆ May be accompanied by vulvar irritation, pain, or pruritus
Wilson's disease ◆ Inherited copper toxicosis	Defective mobilization of copper from hepatocellular lysosomes for excretion via the bile allows ecessive copper retention in the liver, brain, kidneys, and corneas, leading to tissue necrosis and subsequent hepatic and neurologic disorders.	*Kayser-Fleischer ring:* ◆ Rusty brown ring of pigment at periphery of corneas ◆ Signs of hepatitis leading to cirrhosis ◆ Tremors, unsteady gait, muscular rigidity, inappropriate behavior, and psychosis ◆ Hematuria, proteinuria, and uricosuria
Wiskott-Aldrich syndrome ◆ X-linked recessive immunodeficiency disorder ◆ Defective B-cell and T-cell functions	Deficiency in B-cell and T-cell function allows for susceptibility to infection. Metabolic defect in platelet synthesis causes production of small, short-lived platelets, resulting in thrombocytopenia.	*In neonate:* ◆ Hemorrhagic symptoms, such as bloody stools, bleeding from circumcision site, petechiae, and purpura *In older child:* ◆ Recurrent systemic infections and eczema
X-linked infantile hypogammaglobulinemia ◆ Congenital disorder causing recurrent infections starting at about age 6 months	Deficiency or absence of B cells leads to defective immune response and depressed production of all five immunoglobulin types.	◆ Otitis media, pneumonia, dermatitis, bronchitis, meningitis, conjunctivitis, abnormal dental caries, and polyarthritis

RELATED WEB SITES

GENERAL

Agency for Healthcare Research and Quality, *www.ahrq.gov*

American Academy of Pain Medicine, *www.painmed.org*

American Pain Society, *www.ampainsoc.org*

Centers for Disease Control and Prevention, *www.cdc.gov*

Healthfinder (a division of the Agency for Healthcare Research and Quality), *www.healthfinder.gov*

National Guideline Clearinghouse, *www.guideline.gov*

National Institute on Aging, *www.nia.nih.gov*

National Library of Medicine, *www.nlm.nih.gov*

CANCER

American Bone Marrow Donor Registry, *www.abmdr.org*

American Cancer Society, *www.cancer.org*

American Society of Clinical Oncology, *www.asco.org*

CA: A Cancer Journal for Clinicians, *www.caonline.amcancersoc.org*

National Cancer Institute, *www.nci.nih.gov*

National Cervical Cancer Coalition, *www.nccc-online.org*

National Women's Health Information Center, *www.4woman.gov*

Oncology Nursing Society, *www.ons.org*

Women's Cancer Network, *www.wcn.org*

INFECTION

Infectious Diseases Society of America, *www.idsociety.org*

National Center for Infectious Diseases, *www.ncid.cdc.gov*

National Institute of Allergy and Infectious Diseases, *www.niaid.nih.gov*

FLUIDS AND ELECTROLYTES

Infusion Nurses Society, *www.ins1.org*

GENETICS

March of Dimes, *www.modimes.org*

National Society of Genetic Counselors, Inc., *www.nsgc.org*

Online Mendelian Inheritance in Man, *www.ncbi.nlm.nih.gov/Omim*

Sickle Cell Disease Association of America, Inc., *www.sicklecelldisease.org*

CARDIOVASCULAR SYSTEM

American College of Cardiology, *www.acc.org*

American Heart Association, *www.americanheart.org*

National Cholesterol Education Program, *www.nhlbi.nih.gov/about/ncep*

National Heart, Lung, and Blood Institute, *www.nhlbi.nih.gov*

RESPIRATORY SYSTEM

American Association of Neuroscience Nurses, *www.aann.org*

American Lung Association, *www.lungusa.org*

National Asthma Education and Prevention Program Expert Panel Report, *www.nhlbi.nih.gov/guidelines/asthma*

National Heart, Lung, and Blood Institute, *www.nhlbi.nih.gov*

NERVOUS SYSTEM

Alzheimer's Association, *www.alz.org*

American Association of Spinal Cord Injury Nurses, *www.aascin.org*

American Parkinson Disease Association, Inc., *www.apdaparkinson.com*

Brain Injury Association of America, *www.biausa.org*

Epilepsy Foundation, *www.efa.org*

National Institute of Neurological Disorders and Stroke, *www.ninds.nih.gov*

National Multiple Sclerosis Society, *www.nmss.org*

National Resource Center for Traumatic Brain Injury, *www.neuro.pmr.vcu.edu*

Spinal Cord Injury Information Network, *www.spinalcord.uab.edu*

GASTROINTESTINAL SYSTEM

American Dietetic Association, *www.eatright.org*

American College of Gastroenterology, *www.acg.gi.org*

American Gastroenterological Association, *www.gastro.org*

Crohn's and Colitis Foundation of America, *www.ccfa.org*

Food and Nutrition Information Center, *www.nal.usda.gov/fnic*

National Digestive Diseases Information Clearinghouse, *www.niddk.nih.gov/healthinformation/digestive*

National Institute of Diabetes and Digestive and Kidney Diseases, *www.niddk.nih.gov*

Society of Gastroenterology Nurses and Associates, Inc., *www.sgna.org*

MUSCULOSKELETAL SYSTEM

National Association of Orthopaedic Nurses, *www.orthonurse.org*

National Institute of Arthritis and Musculoskeletal and Skin Diseases, *www.niams.nih.gov*

National Institutes of Health Osteoporosis and Related Bone Diseases — National Resource Center, *www.osteo.org*

The Paget Foundation for Paget's Disease of Bone and Related Disorders, *www.paget.org*

HEMATOLOGIC SYSTEM

American Society of Hematology, *www.hematology.org*

National Heart, Lung, and Blood Institute, *www.nhlbi.nih.gov*

IMMUNE SYSTEM

AIDS Treatment News, *www.aidsnews.org*

Arthritis Foundation, *www.arthritis.org*

HIV/AIDS Education and Resource Center, *www.aidsinfo.nih.gov*

Lupus Foundation of America, Inc., *www.lupus.org*

National Institute of Allergy and Infectious Diseases, *www.niaid.nih.gov*

National Institute of Arthritis and Musculoskeletal and Skin Diseases, *www.niams.nih.gov*

ENDOCRINE SYSTEM

American Association of Clinical Endocrinologists, *www.aace.com*

American Diabetes Association, *www.diabetes.org*

American Thyroid Association, *www.thyroid.org*

National Graves' Disease Foundation, *www.ngdf.org*

National Institute of Diabetes and Digestive and Kidney Diseases, *www.niddk.nih.gov*

RENAL SYSTEM

American Foundation for Urologic Disease, *www.afud.org*

American Nephrology Nurses' Association, *www.annanurse.org*

Kidney Information Clearinghouse, *www.renalnet.org*

National Institute of Diabetes and Digestive and Kidney Diseases, *www.niddk.nih.gov*

National Kidney Foundation, *www.kidney.org*

SENSORY SYSTEM

American Academy of Audiology, *www.audiology.org*

American Society of Ophthalmic Registered Nurses, *www.webeye.ophth.uiowa.edu/asorn*

American Speech-Language-Hearing Association, *www.asha.org*

National Association of the Deaf, *www.nad.org*

National Institute on Deafness and
Other Communication Disorders,
www.nidcd.nih.gov

INTEGUMENTARY SYSTEM

American Academy of Dermatology,
www.aad.org
DermaWeb, *www.dermatology.org*
National Pressure Ulcer Advisory Panel,
www.npuap.org
Scleroderma Foundation,
www.scleroderma.org
Wound Care Network,
www.woundcarenet.com
Wound, Ostomy and Continence
Nurses Society, *www.wocn.org*

REPRODUCTIVE SYSTEM

Association of Women's Health,
Obstetric and Neonatal Nurses,
www.awhonn.org
Impotence/Erectile Dysfunction,
*www.emedicinehealth.com/search/imp
otence*
National Women's Health Resource
Center, *www.healthywomen.org*

SELECTED REFERENCES

GENERAL

Assessment Made Incredibly Easy, 3rd ed. Philadelphia: Lippincott Williams & Wilkins, 2005.

Atlas of Human Anatomy. Springhouse, Pa.: Springhouse Corp., 2001.

Atlas of Pathophysiology. Springhouse, Pa.: Springhouse Corp., 2002.

Crowley, L.V. *An Introduction to Human Disease: Pathology and Pathophysiology Correlations,* 5th ed. Sudbury, Mass.: Jones & Bartlett Pubs., Inc., 2001.

Gould, B.E. *Pathophysiology for the Health Professions,* 2nd ed. Philadelphia: W.B. Saunders Co., 2002.

Groer, M.W. *Advanced Pathophysiology: Application to Clinical Practice.* Philadelphia: Lippincott Williams & Wilkins, 2001.

Herlihy, B., and Maebius, N.K. *The Human Body in Health and Illness,* 2nd ed. Philadelphia: W.B. Saunders Co., 2003.

Illustrated Manual of Nursing Practice, 3rd ed. Springhouse, Pa.: Lippincott Williams & Wilkins, 2002.

McCance, K.L., and Huether, S.E. *Pathophysiology: The Biologic Basis for Disease in Adults & Children,* 4th ed. St. Louis: Mosby–Year Book, Inc., 2001.

Nelson, R.J., et al. *Seasonal Patterns of Stress, Immune Function, and Disease.* Cambridge, Mass.: Cambridge University Press, 2002.

Pathophysiology Made Incredibly Easy, 3rd ed. Philadelphia: Lippincott Williams & Wilkins, 2005.

Porth, C. *Pathophysiology: Concepts of Altered Health States,* 7th ed. Philadelphia: Lippincott Williams & Wilkins, 2005.

Porth, C. and Gaspard, K. *Essentials of Pathophysiology: Concepts of Altered Health States.* Philadelphia: Lippincott Williams & Wilkins, 2004.

Prezbindowski, K.S. *Study Guide to Accompany Porth's Pathophysiology: Concepts of Altered Health States.* Philadelphia: Lippincott Williams & Wilkins, 2002.

Price, S. and Wilson, L. *Pathophysiology: Clinical Concepts of Disease Processes,* 6th ed. St. Louis: Mosby–Year Book, Inc., 2002.

Professional Guide to Diseases, 8th ed. Philadelphia: Lippincott Williams & Wilkins, 2005.

Professional Guide to Signs & Symptoms, 4th ed. Philadelphia: Lippincott Williams & Wilkins, 2005.

Smeltzer, S.C. and Bare, B.G. *Brunner and Suddarth's Textbook of Medical-Surgical Nursing,* 10th ed. Philadelphia: Lippincott Williams and Wilkins, 2003.

CANCER

American Cancer Society. *ACS Cancer Detection Guidelines.* Available at: *www.cancer.org/docroot/PED/content/PED_2_3X_ACS_Cancer_Detection_Guidelines.* Accessed 9/24/03.

Choma, K.K. "ASC-US and HPV testing," *AJN* 103(2): 42-50, February 2003.

DeVita, V., et al. *Cancer: Principles and Practice of Oncology,* 7th ed. Philadelphia: Lippincott Williams & Wilkins, 2005.

Dropkin, M.J. "Anxiety, Coping Strategies, and Coping Behaviors in Patients Undergoing Head and Neck Cancer Surgery," *Cancer Nursing* 24(2):143-48, April 2001.

Gates, R., and Fink, R. *Oncology Nursing Secrets,* 2nd ed. Philadelphia: Lippincott Williams & Wilkins, 2001.

Lawlor, P.G. "Delirium and Dehydration: Some Fluid for Thought?" *Supportive Care in Cancer* 10(6):445-54, September 2002.

National Cancer Institute. *Progress shown in death rates from four leading cancers Declin in overall mortality has slowed.*

Available at: *www.cancer.gov/
newscenter/pressreleases/
2003ReportRelease.* Accessed 9/24/03.

Sainio, C., et al. "Patient Participation in
Decision Making about Care," *Cancer
Nursing* 24(3):172-79, June 2001.

Smith, R.A., et al. American Cancer
Society Guidelines for Breast Cancer
Screening: Update 2003. *A Cancer
Journal for Clinicians* 53(3):141-69,
May-June 2003.

Wilmoth, M.C. "The Aftermath of Breast
Cancer: An Altered Sexual Self,"
Cancer Nursing 24(4):278-86, August
2001.

Zoorob, R., et al. "Cancer Screening
Guidelines," *American Family Physician*
63(6):1101-12, March 2001.

INFECTION

Bender, K., and Thompson, F.E. "West
Nile Virus: A Growing Challenge,"
AJN 103(6):32-39, June 2003.

Bartlett, J.G. *2004 Pocket Book of Infectious
Disease Therapy,* 12th ed. Philadelphia:
Lippincott Williams & Wilkins, 2004.

Centers for Disease Control. "Severe Acute
Respiratory Syndrome," FACT Sheet:
Basic Information about SARS.
Department of Health and Human
Services. Available at: *www.cdc.gov/
ncidod/sars.* Accessed 1/13/04.

Conte, J.E. *Manual of Antibiotics and
Infectious Diseases: Treatment and
Prevention,* 9th ed. Philadelphia:
Lippincott Williams & Wilkins, 2002.

Gorbach, S.L., et al., eds. *The 5-Minute
Infectious Diseases Consult.* Philadelphia:
Lippincott Williams & Wilkins, 2002.

Mandell, G.L. *Essential Atlas of Infectious
Diseases,* 2nd ed. Philadelphia:
Lippincott Williams & Wilkins, 2001.

Perry, J. "The Bloodborne Pathogens
Standard, 2001: What's Changed?"
Nursing Management 32(6):25-26,
June 2001.

Tularemia. Available at: *www.nlm.nih.gov/
medlineplus/ency/article/000856.htm.*
Accessed 9/24/03.

Wooten, J.M., and Salkind, A.R., "Super-
bugs. Unmasking the Threat," *RN*
66(3):37-43, March 2003.

FLUIDS AND ELECTROLYTES

Fluids & Electrolytes Made Incredibly Easy,
3rd ed. Philadelphia: Lippincott
Williams & Wilkins, 2005.

Metheny, N.M. *Fluid and Electrolyte
Balance,* 4th ed. Philadelphia:
Lippincott Williams & Wilkins, 2000.

GENETICS

Bachmann, C., and Koletzko, B. *Genetic
Expression and Nutrition.* Philadelphia:
Lippincott Williams & Wilkins, 2002.

Coleman, K.B. "Genetic Counseling in
Congenital Heart Disease," *Critical
Care Nursing Quarterly* 25(3):8-16,
November 2002.

CARDIOVASCULAR SYSTEM

Artinian, N.T. "The Psychosocial Aspects
of Heart Failure," *AJN* 103(12):32-42,
December 2003.

Berne, R.M., and Levy, M.N. *Cardiovascular Physiology,* 8th ed. St. Louis:
Mosby–Year Book, Inc., 2001.

Bosen, D.M. "New Strategies for Treating
Patients with Heart Failure," *Nursing*
33(12):44-47, December 2003.

Bruch, C., et al. "Impact of Disease
Activity on Left Ventricular Perfor-
mance in Patients with Acromegaly,"
American Heart Journal 144(3):538-43,
September 2002.

U.S. Department of Health and Human
Services. *The Seventh Report of the Joint
National Committee on Prevention,
Detection, Evaluation, and Treatment of
High Blood Pressure.* Bethesda, Md.:
National Institutes of Health, National
Heart, Lung, and Blood Institute, May
2003.

Woods, S.L., et al. *Cardiac Nursing,* 5th ed.
Philadelphia: Lippincott Williams &
Wilkins, 2005.

RESPIRATORY SYSTEM

CDC TB Guidelines and Recommendations
Available at: *www.cdcnpin.org/scripts/
tb/cdc.asp#1.* Accessed 2/12/2004.

Des Jardins, T., and Burton, G. *Clinical
Manifestations and Assessment of
Respiratory Disease,* 4th ed. St. Louis:
Mosby–Year Book, Inc., 2002.

Hough, A. *Physiotherapy in Respiratory Care: A Problem-Solving Approach to Respiratory and Cardiac Management.* London: Stanley Thornes Publishing, Ltd., 2001.

Marthaler, M., et al. "SARS What Have We Learned?" *RN* 66(8):58-64, August 2003.

Mishoe, S.C., and Welch, M.A., eds. *Critical Thinking in Respiratory Care.* New York: McGraw-Hill Book Co., 2001.

Schieken, L.S. "Asthma Pathophysiology and the Scientific Rationale for Combination Therapy," *Allergy and Asthma Proceedings* 23(4):247-51, July-August 2002.

NERVOUS SYSTEM

Albers, G.W., et al. "Addendum to the Supplement to the Guidelines for the Management of Transient Ischemic Attacks," *Stroke* 31(4):1001, April 2000.

Barclay, L and Sklar, B., "New Guidelines for Acute Management of Ischemic Stroke," *Medscape Medical News.* April 2003. Available at: *www.medscape.com/viewarticle/451815.* Accessed 1/7/04.

Barker, E. *Neuroscience Nursing,* 2nd ed. St. Louis: Mosby–Year Book, Inc., 2002.

Brodie, M.J., et al. *Epilepsy, Fast Facts,* 2nd ed. Oxford, England: Health Press Limited, 2001.

Gupta, A., et al. "Post-Stroke Depression," *International Journal of Clinical Practice* 56(7):531-37, September 2002.

Kinsman, S.L. "Predicting Gross Motor Function in Cerebral Palsy," *JAMA* 288(11):1399-400, September 2002.

Kirshner, H.S. "Medical Prevention of Stroke," *Southern Medical Journal* 96(4):354-58, April 2003. Available at: *www.medscape.com/viewarticle/452839.* Accessed 1/7/04.

Low, P.A. "Autonomic Neuropathies," *Current Opinion in Neurology* 15(5):605-609, October 2002.

Pena, C.G. "Seizure," *AJN* 103(11):73-81, November 2003.

Zweifler, R.M "Management of Acute Stroke," *Southern Medical Journal* 96(4):380-85, May 2003. Available at: *www.medscape.com/viewarticle/452844.* Accessed 1/7/04.

GASTROINTESTINAL SYSTEM

Florez, D.A., and Aranda-Michel, J. "Nutritional Management of Acute and Chronic Liver Disease," *Seminars in Gastrointestinal Disease* 13(3):169-78, July 2002.

Karlowicz, D. "An Endoscopic Approach to GERD?" *RN* 66(12):56-60, December 2003.

Kohn-Keeth, C. "How to Keep Feeding Tubes Flowing Freely," *Nursing2000* 30(3):58-59, March 2000.

McNally, P.R. *GI/Liver Secrets,* 2nd ed. Philadelphia: Hanley & Belfus, 2001.

O'Malley, P. "Gastric Ulcers and GERD: the New 'plagues' of the 21st Century Update for the Clinical Nurse Specialist," *Clinical Nurse Specialist* 17(6):286-89, November 2003.

Rayhorn, N., et al. "Understanding Gastroesophageal Reflux Disease," *Nursing* 33(10):36-41, October, 2003.

Veronesi, J.F. "Inflammatory Bowel Disease," *RN* 66(5):38-45, May 2003.

Yamada, T., and Kaplowitz, N. *Atlas of Gastroenterology,* 3rd ed. Philadelphia: Lippincott Williams & Wilkins, 2003.

MUSCULOSKELETAL SYSTEM

Anderson, D.L. "TNF Inhibitors: A New Age in Rheumatoid Arthritis Treatment," *AJN* 104(2):60-69, February 2004.

Blakeley, J.A. and Ribeiro, V.E. "Glucosamine and Osteoarthritis," *AJN* 104(2):54-59, February 2004.

Lindgren, V. "When to Suspect this Bone Disorder," *RN* 66(6):32-36, June 2003.

Metules, T. "Osteoporosis," *RN* 66(11): 56-62, November 2003.

National Osteoporosis Foundation. "Medications and Osteoporosis." Washington, D.C.: National Osteoporosis Foundation, 2001. *www.nof.org/patientinfo/medications. htm.*

National Osteoporosis Foundation. Physician's Guide: Pharmacologic Options. Washington, D.C.: National Osteoporosis Foundation, 2001. *www.nof.org/physguide/pharmacologic. htm.*

HEMATOLOGIC SYSTEM

Anderson, S.C., & Poulsen, K.B. *Anderson's Atlas of Hematology.* Philadelphia: Lippincott Williams & Wilkins, 2003.

Beutler, E., et al. *Williams Hematology,* 6th ed. New York: McGraw-Hill Professional, 2001.

Lewis, S.M., et al. *Dacie and Lewis's Practical Haematology*, 9th ed. New York, London: Churchill Livingstone Inc., 2001.

IMMUNE SYSTEM

Gruchalla, R.S. "Drug Metabolism, Danger Signals, and Drug-Induced Hypersensitivity," *Journal of Allergy and Clinical Immunology* 108(4):475-88, October 2001.

Koopman, W.J. *Arthritis and Allied Conditions: A Textbook of Rheumatology,* 15th ed. Philadelphia: Lippincott Williams & Wilkins, 2005.

Rich, R., et al. *Clinical Immunology: Principles and Practice,* 2nd ed. St. Louis: Mosby–Year Book, Inc., 2001.

Sarvis, C.M. "When Lymphedema Takes Hold," *RN* 66(9):32-37, September 2003.

ENDOCRINE SYSTEM

American Diabetes Association. "Nutrition Recommendations and Principles for People with Diabetes Mellitus," *Diabetes Care* 23(Suppl 1):S43-46, January 2001.

Lavin, N. *Manual of Endocrinology and Metabolism,* 3rd ed. Philadelphia: Lippincott Williams & Wilkins, 2002.

Olohan, K., and Zappitelli, D. "The Insulin Pump," *AJN,* 103(4):48-56, April 2003.

Schori-Ahmed, D. "Defenses Gone Awry. Thyroid Disease," *RN* 66(6):38-43, June 2003.

Skyler, J.S. *Atlas of Diabetes,* 2nd ed. Philadelphia: Lippincott Williams & Wilkins, 2002.

RENAL AND URINARY SYSTEM

Campbell, D. "How Acute Renal Failure Puts the Brakes on Kidney Function," *Nursing* 33(1):59-63, January 2003.

D'Amico, M., and Locatelli, F. "Hypertension in Dialysis: Pathophysiology and Treatment," *Journal of Nephrology* 15(4):438-45, July-August 2002.

Johnson, S. "From Incontinence to Confidence," *AJN* 100(2):69-75, February 2000.

Little, C. "Renovascular Hypertension," *AJN* 100(2):46-51, February 2000.

Newman, D.K. "Stress Urinary Incontinence in Women," *AJN* 103(8): 46-55, August 2003.

Ross, C. "Dialysis Disequilibrium Syndrome," *AJN* 100(2):53-54, February 2000.

Saklayen, M., et al. "Pericardial Effusion Leading to Acute Renal Failure: Two Case Reports and Discussion of Pathophysiology," *American Journal of Kidney Diseases* 40(4):837-41, October 2002.

SENSORY SYSTEM

Gold, D.H., and Weingeist, T.A. *Color Atlas of the Eye in Systemic Disease.* Philadelphia: Lippincott Williams & Wilkins, 2000.

Lockwood, A.H., et al. "Tinnitus," *New England Journal of Medicine* 347(12):904-10, September 2002.

Moller, A.R. *Hearing: Its Physiology and Pathophysiology.* San Diego: Academic Press, 2000.

INTEGUMENTARY SYSTEM

American Academy of Dermatology. "New Treatments for Psoriasis Give Dermatologists More Choices for Treating Millions of Americans with the Hard-to-Treat Skin Condition. AAD Press Release, August 2002. Available at: *www.aad.org/PressReleases/psoriasis.html.* Accessed 2/17/04.

Leininger, S. "Scleroderma," *RN* 66(7): 35-42, July 2003.

Ovington, L.G. "Wound Care Products: How to Choose," *Home Health Care Nurse* 19(4):224-31, April 2001.

Trent, J.T. and Kirsner, R.S. "Identifying and Treating Mycotic Skin Infections," *Advances in Skin and Wound Care*, 16(3):122-29, May-June 2003.

U.S. Food and Drug Administration. "FDA Approves First Biologic Therapy for Psoriasis." *FDA Talk Paper,* January 2003. Available at: *www.fda.gov/bbs/topics/ANSWERS/2003/ANS01194.html.* Accessed 2/17/04.

van Onselen, J. *Dermatology Nursing: A Practical Guide.* New York, London: Churchill Livingstone, Inc., 2001.

REPRODUCTIVE SYSTEM

Fink, J.L. "Beyond the Shock of an Abnormal PAP," *RN* 66(6): 56-61, June 2003.

Glasier, A., and Gebbie, A. *Handbook of Family Planning and Reproductive Healthcare,* 4th ed. New York, London: Churchill Livingstone, Inc., 2001.

Korn, A. "Gynecologic Care of Women Infected with HIV," *Clinical Obstetrics and Gynecology* 44(2):226-42, June 2001.

Lewis, J.H., et al. "Erectile Dysfunction," *AJN,* 103(10):48-57, October 2003.

Robboy, S., et al., eds. *Pathology of the Female Reproductive Tract.* New York London: Churchill Livingstone, Inc., 2002.

Scott, J.R., et al. *Danforth's Obstetrics and Gynecology,* 9th ed. Philadelphia: Lippincott Williams & Wilkins, 2003.

INDEX

i refers to an illustration; t refers to a table; **boldface** refers to a full-color illustration page.

---

i refers to an illustration; t refers to a table; **boldface** refers to a full-color illustration page.

---

i refers to an illustration; t refers to a table; **boldface** refers to a full-color illustration page.

---

i refers to an illustration; t refers to a table; **boldface** refers to a full-color illustration page.

i refers to an illustration; t refers to a table; **boldface** refers to a full-color illustration page.

i refers to an illustration; t refers to a table; **boldface** refers to a full-color illustration page.

---

i refers to an illustration; t refers to a table; **boldface** refers to a full-color illustration page.

---

i refers to an illustration; t refers to a table; **boldface** refers to a full-color illustration page.

J

Jaundice, 315, 316i, 317
Joints, 361-362
    arthritic, specific care for, 380
    classification of, 361-362
    movement of, 362
    synovial, structure of, 361-362, 361i
Junctional rhythm, 148-149t. *See also*
    Cardiac arrhythmias.

K

Kaposi's sarcoma, 617t
Kawasaki disease, 452-453t
Keratitis, 617t
Kidney cancer, 48t, 618t
    tumor cell markers for, 29-30t
Kidneys
    compensation by, in acid-base
        imbalance, 96
    function of, 490
    structural variations of, 493
Kidney stones, 519-522, 520i
Kidney transplantation, growth hor-
        mone deficiency and, 471t
Klinefelter syndrome, 124-126, 124i
Kyphosis, 618t

L

Labia majora, 573
Labia minora, 573
Landry-Guillain-Barré syndrome. *See*
    Guillain-Barré syndrome.
Large-bowel obstruction. *See* Intestinal
    obstruction.
Laryngeal cancer, 43t
Lassa fever, 618t
Latex allergy, 443-444
Left atrial pressure, monitoring, 198
Legg-Calvé-Perthes disease, 376-377
Legionnaires' disease, 618t
Leprosy, 618t
Leukemia
    acute, 39t
    chronic lymphocytic, 42t
    tumor cell marker for, 30t
Leukocytes. *See* White blood cells.
Leukocytosis, 397
    as infection symptom, 61

Leukopenia, 397
    as cancer symptom, 25
Lichen simplex chronicus, 558t
Ligaments, 363
Listeriosis, 66t
Lithium as teratogen, 113t
Liver, functions of, 344
Liver cancer, 44t
    tumor cell markers for, 29-30t
Liver failure, 343-345
Lou Gehrig's disease, 269-270
Lund-Browder chart for estimating
        extent of burn, 555i
Lung cancer, 44t
    metastasis sites for, 24t
    tumor cell markers for, 29-30t
Lungs, compensation by, in acid-base
        imbalance, 96
Lupus erythematosus, 444-446
Lyme disease, 67t
Lymphocytes, 398-399i, 400
Lymphoma, 31

M

Macrophages, 426-427
Macular degeneration, age-related, 532
Magnesium, physiologic roles of, 85-86
Magnetic resonance imaging, cancer
        diagnosis and, 28
Major histocompatibility complex,
    424-425
Malabsorption, 345-347
    causes of, 346
Malaria, 80t
Male reproductive system
    anatomy and physiology of, 571-572
    disorders of, 582-585, 588-591,
        593-594, 595-597t, 598-600,
        602
    pathophysiologic changes in,
        575-576, 578-579
Malignant peritoneal infusion as
        oncologic emergency, 34t
Malignant pleural effusion as oncologic
        emergency, 34t
Mammary glands, 572
Marfan syndrome, 126-127
Mast cells, 428
Mastocytosis, 618t

---

i refers to an illustration; t refers to a table; **boldface** refers to a full-color illustration page.

i refers to an illustration; t refers to a table; **boldface** refers to a full-color illustration page.

---

i refers to an illustration; t refers to a table; **boldface** refers to a full-color illustration page.

i refers to an illustration; t refers to a table; **boldface** refers to a full-color illustration page.

i refers to an illustration; t refers to a table; **boldface** refers to a full-color illustration page.

---

i refers to an illustration; t refers to a table; **boldface** refers to a full-color illustration page.

i refers to an illustration; t refers to a table; **boldface** refers to a full-color illustration page.

NOTES